Adapted Physical Activity

Adapted Physical Activity

Robert D. Steadward
Garry D. Wheeler
E. Jane Watkinson
Editors

 The University of Alberta Press

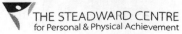 THE STEADWARD CENTRE
for Personal & Physical Achievement

Published by

The University of Alberta Press
Ring House 2
Edmonton, Alberta, Canada T6G 2E1
and
The Steadward Centre
W1-67 Van Vliet Centre
The University of Alberta
Edmonton, Alberta, Canada T6G 2H9

ISBN 0–88864–375–6

**National Library of Canada Cataloguing in
Publication Data**

Main entry under title:

Adapted physical activity/Robert D. Steadward,
Garry D. Wheeler, E. Jane Watkinson, editors.

Includes bibliographical references and index.
ISBN 0–88864–375–6

1. Physical education for people with
disabilities–Textbooks. I. Steadward, R. D.,
II. Watkinson, E. J. (Elizabeth Jane), 1948–
III. Wheeler, Garry David, 1956– IV. Title.
GV482.7.A32 2003   613.7'087
C2003–910885–6

Printed and bound in Canada by
Transcontinental Printing, Inc.,
Louiseville, Quebec.
Edited by Eva Radford.
Book design by Carol Dragich.
Index by Judy Dunlop Information Services.

First edition, first printing, 2003.

The University of Alberta Press is committed
to protecting our natural environment. As part
of our efforts, this book is printed on stock
containing post-consumer recycled fibres and
is acid- and chlorine-free.

The University of Alberta Press gratefully
acknowledges the financial support of the
Government of Canada through the Book
Publishing Industry Development Program
(BPDIP) and from the Alberta Foundation for
the Arts for our publishing activities.

Canada

Contents

I FOCUS ON CRITICAL THINKING

1 Critical Thinking and Professional Preparation 1
Marcel Bouffard and William B. Strean

II PERSPECTIVES

2 Defining Adapted Physical Activity 11
Greg Reid

3 The History of Adapted Physical Activity in Canada 27
A.E. (Ted) Wall

Reaction and Proaction

From Integration to Inclusion

Robert D. Steadward

My encounters with people with disability have spread far and wide; they have encompassed over thirty years of experience in teaching and sport leadership in the ever-expanding field of adapted physical activity. Through all these years, little written material has been available on such an essential matter as the enhancement of quality of life for people with disability through health and physical fitness, and all the benefits derived from them.

It was with great excitement, therefore, that this *Adapted Physical Activity* textbook was finally produced, containing an abundance of knowledge from the respective expertise of each contributing author. Our combined and unanimous purpose was to contribute a series of meaningful, informative, and multifaceted chapters on the miscellany of aspects that will be of interest and value to undergraduate and graduate students of Canadian universities and colleges, and also to community practitioners and all interested readers.

It is predicted that the population of people with disability in Canada alone will amount to over 15 percent of our total national population. Obviously, demographics are destined to change dramatically within the next several years. But let us remember, too, the global impact of this book when we consider the number of countries involved in conflict, and the escalating numbers of traumatic injury that arise from such circumstances. History records centuries of such societal problems. Through the knowledge contained within these pages, the twenty-first century is equipped to find the solutions. It is hoped, therefore, that the chapters within this book will have far-reaching benefits for all humanity.

Previous textbooks pertaining to people with disability have focussed on various disciplines: history, psychology, sociology, physiology, and the like. This book is unique in that it is multidisciplinary, with focus on a specific population, examining the macro from many micro dimensions: instruction, health, sport, and sociology. The purpose of *this* book is to make available to all readers a comprehensive understanding of disability and to provide information on the background and history of adapted physical activity, the socio, economic, and political implications and complexities that are involved in application and service delivery; the entire sphere of independence and inclusion; sport, recreation, leisure, quality of life; and, the relatively current matter of aging with its multifarious consequences on all society.

I hope that our chapters interpret the issues of what is occurring in the world today in such a way that justifies the need for such a book as *Adapted Physical Activity*. As Honorary and Past President of the International Paralympic Committee, and as Founder and Chief Executive Officer of The Steadward Centre for Personal and Physical Achievement, I believe that this textbook is a unique and appropriate resource for global use, as the issues surrounding people with disability are virtually identical, worldwide.

The Development and State of Adapted Physical Activity

Garry D. Wheeler

Persons with disability have come a long way–from concerns with mere survival, to opportunity for Paralympic glory. In many ways, *Adapted Physical Activity* is a testimony to and celebration of the value of physical activity for health and fitness and of sport for social acceptance and opportunity.

Until relatively recently, people with disability have traditionally been viewed as objects of sympathy and charity, dependent on others for their existence. Historically, persons with a disability were disempowered and stripped of autonomous decision-making opportunities. However, during the last half century there has been a strong challenge regarding negative assumptions about the nature of disability and the abilities of persons with disability.

As a result of numerous social, technological, human rights, advocacy, and legislative forces, many–although certainly not all–persons with disability may now look forward to independent lives in which they are treated equally in society and are respected for their abilities rather than their disabilities. Today,

persons with disability have become advocates in solving their own social, economic, and political problems. This change has taken place within the context of human rights movements that have dominated the social agenda of many nations since the end of WWII, the integration and inclusion movements, which have also been facilitated by opportunities in elite sport. However, as the reader will learn, there are still many societal challenges facing persons with a disability in relation to equal access to opportunities. This is particularly true in relation to access to physical education in schools, community recreational opportunities, and competitive and elite sport environments. In fact, there are challenges to the fundamental concept of inclusion.

In introducing *Adapted Physical Activity*, Drs. Bouffard and Strean similarly challenge readers to become independent thinkers and problem solvers, to move away from classic dependency models of education in which the teacher is merely a provider, and the learner the recipient of information that is received unprocessed and, more importantly, unquestioned. In their introduction, the authors encourage readers to challenge the various assumptions underlying disability and the disability movement, to engage in a critical thinking process, and to explore alternatives. The entire text is therefore based on a critical thinking model, as well as on the fundamental principles of inclusion.

In their chapter, Drs. McPherson and Wheeler and co-author Sheri Foster examine many of the influences and forces that have shaped the social reality for persons with disabilities today. Until relatively recently, persons with disability suffered abandonment, persecution, segregation, and marginalization, living with restricted freedoms under institutional philosophies dominated by medical and religious models of care and charity. It was only during the last half of the twentieth century and the first years of the twenty-first century that opportunities and rights for persons with disabilities came to the forefront of the public agenda through a human rights and advocacy agenda that brought about a fundamental shift to humanistic policies and led to the mainstreaming, normalization, integration, and inclusion movements.

The authors point out that the social realities of persons with disabilities, including opportunities for active living and sports, have been shaped by a number of parallel historical forces and influences. These include advances in human rights, war and human conflict, social agencies and humanitarian organizations, specific disability legislation, and technology. These influences have simultaneously shaped the rights of persons with disability in their daily lives as well as increasing opportunities for school-based physical education, community active living, and competitive and elite sports opportunities.

Following the declaration of the Universal Declaration of Human Rights (1948) by the United Nations, numerous disability-specific declarations influenced the rights of persons with disabilities and their access to social opportunities, including recreation and sports. These included the Declaration of the Rights of Mentally Retarded Persons (1971), the Declaration of Rights of Disabled Persons (1975), the World Program of Action Concerning Disabled Persons (1982), the Decade of Disabled Persons (1983–1992), and the proclamation of December 3 as the International Day of Disabled Persons (1991). Finally, the Standard Rules of Equalization of Opportunity (1993) challenged member nations to provide equal access to opportunities in society. Such initiatives provided the environmental context in which opportunities for persons with disabilities have flourished.

Chapters by Drs. Reid and Wall provide the reader with a history of, and insights into, the development of the adapted physical education and adapted physical activity fields. Prior to the 1950s, approaches to physical activity for children in schools and institutions were based on a medical correctives approach as outlined by Dr. Legg in his chapter. In 1952, the term *adapted physical education* was first used and began a challenge to a correctives model, which focussed on rehabilitation rather than the physical education of children with disabilities. This was followed by a half century during which the field of adapted physical activity grew in association with the mainstreaming, integration and inclusion philosophies, the latter being described by Drs. Goodwin, Watkinson, and Fitzpatrick. The growth of adapted physical education opportunities for children was not without its challenges. Legislation, particularly in the United States of America and later in other nations, was an essential tool to ensure the provision of equal access to physical education through legal responsibility. Most notably, Public Law 94–142, also known as the Education of All Handicapped Children Act (1975), created free appropriate education for all handicapped children between three and twenty-one years of age and specifically provided for the provision of physical education in a least restrictive environment.

Instructional strategies in adapted physical activity also developed within the context of changing philosophical stances regarding treatment of persons with disability, and a history of these approaches over the last eighty years is discussed by Dr. Goodwin, concluding with the development of ecological and strategic approaches to instruction. Dr. Nearingburg and her co-author Laurie Clifford explore the value of adapted physical activity consultants as an essential adjunct in support of the inclusive physical education initiative within the schools. Developments in teaching strategies have been complimented by the development of instructional materials grounded in the philosophy of inclusion, including *Moving to Inclusion*, a Canadian publication outlining instructional strategies for including children with disabilities in regular physical education classes.

As adapted physical education and adapted physical activity grew as a practice, adapted physical activity grew as an academic discipline. In turn, this served as a training ground for professionals in the area of research and teaching. Today, adapted physical activity is a burgeoning academic discipline within Canadian universities.

The growth of active living opportunities in the community is examined at the policy level by Dr. Renée Lyons and her co-authors, and at the programming level by Rick Gingras. Policy with regard to community-based physical activity opportunities has traditionally lagged behind school-based developments, and it was not until the federal government announced the National Strategy for Integration of Persons with Disabilities (1991–1996) that a relatively substantial (although short-term) funding base was developed to support community-based and school initiatives. As well, in 1998 the Canadian federal minister of health endorsed *Active Living for Canadians with Disabilities: A Blueprint for Action*. The Canadian initiative to increase access to physical fitness and lifestyle assessment within the community (Canadian Society for Exercise Physiology's INCLUSIVE HEALTH FITNESS AND LIFESTYLE SERVICES FOR ALL DISABILITIES) is discussed by Christine Seidl.

The latter part of *Adapted Physical Activity* is devoted to a discussion of elite disability sports. Prior to WWII, only deaf sports were

organized at the level of an international sports organization (International Committee of Sports for the Deaf 1924). The end of WWII signalled the beginning of a new era of organization in disability sport. As with education, there has been an evolution of philosophy with regard to the organization of disability sport. In education, there was a shift from segregation to integrated and inclusive policies. Changes in philosophy in disability sport mirrored these influences, as sport moved from a medical and organizationally divided model towards an inclusive and united model.

Disability sports were originally based on a medical model. Sports organizations and sporting competition were based on disability type, and classification systems for competition were based on level of injury or classification of disease state. Individual organizations hosted their own events for specific disability types, such as spinal-cord-injured, the blind, and the deaf. Under the stewardship of Dr. Robert Steadward, disability sport strode into the latter decade of the twentieth century under the banner of the International Paralympic Committee (IPC). Gone was the division and diversity that threatened to thwart the growth of disability sport as an international force. With the forming of the IPC in 1989, a new profile emerged, and now the International Paralympic Committee enjoys parallel status with the International Olympic Committee in the bidding process for the games. At the same time, there has been a marked shift from a medical and disability-specific model of sport to a sport-specific model employing a functional integrated classification system.

As with the able-bodied sport system, disability sport faces numerous challenges. Students will learn of them, such as doping and the use of 'boosting' by athletes using wheelchairs. Dr. Lisa Olenik's chapter highlights issues of inequity in participation in relation to women in the Paralympic Games. Other potential sources of inequity may result from the unequal distribution of wealth between nations and the development of new lightweight materials for specialized wheel-chairs or smart prostheses for sprinters. Technological developments are outlined by Stéphane Perreault and provide the student with insights into the athlete technology interface and its contribution to increasing levels of performance of Paralympic athletes. Finally, the issue of athlete retirement is discussed by Dr. Garry Wheeler, as one of the least well-researched areas in Paralympic sport. Important questions are raised with regard to the obligations of the institution of sports in general towards its athletes as they make the transition out of sports.

Having read *Adapted Physical Activity*, the student will be well prepared to discuss a variety of philosophical issues and the development and state of physical activity opportunities across the continuum of school physical education, community recreation, and elite sport within Canada and other areas of the world. Most importantly, the student will have been challenged throughout the text to consider the topics from a critical thinking point of view. Finally, the student will be able to synthesize the materials to gain a perspective of the variety of forces, influences, and movements that have taken persons with disabilities from abandonment, obscurity, persecution, and segregation towards their full inclusion and participation in society and the chance of Paralympic gold.

Acknowledgements

This pioneer project on the broad and complex subject of adapted physical activity would not have been possible without the contribution of all the authors, to whom we are extremely grateful. We are also indebted to Sheri Foster for assisting in the coordination of this endeavour; to Ewen Nelson and Barbara Campbell for their assistance and contribution to the success of this publication; to Mary Mahoney-Robson, Linda Cameron, Cathie Crooks, Leslie Vermeer, and Teresa Krohman of The University of Alberta Press; to Eva Radford, Carol Dragich, and Judy Dunlop for their experience and expertise, and for keeping us on target; to The Steadward Centre for Personal & Physical Achievement for their sponsorship; and, to our families for their continuous support in our efforts.

Robert D. Steadward,
Ph.D., O.C., LL.D (Hons)
Garry D. Wheeler, Ph.D., C. Psych.
E. Jane Watkinson, Ph.D

About the Contributors

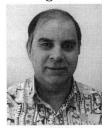

Dr. Yagesh Bhambhani is Professor in the Faculty of Rehabilitation Medicine at the University of Alberta. He is an exercise physiologist by training and has a special interest in studying the acute and chronic physiological responses of exercise in healthy subjects as well as in individuals with disabilities. He has published many articles on wheelchair exercise and sport performance in athletes with spinal cord injury and cerebral palsy. These papers appear in a variety of journals, including *Archives of Physical Medicine and Rehabilitation, Paraplegia, Adapted Physical Activity Quarterly, Clinical Journal of Sports Medicine, Sports Medicine Rehabilitation and Training,* and *Sports Medicine.* He has presented numerous papers at national and international scientific conferences in the field of adapted physical activity including the biennial meetings of the International Federation of Adapted Physical Activity, Vista '93 and Vista '99, and the Paralympic congresses. Dr. Bhambhani is a member of the International Paralympic Committee Research and Education Committee, a standing committee of the International Paralympic Committee, and has played an integral role in its activities since its inception in 1994. He chaired the Leadership Development Initiative for Persons With a Disability Committee, a subcommittee of the Health and Fitness Program of the Canadian Society for Exercise Physiology. This committee has recently developed a supplementary training module entitled *INCLUSIVE FITNESS AND LIFESTYLE APPRAISAL SERVICES FOR ALL disABILITIES.*

Yagesh is a talented badminton and tennis player and plays both these sports on a recreational basis.

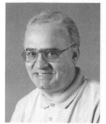

Dr. Marcel Bouffard is Professor in the Faculty of Physical Education and Recreation at the University of Alberta. He completed his undergraduate degree in Physical Education at *l'Université Laval*. He received an M.Sc. degree from *l'Université de Montréal* before completing his doctorate in Adapted Physical Activity and Motor Development under the guidance of Dr. A.E. (Ted) Wall at the University of Alberta. His major research interest is on self-directed learning of movement skills by persons with disability. He is also known for his work on research assumptions and methodological research issues in adapted physical activity.

Marcel is a former fastball pitcher and an avid golfer who took up golf a few years ago. During his leisure time, he enjoys doing some wishful thinking. He believes (most would say foolishly) that he could become a scratch golfer.

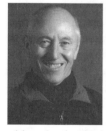

Dr. Arthur (Art) C. Burgess is Professor Emeritus of the University of Alberta. Dr. Burgess developed the Campus Fitness and Lifestyle programme and, in 1988, started Project: Alive and Well, a fitness programme for adults aged fifty-five and older. At the University of Alberta, the faculties of Extension and Physical Education were pioneers in fitness programming for older people. Dr. Burgess was involved with them both. With no guidelines other than sound principles of physical education, a safe but challenging method for group training of older adults was developed. Out of the practical tasks of developing realistic fitness activities suitable for seniors, a philosophy and methodology emerged that is described in Chapter 25 of this book.

Dr. Burgess was born and raised in Victoria, British Columbia. In 1949 he joined the Royal Canadian Air Force serving for five years as a recreation specialist in the areas of sport and athletic training. As a working student, he attended the University of British Columbia from 1954–64, receiving a Bachelor of Physical Education (B.P.E.) degree. He worked with the Vancouver YMCA and the Victoria YM-YWCA from 1958 to 1971 in physical fitness and sport. He attended the University of Alberta from 1971–1984 where he received his M.A. and Ph.D. in Physical Education. In 1977 Dr. Burgess joined the staff of Campus Recreation as Director of Campus Fitness and Lifestyle programmes. Dr. Burgess, now 73, retired to Victoria after fifty-three years as a practicing fitness leader.

He and his wife Dorothy, two years younger, train regularly for fitness three times a week. For recreation, Dorothy and Art are also active in older adult figure skating as an ice dance team. The Burgesses are active as co-presenters and demonstrators of fitness and the active lifestyle with the Canadian Diabetes Association in Victoria.

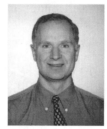

Dr. Robert Burnham was raised and educated in Edmonton. He graduated from the University of Alberta with a Ph.D. in Medicine in 1980. Following a brief period of practice in family medicine, he completed specialty training in the field of physical medicine and rehabilitation in 1986. His areas of interest have included sport medicine, particularly as it applies to athletes with a disability; research; and the diagnosis and rehabilitation of nerve, muscle, and joint disorders. He has gained both local and international sport medicine experience. To further his understanding of research and disability sport, he completed an M.Sc. degree through the Faculty of Physical Education and the Rick Hansen (Steadward) Centre in 1993. His studies have lead to several research publications relating to disability sport medicine.

Robert practices medicine in Lacombe, Alberta, where he lives with his wife and six children.

Dr. Karen Calzonetti is a faculty member in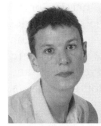
the Department of Physical Education and Kinesiology at Brock University in St. Catharines, Ontario. A graduate of the Adapted Physical Activity programme at the University of Alberta, Dr. Calzonetti is a strong advocate of empowerment and its connection to individuals who have a disability. As a managing partner of Athlete Empowerment for Ontario Special Olympics, she has the opportunity to connect theory with practice on an ongoing basis. Dr. Calzonetti is a long-time supporter of programmes and activities that facilitate and respect the importance of independence, choice, and decision-making for all, and regularly conducts seminars on problem solving and the development of active, self-directed learning.

Dr. Janice Causgrove Dunn was appointed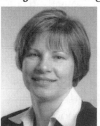
to the Faculty of Physical Education and Recreation at the University of Alberta in 1997, having previously taught at the University of Regina, in Saskatchewan, and Lakehead University, in Thunder Bay, Ontario. She completed her B.P.E. degree in 1984, her M.Sc. degree in 1987, and her Ph.D. degree in 1997, all at the University of Alberta. Dr. Causgrove Dunn's research interests focus on social cognitive processes that impact the motivation and participation of persons with movement difficulties in physical activity, as well as on assessments and interventions for children with developmental coordination disorder (DCD). She has been a member of the editorial board of the *Adapted Physical Activity Quarterly* (*APAQ*) since 1997, has published in journals from the fields of adapted physical activity and sport psychology, and recently contributed to an edited book entitled *Developmental Coordination Disorder.*

Laurie Clifford is an adapted physical edu-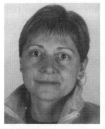
cation consultant with Edmonton Public Schools, Sensory Multi-Handicapped Services. Her work takes her throughout north central Alberta to help teachers include students with disabilities in physical education. She has a B.P.E. degree from Brock University, St. Catharines, Ontario, and an M.A. in Physical Education from the University of Alberta.

Laurie enjoys spending her leisure time with her husband and two sons.

Dr. Sandra O'Brien Cousins is Professor in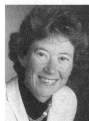
the Faculty of Physical Education and Recreation at the University of Alberta. She began as a lecturer and gymnastics coach in 1971, went on a study leave in 1976 to finish her master's degree at University of British Columbia (UBC), then returned to the University of Alberta where she succeeded in her various roles over the next thirty years. During her fifteen years as Head Coach of the Panda Gymnastics Team, they were unrivalled by any other university gymnastics team. By 1986, her long days in the gym were a challenge to manage along with her two children, Catherine (born 1980) and Kristina (1982). She retired from coaching and began her doctoral studies, receiving her doctorate in Gerontology at UBC in 1991. Since then, Dr. Cousins has developed a successful research programme that focusses on exercise gerontology and, specifically, on motivational issues that act as barriers to older adult healthy lifestyles and active living. Dr. Cousins has published three books, *Coaching the Female Gymnast* (1983), *Exercise, Aging and Health: Overcoming Barriers to an Active Old Age* (1998), and *Active Living Among Older Adults: Health Benefits and Outcomes* (1999). In 2001, she published the results of her study titled *High Quality Aging*

or Gambling with Health? The Lifestyles of Elders Who Play Bingo (2002) for the Alberta Gaming Research Institute on how older people value Bingo play and how it contributes to, or detracts from, their social, mental, and physical well-being. This research will provide some of the first in-depth information in this area.

Maureen J. Dowds retired in 2002 as execu-

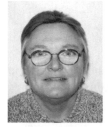

tive director of Manitoba Special Olympics, where she worked since 1986. After graduation from the University of Manitoba with a B.P.E. degree and the University of Western Ontario with a Dip.Ed., Ms. Dowds taught physical education in both junior and senior high schools. Her last teaching position was in a segregated school for adolescents with an intellectual disability. Since the late seventies, Ms. Dowds has volunteered and worked as a professional in the field of sport and physical education for individuals with intellectual disability. As programme director for Manitoba Special Olympics, she instituted several innovative programmes that have positively influenced the sport delivery system for athletes with intellectual disability. With her participation on Canada's national team in athletics, Ms. Dowds has brought that competitive outlook to the Special Olympics movement in Canada. Besides working directly in the Special Olympics field, Ms. Dowds has attempted to increase and open opportunities for athletes with intellectual disability through their participation within the Paralympic movement.

Dr. Claudia G. Emes is Professor in the

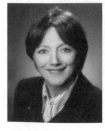

Faculty of Kinesiology at the University of Calgary. Dr. Emes teaches both adapted physical activity and gerontology; her research in these areas focusses more specifically on children with develop-

mental disabilities and on exercise and pain in people who are older. She is a member of the board of directors of Special Olympics Canada and serves on the North American Leadership Council of Special Olympics Inc. Locally, she is an active volunteer and member of the board of directors at the YWCA.

Spending time with her family is Claudia's favourite pastime, but she loves to run and, over the last fifteen years, she has expended a lot of energy planning that elusive second marathon.

Dr. David A. Fitzpatrick instructs motor

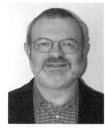

behaviour and pedagogy courses in the Physical Activity and Sport Studies programme at the University of Winnipeg. He earned his Ph.D. from the University of Alberta and his undergraduate and graduate degrees in Physical Education and Education from the University of Manitoba. His teaching interests are in adapted physical activity, physical growth and motor development, motor learning and control, physical activity and aging, and curricular activity courses. He previously taught adapted physical education in a large urban school division and has coached wheelchair basketball, volleyball, and athletics. He has a long-time interest in the study of physical awkwardness, or developmental coordination disorder (DCD), having developed numerous remedial motor skills programmes and formally conducted over 25,000 motor skill observations with over 8,000 children. For one year he was a consultant at Manitoba Education, where he provided curriculum support in fitness and adapted physical education. He was active with the development of the physical education curricular support series Moving to Inclusion, designed to facilitate the inclusion of students with disabilities into school physical education programmes. His academic interests include the observation, assessment, instruction, and programming of basic movement skills during early childhood, physical awkwardness, inclusive physical education, and teaching variables in physical education. Research interests include work on the experiences of people with disabilities in physical education and sport.

David's other interests include music, chess, reading, and jogging.

Sheri L. Foster has been working at The 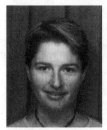Steadward Centre (TSC) for Personal and Physical Achievement since January 1999, coordinating the development of this textbook, co-authoring two chapters, and assisting with editorial work. In addition to these responsibilities, Ms. Foster is a research associate in the Faculty of Medicine and Dentistry (Neurology Division) working with individuals who have Parkinson's or Alzheimer's disease. For the first few years at TSC, Ms. Foster also assisted individuals with multiple sclerosis and spinal cord injuries in the functional electrical stimulation (FES) programme. She holds a B.P.H.E in Health Promotion and an M.Sc. in Exercise Physiology, the latter from the University of Alberta.

In addition to Sheri's professional pursuits, she enjoys participating in many athletic activities. In 1996, when she moved to Edmonton to start her M.Sc., she began training and competing in triathlon. More recently, however, Sheri has taken up additional sports, including mountain biking, kayaking, canoeing, climbing, orienteering, back-country alpine skiing, and has been competing in adventure and mountain bike races for the past three years.

Rick Gingras was awarded a B.Ed. degree in 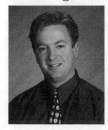Elementary Education from the University of Alberta in the spring of 2001. He also holds a B.P.E. (Adapted), which was awarded to him in 1990. Mr. Gingras held a number of positions within

The Steadward Centre for over ten years before returning to the University of Alberta in 1999. He started at the centre as a fitness programme coordinator and, a few years later, was promoted to Director of Fitness and Lifestyle Programs. Under Mr. Gingras's direction, the centre began implementing unique in-house recreation, fitness, and community outreach programming. Mr. Gingras has been actively involved in provision of physical activity for people with a disability, as a volunteer for a number of years with the Canadian Wheelchair Sports Association (CWSA), as an employee of The Steadward Centre, and most recently as a director on The Steadward Centre's board of directors. Mr. Gingras's most recent endeavour was to coordinate the events for athletes with a disability for the Eighth IAAF World Championships in Athletics held in Edmonton in which he acted as the liaison between the Edmonton 2001 Local Organizing Committee and the International Paralympic Committee. He is currently teaching a special needs junior high class for the Edmonton Public School Board.

Dr. Donna L. Goodwin is Assistant Professor 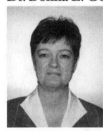with the College of Kinesiology at the University of Saskatchewan. Prior to that she was with the Faculty of Physical Activity Studies at the University of Regina. Dr. Goodwin's research focusses on the experiences of persons with disabilities in physical activity settings. She is particularly interested in the methodological issues surrounding the use of qualitative inquiry with school-aged children. Prior to joining the university community, Dr. Goodwin was an adapted physical education consultant with Edmonton Public Schools. Dr. Goodwin is a University of Alberta Alumni Honour Award winner and a recipient of the Queen's Golden Jubilee Medal for her long-time contribution to the disability community.

Dr. Henriëtte J. Groeneveld completed her
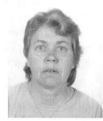
dissertation at Stellenbosch University, South Africa, where she applied Burton and Davis' ecological task analysis (ETA) theory to the knowledge base in disability sport by looking at ETA as a model for the development of functional movement and sport skills of children with physical disabilities while participating in a sports camp. Dr. Groeneveld worked for three years under challenging situations in South Africa in the historically disadvantaged areas. She worked with staff members of elementary and secondary schools to help them provide a physical education programme for their students who have a disability. This included planning, instructing, and evaluating the lessons. In addition, she provided various in-services for community agencies to learn skills and gain access to community programmes. She has since then gained many years of varied, in-depth experience, working to enable people with disabilities reach their maximum potential in the field of sport, recreation, physical activity, and daily living skills. She is now working in Edmonton as a rehabilitation instructor in daily living skills with persons who have a developmental disability. Dr. Groeneveld has been a coach from the grassroots to the elite level for over twenty years. She has travelled with local, provincial, and national teams all over the world, especially in wheelchair athletics and wheelchair basketball. In addition, she has served on various local, provincial, national, and international committees.

Dr. Joannie M. Halas is Associate Professor in
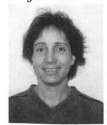
the Faculty of Physical Education and Recreation Studies at the University of Manitoba, in Winnipeg. She is a former physical education teacher who completed her B.P.E. at the University of Manitoba, her M.Sc. at the University of Ottawa, and her Ph.D. at the University of Alberta. As a middle school teacher, Dr. Halas developed physical education programmes that included students who had various physical and intellectual impairments, as well as students who had experienced severe emotional and behaviour difficulties in their lives. Dr. Halas has a tremendous respect for young people, especially those who are challenged to overcome hardship in their day-to-day lives. Her research investigates the quality and cultural relevance of physical education for youth who are marginalized from the mainstream of Canadian society. For example, she recently completed an action research study that involved the construction of a meaningful and relevant physical education programme for adolescent mothers. Currently, she is involved in a study funded by the Social Sciences and Humanities Research Council of Canada that investigates the quality of physical education for Aboriginal youth in Manitoba.

Joannie has a particular interest in outdoor activities; over the years, she has used the natural environment to construct a number of educational and recreational adventures for her students, including winter carnivals, hiking, biking, canoeing, and cross-country ski trips. One of her goals in life is to create a daily balance between work and play, a pursuit that she has yet to fulfill.

Dr. John C. Hudec received his Ph.D. in
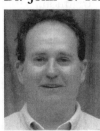
Physical Education and Recreation in 1999. He then focussed his studies on the field of exercise psychology by investigating human motivation for behaviour change. Academically, he has developed a holistic knowledge base, including studies of the biological, social, and behavioural domains of physical education and health promotion. Dr. Hudec has practical experience in fitness evaluation, counselling, certification, and programming. Throughout his career he has worked as a member of interdisciplinary teams, teaching, researching, and providing

rehabilitation and opportunities for many individuals to be physically active. He has worked with people of ranging ability, with many levels of motivation, and from all age groups. Dr. Hudec is currently teaching at Athabasca University in Alberta. Expanding his horizons into interdisciplinary studies, he has instructed team building in health care at the University of Alberta and is on faculty with the Centre for Nursing and Health Studies at Athabasca University in the Master of Health Studies programme.

In addition to outdoor pursuits such as sailing, Nordic skiing, running, and cycling, John remains active in his community as coach in youth sports.

Lynn L. Langille is Research Consultant at 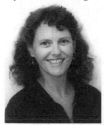 the Atlantic Health Promotion Research Centre (AHPRC) at Dalhousie University, Halifax, Nova Scotia. An anthropologist by training and at heart, Ms. Langille is a co-investigator on many of AHPRC's projects, including the development of a qualitative method to help people with disabilities explore and act on the effects of chronic illness and disability on their relationships. In her work at the AHPRC, Ms. Langille contributes to health promotion research through project development, proposal writing, identification of funding sources, development of data collection tools, facilitation of research partnerships, data analysis, and dissemination of research findings for the purpose of policy and social change.

In her leisure time, Lynn enjoys playing piano and guitar, reading, and a range of physical activities such as walking, dancing, hiking, and swimming.

Dr. David F.H. Legg is the coordinator of the 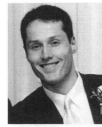 bachelor's degree programme in Applied Business and Entrepreneurship, Sport and Recreation, at Mount Royal College in Calgary. Dr. Legg completed his Ph.D. at the University of Alberta under the tutelage of Dr. Robert D. Steadward and Dr. Gary Wheeler. As a volunteer, Dr. Legg is Vice-president, Finance, for the Canadian Paralympic Committee; Technical Officer for the America's Paralympic Committee; and Past Chair of the board of the Multiple Sclerosis Society, Calgary Chapter. Dr. Legg has also worked professionally with the Canadian Wheelchair Sports Association, coached the national wheelchair rugby team, and volunteered extensively with the Active Living Alliance for Canadians with a Disability.

David lives in Calgary with his wife, Julie, and two sons, Jackson and Isaac.

Patricia E. Longmuir is Research Director for 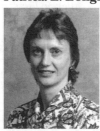 her own consulting company, PEL Consulting. With over twenty years of experience in adapted physical activity, she focusses on providing physical activity opportunities that include individuals of all abilities. Her activities emanate from a strong belief that all individuals have the right to enjoy the active living lifestyle of their choice and that people with disabilities should not be required to seek 'specialists' or 'special facilities or programmes'. The projects of PEL Consulting focus primarily on two areas: education and research. Education initiatives, workshops, and training materials are designed to provide individuals with disabilities and physical activity professionals with the knowledge, skills, and expertise required to ensure that active living opportunities are accessible to all interested individuals. Initiatives include effective advocacy, access to outdoor and natural environments, inclusive fitness services, access to active living in the community, and creating inclusive physical activity environments. Based on a strong love of nature and many outdoor activities as hobbies, Ms. Longmuir has focussed her recent research initiatives on enhancing access to outdoor and natural environments. These projects have included investigations of factors that affect trail accessibility (e.g., grade, type of surface), the ability of individuals with disabilities to access outdoor environments, the suitability of information formats for conveying information about outdoor environments, and the development of design standard, and guidelines for creating accessible natural environments.

Dr. Renée F. Lyons is Professor and Director 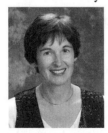 of the Atlantic Health Promotion Research Centre, Dalhousie University in Halifax. The Atlantic Health Promotion Research Centre is a unit of the faculties of Medicine, Dentistry, and Health Professions, and is supported in part by the departments of Health in the four Atlantic provinces. Currently, Dr. Lyons is the principal investigator for $3 million in research grants. She has academic appointments in both the School of Health and Human Performance and the Department of Psychology. She is currently on secondment to the Canadian Institutes of Health Research, Ottawa, where she is the special advisor to the president. A component of this role is the field of rehabilitation and disability research. She has been an advocate and researcher in the area of active living and disability. Dr. Lyons has published widely in the area of coping with significant life challenges, particularly chronic illness and disability. She has been particularly interested in social integration and personal relationships, as well as how social units

share stressors and deal with them collectively. She also has strong interests in rural health and in knowledge translation–how research can be more effectively used in policy and practice.

Renée maintains a very rigorous work life facilitated by morning runs with her long-time running buddy, Dr. Carolyn Savoy.

Dr. Jennifer B. Mactavish is Associate 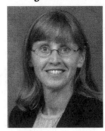 Professor, Faculty of Physical Education and Recreation Studies, and Research Affiliate in the Health, Leisure, and Human Performance Research Institute at the University of Manitoba. She earned a B.P.E. at the University of British Columbia; an M.Sc., with an emphasis in adapted physical activity, at the University of Manitoba; and a Ph.D. at the University of Minnesota, specializing in therapeutic recreation, educational psychology, and developmental disability. Since the early 1980s, Dr. Mactavish has worked extensively with individuals with intellectual disability and their families. This experience has fostered research interests in the social-psychological outcomes associated with participation in recreation and sport across the lifespan, and factors (individual, family, systemic, and programmatic) that support and constrain involvement. More recently, these interests have been extended to include issues broadly related to quality of life (e.g., social integration, independence, later life planning), and methods for enhancing the direct involvement of individuals with intellectual disability in the research process (e.g., participatory action research). In addition to research, Dr. Mactavish is actively involved in teaching future physical education and recreation professionals and volunteering with a number of sport and service organizations dedicated to individuals with intellectual disability.

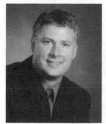

Dr. Michael J. Mahon is Dean of the Faculty of Physical Education and Recreation at the University of Alberta. He was previously at the University of Manitoba where he served as Director of the Health, Leisure, and Human Performance Research Institute. Dr. Mahon's research interests relate to understanding the relationship between people with a disability, leisure, and quality of life. His primary work in this area has dealt with the influence of leisure education on the quality of life of people with disabilities. He has developed and tested a number of leisure education interventions as a part of this work. Most recently, Dr. Mahon has engaged in participatory action research designed to understand and positively influence the lives of older adults with intellectual disabilities through leisure-based later life planning. Dr. Mahon is a past editor of *Therapeutic Recreation Journal*. He is presently an associate editor of *Leisure: The Journal of the Canadian Association of Leisure Studies*. Dr. Mahon has co-authored a text with Dr. Charles C. Bullock entitled *Introduction to Recreation Services for People with Disabilities: A Person Centred Approach*, now in its second edition. He is presently working on two other books focussed on disability, quality of life, and leisure education.

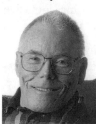

Dr. Gary McPherson, LL.D., has an extensive background in the voluntary sector, having spent more than twenty years in wheelchair sports administration. For eight of those years he served as President of the Canadian Wheelchair Sports Association (CWSA). Dr. McPherson served for ten years as Chair of the Premier's Council on the Status of Persons with Disabilities, providing advice to the Alberta government. He has been recognized for his work with numerous awards and has been inducted as a member of the Edmonton and Alberta sports halls of fame. On November 16, 1995, the University of Alberta Senate recognized his contribution to the community by awarding him an Honorary Doctorate of Laws Degree. He later joined the University of Alberta and was appointed Executive Director of the Canadian Centre for Social Entrepreneurship (CCSE) in the School of Business. He is Adjunct Professor, as well as Special Lecturer and Advisor, in the Faculty of Physical Education and Recreation. Gary is the author and publisher of the book entitled *With Every Breath I Take: One Person's Extraordinary Journey to a Healthy Life, and How You Can Share in it*.

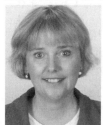

Dr. Patricia C. Nearingburg is an adapted physical education consultant with Edmonton Public Schools and a sessional lecturer at the University of Alberta. The school board position offers her an opportunity to assist teachers with inclusion of students with special needs in a physical education setting. In addition, she has been a member of a number of early education multi-disciplinary teams where her responsibility is to assess, teach, and provide home programming support for families with children with special needs between the ages of two-and-one-half to five years of age. Dr. Nearingburg has been involved as a co-researcher in a study pertaining to fitness levels of adolescents with cerebral palsy. She is presently involved in a multi-disciplinary project pertaining to students with non-verbal learning disabilities.

Patt balances her professional life by being very involved with family and friends.

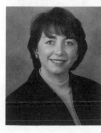

Dr. Lisa M. Olenik is Chair of the Health, Physical Education, Recreation, and Dance Department at Longwood University in Farmville, Virginia. Dr. Olenik received her doctoral degree from the University of Alberta in

Physical Education and Recreation, with an emphasis in disability sport. She has extensive experience in the field of activity and sport programmes for special populations, including providing recreational-based services to people with spinal cord injury, traumatic brain injury, Parkinson's disease, and multiple sclerosis. Moreover, she has facilitated numerous wellness programmes at the local and state level for individuals with disabilities. Dr. Olenik has many publications and has given over eighty professional presentations in her areas of specialization, including women in sport, disability and physical activity, health and wellness, and religion and sport. She serves on numerous national boards and committees. She is Chair of the National Programs Advisory Council for the National Multiple Sclerosis Society and is a member of the International Paralympic Committee Commission on Women and Sport.

Dr. Stéphane Perreault is Professor in the 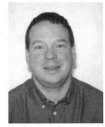 *Département des Sciences du Loisir et de la Communication Sociale at the Université du Québec à Trois-Rivières*, where he teaches team dynamics and social psychology. His research interests include motivation and inter-group relations in sport. Dr. Perreault has been involved in wheelchair basketball as a coach for the past seven years.

During his leisure time, Stéphane enjoys running and playing basketball.

Dr. Greg Reid has been Professor in the 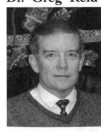 Department of Kinesiology and Physical Education of McGill University for almost thirty years. He received a B.Ed. (P.E.) degree from McGill University, an M.Sc. from UCLA, and a Ph.D. from Pennsylvania State University. His research has dealt with motor learning and performance of individuals with intellectual disabili-

ties, as well as intervention strategies for those with autism. He is investigating self-determination in adapted physical activity, more specifically, self-regulation of learning by children with movement difficulties, with Dr. Marcel Bouffard of the University of Alberta. Dr. Reid is the former editor of the *Adapted Physical Activity Quarterly*, the 1997 recipient of the G. Lawrence Rarick Research Award, and an International Fellow of the American Academy of Kinesiology and Physical Education. Dr. Reid is currently President of the International Federation of Adapted Physical Activity.

Christine M. Seidl has been teaching physical 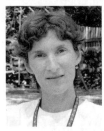 education at Summit School for Developmentally Disabled Children for the past fifteen years. She has also enjoyed part-time involvement with the undergraduate programme in Physical Education at McGill University, where she supervises student teachers and guest lectures in adapted physical activity. As a graduate student, Ms. Seidl was involved in research pertaining to the health-related fitness assessment of people with cognitive disabilities. She has continued to focus on this area since 1994, with her involvement with the Leadership Development Initiative for People With a Disability (LDI-PWAD). This subcommittee of the Canadian Society for Exercise Physiology (CSEP) is committed to providing inclusive fitness appraisal services for all Canadians.

Christine enjoys swimming, skiing, and other outdoor sports. She lives with her husband and three children in Pointe Claire, Quebec.

Dr. Debra Shogan is Professor in the Faculty 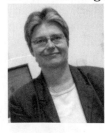 of Physical Education and Recreation at the University of Alberta. She is a social theorist and critic who is interested in how disciplines function to produce conforming subjects and how people resist attempts to make them conform. In her book *The Making of High Performance Athletes: Discipline, Diversity and Ethics* (1999), she looks at these questions in relation to how sport works to produce the conforming athlete. She has also addressed these questions in relation to sexuality, disability, and education.

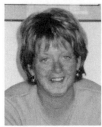 **Leanne Squair** is an issue strategist in the area of accessibility for people with disabilities for the City of Calgary. She is involved in policy planning, development, and implementation of universal design concepts and reviews and makes recommendations on policy issues, accessibility, and services for people with disabilities. Ms. Squair has a strong background in community inclusion and adapted physical activity, having worked for eight years with Calgary Parks and Recreation, Resource Services for People with Disabilities. Her volunteer activities have included serving as president of the Canadian Wheelchair Sports Alberta Section, board member of the Canadian Wheelchair Sports Association, and executive member of the Canadian Wheelchair Basketball Association Development Committee. Her ten-year volunteer commitment to Alberta Recreation and Parks Association has allowed her to be involved in the increased participation by persons with disabilities in recreation and sports activities in Alberta. She initiated the Calgary Rocky Mountain Rollers Women's Wheelchair Basketball team. Ms. Squair believes in breaking down barriers in the community to facilitate inclusion into community programs and facilities. Through the Active Living Alliance for Canadians with Disabilities (ALACD) she has been involved in the development of inclusion training materials that have assisted teachers and students with disabilities in becoming more physically active.

Leanne enjoys reading, running, and coaching and supports her two young children to be physically active and the best that they can be at whatever sport or recreational pursuit in which they are involved.

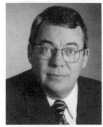 **Dr. Robert (Bob) Steadward**, O.C., LL.D. (Hons), is Past and Founding President of the International Paralympic Committee, the second-largest sport organization in the world and umbrella body for athletes with disability. He is Founder and CEO of The Steadward Centre, a multi-disability fitness, research, and lifestyle facility at the University of Alberta where he is Professor Emeritus. Dr. Steadward co-chaired the successful Bid Committee to host the Edmonton 2001 World Championships in Athletics, held in August 2001. His community service contributions have included posts in sport at all levels, from coach to administrator, from international to local, involving people with and without disability—at Universiade, Commonwealth, Olympic, and Paralympic games.

Dr. Steadward was appointed Officer of the Order of Canada, the nation's highest civilian honour, in recognition of national achievement and merit of a high degree, especially in service to Canada and humanity at large. He is the recipient of two Honorary Doctor of Law degrees, from Leuven University in Belgium and the University of Alberta. Dr. Steadward has received many awards and honours: from the City of Edmonton, Province of Alberta, and the University of Alberta halls of fame; Distinguished Alumni awards from the University of Oregon and the University of Alberta; Provincial and National Volunteer of the Year; and, from the University of Alberta, the Rutherford Teaching Award for Excellence in Undergraduate Teaching. Dr. Steadward is a foremost, acclaimed pioneer and leader in the field of adapted physical activity, having helped to establish related studies at universities nationally and throughout the world. He accepts international students under his tutelage whose academic and research interests and objectives include the promotion of adapted physical activity in their respective homeland. Dr. Steadward has published over 150 books and articles and made uncountable presentations on adapted physical activity and many other issues related to people with disability, in addition to sport environment, women in sport, and sport for severely disabled.

Bob enjoys cycling, golf, skiing and ranching. He and his wife Laura have recently become proud grandparents.

Dr. William B. (Billy) Strean is Associate
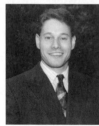
Professor in the Faculty of Physical Education and Recreation at the University of Alberta, specializing in sport psychology. His primary research interests are "play, fun, and games" and coaching. After growing up in Teaneck, New Jersey, Dr. Strean attended Grinnell College in Iowa, where he majored in philosophy, received his elementary education certification, and earned twelve varsity letters in soccer, diving, and track and field. He then obtained his master's degree at the University of Iowa, where he also served as a coach for the Iowa Women's Track and Field Team. Dr. Strean completed his doctoral studies at the University of Illinois. In addition to his research pursuits, Dr. Strean is recognized as an outstanding instructor and presenter. He has conducted a variety of workshops and has been an invited presenter and keynote speaker. He has also served as a sport psychology consultant for elite athletes and national teams, an NCCP Level III ('C' Licence) soccer coach, and coach of many youth sport teams. More recently, Dr. Strean has focussed on professional coaching, and he has completed a variety of coaching courses, including the curriculum and certification programme of the Coaches Training Institute.

Billy is also a proud father and has done extensive work with children.

Bruce Taylor has been a programme coordi-
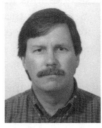
nator with the Physical Activity Unit (formerly Fitness Canada) of Health Canada since 1989. His areas of responsibility and expertise include issues, programmes, and policies pertaining to disability, older adults, and, more recently, Aboriginal people. Prior to his position with the federal government, Mr. Taylor worked in a similar capacity with the Alberta government for seven years, and before that, he taught physical education in a special education setting in Edmonton for a number of years. Mr. Taylor holds a bachelor's degree in Physical Education from the University of New Brunswick and a graduate diploma in Educational Psychology from the University of Alberta.

Bruce's other interests include coaching competitive youth soccer, skiing, and reading. He currently resides in Ottawa.

Dr. A.E. (Ted) Wall joined the Department
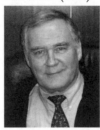
of Physical Education at his alma mater, McGill University, in 1968, after teaching physical education in a local high school. After completing doctoral studies at the University of Alberta, he served there as Professor and Chair of the Department of Physical Education and Sport Studies. In 1986, he returned to McGill as Professor and Department Chair. In 1991, he was appointed Dean of the Faculty of Education, a position he held for seven years. In 1998, he returned to full-time teaching and research within the Department of Kinesiology and Physical Education. In August 2002, he retired from the university. His teaching and research interests have been focussed on two major areas, adapted physical education, with a special interest in children with movement

difficulties, and the psychology of motor performance, with a major interest in the development of sport expertise. In both of these areas, he has used a developmental knowledge-based approach that emphasizes the importance of self-awareness and self-regulation. He is currently completing a text entitled *Understanding Sport Expertise: A Knowledge-based Introduction*, which integrates a variety of expert-novice studies based on a cognitive approach to sport expertise. Dr. Wall has also been involved in a number of important professional initiatives. In 1986, he and Dr. Robert Steadward co-chaired the Jasper Talks Symposium. Subsequently, Dr. Wall served as Founding President of the Active Living Alliance for Canadians with Disabilities. Over the past ten years, he has served as a volunteer board member on a number of organizations that are working with persons with disabilities.

In his spare time, Ted enjoys hiking, sailing, swimming, reading Canadian history, and playing golf.

Dr. E. Jane Watkinson was born in Thunder 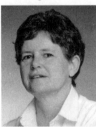 Bay, Ontario, where she attended Fort William Collegiate Institute. She then attended McMaster University in Hamilton, Ontario, from 1966–70, and graduated with her B.P.E. and B.A. (French Literature) degrees. She completed her M.A. in Physical Education at the University of Western Ontario in 1971. She served as a lecturer and volleyball coach in the School of Physical Education, University of Manitoba, during 1973–74. She began her career at the University of Alberta in the fall of 1974, when she accepted a position as an assistant professor. From 1971 through 1977, she also worked on a Ph.D. in Physical Education at Michigan State University and she was awarded the doctoral degree in 1977. Dr. Watkinson has a special interest in developmental disabilities. She has written numerous publications related to physical

activity and children with disabilities. Her current research interests are focussed on the participation of children with mild disabilities especially DCD in physical activity, with a specific interest in recess. In addition to her current role as Associate Dean (Academic), she has served as Associate Dean (Research and Planning), 1988–90; Acing Dean of the Faculty of Physical Education and Recreation (1990–91); Chair of the Department of Physical Education and Sport Studies, June 1992 to December 1994; and Associate Dean (Research and Graduate programmes), 1995-1999. In her new administrative capacity, Dr. Watkinson is responsible for the overall strategic directions of the academic programmes of the Faculty, the well being of students and staff, and the development of the Faculty's teaching and research programmes.

Dr. Garry D. Wheeler was born in England, 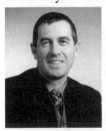 and came to Canada in 1981 to complete his M.Sc. in Physical Education specializing in exercise physiology. He went on to complete his doctorate, a master's degree in counselling, and chartered as a psychologist. Dr. Wheeler is currently the Manager of Research and Counselling at The Steadward Centre, Faculty of Physical Education and Recreation, University of Alberta. His areas of research include FES-assisted exercise, motivation for exercise in persons with disability, and retirement from disability sport. As a volunteer with the Canadian Society of Exercise Physiology and Canadian Fitness Accreditation and Certification Association, he has been involved in the development of the Canadian Physical Activity Fitness and Lifestyle Appraisal and the Inclusive Fitness Appraisal and Counselling Services for Canadians of *All* Abilities system. He is a recipient of the 2000 Dr. Erwin Bako Award for services to the Alberta fitness and health movement, and the 2001 CSEP/FACA National Recognition Award for services to the health, fitness, and lifestyle profession in Canada. He is a member of the International Paralympic Committee, Sport Science Committee.

Garry is married to Carol, his wife of eighteen years and a graduate of the masters of Educational Administration programme at the University of Alberta. He has two children, Ashley, fifteen; Graeme, nine; and a five-year-old Golden Retriever, Baxter Bear. An ardent fitness enthusiast, his hobbies include fishing and a variety of water sports.

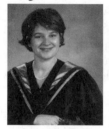

Dr. Joan Matthews White is Head Athletic Therapist, Department of Athletics, and Sessional Instructor, Faculty of Physical Education and Recreation, University of Alberta. She holds a B.P.E., M.Sc., C.A.T.(C), and Ph.D. Dr. Matthews White's research has focussed on sport injuries for athletes with disabilities. Her research and on-field therapy allow her to cross the paths of downhill skiers, cross-country skiers, and sledge hockey players. She enjoyed the experiences of the Lillehammer Winter Paralympics and the Atlanta Summer Paralympics as both an athletic therapist and a researcher. She has also been involved with the Edmonton women's wheelchair basketball team.

Joan enjoys her family, friends, and any activities that combine them.

I ■ FOCUS ON CRITICAL THINKING

Critical Thinking and Professional Preparation

Marcel Bouffard
William B. Strean

The ultimate goal of the educational system is to shift to the individual the burden of pursuing his [or her] own education.
–J.W. GARDNER

Learning Objectives
- To state, in your own words, why the authors claim that exact predictions about one's future professional life are not possible.
- To outline the consequences for professional preparation of not knowing the future.
- To criticize the viewpoint expressed by the authors about university education. Begin to develop a personal philosophy of education and criticize it.
- To state, in their own words, why the authors advocate the development of critical thinking skills. Criticize the viewpoint expressed by the authors.
- To outline a personal definition of critical thinking skills.
- To state what you could personally do to acquire critical thinking skills.

Professional Preparation in Adapted Physical Activity: What Do We Need?

When you first enrolled in university, you might have experienced culture shock. During most of your earlier education, you were most likely asked to memorize lots of facts and then convince your teachers that you knew those facts. During those years, what you were taught was often viewed as certain and unquestionable. You may already have noticed that many of your university teachers have a different attitude towards knowledge. They view knowledge as tentative and uncertain. As university teachers, we also know that questioning the foundations of knowledge is often anxiety producing: not knowing what to think often leads to fear and anxiety (Endler, Edwards, and Vitelli 1991).

Not knowing the future may also produce anxiety. No one, including your university professors, really knows what will happen. Will you find enough money to complete your degree? Will you find a good job that interests you? What practical problems will you be faced with during work? Will you have all the necessary knowledge and skills to provide good professional services? Although we can predict the future to a certain extent (for a discussion see Rescher 1998), nobody can be sure of the accuracy of these predictions.

Although in this introduction we acknowledge that uncertainty about the future might lead to some psychological fear or anxiety, our main intent in this chapter is not to discuss theories of anxiety nor how to cope with it. Instead, we want to underscore that uncertainty about the future has important consequences for the programme in which you are presently enrolled and the adapted physical activity course you are presently taking.

If humans were able to forecast the future, then it would be possible to offer professional preparation programmes based on this knowledge. Ultimately, it would be possible to produce a set of fairly specific condition-action guidelines stating that if such-and-such situation happens, then do that action. In this chapter we will refer to the learning of specific condition-action guidelines as the if-then approach. Theoretically, if we knew the future, it would be possible to prepare people by teaching them exactly what specific conditions they will encounter and what needs to be done when they are met.

Not knowing the future raises important questions and issues about professional preparation. How do we best prepare people for their work when we do not know the details of the situations they will be faced with? We cannot rely on the **if-then** approach. The if-then approach quickly leads to an infinite number of situations, and we are convinced that you want to graduate before you have studied all these situations! At most, only general guidelines can be suggested to face situations. These guidelines will, however, have to be adapted when confronted with the real world.

A fundamental limitation of the if-then approach is that it is based on a dependency model. By dependency, we mean that to know how to act or what to do, you rely on others to tell you how to act or what to do. (At this point, you may ask who told these people how to act or what to do.) Using the if-then approach, you are entirely dependent on what other people tell you in order to justify your actions. Contrary to the if-then model of professional preparation, we contend that university education should empower people to become more independent and capable of justifying their own actions and beliefs.

1 What assumption is made by the authors about human nature?

During your life, and possibly your career as an adapted physical activity professional, you will have to solve numerous problems. By problems, we refer to situations in which the solution is not immediately obvious. In these situations, we contend that you, instead of someone else, should be able to justify your actions and determine what are justified beliefs. This vision is at the heart of the critical thinking movement.

In this chapter, we submit that one of the best ways to prepare adapted physical activity professionals, and physical activity professionals in general, is to empower them with critical thinking skills. The rationale for this position is presented below. While reading this chapter, take time to identify the authors' assumptions and be critical of the ideas presented. You are encouraged to generate a list of pros and cons of the viewpoint embraced by the authors.

UNIVERSITY EDUCATION

It is usually accepted that a major function of the university is to acquire and disseminate knowledge. Although there are still debates about what knowledge is and the different types of knowledge, it usually refers to statements that are supported either through empirical evidence or logic. That is, knowledge refers to statements that are justified. To reduce the uncertainty associated with statements, the university is a place where open-ended research and teaching occurs. This means that faculty and students are critical thinkers. Members of the university community are constantly questioning statements presented to them. "A university does not teach mindlessly. It is supposed to scrutinize its teaching, to criticize, reexamine, and reformulate received ideas. A university is supposed to 'think for itself.' This is essential to our idea of the university. This is what we expect a university to do" (Anderson 1993, p. 43).

Within the university, exposure to critical analysis is the mechanism for testing and validating new data and new ideas. A fundamental belief of the university community is that erroneous ideas, poor research, or flawed conclusions will often fail when openly examined and debated (Anderson 1993). Although the pursuit of knowledge is sometimes accompanied by plateaus, even temporary downturns, on the average there is more or less steady increase in the reduction of uncertainty associated with statements. The constant questioning and criticism of ideas made by the university community is central to this steady increase. A university where the criticism and challenge of ideas is not allowed is no longer a university.

The vision of the university as a place of critical thinking as described above has implications for teaching there. Students should become independent learners capable of understanding, evaluating, and criticizing ideas. If students are not prepared to think for themselves and to make the effort to learn how to do this well, they will always remain slaves to the ideas and values of others and to their own ignorance (Hughes 1992).

Students "should not approach their classes as so many unconnected fields, each with a mass of information to be blindly memorized, but rather organized systems for thinking clearly, accurately, and precisely about interconnected domains of human life and experience" (Paul 1992, p. 21). While attempting to reach this goal, it is important to remember that teachers can only facilitate the learning process. Although some environments are better than others to foster learning, students are ultimately responsible for their own learning and their own development. In fact, we believe that the best education possible is the one that empowers the individual to contribute to his or her own learning: good education not only teaches facts but also instructs people how to learn.

UNIVERSITY EDUCATION IN A PHYSICAL ACTIVITY PROFESSIONAL SCHOOL

Professional schools have a particular role to play at the university and in our society. They should prepare students to deliver services of the highest quality possible. Although the type of professional services delivered by professionals in our field is quite broad, it is essential that professionals use their experience and their knowledge in order to make sensible and reasonable decisions or judgements. An ultimate aim of university education in a professional school should be the improvement of practice in the field. Therefore, we submit that students graduating from physical activity programmes should be able to conduct "critical examination of current usages, techniques, methods, to see if they can be improved and better suited for the purpose they are intended to serve" (Anderson 1993, p. 114). They should also be able to generate new programmes, treatments, and methods. Our students should be capable of distinguishing excellence from error when they deliver services.

As noted earlier, while preparing students to offer quality services and to contribute to the ongoing development of the field, we must recognize that it is practically impossible to prepare them for all the possible situations they will face in the field. This implies that important decisions have to be made about the core of our curriculum. We cannot teach everything or be all things to everybody.

It is useful to categorize three situations that adapted physical activity professionals are likely to face. In the first type, the professional is asked to provide services for which he or she is fully prepared (e.g., develop an aerobic training programme for a person with cerebral palsy who has no medical contraindications). In this case, the professional may provide recommendations based on typical exercise prescription programmes described in textbooks, and with which the professional may have had first-hand experience.

In the second type of situation, the professional may not be adequately prepared (e.g., develop a fitness programme for a person with Down's syndrome who recently had a quadruple bypass). In this case, without more extensive professional preparation, the professional may not have the competencies to offer an adequate programme. In this instance, it would be better to decline further involvement with the person and refer the case to a more qualified practitioner. The important point here is that to offer appropriate services, professionals should also know their limitations.

Between these two extremes, the future professional is likely to be frequently involved in situations where an immediate solution is not available, but the situation is surmountable with further thinking and information-gathering without risks for the participant or the professional. It is for these cases that critical thinking and problem-solving skills are likely to be most relevant and useful.

The situations that professionals in our field are confronted with can frequently be viewed as problems to be solved. A problem exists when a person attempts to reach some goal when no obvious method to solve the problem is available to the problem solver. In some 'ill-defined' problems, the goal to be reached is not even clear. In these messy situations, problem formulation (or representation) is one of the most critical phases of the problem-solving process. To solve problems, it seems logical that our students develop critical thinking skills and be exposed to a problem-based approach to learning. In addition, we submit that the above skills cannot be divorced from moral analysis. Applied ethics is needed to guide both scholarship and professional practice.

During their undergraduate programme our students should acquire the following general competencies (modified after Ennis 1992, p. 76):

- to judge the credibility of sources
- to identify conclusions, reasons, and assumptions

- to judge the quality of an argument, including the truth of its reasons and assumptions
- to develop and defend one's position on an issue
- to ask appropriate searching questions, such as "Why?"
- to plan experiments and evaluations and judge the quality of studies
- to define terms in a way appropriate for the context
- to be both critical and open-minded
- to try to be well-informed on the topic
- to be able to communicate effectively and clearly using speaking and writing skills
- to understand that values often underlie the decision-making process

We are not advocating the development of a curriculum exclusively centred on critical thinking and problem solving. It would be an error to divorce critical thinking from the content area. Studies of expert/novice differences in various domains have continuously revealed the impact of knowledge on problem resolution (Glaser 1991). What should be avoided is the acquisition of 'spotty' knowledge consisting of isolated definitions and superficial understanding.

The result of lower-order learning of this kind is that students leave with a jumble of undigested fragments left over after they have forgotten most of what they had to cram into their memory for particular tests. They rarely grasp the logic of what they learn. Rarely do they relate what they learn to their own experiences and critique their learning and their past experience with respect to each other. Rarely do they ask, "Why is this so? How does this relate to what I already learned? How does this relate to what I am learning in other classes?" In a nutshell, very few students know what it means to rationally organize what they learn" (Paul 1992, p. 7).

BARRIERS

The approach we advocate implies that students have a major role to play in their education. Critical thinking requires intellectual effort and integrity. Unfortunately, some students may come to the university with the expectation that the instructor or the textbook will tell them exactly what to do under all circumstances. In addition, many students may perceive themselves to be inadequately prepared for assignments requiring them to think critically. They may assume that the generation of a solution is not their responsibility. They believe that, one way or another, either the textbook or the professor will tell them what to say or do. Hence, even if the teacher believes that critical thinking should be emphasized in the curriculum, most students may not produce it because they believe it is not expected of them or they do not know how to do it (Paul 1992).

Critical Thinking: What Is It?

Critical thinking is an important part of your education and professional development. Yet it may not be clear what is meant by *critical thinking*. Many people have a first reaction that it relates to 'being critical' or finding fault. You will see below whether or not that fits with how we define critical thinking.

What is critical thinking? If you do not know, you are in good company. A recent large study of college and university professors revealed that although the overwhelming majority (89 percent) claimed critical thinking to be a primary objective of their instruction, only a small minority (19 percent) could give a clear explanation of what critical thinking is (Paul, Elder, and Bartell 1997).

Part of the difficulty may be that there are many definitions of critical thinking in the literature. The experts in the field do not entirely agree on one definition of critical thinking. That may, however, be a good thing. Much of your time in school may have been spent memorizing what a teacher said so that you could write it on a test. The critical thinking approach to teaching suggests that one definition can harness your mind. Answers stop thinking. Questions encourage more thinking. So let us look at a number of definitions of critical thinking and, after reading them, you can try to come to your own definition.

The most basic way to define critical thinking is "thinking that assesses itself" (Paul 1995). This can be elaborated by saying it is thinking about your thinking (with sensitivity to intellectual standards) in order to improve your thinking. This definition adds two key features: standards and a goal, which is to create better thinking (examples of standards include clarity, accuracy, depth, breadth, and logic). This is very different from what you might expect when you first hear the word *critical*. Often we get the sense that if people are being critical, they are telling us what is wrong with us. That really is not the case, which we can see from looking at the root words.

The origin of critical thinking can be found in *criticos* and *criterion*. The first word, *criticos*, has to do with judgement or a person of judgement. The second, *criterion* (which should be familiar, like *criteria*) has to do with standards. Therefore, critical thinking is about judging using standards.

There are some other definitions that are generally consistent with the above, but they may suggest a different focus or flavour. Stephen Brookfield, a leading authority on adult education and critical thinking, focusses on checking assumptions and exploring alternatives as being at the heart of critical thinking. His approach to critical thinking concentrates on identifying different kinds of assumptions, or things we take for granted, checking their validity, and then exploring alternative ways to think and act.

"Reasonable and reflective thinking that is focussed upon deciding what to believe or do" is the foundation of the approach taken by Robert Ennis, who wrote a paper in 1962 that got the critical thinking movement running (Ennis 1962). *Reasonable* is similar to the idea of standards and *reflective* speaks to the idea of stopping and thinking about thinking. This definition focusses on action. Many professionals in adapted physical education are action-oriented people who probably would not want to spend a lot of time sitting around thinking, just for the sake of thinking. Ennis suggested that we bother to think critically because it will help us to make a decision about what we will do in our lives or what we will believe. There are a variety of other definitions that you may come across, but those are some of the major ones from respected thinkers.

Penner (1995) summed it up this way:

> When we first hear the term "critical thinking," our natural inclination is to bring all the connotations of the two words together, and see in which ways the two words might relate. "Thinking" is pretty straight forward; it's everything we do with our minds. But the meaning of "critical" is not so simple. In many ways we associate the word "critical" with negative ideas. "Criticism" is what we experience when someone else judges us negatively. We don't like to be "criticized"; it means that we aren't good enough.

Using these connotations of *critical*, it becomes understandable that people might assume critical thinking is destructive, arrogant, and hurtful; it would seem to be a way to build up one's ego by ridiculing others. But the root word behind *critic*, the Greek *kriths*, has neither positive nor negative connotations; it means simply 'judge', one who evaluates, distinguishes, decides, determines if something is right or wrong. It is in this sense that we use the phrase 'critical thinking'. Thinking in a way that is discerning is properly called 'critical thinking'.

Penner (1995) also offered the following, which is a nice metaphor for us:

> In some ways, developing critical thinking skills is like developing motor skills: both require exercise to develop. Both must also not be imposed by others; there must be some sort of consent involved. Forcing it intimidates and builds resistance. As with physical exercise, there is also more than one way to achieve the goal; in fact, a diversity of methods is needed. The role of an educator wishing to develop critical

thinking skills in learners must therefore be that of a helper, facilitator and motivator. The educator's role is to help learn, not to teach. That's not to say that learner satisfaction is the objective. When deciding what to do or say, a good facilitator will always ask, 'How does this help produce critical thinkers?' Exercise is often temporarily unpleasant, especially when it calls for change.

Critical thinking can take place in virtually any area of life that requires decisions, choices, or considerations. Whenever we are using information, there is an opportunity to think critically. There are a number of occasions for practicing critical thinking when studying adapted physical activity. First, when you are presented with a text, such as this one, you can engage by asking questions, looking for assumptions, or trying to identify the author's point of view. When you are in a discussion, dialogue, or argument, you can bring critical thinking skills to reach a better outcome. As you apply what you learn in a professional setting, you can evaluate current practices and explore what might be better ways to work with people.

Why Should We Develop Critical Thinking Skills?

There are many ways thinkers and researchers have viewed education. Some use the metaphor of the student as a sponge–taking in information and trying to hold as much of it as possible, until such time as one is 'wrung out' for an examination of some sort. In this model, there is little judgement being required on the part of students. A critical thinking approach sees the learner as an active and autonomous participant in the learning process.

Although critical thinking skills and dispositions, as with many things of value, may require signficant time and effort to develop, there are many benefits to working on your critical thinking. As a student, one of the most obvious payoffs is better academic performance. In most of your courses, your success will be determined, at least in part, by your ability to think critically. If you use this book and other strategies to develop your critical thinking skills, you will likely do better in your courses. The value of these skills may become more evident as you move through your education.

You may also find that you develop increased self-confidence in decisions. If you understand your own thinking and your reasons for your decisions, if you have a process to think about your thinking, you will be able to make decisions with more confidence than before. Critical thinking does not mean you have to change what you believe or what you value. You may find that you can hold many of your positions with greater confidence because you can put forth an argument and an explanation of why you think the way you do. You should walk away from your critical thinking efforts with new ways of working your way through practical problems.

Furthermore, you may create more choices about how to think. All of us have some ways to think about things that matter to us. If you weren't already a pretty good thinker, one might guess that you wouldn't be reading this book. Critical thinking training can show you some new options so you have more ways to think about what you care about.

In the grand scheme of things, you can possibly create bigger dreams for yourself. It can get exciting when you see how it can help you to break down barriers that you have built for yourself. By questioning things that you believe to be limiting you, you might be able to expand the exciting opportunities that you can go after. Steven Covey (1989) in his book, *The Seven Habits of Highly Effective People*, put it this way, "People who exercise their embryonic freedom day after day, will little by little, expand that freedom. People who do not will find that it withers until they are literally 'being lived'. They are acting out the scripts written by parents, associates, and society."

Critical thinking can also be considered as an inoculation to protect your health, finances, and self-esteem. There are many potentially damaging messages in our culture. If we accept uncritically what is said by those interests who are after our money, we can suffer in various ways. For example, some advertisers would have us believe things about ourselves that suggest that we are less worthy people unless we spend our money on their products and services. A tendency to ask critical questions can protect you from decisions that will cost you personally or financially. By questioning the assumptions of messages and suspending judgement, we can protect ourselves from bad choices.

In addition to this inoculation, the skills and disposition to question can be of great benefit in deciding what to believe or what to do. When we consume the media, listen to friends and family, or are exposed to 'voices of authority' we do well to question, rather than to accept everything at face value.

Critical thinking also provides an ability to use standards. There are many situations where we have to evaluate or judge ideas. Although we probably have some good intuitive criteria, through work on critical thinking you can develop your ability to use standards explicitly. For example, instead of having a sense that something is 'just not right', you will be able to identify where it is lacking in clarity, precision, and accuracy. You will also be able to go beyond asserting that someone has made a good argument because you liked it; you will be able to show how the speaker has dealt with the issue in sufficient depth and breadth and presented the points logically.

You can also expect to be more effective in your communication–both more critical in how you read and listen, as well as better equipped to deliver messages in speaking and writing. In summary, with more highly developed critical thinking skills and dispositions, you will be better able to decide what matters to you, to go after it, and to obtain what you desire!

How Can You Acquire Critical Thinking Skills?

USING CRITICAL THINKING SKILLS WHILE READING THIS BOOK

Much of what you do as a student involves reading of one kind or another. You can develop critical thinking skills by working on the process of critical reading while you read this book. Then you can apply the skills to the variety of materials that you read. The primary shift is from traditional passive reading to active engagement with the text.

To begin, you may ask questions to become a more active reader. As you go through the book, here are some questions you may ask:

1. **What is the chapter about as a whole?** What is the leading theme?

2. **What is being said in detail and how?** What are the main ideas, assertions, and arguments?

3. **Is the chapter accurate, in whole or part?** You will need the first two questions answered to make up your own mind; knowing the author's mind is not enough. Determining accuracy can be challenging and complex. Using other independent sources of information can help to determine if facts are correct.

4. **What of it?** What is the significance, why is this important to know (according to the author); is it important to you; if it enlightened you, what are the implications? What will you do to pursue the topic or issue further?

5. **What is the author's point of view?** Is a particular perspective taken? How does the way the author is looking at the topic affect what is being communicated?

6. **What are the major assumptions the author is making?** What does the author take for granted about how the world is and how the world should be?

You can shift your approach to reading from simply "taking in the ideas" to "having a conversation" with the author(s) of what you read. By being active and asking questions when you read, you will build your abilities and tendencies to think critically.

USING CRITICAL THINKING AS A PROFESSIONAL

To illustrate how critical thinking can be used in your work, please read the scenario outlined below. Place yourself in the position of the helper. Afterwards, you could consider what it is like to be Todd and what he can add to solving the problem.

> Todd, a twenty-two-year-old male, has been in a coma for two weeks following a car accident. In addition, following his accident Todd had a complete lesion of his spinal cord and is now paraplegic. Todd spent six weeks in a rehabilitation centre before returning home and you see him for the first time one month after he returns home. During your first session with him, he confesses that he is mildly depressed and he is concerned by his perceived inability to move around in his wheelchair. Todd has always been a proud and independent person who does not like to ask people for help. He says he would like to travel longer distances with his wheelchair and as well to climb ramps and hills around his house. At the end of your meeting, Todd asks you to design a programme for him.

2 Given the information you have about Todd, state what you would do as the professional in this situation? (Please answer the question before you read our comments.)

This exercise is an opportunity to sharpen your critical thinking skills **before** you actually intervene. Critical thinking skills are sharpened by thinking about problems and issues. It is in this spirit that we submit the following questions. (These are not the only questions possible. We encourage you to generate your own and outline your answers.) We grouped these questions into five major categories: the participant, you, what you want to do, how will you do it, and overall evaluation.

1. **The participant**

   Do you think it would be appropriate to design a programme for Todd? If yes, given the scenario above, do you have enough information about Todd to design a programme? If your answer is no, what else would you like to know about Todd? What can you do to get this information? If you think it would not be appropriate to design a programme for Todd, what can you do?

2. **You**

   Do you have the necessary knowledge and skills to offer such a programme? If no, what can you do?

3. **What do you want to do?**

   If you think you are qualified to design and implement a programme for Todd, state what you would like to achieve. Do you think that you, as an expert, should make a decision about the goals and objectives of the programme? Or should these ones be decided in consultation with Todd?

4. **How will you do it?**

   How will you structure your interventions? Will you try to determine whether progress is made? If yes, how? If no, state why. What would you do if you observe no progress? What will you do if the programme is too demanding for Todd?

5. **Evaluation**

   Do you think it would be important to document whether your intervention had a positive impact or not? If no, say why. If yes, say why and outline what you would do.

USING CRITICAL THINKING SKILLS DURING YOUR LIFE

We hope you can see that developing critical thinking can help you to be a more effective professional. Critical thinking can occur at any stage during the service delivery process. It can occur before the programme is offered, during its delivery, and after its completion. It is also valuable because it can help you to have a better life. Using your critical thinking skills in a wide variety of areas in your life will not only help you to improve your thinking, but it will allow you to alter the quality of your life.

We go through much of our life without much awareness of our thinking and how it is influencing how life occurs. We make many decisions by habit or by what offers the path of least resistance. When we stop and think about our thinking, we open up new options and see how our automatic ways of operating may not produce the best results.

The most important step in developing critical thinking skills may be your intention to use these skills in your everyday life. Similar to what was said above about reading, the shift occurs with a decision to take on your thinking actively, instead of just letting your thoughts and life come at you. The ability and tendency to ask useful questions and to apply standards can help to create better methods of pursuing what matters to you and more desirable results.

Study Questions

1. What are the consequences of not knowing the future for your professional preparation?
2. In your own words, what is critical thinking?
3. What are some of the costs and benefits of using critical thinking as a professional?
4. What are some of the authors' assumptions about university education? What are some of their implicit values?
5. What do you need personally to overcome to become a critical thinker?

References

Anderson, C.W. (1993). *Prescribing the life of the mind.* Madison, WI: The University of Wisconsin Press.

Covey, S.R. (1989). *The seven habits of highly effective people.* New York: Fireside.

Endler, N.S., Edwards, J.M., and Vitelli, R. (1991). *Endler multidimensional anxiety scale* (EMAS). Los Angeles: Western Psychological Services.

Ennis, R. (1962). A concept of critical thinking. *Harvard Educational Review, 32,* 82–111.

Ennis, R.H. (1992). Assessing higher order thinking for accountability. In J.W. Keefe and H.J. Walberg (Eds.), *Teaching for thinking* (pp. 73–91). Reston, VA: National Association of Secondary Education Principals.

Gardner, J.W. (1963). *Self-renewal.* New York: Harper and Row.

Glaser, R. (1991). Expertise and assessment. In M.C. Wittrock and E.L. Baker (Eds.), *Testing and cognition* (pp. 17–30). Englewood Cliffs, NJ: Prentice-Hall.

Hughes, W. (1992). *Critical thinking: An introduction to the basic skills.* Peterborough, ON: Broadview Press.

Paul, R. (1992). Critical thinking: What, why, and how. In C.A. Barnes (Ed.), *Critical thinking: Educational imperative.* San Francisco: Jossey-Bass.

Paul. R. (1995). *Critical thinking: What every person needs to survive in a rapidly changing world.* Rohnert Park, CA: Foundation for Critical Thinking.

Paul, R.W., Elder, L., and Bartell, T. (1997). California Teacher Preparation for Instruction. In *Critical thinking: research findings and policy recommendations. California Commission on Teacher Credentialing, Sacramento, California, 1997.* Rohnert Park, CA: Foundation for Critical Thinking.

Penner, K. (1995). http://web.ucs.ubc.CA/kpenner/c-think.htm. (Unavailable).

Rescher, N. (1998). *Predicting the future: An introduction to the theory of forecasting.* Albany, NY: State University of New York Press.

II ■ PERSPECTIVES

CHAPTER 2

Defining Adapted Physical Activity

Greg Reid

Learning Objectives
- To write an essay describing the meaning of contemporary adapted physical activity.
- To describe how individuals with a disability were perceived during the facility-based, services-based, supports-based, and empowerment and self-determination paradigms.
- To describe adapted physical activity during the facility-based, services-based, supports-based, and empowerment and self-determination paradigms.
- To explain the meaning of the word *adapted* in adapted physical activity and describe the strengths and limitations of the term.

Introduction

When people ask the question, "What is adapted physical activity?", the difficulty lies with the word *adapted*. Most of us have some idea of what is meant by *physical activity*, but the word *adapted* is problematic. So, our immediate response is often, "It is about physical activity for people with a disability." The questioner usually nods, now knowing what we are talking about, and may add, "That must be very rewarding and you must have a great deal of patience." To describe adapted physical activity in terms of people with a disability is not a huge error; it simply is not the complete story, or a too restricted view. This chapter, in fact this textbook, is designed to provide a more comprehensive and enlightened answer to the question, "What is adapted physical activity?" In our journey to understand a more complete response to the question, we will explore the word *adapted* and even, *physical activity*. Everyone does not view *adapted physical activity* in exactly the same way, which is fine, as long as people can articulate and justify their own meaning.

Students reading this chapter are encouraged to relate the material to their own physical activity and life experiences, other courses, media depiction of people with disabilities, and their knowledge of Canadian history.

---

1 Ask your parents and grandparents about their childhood memories of individuals with a disability. How were people with a disability perceived and depicted? Can you recall individuals with a disability in your school, in your physical education classes? How were they perceived?

Then return to this chapter after reading this complete volume. You will then be ready to answer the question, "What is adapted physical activity?" In doing so, you will realize that much more than patience is required for adapted physical activity to be truly rewarding.

The purpose of this chapter is to sketch the evolution of adapted physical activity terminology and definition over one hundred years. In order to understand these changes, one must place them in a political-social-historical context of how Canadians have viewed individuals with a disability and the notion of disability itself. These have changed remarkably in the past forty years in particular. To provide structure and insight to the chapter, we use the four paradigms, or approaches to disability, identified by Polloway, Smith, Patton, and Smith (1996). Before discussing the views of Polloway et al. (1996), let us look briefly at an earlier history.

Early History

People with a disability have usually been inaccurately perceived and poorly treated through much of history. Individuals with a physical or intellectual disability were considered detrimental to nations at war and economic liabilities in periods of active commerce. During early societies in Greece and Rome, their lives could be terminated by parents, who had other children to feed and clothe and who insisted on work from their offspring. Shapiro (1993) points out that the Bible suggests that disability is a sign of God's disfavour or that it is caused by sin. Ward and Myers (1999) argue that classical literature has often depicted people with a disability as beggars, thieves, or heroes, not average people who are valued, contributing, capable, and maybe average. Thus, throughout much of history, people with a disability have been ill-treated and unfavourably described. Physical activity was not considered.

Yet, some people recognized the importance of physical activity for people with a disability many years ago. In the nineteenth century, Samuel Gridley Howe, the patriarch of blind education, spoke against overprotection and inactivity as a means to prevent potential injury. He stated, "Do not too much regard bumps upon the forehead, rough scratches, or bloody noses, even these may have their good influences. At the worst, they affect only the bark, and do not injure the system, like the rust of inaction" (1841). Even the history of organized sport for individuals with a disability can be traced to the nineteenth century (DePauw and Gavron 1995). R. Tait McKenzie, Canadian physician, sculptor, and physical educator, published a book in 1909, *Exercise in Education and Medicine.* He outlined physical education for those who were deaf, blind, and mentally retarded. However, these were isolated examples from pioneers with extraordinary vision. Unfortunately, neglect of individuals with a disability is a more accurate characterization of the nineteenth and first half of the twentieth century.

Polloway et al. (1996) presented four paradigms, or approaches, to mental retardation and developmental disabilities in the twentieth century, but the paradigms are appropriate for many individuals with a disability. These four paradigms provide a backdrop to the evolution of terminology associated with adapted physical activity, since definitions and viewpoints are always products of cultural beliefs, values, and expectations. Definitions are socially constructed, expressing current opinion, and subsequently change with time. How a society thinks about, and deals with, individuals with a disability will be reflected in the definitions of that specific period of time. Therefore, definitions of, and general approaches to, adapted physical activity reflect general viewpoints of society, as well as more specific thoughts in special education, education, and sport. The four paradigms depict society, as well as practice in education (table 2.1).

Facility-based Paradigm

The first half of the twentieth century can be characterized as a facility-based paradigm (Polloway et al. 1996). People with disabilities were usually found in institutions, residential programmes, and special schools. These facilities were often physically isolated, thus removing any substantive interaction with society. It was even believed that some people with disabilities, such as those with mental retardation, were a menace to society, engaged in vice and crime. Thus, isolation protected society from people with a disability (Bouffard 1997). Those with cerebral palsy or who were deaf might have been incarcerated in institutions because they could not express their intellect. That is, they could not respond to questions because they could not articulate words or write a response, in the case of cerebral palsy, or they did not understand the question, in the case of deafness. Such individuals were assumed to have severe learning problems. Usually, there was no education or treatment, minimal opportunity for recreation, and almost no planned physical activity. In many large institutions there were documented accounts of mistreatment, lack of privacy, and virtually no respect for the "inmates" (Blatt and Kaplan 1967).

There were more enlightened facilities, such as special schools, that did attempt to provide education. However, the prominent belief was that the education needs of the children were very different from 'normal' children, and hence grouping children with disabilities together, and isolating them from others, seemed to make sense. When education was provided, the curriculum was largely based on the label of the group, rather than the needs of individuals. A class of children with intellectual disabilities (or morons and imbeciles as they were called), likely received the same basic lessons, despite some students who needed much practice at simple word recognition, and others who were able to read at the grade six level. Planned physical activity might have been offered as physical education or physical training, but expectations were low indeed. Students were seldom challenged or provided with any form of motivation, and almost no attention was given to physical fitness or participation in lifetime activities. If children with a mild disability had the good fortune to attend a community-based school, exemption from physical education was common. The prevailing belief was that they were unable to profit from physical education; in fact, they might be harmed by vigorous activity.

While the first half of the twentieth century was dominated largely by neglect, medically oriented *corrective therapy* did attempt to alleviate physical or orthopedic problems through prescribed exercise and massage. Corrective therapy was concerned with posture, fitness, or health difficulties (Sherrill 1998) and was common in the US. It attempted to recondition soldiers for return to active duty, rehabilitate more serious injuries, and address posture and poor fitness in school-aged children. Almost all textbooks in adapted physical activity published between 1900–1950 had the word *correctives* in the title (Sherrill and DePauw 1997). *Adapted physical activity* did not enter professional language for many years. The medical perspective of correctives was consistent with the historical fact that early physical education was dominated by physicians who realized that exercise were beneficial in the treatment of some physical disabilities.

2 The medical profession offers so many benefits to society that it is probably the most respected profession today, but have you ever stopped to think about its impact in education? How might it influence our thinking and practice? More specifically, how did the medical profession view disability or physical activity for a person with a disability?

Table 2.1 Special Education Paradigms and Their Relationship to Physical Education

Paradigm	Key Points	Terminology and Ideas in Physical Education
Facilities-based	• isolation • neglect • medical model • person viewed as patient in need of cure • condition resides in the person	Corrective therapy, fix the problem • emphasis on physical rehabilitation • posture and fitness • children with mild disabilities were excused from physical education
Service-based	• special programmes and services • educational model • skill improvement • people defined largely as their disability, rather than as individual first, who happens to have a disability	Adapted physical education Developmental physical education Special physical education • much focus on programmes based on disability level
Supports-based	• disability viewed as a part of human variation • difficulties reside in person-environment interaction • provide support to allow person to function in inclusive environments	Adapted physical activity • sport becomes prominent • programmes become individualized • lifespan notion adopted • definitions based less on disability and more on adaptations
Empowerment and Self-determination	• major decisions move to individual with a disability, not the experts • focus on choice, decision making, self-awareness, and self-regulated learning	Adapted physical activity • self-determined physical activity

SOURCE: From "Historical Changes in Mental Retardation and Developmental Disabilities" by E.A. Pollaway et al., 1996, *Education and Training in Mental Retardation and Developmental Disabilities, 31*, pp. 3–12.

As might be expected from a medical viewpoint, problems were conceptualized as residing in the individual. Disabilities were difficulties or limitations resting with the person, not how the person interacted within an environment, which conceivably might change. The person was a 'victim', or 'patient', with a sickness that required a cure. Even the term *therapy* is medically oriented and suggests that something is very wrong with the individual. Corrective therapy essentially ignored intellectual disability, deafness, and visual impairments, since they could not be 'corrected' or 'cured'.

It was not uncommon for physicians to recommend to parents that the child with a disability should be placed in an institution, arguing there was little hope for functional improvement, or successful management of behaviour. To be fair, most educators were equally pessimistic. Physicians and educators were merely reflecting societal values and beliefs prevalent in the first half of the twentieth century. City planners felt no responsibility to create buildings that were accessible to wheelchairs. No restaurant created a washroom large enough for a wheelchair. A public school could deny registration to a child with

Down's syndrome, or who was deaf, and assume no further educational responsibility for that child. Employers did not hire individuals with a disability for a host of reasons, most of which were based on ignorance. It was quite common for families to deny they had a child with a disability since it was often associated with guilt–the parents had done something wrong and were being punished.

Today, disability is viewed much less in biological terms and more in social-environmental terms. A disability is now conceived as part of all humanity, an individual difference with each person having abundant developmental potential. With increased public awareness and education, significant advocating and lobbying, greater acceptance of diversity, and improvements to the environment, people with disabilities can participate in all aspects of society. We will return to some of these perspectives about disability later in this chapter.

Service-based Paradigm

A service-based paradigm emerged in the 1950s due to several phenomena (Polloway et al. 1996). A public outcry occurred when the plight of individuals in overcrowded institutions was revealed. New respect was apparent for those World War II veterans who returned with spinal cord injuries and amputations. Appropriate treatment, rehabilitation, and opportunity for employment were minimum expectations. Professional papers and research also acclaimed the previously unexpected abilities of those with a disability. For example, in physical activity there were many published reports of programmes that demonstrated that individuals with a disability could actually learn to swim, improve in fitness, participate in sport, and enjoy dance (e.g., Brown 1953; Kelly 1954; Meyer 1955).

In this model, special services were offered to individuals with a disability, with the view that skills would prepare them for integration, or re-integration, into society. There was new optimism in the potential of individuals with a disability. Thus, rehabilitation programmes for veterans with a disability, special classes in regular schools, resource rooms staffed by special educators, and "sheltered" workshops for adults, became prominent. It was believed that societal integration could be achieved through services that improved physical, academic, and social skills. The term *mainstreaming*, which will be explained in Chapter 9 (Reid), became prominent during this era. In physical education there was a shift from 'correcting' disabilities, or simply ignoring them, to an attitude of providing helpful services. The influence of corrective therapy remained firmly entrenched in textbooks, with chapters on posture and exercise, but the benefits of play, games, sport, and dance were now advanced for social, emotional, and psychological reasons. The services-based approach in physical education was largely restricted to school-aged children, and became known as *adapted physical education*.

In 1952, adapted physical education was defined in the US as, "a diversified program of developmental activities, games, sports, and rhythms suited to the interests, capacities, and limitations of students with disabilities who may not safely or successfully engage in unrestricted participation in the vigorous activities of the general physical education programme" (Committee on Adapted Physical Education 1952). This definition was based in education rather than medicine, and had a broader programming focus than correctives, since it dealt with games, sport, and rhythmics. Also, it could easily accommodate a wider range of disabilities such as intellectual disability, which had been largely ignored in corrective therapy. Teaching and programming suggestions in physical education for many disability groups became common.

Terminology other than *adapted physical education* was proposed during these years, including *remedial, developmental, special, individualized, therapeutic,* or *corrective physical education* (Porretta, Nesbitt, and Labanowich 1993; Sherrill and DePauw 1997). Names tended to reflect the emphasis of the programme. Some of these are defined in table 2.2. *Special physical education* remains the preferred terminology for some (e.g., Dunn

1997; Jansma and French 1994), but *adapted physical education* became the most common moniker and was adopted in the title of some early texts (e.g., Clarke and Clarke 1963; Daniels 1954; Fait 1960).

---

3 But let us look again at the 1952 definition, with fifty years of experience. What is stated explicitly, and what is implied by the definition? Do not memorize it, but study its meaning and implications.

The 1952 definition remained focussed on the limitation or disability of the person, much like the earlier 'correctives'. We will see how contemporary definitions do not require the notion of a disability (see also Chapter 5 (Shogan)). Also, it was believed that students with a disability could not safely or successfully participate in the regular physical education programme. This provides insight into the meaning of the word *adapted*. *Adapted* referred to a "programme," presumably quite different from regular physical education, rather than a minor curricular change or teaching modification. Thus, students were often considered to be 'in' adapted physical education.

A special programme of adapted physical education is consistent with removal of children from regular physical education. If a school did not have an adapted physical education teacher, the long-standing exemption from participation was justified. Since almost no Canadian school board hired adapted physical educators, it meant that many children were simply excused from participating in physical education. Viewing adapted physical education or special education as a separate 'programme' stalled serious discussion about placing special education students into regular schools, or promoting integration of students with special needs who were already in regular schools. Presumably, the adapted programme could not be implemented in the regular school. Finally, the link between adapted physical education and disability was so strong that programmes were conceptualized and defined by a disability label rather than by the needs of the individual. Thus

Table 2.2 Terminology

Individualized physical education: programmes that respond to the unique needs of individual. For students with disabilities this includes movement programmes that respond to the physical, mental, and emotional needs of each individual through structured, success-oriented learning experiences.

Therapeutic physical education: programmes that strive to rehabilitate through prescribed exercises those who have temporary disabilities.

Developmental physical education: programmes that develop motor ability and physical fitness in those below the desired level.

Remedial physical education: programmes designed to correct faulty movement patterns through selected activities.

Special physical education: programmes designed to enhance the physical and motor fitness of persons with disabilities through modified and developmentally sequenced sport, game, and movement experiences individualized for each participant.

SOURCE: Modified from *Special Physical Education: Adapted, Individualized, Developmental* (p. 3) by J. Dunn, 1997, Madison, WI: Brown and Benchmark.

community recreation programmes might offer "swimming for the mentally retarded." It was assumed that this was the time for all those with mental retardation to swim, regardless of age, or swimming skills, or social ability. It was programming according to disability label.

Today, we may be critical of this approach and some of the other implications of the 1952 definition, but it was a significant step beyond the neglect of earlier years. Physical education was beginning to recognize the physical activity needs of people with a disability. Also, by achieving recognition as a specialty within physical education, professionals who shared common interests began to meet and discuss issues of adapted physical education at conferences and workshops. Publications documented success stories of individual achievement, programme effectiveness, and research findings. All of these factors led to important changes in conceptualization of disability, terminology, and practice in *adapted physical education.*

Supports-based Paradigm

The services-based approach assumed that appropriate programming would be followed by successful integration. However, it soon became apparent that most people with disabilities remained in special schools, special classes, sheltered workshops, and group homes (Polloway et al. 1996). In response to this inefficiency, a supports-based, inclusion paradigm emerged in the 1980s (Block and Krebs 1992). Supports were technical, natural, or human that assisted individuals with a disability to function in inclusive settings, that is, within natural settings in the community. For example, a teaching assistant or peer might be assigned to support a student with a physical disability to accomplish some tasks and to promote interaction with other peers. The potential of the computer also became apparent as a means of supporting individuals as they functioned in inclusive environments.

Inclusion will be described in more detail in Chapter 9 (Reid), but it means that *all* individuals are welcomed in community settings such as schools, recreation centres, and clubs, regardless of how they might be perceived as different. Inclusion is more than a placement, however, since its philosophy is that everyone belongs, contributes, and develops. Inclusion meant that people with disabilities no longer needed to demonstrate certain skills to 'gain entrance' to school or recreation settings and programmes, for the inclusive setting was now the starting point. "Individuals should be maintained in inclusive settings and supported in those locations in order to insure successful learning, work experience, and/or adjustment (Polloway et al. 1996, p. 6).

The 'older' view of adapted physical education, as a separate programme for school-aged children with disabilities, began to be challenged in the 1970s and 1980s. If inclusion was a desirable goal in a supports-based paradigm, changes were necessary to what was meant by adapted physical education. It could no longer be assumed that special classes or schools were the most appropriate placement for students with disabilities, or that adapted physical education must always be a 'different programme.' Thus, Sherrill (1976, p. 4) defined *adapted physical education* as "the science of analyzing movement, identifying problems in the psychomotor domain, and developing instructional strategies for remediating problems and preserving ego strength."

4 Once again, let us look at the meaning of this definition, rather than memorize it. What are the essential components? How is this definition different from other definitions? There is no mention of disability...can adapted physical education be defined without reference to disability?

It does refer to analysis and identification of problems and remediation, but it does not restrict itself to disabilities. There is no assumption that all people with disabilities will require adapted physical education. For example, an adult with an amputation might enjoy the local fitness facility and pool. He cycles on a stationary bike and stretches for thirty minutes before heading to the pool, where the prosthesis is removed before he hops into the water for a twenty-minute swim. As an independent young adult, the individual is capable of dealing with any unique problems that may arise. There is no attraction to the "Personal Swim and Gym Programme for Adults with a Disability" where individual attention and assistance is provided. This individual does not need or require adapted physical education.

The Sherrill (1976) definition also opened the possibility that an individual *without* a disability might benefit from teaching and equipment adaptations that have been described in many resources (e.g., Block 1994; Downs 1995; Davis and Burton 1991; Active Living Alliance for Canadians with a Disability 1994;

Sherrill 1998). For example, a seven-year-old child has considerable difficulty with ball-catching and his parents express concern at the parent-teacher interview. The teacher who has studied adapted physical education develops some guidelines for teaching and activity suggestions for the parents to use with their child. In addition, the teacher is able to offer individual attention in some physical education classes because the students often work on individually challenging tasks. Thus, adapted physical education in the 1976 Sherrill definition dealt more with adaptations and teaching skills, than with a specific programme for people with a disability. Also, nothing is stated or implied to suggest that students must be removed from regular physical education classes, leaving the potential of the instructional strategies to be provided in regular programmes.

A final implication from this definition was that adapted physical education must recognize how people feel about themselves. Programmes can not be justified if they reduce feelings of self-worth and confidence. Rather, they should augment self-confidence and self-concept.

While the 1976 Sherrill definition advanced the field, two perspectives forced professionals to re-think the meaning of adapted physical education once again in the 1980s. First, the word *education* was considered to be restricted to instruction of school-aged children and adolescents (Broadhead 1990; DePauw and Sherrill 1994). Many subfields in physical education were adopting a lifespan approach, which includes all ages, preschoolers to older adults. After all, physical activity is appropriate for everyone, not just children! Thus, in many contexts, the term *education* seemed to limit rather than to embrace. Second, the sport movement for individuals with a disability, which had grown enormously since World War II, had moved from a strong rehabilitation model to an athletic model (Chapter 26 (Steadward and Foster)). Sport participants no longer saw their involvement as therapeutic or rehabilitative, but rather as a pure athletic performance.

They sought personal performance records and challenging competition. The international disability sport movement made significant organizational strides in the 1980s, leading to the establishment of the International Paralympic Committee. Elite athletes wanted sport-specific coaching and rigorous scientific training regimes to achieve international levels of performance. Also, many individuals with a disability began to engage in sport on a more recreational level, that is, as a fun and social event. Such participation occurs for reasons other than rehabilitation or aspirations of becoming an elite athlete. Terminology was needed to reflect these new realities.

Adapted physical activity was adopted as the umbrella term that included education, recreation, and sport (DePauw and Sherrill 1994; Poretta et al. 1993). Adapted physical *education* is still appropriate in school-based contexts (e.g., Winnick 2000), but there is widespread agreement in the international community for the more encompassing term suggested by *activity*. Activity can include all forms of gross motor activity, from play, to games, to sport, from informal recreation environments to elite sport settings, and across all ages, from infants to older adults. The first formal use of *adapted physical activity* is usually attributed to the International Federation of Adapted Physical Activity (IFAPA), which was created in 1973 by Dr. Clermont Simard, a Laval University professor. In fact, Quebec City was the site of the first International Symposium of Adapted Physical Activity in 1977, which led to additional symposia every two years in various locations throughout the world. In 1984, another significant event supported the term *adapted physical activity*, as a new journal, the *Adapted Physical Activity Quarterly*, began publishing research, reviews, and position papers.

At the Seventh Symposium of the International Federation of Adapted Physical Activity in 1989, there was an attempt to define *adapted physical activity*. It was suggested that "adapted physical activity refers to movement, physical activity, and sports in which special emphasis is placed on the interests and capabilities of individuals with limiting conditions, such as the disabled, health impaired, or aged" (Doll-Tepper, Dahms, Doll, and von Selzam 1990, p. v). This definition included the interest of the participant, which implies some degree of choice or input by the participant in physical activity. It also included sport. The full range of age is made explicit by the term *aged*. However, by using the phrase "limiting conditions" the definition appeared to return to an emphasis of difficulties that reside in the person.

Two definitions of adapted physical activity in the 1990s have produced significant advancement. Sherrill (1993, p. 5) defined *adapted physical activity* as a "cross disciplinary body of knowledge directed toward identification and solution of psychomotor problems throughout the lifespan." Notice how this modifies her 1976 definition to include the lifespan concept, and that adapted physical activity can be conceived as a body of knowledge which is cross-disciplinary. This implies a distinct adapted physical activity body of knowledge that is an integration of knowledge from several other disciplines. This is quite a leap from adapted physical education as just a programme! DePauw and Sherrill (1994, p. 7) expanded Sherrill's 1993 definition to "a cross disciplinary body of knowledge directed toward (a) identification and solution of psychomotor problems throughout the lifespan; (b) advocacy for equal access to healthy, active lifestyle and leisure, high quality physical education instruction, and lifetime involvement in sport, dance, and aquatics; and (c) school-community service delivery that supports integration and inclusion." They argued that this definition placed emphasis not on disabilities but on individual differences and environmental interactions. Again therefore, adapted physical activity is not restricted to disabilities per se. Advocacy, the act of promoting a cause, is also included as an essential component of adapted physical activity. It is explicitly noted that adapted physical activity is also about delivery systems that support integration and inclusion.

Empowerment and Self-determination

The fourth and final paradigm is empowerment and self-determination (Polloway et al. 1996). The facility-based, services-based, and supports-based models assumed that an expert was 'in charge' of the facility, the services, or the supports. All three models can be viewed as models of dependency, where personal control, feelings, and values are not priorities. Self-determination assumes that individuals with a disability should be empowered to make choices, reach decisions, assume responsibilities, take some risks, regulate their own learning, know their strengths and limitations, and to live independently as adults (cf. Hunter 1987; Lord 1987). Thus, self-determination reinforces personal power over one's life, rather than being dependent upon others. **Are any of us totally independent?** The answer is surely no. Also, children are not as independent as adults; in fact, one of the most challenging aspects of parenting is the transfer of decision-making to our children as they develop. So, empowering people to be self-determined is not inconsistent with providing assistance when required and requested and is clearly developmentally related. But we should always strive for appropriate self-determination in adapted physical activity, so those individuals with a disability assume the major responsibility for their physical activity needs. Adapted physical activity must incorporate self-determination (Reid 2000), much as recreation specialists have been advocating for many years (e.g., Lord 1987).

5 Do you accept that self-determination should have a major impact on people with a disability? How does this affect your view of individuals with a disability? What first comes to mind when you think of the word *disability*? Do you think that your view of disability reflects what most people think today?

Taking personal control over one's life is quite inconsistent with the old medical view of disability as 'sickness in need of a cure' where 'experts' were in charge. While disability was often equated with being defective in the past, many people now conceptualize disability as simply being different. If something, or someone, is different, we must then ask ourselves to what extent, if at all, we should promote change in the person just to make them act or appear less different. O'Neill (1999), an individual with autism, writes, "It is quite tiring to read book after book denouncing Autism as a horrible condition. I am qualified to offer an opposite opinion. The theme of this book is to say that difference can be wonderful, and Autism shouldn't be tampered with, or altered. Autistic people shouldn't be changed."

6 Do you agree with this statement? Are there instances when we should attempt to change the person? How can we resolve the dilemma of celebrating individual differences with the need to provide excellent programmes in education and recreation?

In summary, we have seen how adapted physical activity has evolved from a period of neglect (or at best corrective therapy) in the early part of the twentieth century, to special programmes of physical *education* for students with disabilities in segregated settings (1950–80), to promoting self-determined physical *activity* in inclusive settings across the life span (1980+). Table 2.3 includes some of the key points about contemporary adapted physical activity as well as changing views of disability.

7 Can you write your own definition of adapted physical activity? Can you critique and support it with logical arguments? Can you create a list of what adapted physical activity is not? Is there a more effective term to distinguish the field?

Adapted physical activity in the twenty-first century is argued by many to be a cross-disciplinary body of knowledge and practice that enables professionals to interact with people experiencing difficulties with movement. It is about advocacy in physical activity and promoting self-advocacy in people with a

Table 2.3 Contemporary Adapted Physical Activity Is…

- a cross-disciplinary body of knowledge

- a philosophy and attitude of acceptance of diversity

- a focus on individual differences

- a process of advocacy

- programming characterized primarily by adaptations of teaching skills and techniques to accommodate individual motor differences

- a process of promoting independent self-determined physical activity

disability. It is about promoting self-determination in physical activity, providing choice, and teaching self-regulation. It is an attitude about including rather than excluding people, but we can acknowledge a number of activity settings. It is about programme development and delivering services, but it certainly is not just a programme into which people with a disability are placed on the basis of a label. In fact, disability is not necessary to define adapted physical activity, since it is more about dealing with individual differences and human potential. Some people with a disability will not need our services or assistance, and our skills can be effectively employed for those without a disability. However, in reality a significant portion of our work will involve individuals who have a disability. Therefore, we should be familiar with relevant issues and trends in the disability literature as well as information resources about specific disabilities that can be consulted when needed.

What Is Implied by the Term *Adapted*?

8 What does the word *adapted* mean to you? Does it define the field or limit it?

Adapted suggests change, modification, or adjustment of goals, objectives or instruction (e.g., Bernabe and Block 1994; Downs 1995; Active Living Alliance for Canadian with a Disability 1994). A change might include selection and use of a fitness test that has been designed for a specific disability, or having a student participate in a wheelchair race. A modification could be as minor as providing some physical assistance or selecting a different ball size to enhance success. It could be as major as equipping a sailboat for wheelchairs, or as challenging as guiding a downhill skier who is blind from the summit to the base of a mountain. Change and modification will be described throughout this book. These adaptations should not occur for the sake of change, but as means to enhance learning, practice, and enjoyment of independent physical activity for those experiencing some movement difficulty. Adaptations should enhance choice and opportunity, hence empowering people.

It is often noted that all quality physical education is adapted physical education (Sherrill 1998, p. 8; Stein 1987). After all, quality physical education encourages individualization through teacher-student interaction, task selection, choice, and environmental modifications that encourage different ability levels and needs. Also, many scholars of adapted physical activity acknowledge that the basic purpose of adapted physical activity is no different from 'regular' physical activity (e.g., Sherrill 1998, p. 102). In the context of schools, Stein (1987) argued that the adapted physical education curriculum is a myth. That is, the activity content of adapted physical education is no different from activities in "good, appropriate, individualized, and developmental physical education programmes" (Stein 1987, p. 34). In a complementary statement, Jobling and Carlson (1998) suggested that programming for students with disabilities is more about preservation of quality in physical education, not adaptation or modification. While some unique activities have been created, such as the sport of goalball for those with visual impairment, most adaptations are changes of instructional methods or uses of

adapted devices to enable participation and enhance learning, rather than changes in activity per se. This is another reason why adapted physical activity is more about adaptation than a special, or different, programme.

However, promoting adapted physical activity as a highly specialized field of 'adaptation' of activity, method, sport, and exercise leads to several problems with the term *adapted*. Teachers, coaches, and recreation specialists might feel inadequate and ill-prepared to deal with people with disabilities, unless they have ten courses in the specialization! This can be highly divisive and counter-productive to including people with disabilities in society. If the field is a specialty requiring a great deal of advanced education and skill, it might be implied that most professionals are not prepared to interact with individuals with a disability. It has been argued in the field of leisure that too much professionalization can be a detrimental to quality leisure experiences for those with a disability (McGill 1987). In reality, teachers and recreation personnel can promote physical activity for most individuals with a disability with their current knowledge and skills, if they believe in individualization and accommodation. Jobling and Carlson (1998) have strongly argued that we need to look at quality teaching in physical education for children with disabilities and expend less energy discussing adaptations or modification. Of course, the mere existence of the textbook you are now reading indicates that the authors and editors feel that some focus, or specialization, in adapted physical activity is justifiable. Most of them believe that some additional knowledge and skill specific to adaptation is desirable, but how much, and what form, would likely produce a lively debate. Yet, arguments against the term *adapted* physical activity include the position that it implies too much specialization, promotes change or adaptation when none is required, and diverts attention from changes needed in regular physical activity programmes. In turn, this promotes differences, not similarities, and might lead to segregation, rather than integration.

9 Can we use the term *adapted* and maintain a philosophy of including rather than excluding individuals?

Most of the authors of this text believe that we can, but to ignore the issue is not productive. At the least we should acknowledge that some people have questioned the utility of the term *adapted*. As yet, a widely accepted alternative has not emerged.

Every educator, coach, or recreation specialist should be able to use adaptations in method and organization to foster activity of all participants, with or without a disability. The Canadian Association of Health, Physical Education, Recreation, and Dance adopted the position in 1978 that every physical education undergraduate in Canada should receive a compulsory course in adapted physical activity. Most of our university programmes in physical education or kinesiology offer such a course, but it varies among universities whether it is required or not. The intent of the 1978 position was that all physical educators would have some background in dealing with individuals with a disability, many of whom were involved in integrated physical activity. Working with a Canadian group of teachers and professors of adapted physical education, Watkinson (1985) clarified the different roles for adapted (specialist) and regular (generalist) physical educators (table 2.4). It is clear from table 2.4 that regular physical education teachers should be able to include most students with a disability into the regular programme. However, as adaptations become more extensive, creative, and possibly unique to a individual's disability, it is likely that most physical educators would benefit from suggestions of adapted physical activity specialists.

Summary

This chapter has outlined changes in terminology, definition, and philosophy associated with adapted physical activity over the last one hundred years. The paradigms of Polloway et al. (1996) were used to structure the discussion since terminology at any point in history reflects current thinking about the phenomenon. Thus, the facilities-based period was strongly influenced by a medical assumption that disability resided in the person who was ill, and the condition should be cured or corrected. Not surprisingly, the first term for our field was *corrective therapy*. The service-based period saw the emergence of school programmes for individuals with a disability and the term *adapted physical education*. During this period, the goal was to provide helpful instruction so that the individual could acquire skills necessary to function in society and to be included with age peers. Adapted physical education was conceptualized largely as a special programme. The supports-based period focussed on means to include people with disabilities even if they did not possess all the necessary skills. This was achieved by providing the person with human or technical support so that greater independence could be enjoyed. *Adapted physical activity* replaced *adapted physical education* as the internationally accepted term, since it incorporated an age range beyond the school years and it included the growing sport movement. Adapted physical activity was no longer conceptualized only as a special programme for people with a disability, but rather as adaptations that could facilitate physical activity across a wide range of individual differences. Thus, disability was no longer absolutely necessary in a definition of adapted physical activity. The empowerment and self-determination paradigm is the most recent period, largely since the 1990s. The belief is that individuals with a disability should have prime decision-making powers in decisions affecting their life. This last period has not yet had a profound impact in adapted physical activity, although it has had considerable influence in recreation and leisure. The immediate future will see more attention in practice and research being devoted to self-determined physical activity, how to best conceptualize it, how important it is to participants, how it can be promoted, and how to measure its impact.

Table 2.4 Some Differences Between General Physical Educators and Specialists

Competencies in Program Planning

Generalist	Specialist
1. Can plan programs of activities that have the potential for maximum participation of the handicapped or disabled.	1. Has knowledge of existing programs designed for individuals with special needs. This includes national, provincial and local special programs (e.g., Red Cross, Special Olympics school curricula) and special published programs or activities (e.g., PREP, Aqua-Percept, Cooperative Games).
2. Can recognize when a human support is needed to achieve the above.	
3. Has a knowledge of existing service delivery systems for the handicapped and disabled.	2. Can match programs (as above) and population needs.
4. Can recognize when participation in an integrated program is not beneficial or when special services are required.	3. Has knowledge of the continuum of delivery services of programs for the handicapped and disabled in recreation and education. Is familiar with the organizations that exist to support special populations.
5. Has a knowledge of available resources for consulting and referral.	4. Has knowledge of the rules of different professionals working with the handicapped and disabled (e.g., occupational therapist, physical therapist).
	5. Has a knowledge of pertinent legislation concerning the handicapped and disabled.
	6. Can develop (in written form) goals, objectives and evaluation techniques for new programs.
	7. Considers the following factors in planning programs: facilities, equipment.

Table 2.4 provides some examples of skills expected in the repertoire of general physical educators who will teach students with special needs, and adapted physical activity specialists. The specific skills reflect 1985 thinking. Today many authorities might argue that the generalist should have more skills than expected in 1985. Still, the point being made is that there will be a difference, the specifics open to healthy debate.

SOURCE: From "Professional Preparation in Adapted Physical Education," by E.J. Watkinson, 1985, Jan/Feb, CAHPERD *Journal*, *51*, pp. 14–17. Reproduced with permission of the Canadian Association for Health, Physical Education, Recreation, and Dance, 403–2197 Riverside Drive, Ottawa, ON K1H 7X3.

Study Questions

1. Distinguish between corrective therapy, adapted physical education, and adapted physical activity.
2. Select one of the four paradigms (facility-based, services-based, support-based, and empowerment and self-determined-based) and outline the prevailing view toward people with a disabilities, and the terms used during that period for adapted physical activity.
3. Describe a contemporary definition of adapted physical activity by indicating how it different from earlier definitions.
4. What is meant by *adapted* in adapted physical activity, and how has this word been criticized?

References

Active Living Alliance for Canadians with a Disability. (1994). *Moving to inclusion*. Ottawa: Author.

Bernabe, E., and Block, M. (1994). Modifying rules of a regular girls softball league to facilitate the inclusion of a child with severe disabilities. *Journal of the Association for Persons with Severe Handicaps, 19*(1), 24–31.

Blatt, B., and Kaplan, F. (1967). *Christmas in purgatory*. Boston: Allyn and Bacon.

Block, M., and Krebs, P.L. (1992). An alternative to least restrictive environments: A continuum of support to regular physical education. *Adapted Physical Activity Quarterly, 9*, 97–113.

Block, M.E. (1994). *A teacher's guide to including students with disabilities in regular physical education*. Baltimore: Paul H. Brookes.

Bouffard, M. (1997). Using old research ideas to study contemporary problems on adapted physical activity. *Measurement in Physical Education and Sport Science, 1*, 71–87.

Broadhead, G.D. (1990). Adapted physical activity: Terminology and concepts. In G. Doll-Tepper, C. Dahms, B. Doll, and H. von Selzam (Eds.), *Adapted physical activity: An interdisciplinary approach* (pp. 3–9). Berlin: Springer-Verlag.

Brown, R.I. (1953, April). Swimming: Activity for the handicapped. *Journal of Health, Physical Education, and Recreation, 24*, 14–16.

Clarke, H.H., and Clarke, D.H. (1963). *Developmental and adapted physical education*. Englewood Cliffs, NJ: Prentice Hall.

Committee on Adapted Physical Education. (1952, April). Guiding principles for adapted physical education. *Journal of Health, Physical Education, and Recreation, 23*, 15, 28.

Daniels, A.S. (1954). *Adapted physical education*. New York: Harper and Brothers.

Davis, W.E., and Burton, A.W. (1991). Ecological task analysis: Translating movement theory into practice. *Adapted Physical Activity Quarterly, 8*, 154–77.

DePauw, K.P., and Sherrill, C. (1994). Adapted physical activity: Present and future. *Physical Education Review, 17*, 6–13.

DePauw, K.P., and Gavron, S.J. (1995). *Disability and sport*. Champaign, IL: Human Kinetics.

Doll-Tepper, G., Dahms, C., Doll, B., and von Selzam, H. (1990). *Adapted physical activity: An interdisciplinary approach*. Berlin: Springer-Verlag.

Downs, P. (1995). *Willing and able*. Canberra: Australian Sports Commission.

Dunn, J. (1997). *Special physical education: Adapted, individualized, developmental*. (7th ed.). Madison, WI: Brown and Benchmark.

Fait, H.F. (1960). *Adapted physical education*. Philadelphia: W.B. Saunders.

Howe, S.G. (1841). *Perkins report*. Watertown, MA: Perkins Institute for the Blind.

Hunter, D. (1987). Effective programme development for and with persons with disabilities. *Canadian Association for Health, Physical Education and Recreation, 53*(5), 26–30.

Jansma, P., and French, R. (1994). *Special physical education* (2nd ed.). Englewood Cliffs, NJ: Prentice Hall.

Jobling, A. and Carlson, T.B. (1998). "Quality" in physical education for children with disabilities: Are there opportunities to learn? *Brazilian International Journal of Adapted Physical Education Research, 4*, 33–46.

Kelly, E. (1954, April). Swimming for the physically handicapped. *Journal of Health, Physical Education and Recreation, 25*, 12–14.

Lord, J. (1987). Involving disabled persons and communities in leadership training. *Canadian Association for Health, Physical Education and Recreation, 53*(5), 31–32.

McGill, J. (1987). Increased professionalism in the field of leisure and disabled persons: What will it mean? *Leisurability, 13*, 4–17.

McKenzie, R.T. (1909). *Exercise in education and medicine*. Philadelphia: W.B. Saunders.

Meyer, H.C. (1955, May-June). Swimming for the deaf. *Journal of Health, Physical Education and Recreation, 26*, 12.

O'Neill, J.L. (1999). *Through the eyes of aliens*. Philadelphia: Jessica Kingsley.

Polloway, E.A., Smith, J.D., Patton, J.R., and Smith, T.E.C. (1996). Historical changes in mental retardation and developmental disabilities. *Education and Training in Mental Retardation and Developmental Disabilities, 31*, 3–12.

Porretta, D., Nesbitt, J., Labanowich, S. (1993). Terminology usage: A case for clarity. *Adapted Physical Activity Quarterly, 10*, 87–96.

Reid, G. (2000). Future directions of inquiry in adapted physical activity. *Quest, 52*, 370–82.

Shapiro, P.O. (1993). *No pity: People with disabilities forging a new civil rights movement.* New York: Times Books.

Sherrill, C. (1976). *Adapted physical education and recreation: A multidisciplinary approach.* Dubuque, IA: Wm. C. Brown.

Sherrill, C. (1993). *Adapted physical activity, recreation, and sport: Crossdisciplinary and lifespan.* (4th ed.). Madison, WI: Brown and Benchmark.

Sherrill, C. (1998). *Adapted physical activity, recreation, and sport: Crossdisciplinary and lifespan.* (5th ed.). Boston: WCB/McGraw-Hill.

Sherrill, C., and DePauw, K.P. (1997). Adapted physical activity and education. In J.D. Massengale and R.A. Swanson (Eds.), *History of exercise and sport science* (pp.39–108). Champaign, IL: Human Kinetics.

Stein, J. (1987). The myth of the adapted physical education curriculum. *Palaestra, 4*(1), 34–37, 57.

Ward, M.J. and Myers, R.N. (1999). Self-determination for people with developmental disabilities and autism: Two self-advocates' perspectives. *Focus on Autism and other Developmental Disabilities, 14*(3), 133–39.

Watkinson, E.J. (1985). Professional preparation in adapted physical activity. *Canadian Association of Physical Education and Recreation Journal, 51*(3), 14–17.

Winnick, J.P. (2000). An introduction to adapted physical education and sport. In J.P. Winnick (Ed.), *Adapted physical education and sport* (3rd ed.) (pp. 3–17). Champaign, IL: Human Kinetics.

CHAPTER 3

The History of Adapted Physical Activity in Canada

A.E. (Ted) Wall

Learning Objectives

- To discover the people, the ideas, and motivating forces that led to the development of adapted physical activity in Canada. As you read this chapter, it will become increasingly evident that many personal, professional, economic, and social forces played a significant role in the development of our field.
- To understand the impact of the ideas and energy of some of our pioneering leaders.
- To recognize, at the same time, the close professional cooperation and personal interactions with our American and international colleagues.
- To celebrate the emergence and influence of organizations that facilitated people working together on behalf of persons with a disability.
- To understand the profound influence that certain paradigm-shifting ideas, such as the principle of normalization, have had on the way we view persons with a disability and especially on how they view themselves.
- To learn how, due to the influence of this powerful principle, volunteers and professionals moved towards increasingly more collaboration with participants to facilitate their full involvement in physical activity.

Each of these forces will be examined in this chapter; however, it will be very difficult to convey the ongoing interplay among them because the history of adapted physical activity in Canada has been a continuous, interactive process driven by dedicated participants, committed professionals, and enthusiastic volunteers. In an attempt to provide a coherent historical structure, the story of the evolution of adapted physical activity in Canada will be divided into the following periods:

- the early years: the roots of the profession
- the 1940s and 1950s: the rise of adapted physical activity in Canada
- the 1960s: a call for change
- the 1970s: normalization, integration, and new professional organizations
- the 1980s: national collaboration and a blueprint for action
- the 1990s: answering the challenge at the national and international level

The Early Years: The Roots of the Profession

The history of adapted physical activity in Canada may well have begun in 1843 when Frederic K.S. Barnjum established a gymnasium in Montreal. In a very short time, Barnjum developed an excellent reputation as a gymnastics instructor. Thus, when McGill University constructed its first gymnasium in 1862, it was not surprising that university officials approached Barnjum to become the instructor in gymnastics. Barnjum also took an interest in teacher training, for from 1862 he served for many years as an instructor in the School for Teachers at McGill University (Gurney 1990). Two of his better known student-athletes were James Naismith and Robert Tait McKenzie, both of whom went on to become outstanding leaders in the field of physical education. James Naismith is best known for his invention of the game of basketball, which subsequently resulted in the wonderful game of wheelchair basketball, an enormously popular sport in its own right. However, Naismith is only one of the pioneers with deep roots in Canada who have influenced the development of our field; another was Robert Tait McKenzie.

Naismith and McKenzie were born in Almonte, Ontario. McKenzie was slightly younger than Naismith and, after he graduated from high school in 1885, he followed his boyhood hero to McGill. Like Naismith, McKenzie was an outstanding university athlete who competed in gymnastics, football, swimming, and track. In 1890, Frederic Barnjum died and James Naismith was appointed the director of physical education at McGill. Naismith immediately asked McKenzie to serve as his assistant. The year after, Naismith resigned to attend Springfield College and Mckenzie was appointed to replace him. In 1892, McKenzie was granted a medical degree and joined the staff of the Montreal General Hospital, but continued to serve as the director of physical education at McGill.

Soon McKenzie was speaking and writing about the value of physical training in the lives of young people. For example, in 1894 in a paper entitled "The Place of Physical Training in the School System," McKenzie argued strongly for increased opportunities for physical training in the schools. Even in this early paper, it is clear that McKenzie was concerned that the benefits of physical training be available to all individuals within the school, including those with specific medical conditions. He wrote,

> there will always be some whose physique or condition of health debars them from such rough games as football or hockey, but most of whom could take light exercise with great benefit. In other pupils special care is demanded requiring exercises that vary with the particular case, for the danger of overstrain and injury may be greatly increased by the kind of exercise employed. (p. 4)

McKenzie underscored the importance of recognizing the individual differences that exist in every school class and stressed the value of developing programmes under the leadership of well-trained teachers to meet the needs of all students. These ideas are still basic principles of adapted physical activity.

In 1904, McKenzie left McGill to become the director of physical education at the University of Pennsylvania; however, as he would do throughout his life, he maintained close contact with his Canadian colleagues. In 1909, McKenzie published one of the early texts on physical education. *Exercise in Education and Medicine* became one of the most influential professional textbooks of its time. In it, McKenzie continued to place great emphasis on the importance of meeting the physical activity needs of every individual, no matter what his or her level of ability. However, viewed from today's perspective, a careful reading of his chapter on physical education for persons with an intellectual disability shows that he, like most of his colleagues at the time, had a rather limited understanding of the causes of developmental delay. The suggestions he made for remedial programmes were based largely on anecdotal and clinical evidence. Nevertheless, he recognized before many others did that individualized programmes were often needed and were, in fact, the best means to facilitate learning and development. Even so, the recommendations that McKenzie made reflect an assumption that something should be done for or to persons with a disability, rather than what could be done with them or what could they do for themselves.

---

1 As you read this chapter, consider to what extent has our field facilitated the personal empowerment of persons with a disability.

In August 1914, the First World War began and it went on for four tragic years. Even though he was living in the United States, McKenzie immediately volunteered for military service in the British army. His professional background allowed him to play an active role in the delivery of medical and rehabilitative services during and after the war (Ebbs 1971). Based on his medical and rehabilitative work during the war, he wrote his famous physical therapy text, *Reclaiming the Maimed* (1918). In it, McKenzie discussed the benefits of exercise and sport activities for persons with a disability and provided insightful advice for professionals working in the field. Its publication had a profound effect on both the development of adapted physical activity and on the profession of physical therapy (Hermann 1937).

Dr. A.S. Lamb was another pioneering leader who had a major influence on the field of adapted physical activity. A graduate of the International YMCA Training School at Springfield, Massachusetts, he joined the McGill University physical education staff in 1912. In his new position, he soon recognized the importance of completing a medical degree and so, while continuing to teach physical education, he enrolled in the Faculty of Medicine and graduated as a physician in 1917 (Eaton 1970). During his years at McGill, Dr. Lamb organized the first university health service in Canada and was a tireless advocate on behalf of physical and health education for every individual in the community. Throughout his professional life, he encouraged his colleagues to ensure that the physical education and sport programmes they offered provided opportunities for people of all abilities to be as active as possible.

In April 1909, Lord Strathcona established an endowment fund of five hundred thousand dollars to encourage the incorporation of physical training into the school curriculum. The interest from the endowment was to be used to promote physical training and military drill in the schools as well as to support the training of teachers of physical education. Unfortunately, the Strathcona Trust programme placed special emphasis on military drill and, within a short time, it began to have a major influence on the school physical education curriculum. However, not everyone was in favour of this emphasis on military drill. In 1916, Ethel Mary Cartwright, a member of the McGill University physical education staff, published an article criticizing the narrow objectives of the Strathcona Trust programme (Cartwright 1916). Approximately five years later, at a meeting of the Strathcona Trust Executive, representatives from Alberta and Ontario also strongly criticized the objectives of the programme. The Alberta representative charged that the programme was too rigid and that its formal nature made it monotonous for the students. The provincial representatives called for much greater emphasis on health education, physical training, and corrective exercises. These suggestions resulted in the development of the Strathcona Trust Syllabus of 1929. It was more positively accepted by professionals in the field; within a short time, the revised programme became more widely used by class teachers who were responsible for teaching physical education in their schools (McDiarmid 1970).

Throughout the twenties, interest in physical education as a profession continued to grow. In 1931, Dr. Lamb and Miss Jessie Herriott wrote to physical education leaders working in every province suggesting that a national association be created. Nearly two hundred favourable replies were received. Under the leadership of F.L. Bartlett and Mary Hamilton, the founding meeting of the Canadian Physical Education Association

(CPEA) was convened in Toronto in April 1933 (Gurney 1983). A precursor of the Canadian Association of Health, Physical Education, Recreation and Dance (CAHPERD), the 160 founding members of CPEA began a proud legacy of professional contributions. From the beginning, one of CAHPERD's basic professional principles was the importance of serving the needs of all individuals, with a special focus on children and youth (Blackstock 1965). As we shall see, that principle has been a major goal throughout the history of our field.

The economic depression of the 1930s was a turning point in the development of physical education in Canada, as important changes to the physical education curriculum were adopted and, as noted above, our first national professional association was formed. Moreover, it was during those years that the name of the profession changed from the popular 'training' or 'culture' to the more appropriate 'physical education' (Consentino and Howell 1971, p. 49). At the same time, during those economically difficult years, municipal recreation became increasingly important in meeting the social and recreational needs of the many individuals who were unemployed. However, it would be a number of years before municipal recreation services would become a powerful vehicle for the provision of physical activity and recreation opportunities for persons with a disability.

The 1940s and 1950s: The Initial Rise of Adapted Physical Activity in Canada

World War Two had far-reaching effects on Canada, as an enormous amount of its human and physical resources were focussed on the war effort. However, even though the war was underway, there were a number of important developments that contributed to the growth of adapted physical activity in Canada. The first Canadian degree programme in physical education was offered in the fall of 1940 at the University of Toronto, followed by the offering of degree programmes at McGill University and the University of British Columbia, in 1945 and 1946 respectively.

Many returning veterans entered university programmes, which dramatically increased university enrolment including physical education. By the end of the decade, seven Canadian universities were offering degree programmes in physical education, and by 1965, no less than seventeen degree programmes were offered in eight provinces (Meagher 1965).

In addition to these initiatives on the educational front, at the national level the Canadian government passed the *National Physical Fitness Act* in July 1943. Just two years later, professionals and volunteers working at the community level established the Parks and Recreation Association of Canada, which in 1970 changed its name to the Canadian Parks and Recreation Association (McFarland 1970).

As they had done after the First World War, the tragic results of combat provided a further stimulus for change. Dr. Ludwig Guttmann, the legendary neurosurgeon, observed prior to the end of the Second World War that persons with physical handicaps were rarely involved in physical activity and sport. In a classic paper published in 1945 entitled "New Hope for Spinal Cord Sufferers," Guttmann described the value of games and sport for paraplegics and recommended a variety of physical activities that persons with a disability might enjoy. In July 1948, motivated by his belief that "active exercises play a cardinal part in the rehabilitation of spinal injured people," Guttmann organized the first Stoke Mandeville Games for the Paralyzed at Aylesbury, England. Only sixteen athletes participated in those games; however, since that time paraplegics and tetraplegics have competed each year at Stoke Mandeville. The dramatic increase in the number of athletes with a disability attending the International Stoke Mandeville Games (held every fourth year in the country that is hosting the Olympic Games) stems from those initial games (Guttmann 1976).

Immediately after World War II, the Therapeutics Section of the American Association for Health, Physical Education and Recreation (AAHPER) struck a committee

... the programme needs of persons ... ability. It was at this meeting that ... educators in the United States began ... ocess of changing the name of the field ... correctives to *adapted physical education*. ... act, in 1952 the recommendation to use ... term *adapted physical education* was ... accepted by AAHPER (DePauw and Sherrill 1994). The use of this new term meant that a broader and more inclusive view of physical activity for persons with a disability was becoming more widely accepted.

During this period, rapid developments in the United States had a significant influence on the growth of the field in Canada. The publication of the text *Adapted Physical Education* by Arthur Daniels in 1954 encouraged those working with persons with a sensory and/or a physical disability to provide more challenging activities for participants. However, it is interesting to note that Dr. Daniels did not address the question of the needs of individuals with an intellectual or learning disability in his text. Important developments were also occurring in the area of physical activity for persons with a physical disability, for in 1957, the first United States National Wheelchair Games was successfully held at Adelphi College, New York, approximately a decade after the first Stoke Mandeville Games had been organized by Sir Ludwig Guttmann.

In Canada, the 1950s saw a number of important advances in physical education and recreation. The appointment of Dr. Doris Plewes as fitness and recreation consultant in the Fitness Division of the Department of Health and Welfare in Ottawa positively influenced the emergence of the physical fitness movement in Canada. In order to provide scientific support for an increased emphasis on physical fitness, she encouraged Dr. William Orban to develop the Canadian Physical Efficiency Test. Within a short time, he had designed a battery of seven tests and, with the help of teachers and leaders in the field, it was administered to children and adults in several provinces (Orban 1965, p. 241). The publication of the test results indicated "that Canadians were not as physically fit as

had been thought" and, more importantly, the findings "prompted an increased demand to know what actually could be done" (Orban 1965, p. 241). One of the experts who worked closely with Dr. Orban on the 5BX Programme during the fall of 1957 was Dr. Frank Hayden who, like Orban, was a Ph.D. graduate from the University of Illinois. As we shall see, Dr. Hayden's expertise in physical fitness would allow him to make an immense contribution to adapted physical activity through his leadership in the Special Olympics movement.

The 1960s: A Call for Change

The decade of the sixties was a turbulent one that initiated considerable social unrest. It was also a decade that witnessed a call for change and many advances in the field of adapted physical activity. One of the most important advances was the establishment of the International Stoke Mandeville Games Federation under the leadership of Sir Ludwig Guttmann in England and the hosting in Rome, Italy, of the first Paralympic Summer Games, with twenty-three participating countries. The growing response to these games indicated that participants, professionals, and volunteers were becoming more aware of the value of physical activity for persons with a disability.

In the United States, Dr. Julien U. Stein published a number of informative articles on the motor performance of persons with an intellectual disability and, in 1966, he became the director of the AAHPER Project on Recreation and Fitness for the Mentally Retarded. For the next sixteen years, Stein and his colleagues made an enormous contribution to the field by encouraging the development of programmes and services for persons with a disability, not only in the United States, but also in Canada.

In 1947, Patricia Austin, after teaching high school physical education in Toronto for three years, was asked by Dr. Maury Van Vliet, the director of physical education and athletics at the University of Alberta, to join the university's teaching staff in physical education. Her deep interest in the needs of individuals with a disability led Dr. Austin to pursue doctoral studies under the direction of Dr. Janet Wessel at Michigan State University, which she completed in 1965. In a series of major addresses and papers, Dr. Austin began to advocate on behalf of children with a disability, especially those with developmental disabilities. In an article published in the *CAHPER Journal* in 1968, entitled "Bridging the Gap Between Theory and Practice," she challenged her university colleagues to increase their research efforts, especially in the applied field. Her vision of research in physical education was a bold one. It called for "a shift from the practice of isolationism in universities to one of cooperation and interdependence with the social institutions of the larger community" (p. 27). As we will see in this chapter, the field of adapted physical activity in Canada did indeed eventually follow the collaborative vision that she so wisely articulated.

In 1969, in her Robert Tait Mackenzie Memorial address entitled "The Forgotten Child," delivered at the CAHPER convention in Victoria, Dr. Austin again urged her fellow professionals not to forget to focus on the needs of the individual child in physical education settings. Discussing the curriculum implications of the wide individual differences that teachers face in their classes, she emphasized that "there is a need to shift our position from one which approaches physical education as a content to be mastered to one which sees it as a personalized learning experience" (Austin 1969, p. 38). Moreover, she went on to argue that "it is the conditions under which this content is to be learned that must be flexible to accommodate each child. It is not the child who accommodates to fit the conditions" (Austin 1969, p. 38). In this article, she encouraged physical educators to pay more attention to the "forgotten child," that is, the child at play rather than the child being assessed or measured. And, most importantly, she specifically challenged professional physical educators to meet the physical activity needs of all children. Dr. Austin's challenge was an important one as it signalled the need for professionals to more fully appreciate the

capabilities, interests, and needs of all individuals, including those with a disability.

In the late 1950s and early 1960s, research studies began to show that children with intellectual handicaps were much less fit than their non-disabled peers. Armed with his academic training in the fitness field, Dr. Frank Hayden began to question why children with an intellectual disability performed so poorly on tests of physical fitness and motor performance. Within a few years, his research showed that given the right opportunities people with an intellectual disability could develop the physical skills they needed to participate more fully in physical activity and, by doing so, become more physically fit. As he later recalled, his research findings led him on a lifelong quest to find the means to facilitate the participation of persons with an intellectual disability in physical activity and sport (Hayden 1998).

When officials at the Kennedy Foundation in Washington, DC, became aware of Dr. Hayden's work they encouraged him to join their staff. Shortly thereafter, he became a director at the Kennedy Foundation where he worked closely with Eunice Kennedy Shriver in shaping the vision and values of the Special Olympics Movement. During his seven years in Washington, Dr. Hayden facilitated the establishment of federal legislation to assist persons with a disability, developed new concepts of playground design, and initiated the development of innovative methods for the teaching of sport skills to persons with an intellectual disability.

The first Special Olympics sport competitions were held at Soldier Field in Chicago in 1968. A floor hockey team from Toronto represented Canada at those competitions, which meant that Canada became the first nation, aside from the United States, to participate in the Special Olympics. During the next year, the first Canadian Special Olympics (CSO) Games were held in Toronto with the enthusiastic support of Harry "Red" Foster, a noted Toronto businessman and philanthropist, who for many years served as the chair of the

Canadian Special Olympics Foundation (Canadian Special Olympics 1999).

Positive developments were also occurring for persons with a physical disability. In 1968 Edmonton hosted the first National Games for Athletes with Disabilities, held under the auspices of the Canadian Wheelchair Sports Association. Dr. Gary McPherson, an outstanding disabled sport administrator and leader in the field, recalls that, as a resident of the polio ward at the University of Alberta Hospital, he and his friends who were ham radio enthusiasts saved the day for the organizing committee. At the time, a national mail strike presented a serious communication problem, as the high cost of long-distance telephone calls made it nearly impossible to get the games off the ground. Gary recalls that every Saturday morning, Robert Steadward met with him and his friends at VE6RD station in the hospital in order to communicate with other ham radio stations across Canada on matters related to transportation, funding, accommodation, and entries in the various events. The games went off without a hitch. This wonderful story underscores the close cooperation among participants, volunteers, and professionals that eventually characterized the development of adapted physical activity in Canada (Steadward, Nelson, and Wheeler 1994).

In the late 1960s other Canadian adapted physical activity leaders such as Prof. Brian Cleary at McGill University addressed the physical education needs of children with a learning disability based on the work of Dr. Newell Kephart and Dr. Marianne Frostig. At the same time, Dr. James Widdop, after completing his Ph.D. under the direction of Dr. Lawrence Rarick at the University of Wisconsin, began a series of programme development studies at McGill and later at Lakehead University of children with an intellectual disability. Through their work and writing, Cleary and Widdop stimulated interest in the needs of persons with a disability in their local area, but also re-emphasized the importance of considering the physical activity needs of all students.

The call for change by these early leaders certainly had a significant effect. During the next decade, Canada would experience a significant mobilization of professional and voluntary effort in the field of adapted physical activity. Nevertheless, it is interesting to note that Van Vliet's (1965) *History of Physical Education in Canada* includes twenty chapters ranging from the early years of physical education to the emergence of the fitness movement in Canada, and yet there is no mention of the field of adapted physical activity. Moreover, in the chapter written by Dr. Max Howell (1965) entitled "Physical Education Research in Canada" there are no citations of research in adapted physical activity, nor are there any theses on the subject reported in the list of 171 titles included in "Appendix G: Graduate Theses and Projects in Canada." Clearly, the influence of those interested in adapted physical activity only began to be felt after 1970 in answer to the call of our leaders in the preceding decade.

The 1970s: Normalization, Integration, and New Professional Organizations

During the 1970s, the articulation of the principle of normalization revolutionized the field of adapted physical activity. In his thought-provoking book, *The Principle of Normalization in Human Service* (1972), Wolf Wolfensberger defined normalization as performing culturally normative activities in as culturally normative a way as possible. People with disabilities and those who cared for them were profoundly influenced by this simple yet powerful concept.

During the seventies, efforts to apply the concept of normalization in schools, community organizations, and the workplace initiated heated debates between those who favoured traditional segregated programmes and those who wanted to move quickly towards integrated programmes. Moreover, the application of the principle of normalization went far beyond the programme level. It generated a new way of viewing persons with a disability and spoke to fundamental issues related to the social organization of our communities and the agencies involved in them. The movement to integration and the development of the concept of inclusive communities that emerged from those debates would ultimately change the way in which volunteers and professionals viewed and worked with persons with a disability. In fact, as the nature of the debates shifted more towards a dialogue on normalization and the integration process, new government policies and legislation emerged that positively influenced the lives of countless Canadians with a disability.

The 1970s saw other major developments in addition to the articulation and application of the principle of normalization. The passing of the Education for All Handicapped Children Act (PL 94–142) in 1975 had a profound impact on the educational and school services provided to persons with a disability in the United States. It mandated that all students have the right to nondiscriminatory evaluation and placement procedures, and they must be educated in the least restrictive environment. This law had a significant influence on educational and recreational services in Canada; but it also signalled that a new set of values must guide our interactions with persons with a disability.

Since the first Stoke Mandeville Games, the role of international sporting events for persons with a disability has been a major vehicle for the promotion of social change at the national and international level. The outstanding success of the Torontolympiad for the Physically Disabled, organized by Dr. Robert Jackson and Dick Loiselle in 1976, certainly had a major impact on the delivery of sport for persons with a disability in Canada. Since that time, just less than a quarter of a century ago, Canada has continued to produce many fine athletes who have won the highest of honours at these games. At the Torontolympiad for the Physically Disabled, Dr. Robert Steadward, a professor of physical education at the University of Alberta, was the manager of the Canadian Team. Within a decade he would play a key role in the worldwide development of sport for persons with a disability.

In 1976, an ad hoc CAHPER Committee on Adapted Programmes, chaired by Dr. Claudia Emes, a professor of physical education at the University of Calgary, began to discuss the creation of the Adapted Programmes Special Interest Group, which held its first meeting in Wolfville, Nova Scotia, in 1977, and which, for over twenty years, provided professional leadership in the field (Gurney 1983).

In a paper presented at the CAHPER conference in Wolfville, Dr. Don Newton (1977) reported on a survey of graduates of the BPE programme at the University of Calgary. The graduates were provided a list of thirteen theory courses and asked to indicate which of them should be part of the core curriculum. The graduates rated Development and Adaptive Physical Education eighth in the list of required courses, with 77 percent indicating that it should be a required core course. Based on the results of this survey, it seems that by the late seventies the need for professionals to acquire expertise in this important area was becoming more widely accepted. In fact the very next year, the Adapted Programme Special Interest Group published a position paper calling for the establishment of a compulsory course in adapted physical activity and called on professionals "to upgrade the motor, play, social and life skills of disabled persons so as to foster the normalization process" (CAHPER 1978, p. 3).

The year 1977 was a particularly important one in the history of the field. That year, the first International Federation of Adapted Physical Activity (IFAPA) Conference was held in Quebec City under the leadership of Dr. Clermont Simard of Laval University. Dr. Simard and his colleagues began IFAPA in 1973, and after four years of organizational effort, they hosted a very successful symposium that attracted international scholars and practitioners. Since 1977, a biennial symposium has been hosted by cities around the world. The high quality of the presentations and the opportunity for Canadians to interact and share ideas with their international colleagues have been a very tangible outcome of the vision of Dr. Simard and those who worked with him.

In 1979, Peggy Hutchison and John Lord published a book entitled *Recreation Integration* that described the importance of three interacting processes in the integration process: upgrading, educating, and participating. The upgrading component referred to the physical and social skills that persons with a disability need to develop to have the confidence and self-esteem to participate in physical activity and recreation activities in their community. The educating component identified the need of persons with a disability as well as advocates, parents, physical activity and recreation staff, volunteers, and the general public to become more informed about persons with disabilities and the integration process. Finally, the participating component argued that, with appropriate advocacy and support and with careful programming, persons with disabilities will be able to participate in physical and leisure activities, especially if each community offers a continuum of opportunities ranging from supportive segregated programmes to ones that are fully integrated.

In the introduction to their book, Hutchison and Lord (1979) recognize that the initial years of the recreation integration movement were not easy ones. As they put it,

> Despite resistance, we have noticed a tremendous interest in integration in recent years. Through our involvement with community groups, we have talked with many consumers, parents, and individuals in leisure and human services, who are searching for alternatives to traditional ways of providing services for devalued persons. This struggle to discover and act upon principles which improve the lives of individuals with a disability, served as a strong impetus for writing this book (p. 3).

Throughout that momentous decade, leaders in the field called for increased participation opportunities for persons with a disability. Moreover, the Canadian Parks and Recreation Association and the National Institute on Mental Retardation began to encourage generic sport agencies, service organizations, and municipal, provincial, and federal governments to provide greater access to physical activity opportunities for everyone in the community. In fact, at the end of their book, Hutchison and Lord identified no less than eleven provincial councils/committees that were involved in guiding the recreation integration movement in each of Canada's ten provinces and the Northwest Territories. In less than a decade, the principle of normalization and the recreation integration movement that it generated had touched the lives of countless Canadians.

In 1979, the Canadian Council of University Physical Education Administrators sponsored a national conference entitled "Body and Mind in the 1990s" at Brock University in St. Catherines, Ontario. At that conference, Dr. Clermont Simard and I presented a paper entitled "A Prospective View of University Preparation in Adapted Physical Activity for the 90s." It is interesting to note the issues that were of concern just over twenty years ago and especially to reflect on the thoughtful, yet quite critical, response of Dr. John Lord that followed our presentation (Simard and Wall 1980).

Essentially, our position paper argued that if the field was to make a significant impact on the lives of Canadians with a disability, then all undergraduate professional preparation programmes would have to include a compulsory core course in adapted physical activity. Moreover, given the diverse needs of persons with a disability within the schools and community, the paper called for the creation of specialized programmes to train specialists in the field. Furthermore, it was argued that opportunities for graduate study should be increased to enhance research activities and professional leadership capabilities. The paper also called for the establishment of a central clearinghouse to facilitate the distribution of resource materials to professionals and volunteers in communities across Canada.

Another major recommendation was the development of an adapted physical activity delivery system that underscored the importance of providing a much wider range of physical activity participation options for persons with a disability. The proposed system described options from those with a relatively high degree of emphasis on rehabilitation and/or instruction that would take place in relatively segregated settings, to those that placed much greater emphasis on participation and socialization within community settings.

In his thoughtful response, John Lord outlined the problems that the use of inappropriate labels can have on people and those who are involved with them. Quite rightly, he noted "the language we use to describe our concerns and our activity indicates a value orientation" (Simard and Wall 1980, p. 239). Most importantly, he challenged those in attendance to examine the dominant ideology, that is, the beliefs, attitudes, and values that are often, quite unconsciously, accepted by society and that can support the use of inappropriate actions and practices that devalue differences in the community. For example, he asked those in attendance to "consider 'adapted physical activity' or 'therapeutic recreation' as examples of how language reflects values" (Simard and Wall 1980, p. 239). He went on to suggest that:

> these notions often serve as rationales for maintaining segregated and overprotective experiences even though participants are ready for more stimulating, integrated settings. Even talking about *the* handicapped or *the* disabled further perpetuates the idea that there is a homogeneous group of *them*. (p. 239)

In concluding his critique, Lord recognized that considerable progress had been made; however, much more work had to be done if professionals, volunteers, and participants were to reach the goals that the principle of normalization set out for all of us. Certainly, the challenges Lord posed in his critique would be more fully addressed in the next decade.

---

2 To what extent do members currently in our field follow the recommendations that John Lord so clearly articulated in his critique over twenty years ago?

The 1980s: National Collaboration and a Blueprint for Action

This decade saw many changes in the lives of individuals with a disability and those who cared about them. In 1980, Canadians were deeply moved by the personal heroism of Terry Fox, who decided to run across Canada to raise money and awareness for cancer research, even though his right leg had been amputated due to a rare form of bone cancer. Terry Fox began his Marathon of Hope in St. John's, Newfoundland, on April 1 and ended it in Thunder Bay, Ontario, on September 1 after running a total distance of 5373 kilometres. Canadians from coast to coast were deeply moved by his heroic effort and contributed over $24 million to the Terry Fox Foundation. Each year, in cities across Canada, thousands of people remember Terry Fox's courage by participating in community runs that generate funds for cancer research. As the athletes at the Torontolympiad had done, Terry Fox brought Canadians closer to an individual with a disability, which allowed them to appreciate his abilities more fully and, in doing so, empowered persons with a disability to view themselves in a positive way.

The very next year, the United Nations General Assembly appropriately proclaimed 1981 the International Year of Disabled Persons and its theme was Full Participation and Equality. During the next ten years, tremendous strides were made in Canada in the provision of programmes and physical activity participation opportunities for persons with a disability. Public and private agencies began to recognize the need to eliminate architectural barriers so individuals with a physical disability could more readily enter arenas, gymnasia, and swimming facilities. Sporting goods firms began to manufacture more sophisticated equipment to facilitate the participation of persons with a disability in aquatics, outdoor recreation, and team sport activities. In addition to the reduction of architectural barriers, public education programmes within schools, the workplace, and the media began to reduce the attitudinal barriers that for years had prevented persons with a disability from participating in physical activities in public settings.

In 1980, with the support of Fitness Canada, the Canadian Fitness and Lifestyle Research Institute (CFLRI) was created. One of its first tasks was to conduct the Canada Fitness Survey, which was the first such national survey ever completed. Under the guidance of a distinguished set of chairs of the CFLRI board, the institute has conducted and supported many excellent studies related to the fitness of all Canadians and the factors that affect their participation in physical activity. Since 1986, the CFLRI has supported no less than fifteen research projects related to the physical activity of persons with a disability. Most importantly, the results of these studies have been widely distributed through the auspices of the institute. Canada's role as a leader in adapted physical activity research was surely enhanced by the inclusive vision that the CFLRI has followed for the past twenty years.

The field of adapted physical activity received a major stimulus with the initial publication of the *Adapted Physical Activity Quarterly* (*APAQ*) in 1984. In its first ten years, the articles ranged from book reviews and professional viewpoints to research and programme development studies. In 1995, Dr. Geoffrey Broadhead and Dr. Greg Reid, the first two editors of *APAQ*, completed a documentary analysis of the articles published in its first decade. A significant number had a professional focus on pedagogy, assessment, and integration; at the same time, a large number were written from biomechanics, physiology, motor learning, and motor development perspectives. It is also interesting to note that sixty-four Canadian authors contributed to *APAQ*'s initial ten volumes. There is no doubt that the publication of this important journal has had a positive impact on research and practice in our field (Reid and Broadhead 1995).

In the mid-eighties, Canadians were moved by the courage and abilities of Rick Hansen who from March 21, 1985, to May 22, 1987, wheeled through thirty-four countries on his Man in Motion tour on behalf of enhanced rehabilitation, research, and wheelchair sport opportunities. As with Terry Fox, a major goal of Rick Hansen's efforts was to increase public awareness of the abilities of persons with a disability and to move Canadians to encourage and support the full inclusion of all individuals in our communities.

In October 1986, the Adapted Programmes Special Interest Group of CAHPER, in cooperation with the University of Alberta and with the support of Fitness Canada, sponsored the Jasper Talks symposium in one of the most beautiful settings in the Canadian Rockies, Jasper Park Lodge. The symposium brought together delegates from across Canada to acknowledge past achievements, examine the current situation, and generate strategies for change in adapted physical activity in Canada. The delegates who attended the symposium represented a broad spectrum of participants, professionals, and volunteers who ranged from those involved with persons with a developmental disability to those with a physical and/or sensory disability.

A brief consideration of the themes discussed at the Jasper Talks symposium (1988) and the recommendations that emerged from it can provide a relatively realistic indication of the state-of-the-art in adapted physical activity midway through the 1980s. At the same time, a brief review of some of the major ideas that were shared at the symposium will provide a framework for understanding the content and relevance of the *Blueprint for Action* which stemmed from it.

Delegates to the Jasper Talks symposium discussed three major themes:

- programme development and evaluation
- professional education and leadership training
- delivery systems

Acknowledged leaders in the field presented position papers on each of the themes to help frame the delegates' follow-up discussion and recommendation sessions. Under the initial theme of programme development and evaluation, Greg Reid addressed issues related to skill upgrading, while Jane Watkinson discussed the value and challenges of implementing effective integrated programmes. Jane Taylor addressed the need for leisure counselling, and Don Hunter presented programme development guidelines for the implementation of inclusive municipal recreation programmes. The second major theme focussed on professional education and leadership training. In this session, John Lord observed that the current use of traditional leadership methods emphasized the control of participants, labelled individuals with a disability, and provided services that were not typically available within the community. He called for value-based leadership training that emphasized equality, integration, and consumer involvement. Donna Goodwin reported that, based on her experience in public school settings, teachers were aware of the need for mainstreaming and they were willing to attempt it; however, many of them believed that they needed more training if they were to facilitate effective integration in physical education settings confidently. Robert Steadward shared some of the recent advances related to the training, instruction, and participation of individuals with a physical disability and called for government action at all levels to increase support for research and, especially, to improve the dissemination of new knowledge to practitioners in the field.

The recognition the delegates gave to the importance of developing and implementing an effective delivery system was perhaps one of the most important aspects of the Jasper Talks symposium. Dr. Murray Smith outlined a generic physical activity delivery system model developed by Jim Ball and his colleagues at Fitness Canada. The proposed model included two main factors: the nature of different participation options and the developmental processes that would allow individuals to develop the expertise to participate in them. As early leaders in the field had done, Smith emphasized that a person's developmental level determined his or her level of involvement in physical activity; hence, he called for a continued emphasis on developmental skill upgrading processes.

The final keynote speaker was Dr. Jim McClements who stressed that the importance of providing generic participation options was a fundamental principle of the integration process. He reported on the positive social interactions that took place among athletes, officials, and organizers and the pleasure that the athletes experienced from participating in integrated sport opportunities. He concluded by recommending strategies to encourage improved access to generic programmes.

After hearing the position papers that introduced each of the three themes, the delegates moved into small, broadly representative groups to discuss the implications of the state-of-the-art ideas which had been shared and to develop recommendations for action that would be considered by an assembly of all of the delegates. The recommendations generated by the delegates were published in the *Proceedings of the Jasper Talks* (1988).

Immediately following the Jasper Talks, Fitness Canada established a National Advisory Committee on Physical Activity for Canadians with a Disability to develop an action plan designed to enhance the development of physical activity opportunities for Canadians with a disability. An exhaustive situational analysis was conducted that included a profile of persons with a disability, an examination of environmental factors and trends, an analysis of the needs of stakeholders, and potential blocks to improvements in the field. After extensive consultation and discussions, the advisory committee published and distributed the *Blueprint for Action* to over a thousand Canadians.

The *Blueprint for Action* (1988) endorsed the comprehensive societal vision that was adopted at the Canadian Fitness Summit in June 1986, which stated:

> The vision of fitness by the year 2000 depicts a society that values well-being as fundamental and as an integral part of day-to-day life. Canadian social structures, the family, the schools, the workplace, the health care system, will all enthusiastically embrace and reward daily physical activity

and behaviours which contribute significantly to health and well-being. Regular physical activity and optimal well-being will be ingrained as important and widely accepted values in Canadian society (in effect, a Canadian "cultural trademark"). (p. 16)

In addition to endorsing the vision of the fitness movement developed at the Canadian Fitness Summit in June 1986, the advisory committee also recommended that the following key elements be added to that vision statement:

- The education of self-empowered individuals who have the knowledge, skill, and support to accept responsibility and make independent decisions for full and satisfying lifestyles is the central focus of the vision.
- The creation of equal opportunities and access to quality programmes, services, and resources is also fundamental. Each community should have a full continuum of participant-centred programmes based on the needs and choices of the individual.
- The establishment of a network of competent and enabling advocates, support persons, and leaders.
- The development of a community-based infrastructure that facilitates collaboration and communication among all levels and sectors of Canadian society.
- The heightening of awareness of and support for persons with disabilities among all Canadians.
- The provision of readily available support resources, research, and current information.

In order to realize this national vision, the *Blueprint for Action* (1988) challenged Canadians to reach the following seven goals and priorities designed to foster increased physical activity among Canadians with a disability by:

1. facilitating the growth of self-empowered individuals through awareness, education, and support
2. developing quality delivery systems and networks with clearly defined roles, responsibilities, and communication links at all levels
3. enhancing organizational planning and policy development by providing resources and support mechanisms
4. identifying, developing, and promoting effective programmes and services
5. developing and promoting leadership by providing the programmes and support necessary to meet the needs
6. developing public awareness through promotional strategies involving community action and education
7. identifying, promoting, and supporting research priorities and state-of-the-art information (p. 17)

In a very real sense, the *Blueprint for Action* was a call to action; at the same time, it was a portrait, perhaps better termed a snapshot, of where adapted physical activity was at the end of the 1980s. Many achievements could and should have been celebrated; however, as the *Blueprint for Action* so clearly documented, much more work had to be done. As the next section of this chapter will show, since its publication, the *Blueprint for Action* has provided considerable guidance for initiatives at the local, provincial, and national levels.

Before closing this brief overview of developments in the 1980s, we must turn our attention to further developments at the international level. In 1989, in a paper entitled "Sports for Athletes with Disabilities: Future Considerations" presented at the Seventh International Symposium of Adapted Physical Activity in Berlin, Germany, Dr. Robert Steadward addressed a number of major organizational issues related to sport for persons with a disability at the national and international levels (Steadward 1990). In a thoughtful presentation, Dr. Steadward presented a summary of principles recommended by the Canadian Federation of Sports

Organizations for the Disabled which described in a visionary way the importance of creating a worldwide organization called the International Paralympic Committee and how such an organization might effectively govern itself. The ideas that he expressed garnered wide support and, in September 1989, Dr. Steadward was elected the first president of the newly formed International Paralympic Committee. Since that time, he has continued to play a dynamic leadership role as the president of this important organization for the promotion of sport for persons with a disability.

There can be little doubt that much organizational progress was made in support of adapted physical activity at the national and international levels during the 1980s. Perhaps the greatest change came from persons with a disability themselves. Many of them were becoming more fully involved in physical activity in their own communities and were, in fact, demanding and expecting to participate in sport activities ranging from alpine skiing to scuba and sky diving! However, the pioneers in our field would also want us to ask:

3 What percentage of persons with a disability are physically active in our communities, and are our communities sufficiently inclusive that all individuals feel that they can take part?

The 1990s: Answering the Challenge at the National and International Levels

Following the release of the *Blueprint for Action* in 1988, Fitness Canada continued to play a significant role in addressing the physical activity needs of persons with a disability. In fact, in September 1991, the Canadian government announced the five-year National Strategy for the Integration of Persons with a Disability. Approximately $3.5 million over five years was provided to Fitness Canada to continue its efforts to enhance active living opportunities for Canadians with a disability.

After receiving feedback from interested individuals and organizations across Canada, the National Advisory Committee, with the financial and professional support of Fitness Canada, was instrumental in the creation of the Active Living Alliance for Canadians with a Disability. A unique feature of the alliance was that it brought together generic and disability specific organizations that were dedicated to reaching the goals outlined in the *Blueprint for Action*. Since its inception, the alliance has played an important role in the development of adapted physical activity in Canada.

In 1995, Health Canada completed a comprehensive assessment of the activities of the Active Living Alliance for Canadians with a Disability and the initiatives of the National Integration Strategy. The thoroughly documented report indicated that substantial progress had been made towards the goals which had been collaboratively established in the *Blueprint for Action*. More recently, in a special issue on inclusive physical education in the *CAHPERD Journal*, Dr. Robert Steadward and five of his colleagues at the University of Alberta published an article documenting the contributions that the alliance had made since its inception (Steadward, Legg, Bornemann, Weiss, Jeon, and Wheeler 1997). Their four-month study provides a thoughtful analysis of the many initiatives that have been undertaken by the alliance during the past decade. Space does not permit a full listing of the major initiatives that have been successfully implemented by the alliance; however, some of the most notable ones that Dr. Steadward and his colleagues described are briefly discussed below. (See also Chapter 8 (Legg) for a profile of the alliance.)

Self-empowerment was one of the most important goals established in the original *Blueprint for Action*. In order to facilitate the self-empowerment process, the alliance developed workshop materials and a video describing how advocacy groups could be developed and used effectively at the community level. In addition, three excellent resource packages, entitled *Words with Dignity*, *Fit for All*, and *Positive Images*, were developed and distributed in communities across the country. Designed to foster the use of appropriate words and images among those referring to persons with a disability, these very impressive resources penetrated "beyond the active living market into the realm of business and the media" (Steadward et al. 1997, p. 11). Clearly, they have had a positive impact at the community level and beyond.

Another major initiative to facilitate self-empowerment and increased physical activity was the development of the Moving to Inclusion series of resource manuals designed to help teachers enhance the participation of students with a disability in physical education, intramurals, and other school physical activity opportunities. Funded by the Health Canada Fitness Programme, volunteers from ten of the alliance's national partners and twelve provincial and territorial ministries of education were involved in the development of the following resource packages:

- The Student with a Visual Impairment
- The Student with Cerebral Palsy
- The Student who Uses a Wheelchair
- The Student who is Deaf or Hard of Hearing
- The Student with an Intellectual Disability
- The Student with an Amputation
- The Student with Multiple Disabilities
- Skiing for Students with a Disability
- Students who are Physically Awkward

The Moving to Inclusion manuals provide up-to-date information on programme planning, the adaptation of tasks and equipment, as well as suggestions on how to modify the rules and settings for different games and physical activities. In order to ensure that these resource materials had an impact at the school level, in 1994, Health Canada distributed copies of the manuals to over fifteen thousand schools across Canada. At the present time, over twenty-five thousand copies have been circulated. In addition, to help facilitate the use of these materials, over four hundred volunteer leaders were trained to provide advice and support at the school and community level. The impact of the series has reached far beyond Canada's borders, as school and recreation personnel in many other countries are currently using them. However, advocates for persons with a disability are currently asking the following question:

---

4 To what extent are teachers and other professionals and paraprofessionals actually using the materials and strategies in the Moving to Inclusion series?

In addition to working at the school level, the alliance, under the active leadership of members of the Canadian Parks and Recreation Association, developed an important policy development document. "Municipal Government Policy Guidelines for Persons with a Disability" was designed to encourage municipalities to assess the services they provide in relation to the needs and wishes of persons with a disability. This material was widely disseminated to help people at the local level establish inclusive community recreation policies and practices.

Since its inception, the alliance has recognized the importance of developing leaders and resource persons to help it reach its goals. As early as 1991, the Leadership Development Model Package was developed to help organizations move forward in their leadership training efforts. In 1992, with the help of funds from the National Inclusion Strategy, the alliance undertook the Leadership Development Initiative, which placed special emphasis on the development of leadership skills designed to meet the physical activity needs and concerns of persons with a disability. As part of this initiative, the alliance and its national partners created the Inclusion Assessment Tool, to help communities assess the degree to which they are establishing truly inclusive communities. Shortly thereafter, the Inclusion Action Pack was developed to provide a practical resource guide for leaders in the establishment of inclusive active living programmes. Again, these initiatives were well-received in communities across the country (Steadward et al. 1997).

In addition to the above achievements, the holding of an annual forum has been one of the most important contributions that the alliance has made to the development of adapted physical activity in Canada. Held in different cities across the country, the yearly forum has provided an excellent venue for sharing success stories, addressing major concerns, and organizing personal and professional development opportunities. The forums have been especially valuable in developing local, regional, and national networks. Very often, it is the enormous amount of effort involved in organizing the forum at the local level that mobilizes people from agencies within a city or region to meet and work together for the first time. The networking opportunities that are provided in the work leading up to these events, as well as at them, have been very beneficial at both the individual and organizational level.

As these observations on the activities of the Active Living Alliance for Canadians with a Disability show, the last decade of the twentieth century saw an explosion of activity in the area of adapted physical activity. Another whole chapter would be needed to begin to do justice to the increase in undergraduate courses and programmes in the area. The extensive research work within and outside of universities would provide material for another entire book (Reid and Broadhead 1995; Reid and Prupas 1998). The movement to inclusive programming within the schools and at the municipal level has been especially heartening. While leadership has been provided by research and activity centres such as the Robert Steadward Centre at the University of Alberta, the fine work done at Variety Village in Toronto must also be mentioned. In addition, the ongoing leadership and support provided by the Canadian Special Olympics, the Association for Community Living, and the many disability-specific organizations working on behalf of persons with a disability should not be forgotten. However, before closing this chapter, I would like to mention briefly the international role that Canada is continuing to play in the field of adapted physical activity.

In 1993, Dr. Robert Steadward hosted an international conference on high performance sport for athletes with disabilities, called "Vista '93". One hundred and sixty-three athletes, coaches, sport scientists, and sport administrators met in the scenic Rocky Mountain setting of Jasper to share information and discuss the latest views on topics ranging from scientific and technical matters to the ethics of sport and the future of the paralympic sport movement.

During his keynote address to the conference, Dr. Gary McPherson celebrated the fact that "disability and sport have come full circle–from being based on a medical rehabilitation model, to being athlete and performance centred. We should take a measure of pride in these milestones. Each and every one of us has made a contribution" (Steadward, Nelson and Wheeler 1994, p. 12). Dr. McPherson pointed to the benefits that have accrued through increased awareness of the importance of physical activity and nutrition on the health of everyone. Most importantly, he went on to say that "your efforts have raised the self-esteem of, I would suggest, thousands of athletes with disabilities. They have in turn taken this confidence into their private lives–their families, jobs, communities. They have influenced their peers, parents, children, and co-workers. And as role models, they are influencing millions more" (McPherson 1994, p. 14).

In closing, Dr. McPherson stated:

I would like to leave you with this. To maintain, retain, or obtain the moral and financial support of others, it is crucial to remember the effect it has on all people. It is also crucial to expand the focus of the work. We need to see our work not so much as a narrow context of pure and applied research, but rather in a broader and more global sense. (Steadward, Nelson and Wheeler 1994, p.14)

The outstanding leadership provided by Dr. Robert Steadward as the president of the International Paralympic Committee and the fine work of Dr. Clermont Simard as the founding president and of Dr. Greg Reid as the current president of the International Federation of Adapted Physical Activity shows that Canadians continue to take up the challenge that Dr. McPherson posed to all of us.

The above history of adapted physical activity in Canada has been a rather lengthy one. However, in writing each section of it, I have been aware of just how many significant events, programmes, and individual contributions have not been mentioned. The wonderful partnership that has evolved among participants, volunteers, and professionals in the field is at the heart of the story. It has been this willingness for different people, agencies, and governments to support the movement to inclusion and full participation in physical activity that has been the most impressive aspect of this story. Canadians have much to celebrate in the field of adapted physical activity; however, there are still many significant challenges that must be met before we can honestly state that the goals set forth in the *Blueprint for Action* have truly been reached.

Study Questions

1. A number of major factors have influenced the history of adapted physical activity in Canada, identify the three most important factors and briefly justify your selection of them.
2. Based on your own experience, how successful have we been in developing "inclusive" communities that facilitate "active living" by all Canadians?
3. Select one of the people referred to in this chapter and using internet or library resources develop a more complete biographical sketch of their role in the development of adapted physical activity in Canada.

References

Austin, P.L. (1968). Bridging the gap between theory and practice. *CAHPER Journal, 34*(4), 21–27.

Austin, P.L. (1969). The forgotten child. *CAHPER Journal, 35*(6), 11–15, 338.

Austin, P.L. (1969). The Canadian Special Olympics. *CAHPER Journal, 36*(2), 16–17.

Austin, P.L. (1971). An experimental dance study for children with learning disabilities. In J. Boorman and D. Harris (Eds.), *Dance: Verities, values, visions* (pp. 39–43). Waterloo, ON: Binational Dance Conference.

Blackstock, C.R. (1965). The Canadian association for health, physical education and recreation. In M.L. Van Vliet (Ed.), *Physical education in Canada* (pp. 276–91). Scarborough, ON: Prentice-Hall.

Canadian Association for Health, Physical Education and Recreation. (1978). *Position paper on adapted programmes.* Ottawa: Author.

Canadian Special Olympics. (1999). *History of major Canadian Special Olympics events.* Toronto: Author.

Cartwright, E.W. (1916). Physical education and the Strathcona Trust. *The School, IV*(4), 306–10.

Consentino, F., and Howell, M.L. (1971). *A history of physical education in Canada.* Toronto: General Publishing.

Daniels, A. (1954). *Adapted physical education: Principles and practices of physical education for exceptional students.* Englewood Cliffs, NJ: Prentice-Hall.

DePauw, K.P., and Sherill, C. (1994). Adapted physical activity: Present and future. *Physical Education Review, 17*, 6–13.

Eaton, John D. (1970). Arthur Stanley Lamb, M.D.: His influence on Canadian sport. *Proceedings of the First Canadian Symposium on the History of Sport and Physical Education, 1*, 417–30.

Ebbs, J. Harry. (1971). R. Tait McKenzie: Medical contributions. In S.A. Davidson and P. Blackstock (Eds.), *The R. Tait McKenzie Memorial Addresses* (pp. 42–44), Ottawa: Canadian Association of Health, Physical Education and Recreation.

Gurney, Helen. (1983). *The CAHPER story.* Vanier, ON: Canadian Association for Health, Physical Education and Recreation.

Guttmann, L. (1976). *Textbook of sport for the disabled.* Oxford: Alden Press.

Hayden, Frank J. (1998). *"Pure sport."* Convocation Address, University of Calgary, Calgary, Alberta.

Hermann, Ernst. (1937, June). Physical education and physical therapy: Past and present. *Journal of Health and Physical Education,* 349–51 and 395.

Howell, M.L. (1965).Physical education research in Canada. In M.L. Van Vliet (Ed.), *Physical education in Canada* (pp. 249–75). Scarborough, ON: Prentice-Hall.

Howell, M.L. and Consentino, F. (1970). The history of physical education in Canada. *Proceedings of the First Canadian Symposium on the History of Sport and Physical Education, 1,* 343–59.

Hutchison, P., and Lord, J. (1979). *Recreation integration.* Ottawa: Leisurability Publications.

Jasper Talks. (1988). *Proceedings of the Jasper Talks: Strategies for change in adapted physical activity in Canada.* Ottawa: CAHPER.

McDiarmid, J. (1970). The Strathcona Trust: Its influence on physical education. *Proceedings of the First Canadian Symposium on the History of Sport and Physical Education, 1,* 397–413.

McFarland, E. (1970). A historical analysis of the development of public recreation in Canadian communities. *Proceedings of the First Canadian Symposium on the History of Sport and Physical Education, 1,* 59–67.

McKenzie, R. Tait. (1894, February). The place of physical education in the school system. *Montreal Medical Journal,* 1–4.

McKenzie, R. Tait. (1909). *Exercise in education and medicine.* Philadelphia: W.B. Saunders.

McKenzie, R. Tait. (1918). *Reclaiming the maimed.* Philadelphia: W.B. Saunders.

Meagher, John W. (1965). Professional preparation. In M.L. Van Vliet (Ed.), *Physical education in Canada* (pp. 64–81). Scarborough, ON: Prentice-Hall.

National Advisory Committee on Physical Activity for Canadians with a Disability. (1988). *Blueprint for action: Physical activity for Canadians with a disability.* Ottawa: Fitness Canada.

Newton, D.M. (1977). Professional preparation: Where do we go from here? *Proceedings of the CAHPER Conference,* 106–15. Wolfville, NS: CAHPER.

Orban, William A.R. (1965). The fitness movement. In M.L. Van Vliet (Ed.), *Physical education in Canada* (pp. 238–48). Scarborough, ON: Prentice-Hall.

Reid, G., and Broadhead, G.D. (1995). *APAQ* at ten: A documentary analysis. *Adapted Physical Activity Quarterly, 12,* 103–12.

Reid, G., and Prupas, A. (1998). A documentary analysis of research priorities in disability sport. *Adapted Physical Activity Quarterly, 15,* 168–78.

Sherrill, C., and DePauw, K.P. (1994). History of adapted physical activity and education. In J. Massengale and R. Swanson, (Eds.). *History of exercise and sport science.* Champaign, IL: Human Kinetics.

Simard, C., and Wall, A.E. (1980). A prospective view of university preparation in adapted physical activity for the '90s. In Frank J. Hayden (Ed.), *Body and mind in the 90s* (pp. 225–37). Hamilton, ON: Canadian Council of University Administrators.

Steadward, Robert D. (1990). Sports for athletes with disabilities: Future considerations. In G. Doll-Tepper, C. Dahms, B. Doll, and H.V. Selzam (Eds.), *Adapted physical activity: An interdisciplinary approach* (pp. 65–73). Berlin: Springer-Verlag.

Steadward, R.D., Nelson, E.R., and Wheeler, G.D. (Eds.). (1994). *Vista '93: The outlook.* Edmonton, AB: Rick Hansen Centre.

Steadward, R.D., Legg, David F.H., Bornemann, Rebeccah A., Wiss, Chistina B., Jeon, Justin Y., and Wheeler, Garry D. (1997). Active Living Alliance for Canadians with a Disability: A ten year retrospective analysis. *CAHPERD Journal, 63*(3), 10–15.

Wolfensberger, W. (1972). *The normalization principle in human service.* Toronto: National Institute on Mental Retardation.

CHAPTER 4

Disability Definitions

Leanne Squair
Henriëtte J. Groeneveld

Learning Objectives
- To enhance students' knowledge of physical and developmental disabilities, mental health concerns, and sensory impairments.
- To enhance students' knowledge of the disability definition, the cause, symptoms, characteristics, treatment/management, and some physical activity implications related to the disability.

Introduction

Society's understanding of disability has been shaped by a medical community that emphasizes the physical and mental functioning of the individual. With this approach, people with a disability are grouped according to their etiology (the medical cause, or description of their condition). Thus, we speak of children "with spina bifida," implying that such children are more or less alike in some respect, that they share "characteristics" that define them. For decades, our society actually spoke of the condition first ("physically handicapped boy", "mentally retarded student") communicating an assumption that the condition itself defined the person, but this practice has been largely abandoned in professional and educational settings (see *Words with Dignity*, from the Active Living Alliance for Canadians with a Disability 1992).

It has been suggested that the medical approach has led to a lack of appreciation of individual difference and to the adoption of treatments, or programmes, aimed at the condition rather than the person. Critics of this approach say that this medical model of disability has led to the assumption that people with a disability are sick, require care, need protection, sympathy, and charity. As a result, people with a disability have been marginalized, denied respect, and prevented from experiencing opportunities to succeed on the basis of their own merits. Recently, concerns about the medical 'categorization' of conditions have prompted professionals to look for other ways of describing people and to non-categorical approaches to the provision of services.

Disability can also be characterized on the basis of limitations in function, an approach that puts an emphasis on the systematic appraisal of functional impairment and functional ability in order to provide suitable interventions for fitness and skill development for each individual. Chapters throughout this book (see Chapter 22 (Seidl) and Chapter 15 (Watkinson and Causgrove-Dunn) for example) are consistent with this second approach, in that programme development is based on individual assessment of need rather than on the basis of etiology. Two individuals with the same disability may have significantly different needs, characteristics, interests, and functional abilities. Two individuals with quite different 'conditions' may have similar movement function and similar programme needs. Motivation, experience, technological aids, communication skills may all contribute to these similarities and differences. The functional approach on which most of this book is based attempts to look at individual need for service, regardless of disability. It is an attempt to put the person first and the disability second.

CLASSIFICATION AND CATEGORIZATION

Typically, people communicate by using a language that contains numerous categories (e.g., car, cat, oxygen, photocopier, etc.). In a broad sense, a category refers to a set of people, actions, or objects which all have at least a particular characteristic or quality in common. For example, the definition of *car* could be "a road vehicle which has four wheels and is self-powered by an engine." When someone uses this definition of a car, the person is stating that any object that is (a) a road vehicle, (b) has four wheels, and (c) is self-powered by an engine is a car. The definition, or category, states what is common across all cars. It is important to note that many possible characteristics of a particular car are not included in the definition (e.g., colour, weight, seats, horsepower, etc.).

Categorization by sorting individuals according to boundary conditions is also frequently made. For example, a person with an intellectual disability must have an estimated IQ of seventy or less on an intelligence test. In this case, experts choose, after careful consideration, the IQ boundary to be seventy. One common characteristic of persons with intellectual disability is that their IQ is seventy or less. However, commonality does not imply homogeneity; two persons with intellectual disabilities can have different IQs. In addition, they can have fairly different functioning levels.

The medical profession, with its emphasis on disease, has developed an extensive classification system. You are likely familiar with terminology such as *cerebral palsy*, *muscular dystrophy*, *spina bifida*, *autism*, etc. Each term refers to a category. It is important to understand that these categories emphasize some features and de-emphasize some others. Instead of using a classification system based on a 'medical model', many adapted physical educators nowadays recommend the adoption of a classification system based on functional level (i.e., what people can do with or without assistance). It is recognized that two persons may have the same medical classification but they can have different functional levels. On the other hand, two persons with different medical classifications may have the same functional level. Stated differently, there is no direct relationship between a classification based on the medical model and a functional level classification system.

In a sense, each classification system is imperfect and incomplete because many dimensions are needed to characterize an individual. Although we recognize the importance of knowing what people can do, with and without assistance, there can be important information conveyed by the etiology of a person's 'condition' that may have implications for our interactions with them. We learn something about a person when we are told that person has Down's syndrome, or multiple sclerosis. These terms can inform us, and thus it is essential that we, as professionals, have a basic understanding of disabilities and the terms that are used to describe them.

The following chapter will provide you with a basic understanding of disability from the perspective of its etiology or its common description, in other words, according to the medical model. The terms included here are used by many professionals to describe certain features of groups, and for this reason alone they need to be understood. Indeed, much communication in adapted physical activity begins with an understanding of the etiology of disability. Our vocabulary can contribute to the perpetuation of prejudice against participants with disabilities (*Words with Dignity* 1992), reinforce the beliefs of imperfection, and increase the polarity between able-bodied and persons with disabilities. Therefore, it is now customary to describe the person first and the disability second. Hence we say "a child with developmental coordination disorder," "a participant who has multiple sclerosis," rather than "a hemiplegic." You should also remember as you read this material that there are wide individual differences within each 'group', and it is these individual differences that most likely determine a person's physical activity and recreation needs and interests.

> **1** What makes it important for society to describe the person first, then his or her abilities, and finally his or her disability?

Mental Health

Mental health is a state of being. It refers to how one is able to cope with the demands and stress of daily living. We all may experience times when we feel depressed, get unreasonably angry or over excited. We even have periods when we think that everything and everybody is out to get us and that we cannot handle regular life issues. These are normal reactions to particular situations. If one has positive mental health one is able to assess the circumstances and move on.

Mental Illness

Statistics show that one in every six Canadians will have a mental health problem at some point in their lives (Canadian Mental Health Association 1993). Mental illness includes a broad range of psychological or behavioural symptoms that reduce an individual's capacity to cope with daily life: a person may lose contact with him- or herself, emotions may be uncontrollable, behaviour may be inappropriate, or the ability to communicate with other people may be lost (Canadian Mental Health Association 1993). Causes may include the amount of stress in their lives, the patterns of communication they develop within their families, poverty and poor housing, the number of close family and friends whom they have to support them through difficulty, and their level of self-esteem. Mental illnesses account for a large number of hospital stays each year. Since it is human nature to fear what we do not understand, mental illness is feared by many and, unfortunately, still carries a stigma (a mark or sign of disgrace). Many people hesitate to get help for a mental health problem because of this stigma. This is unfortunate because effective treatment exists for almost all mental illnesses.

MOOD DISORDERS (DEPRESSION AND/OR MANIC DEPRESSION)

Everyone experiences 'highs' and 'lows' in life, but individuals with mood disorders experience them with greater intensity and for longer periods of time than most people.

Depression is the most common mood disorder (American Psychiatric Association 1994). A depressed individual may experience feelings of hopelessness, changes in eating patterns, disturbed sleep, constant tiredness, an inability to have fun, and thoughts of death or suicide. Stressful or discouraging situations may overwhelm certain people on a continual basis and have the potential to become serious. Experiences of failure commonly result in temporary feelings of worthlessness and self-blame, while personal loss causes feelings of sadness, disappointment, and emptiness.

Researchers believe that a deficiency of certain chemicals in the brain and/or genetics may also affect how likely we are to develop an ongoing or serious depression (Canadian Mental Health Association 1993). The most common and successfully used treatments are psychological counselling and/or antidepressant medication.

MANIC DEPRESSION (BIPOLAR DISORDER)

Manic depression is known as bipolar disorder due to the opposing moods that accompany the mental illness. People with bipolar experience unusually great highs and elation (manic stage) and great lows and depression (depressive stage). When the 'highs' get out of hand, the manic person can behave in a reckless manner, sometimes to the point of financial ruin or getting in trouble with the law.

Researchers believe that biological factors such as the brain's chemistry seem to play a major role in producing the illness. One's personality and/or stresses in the environment may also play a part in bringing on an acute episode of mania or depression. Stress management and medication are helpful in controlling manic and depressive episodes.

ANXIETY DISORDERS

Everyone experiences anxiety at some point in life. People become anxious when they have to face a highly stressful situation. When one is anxious and under stress the body reacts—hands become clammy, the heart beats faster, one can even feel lightheaded or dizzy. Some people become preoccupied with fear and worry, causing the intense feelings of anxiety to continue. If this occurs, an individual may have an anxiety disorder. Anxiety can take the form of panic disorder, phobia, or obsessive-compulsive disorder. Without treatment, an individual's physical, mental, and emotional health may be in jeopardy (American

Psychiatric Association 1994). Anxiety disorders can also lead to alcohol and/or drug abuse, family problems, depression, and in some cases, suicide.

People may develop phobias (unreasonable fear of objects, animals, or situations), panic disorders (episodes of intense, sudden fear, and physical symptoms such as difficulty breathing), or obsessive-compulsive disorders (unable to control the repetition of unwanted thoughts or actions).

PHOBIAS

It is unclear how phobias start. However, if an individual is prone to excessive anxiety and stress, he or she is more likely to be vulnerable to panic attacks and phobias. People with phobias have irrational and uncontrollable fears of objects and/or situations. They experience feelings of intense panic when confronted by whatever it is that frightens them and go to considerable lengths to avoid the object or the situation. An individual with a phobia may experience physical feelings, such as anxiety, when confronted with a feared situation. The most effective forms of therapy are based on cognitive and behavioural approaches. Individuals may also learn calming techniques; meditative therapy and antidepressant medication can be prescribed to assist their anxiety.

PANIC DISORDERS

On average, one out of every three young adults reports having had a panic attack (Canadian Mental Health Association 1993). During a panic attack, sensations such as sweating, nausea, trembling and numbness in the legs or hands, dizziness, hot or cold flashes, a feeling of tightness or pressure in the chest, hyperventilation, 'jelly' legs, or blurred vision can develop. Individuals may even feel as if they are going to die of a heart attack or lose control of their body functions. These intense feelings of panic usually do not last for very long and most people brush off the episode as a momentary panic situation. However, some people become very agitated and develop a fear that it will happen again. If an individual has more than four panic attacks within one month, or a panic attack occurs when the individual is not in an anxious or stressful situation, it is probable that they have a panic disorder. Panic disorders usually begin before an individual is thirty years old.

OBSESSIVE-COMPULSIVE DISORDER

People with this disorder experience unwanted thoughts that make no sense, but that nevertheless cause the individual to feel anxious. Irrational thoughts may concern contaminating themselves or others with dirt or germs, or they may be obsessed about their own safety or the safety of a loved one. In response to their obsessive thoughts, the individual may need to think neutralizing thoughts or perform certain compulsive rituals, including repetitive hand-washing or counting. As with phobias, a traumatic event can trigger obsessive thoughts or behaviours. People who are described as perfectionists seem more prone than others to develop obsessions.

SCHIZOPHRENIA

Schizophrenia tends to appear when the body is undergoing the hormonal and physical changes of adolescence. It is a chemical imbalance in the brain, which results in splitting thoughts from reality, thoughts from feeling, and thoughts from expression. People who have schizophrenia may have mixed-up thoughts, delusions (false or irrational beliefs), hallucinations (seeing or hearing things that do not exist), and exhibit bizarre behaviours. It is difficult for an individual with schizophrenia to discern what is real and what is not real, and this significantly affects ability to function on a daily basis.

Schizophrenia usually strikes in the late teen years or the twenties. Some people have only one episode of very severe symptoms (psychosis). Others have many throughout their lives but manage to live relatively normal lives between episodes of psychosis. However, some people are more or less continuously bothered by this illness. Antipsychotic medication is the main treatment for the symptoms the individual may experience.

EATING DISORDERS

Eating disorders are most common in men and women under the age of thirty. They are most common in young girls. Anorexia nervosa is a very serious illness that involves drastic weight loss due to fasting when an individual's body image is disturbed and an intense fear of becoming obese takes over. This can lead to emaciation, with failing physical and psychological health. Without treatment, a person with this disorder can die. Bulimia is an eating disorder that is characterized by secretive episodes of binge-eating followed by self-induced vomiting and/or abuse of laxatives or diuretics, and/or excessive exercise and fasting. The main treatment for eating disorders is psychotherapy. Medication may also be prescribed.

PERSONALITY DISORDERS

Individuals with personality disorders usually have a difficult time getting along with others. In general, people with personality disorders have a lot of difficulty understanding themselves and others. As a result, they may be irritable, demanding, hostile, fearful, or manipulative. Personality disorders are the most difficult disorders to treat. Individuals, in many cases, do not seek help because they are able to live normally in some ways. It is in the area of relationships with other people that they experience difficulty. They tend to blame others rather than consider that the problem may be within themselves. Treatment consists of intensive psychotherapy, sometimes supplemented with medication.

MULTIPLE PERSONALITY DISORDER

Multiple personality disorder is characterized as a severe dissociative disorder that involves a disturbance in both the memory and identity of an individual. The individual uses primitive defense mechanisms involving devaluation, denial, and/or taking on the personality of another in order to cope with trauma experienced in childhood.

There are three factors that determine if a person has a multiple personality disorder:

1. Two or more personalities exist within the individual, each being dominant at certain times.
2. The dominant personality determines the individual's behaviour.
3. Each individual personality is complex and integrated with its own unique behaviour patterns.

Individuals with mental illness may have difficulty in physical activity situations because they are feeling worthless, helpless, or hopeless. As an adapted physical activity specialist, there are many challenges in motivating people with mental illnesses to participate in activities. They may have difficulty concentrating or making decisions in a game situation. Individuals may need to be reminded to attend a programme or activity, and might need to be accompanied by someone and transported to the activity location. Individuals with mental illness need to feel comfortable in a physical activity setting in order to participate. Medication and feelings of inadequacy may cause persons to have a loss of energy and feel very tired, which would affect their involvement in a number of physical activity settings. One of the side-effects of medication is over-eating, which results in an increase in weight gain; such individuals feel very self-conscious about their bodies and they may not wish to participate in physical activities. Further side-effects of medication are feeling physically unwell and tiredness. Individuals may have a lack of money, and so require no-cost or low-cost programme opportunities.

Physical Disabilities

AMPUTATION

The term *amputation* is used when an individual loses a limb(s) or portion of a limb(s). Not all amputees are alike. Some individuals have congenital amputations, which means the individual was born without a limb(s) or part of a limb(s). There are two types of congenital amputations, namely *phocomelia*, where the middle part of the limb is absent, though the distal and proximal segments are still intact. The second type is similar to a surgical amputation whereby no normal structures (i.e., hands or fingers) are present below the missing part (Porretta 2000a). People who have had amputations have lost a limb(s) or part of a limb(s) through diseases such as diabetes or cancer, or through accidents. Individuals with amputations can be fitted with prostheses, although caution is needed to make sure the prosthetic device does not cause injury to the remainder of the limb. In general, an amputation alters the centre of gravity and coordination of the individual (Canadian Amputee Sports Association 1993). Some individuals with lower limb amputations choose not to use their prosthesis, but rather prefer to use wheelchairs for mobility.

---

2 Generally, the use of prostheses would be considered beneficial. Can you think of any situations in which the use of a prosthesis might confer a disadvantage for a person with disability, or for a person without disability, and result in claims of unfairness or discrimination?

AMYOTROPHIC LATERAL SCLEROSIS (ALS)

Usually referred to as Lou Gehrig's Disease, ALS is a neuromuscular disease that attacks the nerve cells and pathways in the brain and spinal cord. ALS is progressive and fatal. Symptoms often start with lack of fine motor movements in the hands and feet and work toward the centre of the body and progress to lack of gross motor skills. One side of the body is usually more affected than the other. Physical activity should be participated in to the extent possible for quality of life. Eventually, paralysis will move throughout the entire body, except the eye muscles and the muscles of the bladder and anus. The brain is not affected. There is no cure for this disease. Individuals with ALS should be encouraged to do a general maintenance programme, specifically to strengthen the unaffected and/or less-affected muscles. Vigorous and tiring exercises should be avoided. Individuals with ALS should stop exercising before they become fatigued (http://www.caregiver.org).

ARTHRITIS

Arthritis means "inflammation of the joints" that causes swelling, pain, and restricted movement in the affected area. Inflamed joints can lead to a decrease in range of motion and, in some cases, may result in permanent joint contractures and/or muscle atrophy (Porretta 2000a). There are many different kinds of arthritis; some respond to treatment, while others are chronic. Chronic arthritis frequently goes in and out of remission (http://gocarolinas.adam.com; Sherrill 1998). One attempts to reduce the pain and discomfort to the individual by treatment.

The cause of arthritis is unknown; it is not inherited nor the result of diet or climate. There is no cure (Porretta 2000a). Individuals with arthritis should participate in a physical activity programme to maintain bone density and range of motion in the joints, which will alleviate permanent contractures. In addition, muscular strength and pain relief may occur when participating in an exercise programme. Make sure that sufficient rest periods are incorporated to prevent fatigue. Modifications in the activities should be encouraged when individuals have severe joint limitations, to ensure protection of the joints and/or undue stress (i.e., avoid leaping, jumping, twisting, or hopping activities) (http://gocarolinas.adam.com; Porretta 2000a; Sherrill 1998).

ARTHROGRYPOSIS

Arthrogryposis is a non-progressive, congenital impairment, where fatty and connective tissue surrounds the joints instead of normal muscle tissue. This results in restrictive range of motion in the joints. There are varying degrees of arthrogryposis; some individuals are minimally affected, while others have to use wheelchairs (Porretta 2000a; Sherrill 1998). Participation in physical activities is encouraged, especially range of motion activities (Porretta 2000a).

ASTHMA

Asthma is a chronic lung disorder characterized by periodic attacks of wheezing alternating with normal breathing. The cause may be intrinsic (inside the body) or extrinsic (caused by an allergy). Asthma can be treated by medication such as anti-inflammatory drugs, and/or broncho-dilators (http://gocarolinas.adam.com; Sherrill 1998). Individuals who manage their asthma can fully participate in unrestricted physical activity. However, persons with asthma who exercise at high intensity or for a long duration may have an asthma attack. This condition is called exercise-induced asthma. To prevent an exercise-induced asthma attack, the individual should pay attention to the following factors: proper warm-up, air condition, interval training versus sustained exercise, and use of medication prior to exercise (Surburg 2000; Sherrill 1998). They should drink plenty of fluids while exercising. The drinks should be at room temperature, since cold drinks may trigger an attack.

BRAIN INJURY

A traumatic brain injury refers to permanent damage to the brain caused by an external blow to the head. This injury can result in short- and long-term memory loss; impairment of language, hearing, vision, sensation; or coma, depending which part of the brain was injured (Canadian Wheelchair Sports Association 1994). The extent and the location of the brain damage and the success of the rehabilitation depend on whether the impairments are mild or severe. According to Appleton (1998) the majority of head injuries in children are caused by child abuse; falls from buildings, play equipment, or trees; injuries from objects (i.e., ball, stones); road traffic accidents; seizures and other causes of loss of consciousness; sport-related injuries (i.e., skate-boarding, skiing, football).

In some cases, individuals with brain injury wear helmets to prevent further injury when the individual has poor balance and/or lacks coordination. Other physical impairments may require the individual with brain injury to use crutches and/or a wheelchair (Auxter et. al. 1993; Porretta 2000a).

CEREBRAL PALSY

The word *cerebral* relates to the brain, and *palsy* means "disordered movement or posture." Cerebral palsy is a nonprogressive condition caused by damage to the motor control areas of the brain before, during, or soon after birth. The disability affects the control of movement and posture. The effects vary from no visible signs to multiple signs, based on the location and the amount of damage to the brain, and involve lack of control of facial and limb movements and speech difficulties (Auxter et al. 1993; Porretta 2000b).

Abnormal muscle tone varies from individual to individual, and is described in three main categories:

Spastic cerebral palsy–damage has occurred to the motor areas of the cerebrum, which results in stiff muscles and restricts movement. Muscle tone is hypertonic or spastic.

Athetoid cerebral palsy–damage has occurred to the basal ganglia, which is located deep in the cerebral hemispheres of the brain, and results in uncontrollable movements. Muscle tone is low or fluctuates.

Ataxic cerebral palsy–damage has occurred to the cerebellum, which results in unbalanced movement. Muscle tone fluctuates (Porretta 2000b; Canadian Cerebral Palsy Sports Association 1994; Sherrill 1998).

Sometimes individuals who have cerebral palsy, especially spasticity, use braces or orthotic devices to prevent permanent contractures or to support affected muscles. Surgery can be performed to lengthen contracted tendons (Porretta 2000b).

Some individuals with cerebral palsy startle when a loud noise or sudden jarring movements occur. This is called a moro, or startle, reflex. Therefore, in sport, the use of an alternative-signalling device, instead of using a starting gun or whistle, is recommended. In addition, some individuals are prone to seizures, and most use drugs to prevent the occurrence of a seizure. The flexor muscles in individuals who have cerebral palsy may be disproportionately stronger than the extensor muscles (Canadian Cerebral Palsy Sports Association 1994; Sherrill 1998; Porretta 2000).

CONGENITAL HIP DISLOCATION

Congenital hip dislocation is a malformation and dislocation of the hip. Specifically, the acetabulum of the iliac is shallower which displaces the femoral head. The cause is unknown. Surgery is needed to correct the problem. Individuals who are treated for hip dislocation should be careful with full range of motion movements that might cause them to dislocate the hip (http://gocarolinas.adam.com; Auxter et al. 1993).

CYSTIC FIBROSIS

Cystic fibrosis is a hereditary condition that affects the respiratory and digestive systems. Thick mucus is formed that clogs the bronchial tubes, resulting in lung infections. The thick mucus can also obstruct the pancreatic ducts, preventing enzymes from reaching the intestines and resulting in malnutrition. There is no known cure. The lifespan of individuals with cystic fibrosis is increasing although many still die before the age of ten and 80 percent before the age of thirty. Treatment for an individual who has cystic fibrosis can be antibiotics for prevention of respiratory infections and replacement of pancreatic enzymes for the missing enzymes (http://gocarolinas.adam.com; Eichstaedt and Kalakian 1993). Individuals with cystic fibrosis can fully participate in physical activity but they should make sure that they drink plenty of fluids.

DIABETES MELLITUS

The common term used is *diabetes*, which means "passing through." It is a condition whereby the pancreas does not produce enough insulin to meet the body's needs (Type I) or produces enough insulin, but the cells in the body are unable to use the insulin efficiently (Type II). Although the cause of diabetes is unknown, there is a belief that heredity and diet play a role in its development.

Type I, or insulin dependent diabetes, also known as juvenile diabetes, occurs before the age of thirty in both genders. Individuals with Type I diabetes have to inject themselves with insulin daily. In addition, glucose levels have to be carefully monitored and a disciplined balance of food intake and exercise has to be managed. This condition is not curable and is a lifelong condition. Recent advancements in research have occurred whereby islet cells of human cadavers are being transplanted into a Type I diabetic. After this procedure is completed, the individual is no longer dependent on insulin injections but has to take medication. So far, this procedure has only been done on a few individuals.

Type II, or noninsulin-dependent diabetes, occurs mainly in adults who are overweight or obese. Type II diabetes is more common in females than males. The treatment of Type II diabetes is usually proper diet and exercise (http://gocarolinas.adam.com; Surburg 2000; Sherrill 1998).

Regular exercise is essential to assist in controlling the amount of sugar in the blood and burn excessive calories and fat to maintain a desired weight. Before and after exercise, an individual with diabetes should test and monitor blood-glucose levels. One should drink plenty of fluids without sugar while exercising. In case the blood-glucose levels get low during and after exercise, individuals should always carry sugar-contained food (http://gocarolinas.adam.com; Sherrill 1998).

EPILEPSY

Epilepsy is a chronic brain disorder characterized by reoccurring seizures. It affects individuals of any age and the cause is not known. There are various types of seizures, such as:

Tonic-clonic seizures, also known as grand-mal seizures, last for several minutes. The symptoms are continuous muscle contractions in major parts of the body, loss of consciousness, biting of tongue and/or cheek, temporary stoppage of breath, and incontinence of the bowel and/or bladder.

Absence seizures, also known as petit-mal seizures. Minimal movement involved, there is a short period of time that unconsciousness occurs though this does not last longer than thirty seconds. This seizure most often only occurs in children.

Partial seizures: include symptoms that are short-term inappropriate behaviour and abnormal sensations. Loss of consciousness usually does not occur.

Most seizures are controlled through medication. In some cases brain surgery is performed to eliminate the seizures. Individuals who have epilepsy can fully participate in physical activity; however, they should make sure that they take their medication. Participation in physical activity should be done with a partner or in a group in case a seizure occurs (http://gocarolinas.adam.com; Sherrill 1998).

FRIEDREICH'S ATAXIA

Friedreich's ataxia is an inherited form of progressive degeneration of the cerebellum, spinal cord, and sensory nerves. This generally occurs in childhood before puberty. Nikolaus Friedreich, a German neurologist, first diagnosed this condition in the 1860s.

Symptoms are unsteady gait, coordination and balance difficulties, changes in speech, vision abnormalities, abnormal muscle control and tone, and skeletal deformities. There is no cure for Friedreich's ataxia; however, research is being done to find the gene responsible for this disease (http://gocarolinas.adam.com; Porretta 2000a; Sherrill 1998).

Individuals with Friedreich's ataxia are encouraged to participate in regular physical activity to control symptoms and maintain general health. This may include exercises of muscular strength and endurance, body coordination, and the development of grip strength.

GUILLAIN-BARRE SYNDROME

Guillain-Barre syndrome is also known as infectious polyneuritis. Guillain-Barre syndrome is a progressive muscle weakness caused by an acute inflammation of the nerves. The syndrome affects both genders and can occur at any age although it is most common in individuals between thirty and fifty years of age. Parry and Pollard (1993) indicated that one to two persons per one hundred thousand per year are affected worldwide.

Symptoms are primarily uncoordinated movements, muscle weakness, and sensation changes. In most cases, there is a complete recovery from the symptoms. Individuals with Guillain-Barre syndrome can fully participate in physical activity (http://gocarolinas. adam.com; Porretta 2000a; Sherrill 1998).

HEMOPHILIA

Hemophilia is a bleeding disorder in which it takes a longer time than usual for the blood to clot, resulting in abnormal bleeding. It is hereditary and is a common X chromosome-linked disease. It mostly affects males, while females are carriers. The individual who has hemophilia can fully participate in physical activity, if appropriate precautions and modifications are put in place (Surburg 2000; Sherrill 1998; Eichstaedt and Kalakian 1993).

MULTIPLE SCLEROSIS (MS)

MS is a disease of the central nervous system involving decreased nerve function by disintegration of the myelin sheath, which covers the nerve cells. The cause of the destruction of the myelin sheath is not known. Some research indicates that there is a combination of hereditary, viral, and environmental factors associated with the disorder. MS usually affects adults between the ages of twenty to forty. Some of the symptoms are weakness and/or paralysis of extremities, fatigue, numbness, loss of bladder or bowel control, and problems with speech, vision, swallowing, and balance. There is no known cure, but the MS may go into remission.

A regular exercise programme maintains muscle tone. Strenuous activity should be avoided. To maintain energy levels, the individual has to take adequate rest periods. Individuals with multiple sclerosis tend to exercise in the morning, since their energy levels are down in the afternoon (http://gocarolinas.adam.com; Surburg 2000; Sherrill 1998).

MUSCULAR DYSTROPHY

Muscular dystrophy is a hereditary disease characterized by progressive muscle weakness and atrophy of the muscle fibres. It only affects males. There are various types of muscular dystrophy, of which Duchenne muscular dystrophy is the most common and severe childhood form of the disease. Dystrophin, a protein that allows the muscle cells to function properly, is absent in individuals who have Duchenne muscular dystrophy. There is no cure for muscular dystrophy. Strengthening, endurance, and range of motion activities on a regular basis are recommended to maintain muscular development. Rest periods should be incorporated into programmes to avoid fatigue, which may actually aid in the progression of the condition. Since obesity is common in persons with muscular dystrophy, low-intensity aerobic activities are beneficial (http://gocarolinas.adam.com; Porretta 2000a; Sherrill 1998).

OSTEOGENESIS IMPERFECTA

Osteogenesis imperfecta is also referred to as brittle bone disease. *Osteo* meaning "bone," *genesis* meaning "origin" and *imperfecta* meaning "something is wrong." It is a hereditary condition characterized by weak bones and elasticity of the joints, ligaments, and skin. An unknown cause produces a decrease in the production of calcium and phosphorus, which results in a weak bone structure. Many individuals who have osteogenesis imperfecta must use wheelchairs. There are two types of the disease, congenital and tarda. Congenital is severe and could be fatal. *Tarda*, which means "later onset," is mild and the person may have a good life expectancy. Individuals with osteogenesis imperfecta should be encouraged to participate fully in physical activity (http://gocarolinas.adam.com; Porretta 2000a; Sherrill 1998).

OSTEOMYELITIS

Osteomyelitis is an acute or chronic infection in the bones. It can occur at any age. The infection spreads through the blood to the bone, since the original site of infection is usually located somewhere else in the body. The infection might be the result of the presence of bacteria or fungus. Pus forms within the bone, which may result in a bone abscess. In children, the long bones (i.e., humerus, femur, tibia) are usually affected, while in adults the pelvis and vertebrae are commonly affected.

Symptoms are pain in the bone and bone tenderness, heat and local swelling, drainage of pus through the skin in chronic infection, and general discomfort. Medical treatment should start immediately to eliminate the infection. When chronic infection occurs, surgery will have to be performed to remove the pus and dead bone tissue. Individuals with osteomyelitis can fully participate in physical activity providing they do not have any infection (http://gocarolinas.adam.com; Sherrill 1998).

OSTEOPOROSIS

Osteoporosis is a condition whereby the bones in the body lose density and bone tissues become thinner. Phosphate and calcium are the two components necessary to produce bone and bone tissue. When an individual does not take enough calcium or when the bone does not absorb enough calcium from the diet, bone production and bone tissue

may suffer. The body may reabsorb calcium and phosphate back into the body by taking it from the bones; this will result in weakening of the bone tissue. This ultimately results in brittle bones, which are subject to fracturing.

At the time of menopause, many women can suffer from this disease due to a reduction in the production of estrogen. In men, there is usually a deficiency of the androgen hormone. Participation in regular physical activity might reduce the risk of bone fractures. Activities where falls might occur should be avoided (http://gocarolinas.adam.com; Sherrill 1998).

PARKINSON'S DISEASE

Parkinson's disease is a disorder in the part of the brain that controls muscle movement and is associated with a decrease of neurotransmitter dopamine. Dopamine is necessary for transmitting impulses. Due to insufficient dopamine the nerve cells are unable to transmit impulses properly and this results in loss of muscle function. The exact reason why the brain cells deteriorate is not known. Parkinson's is a slow, progressive disease, which results in tremors, problems with walking, coordination, and movement. It affects both genders and often develops after the age of fifty. There is no known cure for Parkinson's disease. Participation in physical activity is encouraged as long as there are enough rest periods incorporated to avoid the individual becoming fatigued, as this may actually further the progression of the condition (http://gocarolinas.adam.com; Sherrill 1998; Auxter et al. 1993).

POLIOMYELITIS (POLIO)

The Greek word *polios* means "grey," referring to the colour of the nerve cell bodies it attacks. *Myelitis* means "infection of the protective layer around the nerve cells." Poliomyelitis is a viral infection that attacks the motor cells in the anterior horn of the spinal cord resulting in flaccid muscular paralysis and atrophy of the muscle. Individuals who have had polio have full sensation. Since 1955 a vaccine has been available to immunize individuals against polio. Today, polio rarely occurs in many industrial countries, whereas in third-world countries it still affects many individuals.

To avoid abnormal shortening of muscles (called contractures) due to lack of exercise, range of motion and stretching exercises should be performed. Individuals who have polio may perform activities with the use of crutches or in a wheelchair, as long as there is no safety problem while participating for everyone involved (Canadian Wheelchair Sports Association 1994; Sherrill 1998; Kelly 2000).

---

5 How would you respond to criticism from a group that participation by an individual who uses crutches and/or a wheelchair poses a health and/or safety threat to others?

Post-polio Syndrome
Individuals who have had polio can develop similar symptoms such as weaknesses, muscle atrophy, fatigue, and joint problems later in life (http://www.petrofsky.com).

SPINA BIFIDA
The Latin word *bifid* means "cleft or split into two parts." Spina bifida is a congenital birth defect of the spinal column caused by failure of the neural arch of a vertebra to properly develop and enclose the spinal cord. There are three forms of spina bifida,

Myelomeningocele. This is the most severe form of spina bifida. The spinal cord, the cord membrane, and the spinal fluid protrude through the vertebral arch into a sac. It can only be corrected through surgery.

Meningocele. The cord membrane and spinal fluid protrude through the vertebral arch into a sac. The spinal cord is not affected. Only surgery can correct this problem.

Occulta. One or more vertebrae are not developed properly. Because this condition is hidden under the skin, it is usually not detected until an x-ray is taken.

Many children with myelomeningocele have hydrocephalus, which is increased spinal fluid in the cranial cavity. This can be surgically corrected by implanting a shunt from the ventricles to the abdominal or thoracic cavity, to allow for proper drainage. Sometimes individuals who have had a shunt implanted might experience blockage in the device, resulting in symptoms such as headaches, swelling along the line of the shunt, loss of appetite, and irritability. When this occurs, a medical doctor will repair or replace the shunt. Any activity that may result in blows to the head should be avoided.

The cause of spina bifida is not known; however, in the late 1980s researchers discovered that folic acid could help reduce the risk of having a child with spina bifida. There is no cure for this disability (Canadian Wheelchair Sports Association 1994; Sherrill 1998; The Spina Bifida Programme 1995; Kelly 2000).

A variety of orthotic devices can be used by individuals who have spina bifida, including HKAFO (hip-knee-ankle-foot), AFO (ankle-foot), and KAFO (knee-ankle-foot), to provide support, improve positioning, correct or prevent deformities, and reduce or alleviate pain.

Due to paralysis there might be little or no sensation in certain parts of the body, therefore, an individual should shift his or her weight when using a wheelchair to avoid developing pressure sores. Also, the individual should check for cuts and/or abrasions on the skin where there is no sensation.

Some individuals might have loss of bladder and/or bowel function. Leg bags for the collection of urine must be emptied on a regular basis. In other cases, individuals who use catheters empty their bladders every three to five hours.

People with spina bifida might have metal rods in their backs, which are surgically attached to their spine to stabilize it. The rods will restrict some bending and rotating movements (Canadian Wheelchair Sports Association 1994; Sherrill 1998; The Spina Bifida Programme 1995; Kelly 2000).

SPINAL CORD INJURIES (SCI)

SCI refers to paralysis of the upper and/or lower extremities and the trunk resulting in impaired function and sensation. *Paraplegia* refers to a lesion level of the spinal cord in or below the thoracic region resulting in paralysis of the lower extremities and part of the trunk. The degree of paralysis depends on the location of the injury of the spinal column and the amount of destruction of the neural fibers. *Quadriplegia* refers to a lesion level of the spinal cord in the cervical region resulting in paralysis of the lower and upper extremities including the trunk. The higher the lesion on the spinal cord the more severe the paralysis. Spinal cord injuries are acquired from injury or disease to the vertebrae and/or nerves of the spinal column (for example, through motor vehicle or diving accidents, falls, and sport injuries).

Many considerations are similar to individuals who have spina bifida. In addition, some individuals with a spinal cord injury have difficulties controlling their body temperature, especially quadriplegics. Therefore, to avoid over-heating they should drink plenty of fluids, sit in shaded areas, and cool their body by using wet towels or water spray bottles (Canadian Wheelchair Sports Association 1994; Sherrill 1998; Kelly 2000). Autonomic dysreflexia may occur in individuals with a lesion level above T6. Characteristics are a rapid increase in heart rate and blood pressure, sweating, goose bumps, and headache. Bowel and bladder distension, skin irritation, or restrictive clothing can trigger autonomic dysreflexia (Kelly 2000; Sherrill 1998; Burnham et al. 1994).

6 Some spinal-cord-injured athletes deliberately induce autonomic dysreflexia to enhance racing performance. Given that autonomic dysreflexia occurs at random in lesions above the sixth thoracic vertebrae and that it may be induced by simply hyper-hydrating, how might it be dealt with by officials who monitor performance-enhancing strategies in athletes?

TOURETTE SYNDROME

Tourette syndrome is a rare disruptive condition with repetitive muscle movements (tics) and vocal outbursts. The cause is unknown. The tics are worse during emotional stress. Tourette syndrome most often occurs in boys. Medications can reduce this condition. Also, various alternative methods of stress reduction can be helpful such as exercise, counselling, and music. Involvement in physical activity reduces stress and may minimize the symptoms (http://gocarolinas.adam.com).

TUBERCULOSIS (TB)

Tuberculosis is an infectious disease caused by bacteria. There is a vaccine that is highly effective, so TB is no longer fatal. Factors that may cause an increase in contracting tuberculosis are unsanitary living conditions, poor nutrition, people with AIDS, and HIV infection. Participation in regular physical activity can be continued after the infectious period is over (http://gocarolinas.adam.com; Sherrill 1998).

Sensory Disabilities

HEARING DISABILITY

Any impairment that affects the ability to perceive and process audio information is considered to be a hearing disability. Hearing loss can occur at any age and can be congenital or acquired from disease, excessive noise, and accidents.

Persons who have a hearing disability can be either hard of hearing or deaf. The Canadian Hard of Hearing Association defines an individual who is hard of hearing as one who may have a level of hearing loss ranging from mild to profound and whose primary method of communication is the spoken language. According to the Canadian Association of the Deaf, an individual who is deaf is defined as a person in whom the sense of hearing is nonfunctional for the ordinary purposes of living and whose mode of communication is visual rather than auditory in nature. Individuals who are deaf use sign language or lip-read to communicate (Canadian Deaf Sports Association 1994; Sherrill 1998).

Table 4.1 Continuum of Hearing Impairment

Classification	Hearing threshold	Degrees of hearing loss	Difficulty understanding the following speech/levels of loudness
Hard of hearing	27–40 dB	slight - conductive loss	faint speech
Hard of hearing	41–55 dB	mild - use of hearing aid	normal speech
Hard of hearing	56–70 dB	marked	loud speech
Hard of hearing/deaf	71–90 dB	severe - sensory - neural loss	shouted speech
Deaf	> 90 dB	profound - use of sign	any speech, even amplified

Hearing loss can be divided into three categories:

- *conductive*, which means that sound is not being transmitted to the inner ear
- *sensory-neural*, which is hearing loss due to nerve damage
- *mixed hearing loss*, which is a combination of conductive and sensory-neural hearing loss

Sensory-neural loss is more severe and more likely to be permanent. Some individuals with hearing loss might be using hearing aids to amplify the sound. Balance might be affected in persons who have damage in the semicircular canals of the inner ear (Craft and Lieberman 2000).

Individuals who have a hearing disability can fully participate in physical activity. When giving instruction, the instructor should face the person who has a hearing disability. Visible signals should be used (for example, a flag instead of a whistle) as well as demonstrations. Balance might be affected in persons who have damage in the semicircular canals of the inner ear (Craft and Lieberman 2000). Hearing aids are usually removed when participating in water activities. Some individuals might have ventilation tubes in their ears, therefore underwater activities should be avoided (Canadian Deaf Sports Association 1994; Sherrill 1998).

VISUAL DISABILITY

The eye is responsible for sensing stimuli in the form of light waves, which pass through the cornea (outside covering of the eye), are focussed by the lens, and are then projected onto the retina (rear inside surface of eye). The retina converts these light rays into nerve impulses to be carried to the brain. When this pathway is disturbed, visual impairment results.

Individuals who are legally blind are described as totally blind or partially sighted. Persons who are legally blind have a visual field of less than twenty degrees, or their visual acuity is less than 6/60 in the best eye with corrective lenses. A visual disability can be congenital or acquired through disease or an accident (Canadian Council for the Blind 1993; Sherrill 1998). There are various causes of visual impairments, such as the following:

Albinism–a genetic condition where there is a lack of normal pigmentation in the iris and throughout the body. The person's eyes are sensitive to light.

Cataracts–an eye disease where, instead of having a clear lens, the lens is opaque. The eyes may be sensitive to light and glare and squint to compensate for impaired vision. Cataracts can be caused by rubella.

Glaucoma–the inability of the intra-ocular fluid to drain properly. This results in an increase in pressure and can lead to total blindness.

Retinal blastoma–a form of cancer, which often leads to removal of the eyeball. When this occurs, individuals often wear a prosthetic eyeball.

Rubella–limited vision may occur when an individual's mother has rubella during her third trimester of pregnancy (Craft and Lieberman 2000; Eichstaedt and Kalakian 1993).

To foster independence, individuals who have a visual disability may need an orientation of the area where the activity is taking place. In equipment or field markings, colour contrast might be appropriate for an individual who is partially sighted. Providing auditory cues such as beepers, clapping, or calling to locate the targets assist the person. Provide peer helpers and/or make sure the individual with the visual disability is close to the instructor.

When instructing one can use:

a) descriptive language (clearly describe an activity)

b) hand-body manipulation (guide or move the individual's body through the movement)

c) 'brailling' (the individual with a visual disability, usually totally blind, either touches the instructor who is demonstrating the movement to be used or a doll that is put through the motion) (Canadian Council of the Blind 1993; Craft and Lieberman 2000; Sherrill 1998).

Learning Disabilities

Learning disabilities arise when one or more of the basic psychological processes involving understanding or using spoken or written language exist. Rief (1993) states that learning disabilities have the potential to create an imperfect ability to listen, think, speak, read, write, spell, or do mathematical calculations.

Each individual has challenges with only certain aspects of learning. The nature of learning disabilities is unclear. There seems to be a discrepancy between a child's intellectual potential and actual learning achievement.

Individuals with a learning disability may have difficulty in any of the four learning steps:

1) input of information in the brain
2) organizing and understanding information
3) storing information in memory
4) communicating through language or motor output

Input refers to how the brain processes what is heard or seen. For example, reversing letters or difficulty distinguishing letters such as *d* and *b*, and *p* and *q*. Some people might have trouble organizing their position in space or might confuse left and right. Some individuals may have difficulty distinguishing subtle differences in sounds and misunderstand what one may say and therefore respond incorrectly (Learning Disabilities Association of Alberta Calgary Chapter 1994).

Organizing and understanding involves sequencing of information in the correct order, understanding it in the context used, and integrating it with other information being processed. For example, one may confuse the sequence of thoughts or events and, after hitting a ball, run to third base rather than first base.

Memory refers to storing information so that it can be retrieved later. There are two types of memory that might be affected: short-term and long-term memory. *Output* is how information is communicated through words (language output) or through muscle activities (motor output). One might have difficulty answering specific questions or have difficulty with gross or fine motor movements. For example, one may be clumsy, stumble, and have trouble walking, running, or riding a bike.

In a physical activity setting, the learning of cognitive information is difficult and there may be some motor coordination difficulties. Parents or guardians should be consulted on effective ways to teach their children.

ATTENTION DEFICIT-HYPERACTIVITY DISORDER (ADHD)

Attention Deficit-Hyperactivity Disorder (ADHD) is a clinically diagnosed disorder characterized by three types of behaviours, which include hyperactivity, distractibility, and impulsivity. Individuals may exhibit one, two, or all three characteristics. ADHD is caused by neurological differences in the brain and extends beyond hyperactivity caused by anxiety.

An individual who exhibits hyperactivity appears to be in constant motion (for example, fingers or feet tapping, leg swinging, or body wiggling). Children may be doing several things at once when playing.

The individual with distractibility has difficulty filtering out unnecessary information. Individuals with distractibility are easily distracted and have a short attention span. Visual input, such as movements of people or equipment all over the gymnasium, may be distracting. People talking, a music system, or extraneous playground noise, are challenging sound input situations for these individuals.

Individuals with impulsivity will seem to have very little patience. They do not stop to think before they act and may answer questions before one finishes asking one. They may get angry, and yell, throw, or hit. They may not learn from experience if they cannot pause long enough to reflect before they act. In a physical activity situation, an environment with the fewest distractions is the most effective. The activity/programme should be consistent and structured.

DEVELOPMENTAL COORDINATION DISORDER (DCD)

DCD is a disorder resulting from developmental delays or practice deficits in motor skills that is demonstrated in poor movement skills and interference in activities of daily living. Individuals can withdraw from physical activity, which leads to low fitness levels and reduced skill acquisition since the individual does not practice. Psychosocial difficulties such as poor self-esteem and social isolation can develop when no intervention occurs (http://gocarolinas.adam.com; CAHPERD 1994).

Developmental Disabilities

ALZHEIMER'S DISEASE/DEMENTIA/SENILITY

Alzheimer's disease/dementia/senility are the loss of intellectual functions in an alert and awake individual. The progression of these diseases vary with each individual. Cognitive ability and judgement get progressively worse; there is the loss of language functions and memory, the inability to think abstractly or care for oneself, personality changes, emotional instability, and loss of sense of time and place in these individuals.

All activities can be performed with full instruction and guidance from another person.

ASPERGER'S DISORDER

Experts now use terms such as *Asperger's disorder* and *pervasive development disorder* to describe a form of higher functioning autism. With this condition, there tends to be social isolation and eccentric behaviour in childhood. There are difficulties in two-sided social interaction and nonverbal communication. Children with Asperger's have been described as 'little professors', with quick tongues and sharp minds. These youngsters may stand too close and speak in loud monotones, but they can hold forth eloquently on their pet interests.

AUTISM

While the cause of autism is still unknown, most research indicates some type of brain-based developmental disorder. Autism impacts on the normal development of the brain in the areas of social interaction and communication skills. It impairs social relationships or can be seen in a lack of response to other people (e.g., treating others as objects, appearing to look through people, or having poor eye contact). It is sometimes described as 'mindblindness', which means social behaviour does not come naturally. Individuals with autism have difficulty interpreting facial expressions or emotions, and they do not know how to share or make friends. People with autism often excel at certain tasks.

Individuals may be deficient in language development and exhibit peculiar speech patterns. There may be difficulties in the use of abstract terms or they may simply echo words without understanding the meaning. Children with autism become distressed when minor changes occur in the environment or with the child's routine. Self-stimulating behaviours such as hand-flapping, twirling, rocking, or self-injurious behaviours such as head-banging or biting may occur. A lack of normal fear of dangers is exhibited in children with autism, so they may run in front of cars or climb onto high ledges. Most of us use context and categories to sort out our perceptions; people with autism tend to view the world as an array of discrete particulars. They have poor concentration skills, short attention spans, and are easily distracted. These all need to be taken into consideration in a physical activity setting.

Effective strategies include creating a daily routine to lesson/activity plans (e.g., starting in a circle each time) and making smooth transitions from one activity to another. Instructors can provide warnings/clues to when transitions may occur and should try to keep the programme consistent and very structured. Instructions should be clear and simple. Activities should be planned with shorter duration to keep the child's attention. The use of visual, rather than auditory, cues may work more effectively with these children. Individuals with autism typically do not respond well to being touched, held, or cuddled.

DOWN'S SYNDROME

Down's syndrome is the most common chromosomal error in human beings. It is not known exactly why it happens. There are twenty-three pairs of chromosomes in each cell, making a total of forty-six. A person with Down's syndrome has an extra twenty-first chromosome, therefore having forty-seven chromosomes in total.

People with Down's syndrome have many similarities in their physical features including a round face, lack of a defined fold in the eyelid, large tongue, and short, stubby fingers. Their speech may be difficult to understand and they may exhibit varying degrees of developmental disabilities. These characteristics may affect their participation in physical activities.

Instructions need to be clear, simple, and concise, and activity skills should be broken into small, sequential steps. Repetition and demonstration are effective in the learning of skill sets for activities. The use of a buddy system has been demonstrated to be an effective learning strategy. Some individuals may have difficulty keeping up to the other participants in the programme due to hypotonia (low muscle tone) and low levels of cardiovascular fitness.

About 15 percent of all individuals with Down's syndrome are affected by atlanto-axial instability (Canadian Special Olympics 1994). These individuals should not engage in activities that could potentially injure the neck area (e.g., gymnastics, wrestling, diving, trampolining, etc.).

FETAL ALCOHOL SYNDROME (FAS) AND FETAL ALCOHOL EFFECTS (FAE)

Fetal alcohol syndrome is the outcome of the effects of heavy and persistent maternal alcohol consumption during pregnancy. FAS is estimated as the most common, preventable cause of developmental disability in North America.

Clinically, three areas are affected:

1. Prenatal and/or postnatal growth delay (low birth weight and height)
2. Central nervous system damage including permanent brain damage, learning and behavioural disorders, memory/attention deficits, hyperactivity, speech/language delays, and poor coordination
3. Head and facial abnormalities (e.g., small head circumference and abnormally small eyes)

FAE describes individuals who were exposed to alcohol prenatally, but who lack the full set of characteristics of FAS. FAE individuals have deficits in one or more of the above three areas. FAE is more common than FAS.

INTELLECTUAL DISABILITY

Individuals with intellectual disabilities often have delayed processing abilities that relate to their learning capacity. Both mental and physical abilities are affected to varying levels. Eichstaedt and Kalakian (1993) state that developmental disabilities may result in abnormal reflex behaviour, delays in various sensory systems, and specific challenges in motor sensory responses, motor patterns, or motor skills. The effects are usually severe and chronic.

Directions should be clear, brief, concise, with appropriate vocabulary and common language that suits the level of understanding. You may want the participants either to repeat the instructions in their own words or to demonstrate. When learning skills and games, repetition and demonstrations are very effective. The use of verbal prompts, pictures, videos, and other visual aids are effective. Instructors can break down steps of an activity into small sequential steps for successful learning. The use of a buddy system works well in most situations. Offer a variety of activities to accommodate short attention spans and to make learning more interesting and challenging.

Disability, Function, and Physical Activity Recommendations

At the outset of this chapter, the point was made that it is important that we focus on the functional abilities of persons with disability rather than on the disability or disease process when providing physical activity programming or services and/or prescribing physical activity. However, it is important to recognize that different disability types may present with similar impairments (similar functional abilities) but require different considerations with regard to fitness assessment and/or physical activity prescription. Let us look at three disability examples and consider how we might classify according to functional abilities: spinal cord injury (SCI), multiple sclerosis (MS), and an upper and lower limb amputee. In Chapter 22 (Seidl), you will learn that functional impairments and abilities may be examined under a number of headings: mobility, object manipulation (including grasping), behaviour and/or social skills, cognition, communication and perception, and fitness.

First let us use this approach to compare a person with a high-lesion SCI (quadriplegia) and an individual with MS. In both cases our clients present with functional limitations in mobility, object manipulation, and communication. These functional limitations suggest similar accommodations to the assessment and prescription process. In addition, both clients may experience problems with body-heating during exercise. In both cases, this is due to alterations in functioning of the autonomic nervous system, though the source of this alteration is physical trauma in the case of SCI and the scleroses process in MS. Neural damage affects grasping in both cases. The fitness appraiser accommodates both cases with an arm crank healthy-aerobic fitness test. However, there are unique considerations that must be taken into account. In high-lesion SCI, autonomic dysreflexia–a severe hypertension condition–is possible, and caution must be exercised regarding lower limb trauma and time in a wheelchair. In the individual with MS, muscle weakness and severe fatigue suggests caution in the volume and intensity of exercise. Due to complete paralysis, the hip flexibility measure is not performed in the individual with SCI, but is attempted in the individual with MS whose paralysis is not complete. For these individuals with SCI and MS, the functional limitations may appear to be similar, but the condition itself must be understood by the professional so that due care and attention can be paid to problems that might arise during activity.

Now consider an individual with a single below elbow and double below knee amputation. Object manipulation represents functional limitations for this individual. However, the nature of these limitations is much different, and caution regarding autonomic dysreflexia and fatigue are unlikely to be major issues in this case based on the cause of the mobility and object manipulation functional impairments. A grip-strength test is performed on the complete arm. The aerobic step test is possible if a wheelchair is not required and if caution is paid to balance problems. There are no major flexibility issues. Stump care is likely of more importance in this case.

The point is that disability and associated functional limitations must be considered in concert with unique factors associated with that disability. The unique characteristics, some of which may be physiological, while others are psychological, may represent different levels of risk for each individual. Therefore, whereas the person-first, functional approach to providing services to persons with disability is important, it remains essential that you are aware of the fundamental characteristics of conditions as described in traditional disability classifications.

Study Questions

1. According to Appleton, what are the major causes of head injuries in children?
2. What is the difference between spastic, athetoid, and ataxic cerebral palsy?
3. Explain what a moro, or startle, reflex is?
4. What is the cause of epilepsy?
5. What is the difference between tonic-clonic and absence seizure?
6. What do we mean by DCD?
7. What is the most severe type of spina bifida?
8. Who was Lou Gehrig?
9. Explain what an invisible disability is?
10. What are the characteristics exhibited by a child with ADHD?

References

Active Living Alliance for Canadians with a Disability. (1992). *Words with Dignity*. Ottawa: Health Canada.

American Psychiatric Association. (1994). *Diagnostic and Statistical Manual of Mental Disorders*, (4th ed.). DSM-IV.

Appleton, R.E. (1998). Epidemiology: Incidence, causes, and severity. In R.E. Appleton and T. Baldwin (Eds.). *Management of brain-injured children*. New York: Oxford University Press.

Auxter, D., Pyfer, J. and Huettig, C. (1993). *Adapted physical education and recreation* (7th ed.). St. Louis: Mosby.

Burnham, R., Wheeler, G., Bhambani, Y., Belanger, M., Eriksson, P., and Steadward, R. (1994). Intentional induction of autonomic dysreflexia among quadriplegic athletes for performance enhancement: Efficacy, safety, and mechanism of action. In R. Steadward, E. Nelson, and G. Wheeler (Eds.). *Vista '93: The outlook* (pp. 224–41). Edmonton, AB: Rick Hansen Centre.

Canadian Amputee Sports Association, in cooperation with Active Living Alliance for Canadians with a Disability. (1993). *Moving to Inclusion: Active living through physical education: Maximizing opportunities for students with an amputation*. Gloucester, ON: CASA.

Canadian Association for Health, Physical Education and Recreation in cooperation with Active Living Alliance for Canadians with a Disability. (1994). *Moving to Inclusion, Active living through physical education: Maximizing opportunities for students who are physically awkward*. Gloucester, ON: CAHPERD.

Canadian Cerebral Palsy Sports Association, in cooperation with Active Living Alliance for Canadians with a Disability. (1994). *Moving to Inclusion: Active living through physical education: Maximizing opportunities for students with cerebral palsy*. Gloucester, ON: CCPSA.

Canadian Council for the Blind, in cooperation with Active Living Alliance for Canadians with a Disability. (1993). *Moving to Inclusion, Active living through physical education: Maximizing opportunities for students with a visual impairment* (2nd ed.). Ottawa: Canadian Council for the Blind.

Canadian Deaf Sports Association, in cooperation with Active Living Alliance for Canadians with a Disability. (1993). *Moving to Inclusion, Active living through physical education: Maximizing opportunities for students who are deaf or hard of hearing*. Gloucester, ON: CDSA.

Canadian Mental Health Association. (1993). National office pamphlets.

Canadian Special Olympics, in cooperation with Active Living Alliance for Canadians with a Disability. (1994). *Moving to inclusion: Active living through physical education: Maximizing opportunities for students with an intellectual disability*. Toronto: Canadian Special Olympics.

Canadian Wheelchair Sports Association. (1994). *Physical activity for all* (2nd ed.). Ottawa: CWSA.

Craft, D.H. and Lieberman, L. (2000). Visual Impairments and deafness. In J.P. Winnick (Ed.). *Adapted physical education and sport* (3rd ed.). (pp. 159–80). Champaign, IL: Human Kinetics.

Eichstaedt, C.B., and Kalakian, L.H. (1993). *Developmental/adapted physical education: Making ability count* (3rd ed.). Toronto: Maxwell Macmillan Canada.

Kelly, L. (2000). Spinal cord disabilities. In J.P. Winnick (Ed.), *Adapted physical education and sport* (3rd ed.). (pp. 215–34). Champaign, IL: Human Kinetics.

Learning Disabilities Association of Alberta, Calgary Chapter. (1994). *Moving to Inclusion, Active living through physical education: Maximizing opportunities for students who have multiple disabilities.* CAHPERD.

Parry, G.J., and Pollard, J.D. (1993). *Guillan-Barre syndrome.* New York: Thieme Medical.

Porretta, D.L. (2000 a). Amputations, dwarfism and les autres. In J.P. Winnick (Ed.), *Adapted physical education and sport* (3rd ed.) (pp. 199–214). Champaign, IL: Human Kinetics.

Porretta, D.L. (2000 b). Cerebral palsy, stroke and traumatic brain injury. In J.P. Winnick (Ed.), *Adapted physical education and sport* (3rd ed.) (pp. 181–98). Champaign, IL: Human Kinetics.

Rief, S.F. (1993). *How to reach and teach ADD/ADHD children: Practical techniques, strategies, and interventions for helping children with attention problems and hyperactivity.* The Center for Applied Research in Education.

Sherrill, C. (1998). *Adapted physical activity, recreation and sport: Crossdisciplinary and lifespan* (5th ed.). Boston: WCB/McGraw-Hill.

Spina Bifida Programme. (1995). *Answering your questions about spina bifida.* Washington, DC: Department of General Pediatrics, Children's National Medical Centre.

Surburg, P.R. (2000). Other health-impaired students. In J.P. Winnick (Ed.), *Adapted physical education and sport* (3rd ed.) (pp. 235–49). Champaign, IL: Human Kinetics.

WEB SITES

Archimedics.com. Rx: Medical info in a capsule. http://gocarolinas.adam.com

Family Caregiver Alliance Website. An Information Resource on Long-Term Care. http://www.caregiver.org

Petrofsky Research at Loma Linda University. http://www.petrofsky.com

III ■ THE SOCIAL, POLITICAL, AND LEGAL LANDSCAPE

CHAPTER 5

The Social Construction of Disability in a Society of Normalization

Debra Shogan

Learning Objectives

- To assess critically the place of adapted physical activity in what French intellectual Michel Foucault called a "society of normalization" (Foucault 1980a, p. 107). In a society of normalization people are expected to conform to the standards of designated tasks; they are expected to submit to these interventions, designed by experts, in order to achieve or surpass 'normal skill' levels.
- To learn how disciplines define normal human conduct and how this knowledge is then used to achieve social control through expert interventions.
- To discover how the discourse of statistics has served to reinforce the importance of 'normal human behaviour' and 'normal human bodies'.
- To consider how those in adapted physical activity might negotiate their work in such a society of normalization.

Introduction

To understand disability in relation to socially established standards for socially created tasks is to provide a social constructionist account of disability. This account does not deny the physicality of discomfort, pain, and impairment. Instead, it recognizes that notions such as success and failure, good and bad performance, ability and disability acquire meaning in relation to what has been established as normal within a social context, including what are considered to be normal tasks and the skills necessary for these tasks. A social constructionist account recognizes that those who do not achieve the standards established for the tasks of a discipline are labelled as, among other things, 'deficient', 'lacking', or 'disabled' and that they become the focus of expert interventions designed to change them so they can participate in these tasks.

A Society of Normalization

> An essential component of technologies of normalization is the key role they play in the systematic creation, classification, and control of anomalies in the social body...certain technologies serve to isolate anomalies...[O]ne can then normalize anomalies through corrective or therapeutic procedures, determined by other related technologies. In both cases, the technologies of normalization are purportedly impartial techniques for dealing with dangerous social deviations. (Rabinow 1984, p. 21)

Foucault was interested in the emergence of modern institutions and how they placed constraints on ways of participating in modern life. Modern institutions began to emerge in the seventeenth and eighteenth centuries as a way to contend with the efficient management of growing populations. Control of large numbers of people in factories, schools, workplaces, armies, hospitals, and prisons was made possible through disciplines that organized the time and space within which people performed designated tasks.

We commonly understand the notion of discipline in two ways. One is in reference to a body of knowledge; for example, the knowledge that is produced by researchers and practitioners in psychology, medicine, or adapted physical activity. Discipline also refers to the control or management of people; for example, the discipline of students by a teacher, or athletes by a coach. For Foucault, discipline simultaneously entails both of these meanings. Foucault's work documented how practices of controlling people develop as the subject matter, or knowledge base, of a discipline develops. In the discipline of sport performance, for example, coaches utilize knowledge generated by sport performance and translate this information into evermore exacting technologies of intervention to produce disciplined athletes (Shogan 1999, p. 39). By monitoring and examining the consequences of these disciplinary interventions, more knowledge (discipline) is produced which, in turn, makes control (discipline) even more meticulous.

How does a discipline produce knowledge about people, and what are the procedures by which this knowledge comes to control socially? Disciplines establish standards of achievement, behaviour, or performance for specified tasks in relation to the physical and social spaces within which these can occur. Everyone engaged in or by a discipline is measured in relation to these standards and ranked in relation to each other.

Abilities or behaviours are assessed by experts who observe and judge participants in relation to the standards established for the discipline. Observation and judgement by experts are part of an examination process that produces information about an individual's placement in relation to the standards of the discipline and in relation to others. This information makes it possible to isolate individuals so that their weaknesses can be corrected. Participants are subjected to interventions designed by experts in order to close the gap between the deficient skill or behaviour and that imposed by the standard. As Foucault (1979) indicated, examinations make it possible "to know them; to alter them" (p. 172). As deviations from the standard are corrected and an individual's behaviour or skills come closer to the standard, she or he becomes more like others, both in terms of the tasks in which they all engage and their abilities to perform these tasks. Through repeated interventions, everyone is moved closer to the standard, although it is also true that standards "climb slowly up the scale to accommodate a shifting mean of performance" (Ransom 1997, p. 50).

Schooling at all levels is a good example of the way in which discipline works. Education is conceived of as a series of tasks to engage in and behaviours and skills to attain in relation to these tasks. Attainment of behaviours and skills is measured in relation to standards established by the discipline and assessed by teachers or professors whose job it is to gain detailed information about each individual's abilities so that strategies of correction can be introduced. A successful classroom, school, or school district is one in which students are engaged in 'normal' tasks and meet the standards of these tasks. To the extent that students meet the standards of tasks in which they all engage, they become more alike. Not all students do meet or surpass the standards. Those who do not are subject to ever more exact interventions to attempt to close the gap between the deficiency and the standards.

Another effect of the examination is the production of information about how participants behave or perform in relation to standards and how they respond to corrective measures. This information contributes to the body of knowledge of the discipline and serves to reposition what counts as standard behaviours or skills for the discipline. The examination also produces ways to identify people by labelling them. John Fiske (1993) provides an example of how gathering information about workers in an airline reservation centre is used to establish 'normal' work efficiency as well as the categorization of workers. One worker had a 93.55 percent 'utilization' by virtue of handling 79 calls in the day, spending 3.53 minutes on each call, and completing her after call work in about twenty-three seconds. Since the normal utilization for workers at the reservation centre was 96.5 percent, normal calls per day were between 150 and 200, and time spent on after-calls was not more than 0.3 of a minute, this worker was labelled as inefficient. As Fiske indicates, standards are established by "a monitoring knowledge system. [Without standards] the knowledge of any one individual can be neither evaluated nor ranked, and thus cannot be applied...as rewards or sanctions" (1993, p. 74).

The examination re-establishes or repositions the standards of a discipline and produces documented information about individuals and the differences between them. Another way in which disciplines produce knowledge about individuals in relation to standards occurs when participants in a discipline are required to talk about their experiences within the discipline. In what Foucault refers to as "the confessional," participants tell or perhaps write their experiences and an authority records the information along with his or her expert interpretation of the information. This is followed by an intervention "in order to judge, punish, forgive, console, and reconcile...and [to]...produce...intrinsic modifications in the person who articulate[d] it" (Foucault 1980b, pp. 61–62). Sport psychologists, for example, make use of confessionals in a number of ways including paper-and-pencil tests in which athletes indicate (confess) their responses to a variety of possibly stressful situations. For example, consider this introduction to a paper-and-pencil test of attentional control, a technique which many sport psychologists used in the 1980s and 1990s to focus athletes' attention on key situations in their sport.

> By your answering a number of questions about how you have functioned in the past, it's possible for us to conclude to some degree of accuracy what your attentional strengths and weaknesses are...If...you indicate that you make mistakes because you concentrate on one player and forget about what other players are doing, I know that you can narrow attention, but are unable to broaden it, and when a broad focus is demanded, you have difficulty. With this kind of information, plus additional knowledge about your level of anxiety, I can suggest procedures for you to use to learn to broaden your attention. (Nideffer 1980, p. 281)

Attention-control training relies on expert interpretation of these questionnaires, followed by remedial techniques. These techniques include exercises to control focus of attention, so that athletes can achieve and surpass expectations for attention that have been produced as normal for a particular situation (Shogan 1999, p. 42). Implicit in the confession is the assumption that individuals attain self-knowledge by confessing to experts who interpret the confession for them. It is also assumed that it is possible to improve the confessor by interventions designed to bring the individual closer to standards for the discipline. In the case of attentional control confessionals, athletes come to know themselves and be known by others through the following labels: confident, hesitant, aggressive, and/or 'choker'. In a similar way, those who confess their experiences of being unable to meet the standards of normalized movement tasks or activities are labelled by experts as awkward, clumsy, unskilled, incompetent, and/or disabled.

Fiske notes that the more examinations we pass, the more normal we become (1993, p. 75). Likewise, the more we confess, the more normal we become because, like the examination, the confessional entails interventions by experts to change individuals so that they meet the standards of a discipline. When the interventions are successful, normalization is a consequence. Normalization is an effect of the "constant pressure to conform to the same model, so that they might all be…like one another" (Foucault 1979, p. 182).

---

1 What is assumed when a label is used as a way to know someone?

---

2 What do the use of standards and interventions take for granted about the value of sameness?

Normalization and the Social Construction of Disability

Modern institutions emerged in the West in the seventeenth and eighteenth centuries as a way to control large numbers of people in public institutions. Social control was made possible by procedures produced by disciplines that attempted to normalize and homogenize people by controlling the space and time in which tasks were performed. A notion of 'the normal' to signify that which conforms to and does not deviate from a standard coincided with the emergence of the disciplines and gained sophistication with developments in statistics and probability theory during the nineteenth century (MacKenzie 1981; Hacking 1987; Hacking

1990; Davis 1995).[1] Historical records show that people with physical and mental impairments have lived in every age and that their status has shifted according to how these impairments have been understood (Winzer 1997). However, prior to the nineteenth century there was no concept of normal and abnormal nor was there a concept of the disabled in relation to a standard (Davis 1995, p. 24).

The work of statistician Adolphe Quetelet (1796–1847) was central to the conceptualization of 'the normal' to signify what is usual or typical. Quetelet proposed that the method astronomers used to locate a star–the "law of error"–could be applied to frequency distributions of human and social phenomena. Astronomers found that most sightings of a star fell in the centre of a bell curve. They considered those sightings that fell to the sides of the curve to be errors. According to Quetelet, physical characteristics as well as moral and social behaviours could be plotted and determined utilizing this law of error. Quetelet constructed the notion of the 'average man' from the 'true mean' of human attributes (Hacking 1990; Davis 1995). He thought the average or 'the normal' signifies what is usual or typical, as well as the way things ought to be. In contrast, 'errors' were abnormalities, deviations, or extremes (Hacking 1990; Davis 1995).

The norm divides the population into standard and non-standard sub-populations. Quetelet wrote, for example, that "deviations more or less great from the mean have constituted …ugliness in body as well as vice in morals and a state of sickness with regard to the constitution" (cited in Porter 1986, p. 103). In Lennard Davis's (1995) words, "the idea of the norm pushes…variation of the body through a stricter template guiding the way the body 'should' be" (p. 34). The emergence of a notion of normalcy is what, then, creates the 'problem' of the disabled person (Davis 1995, p. 24). Indeed, the very meaning or signification of the normal has become tied to a concept of disability (Davis 1995, p. 2). Adapted physical activity has not been immune to this conceptualization of disability. The American *Adapted Physical Activity National Standards* (1995) indicates, as an example, that practitioners are to understand that "the meaning of obtained test scores that range two or more standard deviations below the mean [are] related to individuals with disabilities" (p. 63).

While Quetelet's focus was on central tendencies, Sir Francis Galton (1822–1911), founder of the biometric school of statistical research, was interested in distributions and deviations from the mean (Hacking 1990). And, while Quetelet considered average or normal human characteristics to be how things ought to be, Galton regarded the normal as an indication of mediocrity requiring improvement (Hacking 1990). Galton thought it problematic to consider all extremes in human characteristics as errors or abnormalities (MacKenzie 1981; Davis 1995). He claimed that certain attributes he valued, such as tallness, intelligence, ambitiousness, strength, and fertility, were positive distributions of a trait and not errors. Galton divided the bell curve (renamed the normal distribution curve) into quartiles that established a ranking system for characteristics. Distributions around the norm were no longer regarded as equal: the average, now referred to as the median, represented mediocrity. Those in the lower quartile were posited as deviant or abnormal and as objects of intervention, while those in the upper quartile represented progress, perfectibility, and normality (Davis 1995).

Quetelet's appropriation of the law of error to explain stability in social statistics and Galton's imposition of his values about human development onto the bell curve have had profound effects on how ability and disability are understood. Far from being a neutral, objective enterprise, statistics as practiced by Galton and Quetelet produced social meaning about 'the normal' and 'the abnormal', 'ability' and 'disability', and created categories such as 'the intelligent', 'the deviant', and 'the disabled' that had implications for tasks in many different social contexts from classrooms to playgrounds, from boardrooms to factory floors. Labels set out in advance how people can take up these tasks and how they will be judged when they do.

The belief that people must alter themselves to achieve standards established for a task, or that they must change to participate in tasks designated as normal for a culture, is another way to understand how ability and disability are socially constructed. When social structures support those who participate in tasks which have been designated as normal or mainstream, and reward those who reach or exceed the standards for performance in these tasks, those who value different tasks or who do not meet the standards of mainstream tasks are disabled by these social structures. Central to this point is understanding distinctions that have been made between impairment, disability, and handicap. The United Nations until very recently defined these terms as follows:

- *Impairment:* Any loss or *abnormality* of psychological, physiological, or anatomical structure or function.
- *Disability:* Any restriction or lack (resulting from impairment) of ability to perform an activity in the manner or within the range considered *normal* for a human being.
- *Handicap:* A disadvantage for a given individual, resulting from impairment or disability, that limits or prevents the fulfillment of a role that is *normal*, depending on age, sex, social, and cultural factors, for that individual.

Handicap is therefore a function of the relationship between disabled persons and their environment. It occurs when they encounter cultural, physical, or social barriers which prevent their access to the various systems of society that are available to other citizens. Thus, handicap is the loss or limitation of opportunities to take part in the life of the community on an equal level with others (1983, pp. 6–7, emphasis added).

While these distinctions made possible the consideration of debilitating chronic illnesses (Wendell 1989, p. 107) by defining impairment and disability in physical terms and handicap in cultural, physical, and social terms, the 1983 UN document made an arbitrary distinction between physical and social aspects of disability. In contrast, activists from the disability movement distinguish between impairment and disability but see no need to distinguish further between disability and handicap. As Oliver (1996) indicates, to be impaired is to lack "part of or all of a limb, or have a defective limb, organ or mechanism of the body... [whereas] disability [is] the disadvantage or restriction of activity caused by a contemporary social organization which takes little or no account of people who have...physical impairments" (p. 22). Recently, the World Health Organization of the United Nations has heeded concerns about effects of the social environment on how we understand disability and it now defines disability as "the outcome or result of a complex relationship between an individual's health condition and personal factors, and of the external factors that represent the circumstances in which the individual lives" (World Health Organization 2000, p. 20). Rather than classify people, this new approach to disability seeks to describe the situation of each person "within the context of environmental and personal factors" (p. 11).

> An environment with barriers, or without facilitators, will restrict the individual's performance; other environments that are more facilitating may increase that performance. Society may hinder an individual's performance because either it creates barriers (e.g., inaccessible buildings) or it does not provide facilitators (e.g., unavailability of assistive devices). (World Health Organization 2000, p. 20)

This new position of the World Health Organization coincides with those writing within the disability movement who have indicated that "not only the 'normal' roles for one's age, sex, society, and culture, but also 'normal' structure and function and 'normal' ability to perform an activity, depend on the society in which the standards of normality are generated" (Wendell 1989, p. 107). Such

factors as "social expectations, the state of technology and its availability to people in that condition, the educational system, architecture, attitudes toward physical appearance, and the pace of life" affect the point at which variation from the norm becomes a disability (Wendell 1989, pp. 107, 109). Notions such as 'success', 'competence', 'excellence', 'merit', and 'ability' acquire meaning only in contexts in which some tasks and their associated skills, attributes, or characteristics are valued more than are others. As Ransom comments, what counts as normal "'falling short of the norm', 'subnormal', shades off into the value judgement 'bad', 'abnormal', 'retarded'. The 'normal' becomes normative" (1997, p. 51).

How and whether one is disabled or enabled by a social context depends on "the relationship of a[n]...impairment and the political, social, even spatial environment that places that impairment in a matrix of meanings and significations" (Davis 1995, p. 3). Indeed, as McDermott and Varenne (1995) indicate, cultures "actively organize ways for persons to be disabled" (p. 337). "The difficulties that people in wheelchairs (or city shoppers with carts...) face with curbs and stairs tell us little about the physical conditions requiring wheelchairs or carts," according to McDermott and Varenne, "but a great deal about the rigid institutionalization of particular ways of handling gravity and boundaries between street and sidewalk as different zones of social interaction" (pp. 327–28).

When some are at a disadvantage as a result of how a social context is organized, it is possible to claim that disability is an *effect* of the social context or, in other words, that disability is socially constructed. Martha's Vineyard of the eighteenth and nineteenth centuries is a striking example of an absence of disability in a community, even though there were a number of people with physical impairments. What was unusual about this community was not only that many people in the community were deaf but also that almost everyone in the community used sign language (Groce reported in McDermott and Varenne 1995, p. 328). Surviving members of the community could not always remember who had been deaf because almost everyone in Martha's Vineyard used sign language, including hearing people with other hearing people (Groce reported in McDermott and Varenne 1995, p. 328). This is an example of how it may be possible in some situations to "eliminate the category of the disabled altogether, and simply talk about individuals' physical abilities in their social context" (Wendell 1989, p. 108).

What is apparent from the discussion to this point is that someone can be disabled in relation to the standards established for certain tasks supported by social structures, yet not have a physical impairment. Impairment is not a necessary condition for someone to be judged as incompetent, unsuccessful, unskilled, unfit, inadequate, or, in short, abnormal. To be judged in this way requires only that one has failed to meet the expectations or standards of tasks which are socially supported. In the section which follows, I am interested in the extent to which the discipline of adapted physical activity is committed to normalizing behaviours and skills in what have been constructed as normal tasks.

3 When someone is labelled as disabled, what is taken for granted about his or her social context?

4 What needs to be taken into account in order to understand an assessment that someone is successful or competent?

Normalization, Disability, and the Discipline of Adapted Physical Activity

Adapted physical activity, like other disciplines, entails both meanings of discipline–discipline as a body of knowledge and discipline as social control. The discipline of adapted physical activity produces knowledge about people who are considered to be lacking in some way. These people may or may not have impairments (refer to Chapter 2 (Reid)). Like other disciplines, the work of adapted physical

activity involves evaluation, ranking, and interventions to change people. It is important to emphasize that the discipline of adapted physical activity is not unique in its relationship to normalization. The impetus to normalize is central to all modern institutions and their related disciplines. The issue of normalization may be more focussed in adapted physical activity than some other disciplines, however, because an emphasis of many adapted physical activity programmes is to normalize participants by including them in mainstream tasks.

What distinguishes adapted physical activity from many other disciplines is that expert intervention is not designed to make everyone equally skilful. Rather, interventions are intended to make it possible for everyone to engage in a range of similar tasks–those designated normal for a culture. However, it is important to understand that attempting to include people in the *same* activities is a type of normalization.

The goal of normalization in adapted physical activity is to "make available to differently abled individuals conditions as close as possible to that of the group norm (average)" (Sherrill 1993, p. 68). Normalization theory is used in adapted physical activity in relation to "disabilities in which persons are perceived as looking or behaving differently" (1993, p. 132). The following three principles are central to normalization theory as proposed by Wolf Wolfensberger in 1972:

1. Behavioural and appearance deviancy can be reduced by minimizing the degree to which persons with disabilities are treated differently from able-bodied persons.
2. Conversely, deviancy is enhanced by treating persons as if they were deviant.
3. To the degree that they are grouped together and segregated from the mainstream of society, individuals will be perceived as different from others and will tend to behave differently. (Wolfensberger in Sherrill 1993, p. 132.)

The goal is to make disability or difference less noticeable by having everyone participate in 'normal' activities or tasks. Sherrill argues that normalization is not intended to make a person like everyone else (1993, p. 68). What it does mean, she says, is that everyone is expected to adapt so that games resemble those played by the able-bodied as much as possible (1993, p. 68). Whether segregated from or included in regular classrooms, the goal is to have everyone engage in the same tasks and share the same values about what these tasks should be.

Wolfensberger developed an instrument called PASSING to evaluate how well services normalize participants into what are considered to be normal tasks (Sherrill 1993, p. 132). We should remember, however, that the use of the term *passing* in other cultural contexts is used to signify that someone in a minority attempts to be mistaken as someone in the majority—the attempt, for example, of a Native to pass as white, or a gay man to pass as straight. In these contexts, however, passing is a double-edged sword which allows the passing person to participate in the privileges of the mainstream culture but only by denying one's own identity.

There is an assumption predominant in adapted physical activity that everyone should participate in the same tasks or activities even if there is not an expectation that they attempt to meet 'normal' standards for these tasks. 'Normal' tasks or activities are those that most people do. However, when the tasks that most people do is the measure of whether someone is normal, not only are categories that deviate from the norm created (such as the disabled), it is difficult to notice other ways of participating in the world. As McDermott and Varenne (1995) point out, "mainstream or 'normal' criterion becomes gradually accepted for assessing members of minorities as deprived and disabled because they do not take part in mainstream activities" (p. 336).

How might the discipline of adapted physical activity negotiate the tension between a commitment to improving the lives of people and the homogenizing effects of normalizing tasks? Furthermore, how can adapted physical activity resist or disrupt the impulse to normalize while making it possible for a range of people to participate in a range of physical activities? One way that the discipline of adapted physical activity is already doing this is through the recognition that not all people who are 'different', including those with impairments, require adapted physical activity (personal communication, G. Reid, Nov. 1, 1999). They are doing just fine without interventions perhaps because they live in a social context, such as Martha's Vineyard, where impairment or other 'differences' do not disable them.

Since Michel Foucault was the person who called our attention to the emergence of a society of normalization, it might be helpful to note how Foucault thought normalization might be countered. Foucault thought that to be engaged in ethical practice is to become aware of *how* one's actions and behaviours are shaped by standards. This awareness provides information from which one can either refuse a particular set of standards or refuse a passive acceptance of them (Foucault 1984). Refusing passive acceptance of rules, codes, and standards allows one to push the limits of what is considered to be normal and create new ways of living in the world.

In the case of adapted physical activity, one might refuse the assumption that certain tasks are acceptable for everyone. Refusal might also include asking whether human life is appropriately understood as the accomplishment of a set of prescribed tasks and noticing instead that human living "requires dealing with indefinite and unbounded tasks while struggling with the particular manner in which they have been shaped by the cultural process." This might lead to a recognition that what comes to count as competence in the tasks created by discipline "is a fabrication, a mock-up, and…[that] the most arbitrary tasks can be the measure of individual development" (McDermott and Varenne 1995, p. 337).

Refusing normalization is not easy work because a society of normalization is comprised of other disciplines that are also intent on normalization. Everything in modern society conspires to normalize. However, if you believe as I do, that the impulse to normalize is one of the major ethical issue of these times, it is important to refuse the ways in which normalization eliminates difference and diversity. And, while it is necessary to acknowledge and celebrate difference, we must also notice that what comes to be accepted as different behaviour, skill, or even bodies is socially constructed when we establish and maintain some tasks as normal tasks for a culture.

---

5 What is assumed when there is an expectation that everyone should be engaged in the same activities?

Summary

This chapter examined the features of a 'society of normalization' and explored implications for adapted physical activity of the impetus to normalize. It was shown how someone becomes disabled when the cultural context in which he or she lives does not accommodate his or her difference from the norm, and it was pointed out that differences that disabled people have may or may not be because of impairments. Unlike other disciplines that intervene to eliminate difference in order to make participants equally skilful, practitioners of adapted physical activity intervene to make it possible for everyone to be included in similar tasks. This, however, is also to normalize participants. Perhaps, a future direction for researchers and practitioners of adapted physical activity is to consider how to make it possible for people with impairments to gain the benefits of physical activity without also privileging those activities that are regarded as standard, or normal, for people to enjoy.

Study Questions

1. Does inclusion allow adapted physical activity to refuse a 'society of normalization'?
2. How can adapted physical activity improve the lives of people without presuming that there are normal tasks to engage?
3. Is disability sport an example of normalization or refusal?
4. Is it possible in contemporary physical activity and sport to create situations in which people with impairments are not disabled?

Acknowledgement

Some of the material in this section has previously appeared in D. Shogan (1998). I would like to thank the *Adapted Physical Activity Quarterly* for allowing me to use this material. In that essay I acknowledged Sheryl McInnes for introducing me to the history of statistics and probability theory.

References

Davis, L.J. (1995). *Enforcing normalcy: Disability, deafness and the body.* London and New York: Verso.

Fiske, J. (1993). *Power plays power works.* London and New York: Verso.

Foucault, M. (1979). *Discipline and punish: The birth of the prison.* (A. Sheridan, Trans.). New York: Vintage.

Foucault, M. (1980a). Two lectures. In Gordon, C. (Ed.), *Power/knowledge: Selected interviews and other writings 1972-1977* (pp. 78-108). New York: Pantheon.

Foucault, M. (1980b). *The history of sexuality: Vol. 1. An introduction* (R. Hurley, Trans.). New York: Vintage.

Foucault, M. (1984) "What is Enlightenment?" In P. Rabinow (Ed.), *The Foucault Reader.* New York: Pantheon.

Hacking, I. (1987). Was there a probabilistic revolution, 1800-1930? In L. Kruger , L. Daston, and M. Heidelberger (Eds.), *The Probabilistic revolution: Vol. 1. Ideas in history* (pp. 45-55). Cambridge, MA: MIT Press.

Hacking, I. (1990). *The taming of chance.* Cambridge: Cambridge University Press.

MacKenzie, D.A. (1981). *Statistics in Britain 1865-1930: The social construction of scientific knowledge.* Edinburgh: Edinburgh University Press.

McDermott, R. and Varenne, H. (1995). Culture as disability. *Anthropology and Education Quarterly 26* (3), 324-48.

Nideffer, R. (1980). Attentional focus: Self assessment. In R. Suinn (Ed.), *Psychology in sports: Methods and applications* (pp. 281-90). Minneapolis: Burgess.

Oliver, M. (1996). *Understanding disability: From theory to practice.* New York: St. Martin's Press.

Porter, T.M. (1986). *The rise of statistical thinking 1820–1900.* Princeton: Princeton University Press.

Rabinow, P. (1984). *The Foucault reader.* New York: Pantheon.

Ransom, J.S. (1997). *Foucault's discipline: The politics of subjectivity.* Durham and London: Duke University Press.

Reid, G. (1999). Personal communication, 1 November.

Sherrill, C. (1993). *Adapted physical activity, recreation and sport: Crossdisciplinary and lifespan* (4th ed.). Madison, IA: WCB Brown and Benchmark.

Shogan, D. (1998). The social construction of disability: The impact of statistics and technology. *Adapted Physical Activity Quarterly 15,* 269–77.

Shogan, D. (1999). *The making of high performance athletes: Discipline, diversity, and ethics.* Toronto: University of Toronto Press.

United Nations Decade of Disabled Persons 1983–1992. (1983). *World program of action concerning disabled persons.* New York: United Nations.

Wendell, S. (1989). Toward a feminist theory of disability. *Hypatia: A Journal of Feminist Philosophy 4*(2), 104–24.

Winzer, M.A. (1997). Disability and society before the eighteenth century. In L.J. Davis (Ed.), *The disability studies reader* (pp. 75–109). New York: Routledge.

Wolfensberger, W. (1972). *The principle of normalization in human services.* Toronto: National Institute of Mental Retardation through Leonard Crainford.

World Health Organization. (2000). *ICIDH-2: Internal classification of functioning, disability, and health.* Prefinal draft full version. Geneva: Author.

CHAPTER 6

Socio-political Influences on Adapted Physical Activity

Gary McPherson
Garry D. Wheeler
Sheri L. Foster

Learning Objectives

- To trace changes in societal perceptions and attitudes towards disability itself and in persons with a disability.
- To describe the development and impact of human rights and the effect that humanitarian and advocacy organizations have had in changing attitudes and increasing the opportunity for persons with a disability.
- To cite key legislation and charters in the area of disability, particularly as it relates to North America.
- To appreciate the impact of these factors on the provision of active living opportunities, inclusive physical education, and elite disability sporting opportunities for persons with a disability.

Note that the learning objectives are by no means exhaustive, and we leave it to you the reader, to elaborate on our thoughts and to develop conjectural relationships between these factors and the historical events that have led to the development of physical activity, recreation, physical education, and sports opportunities for persons with disabilities.

An Overview

This chapter demonstrates how opportunities for recreation and active living in the community have increased for persons with a disability, how disability sport has evolved, and how it has shifted from predominantly a medical rehabilitative model to an elite sport model in as little as fifty years.

We, as a society, have progressed from the view of disability as a function of demonic possession and the work of the gods to a viewpoint that emphasizes physical, sensory, and intellectual functioning and abilities. We have moved from a total lack of legal protection for persons with disabilities to a legislated provision of services that support individuals in their daily life and in their quest for employment and educational opportunities. We have shifted from views of termination, abandonment, isolation, exclusion, institutionalization, segregation, and marginalization to mainstreaming, integration, inclusion, participation, and interdependence. We have changed our view of disability as abnormal to a view of differences in ability. We have shifted from the concept of being unable to one of being able, from dependence to independence, from sympathy and pity to empathy and understanding. Alternatively, others have argued that, although attitudes towards disability and treatment of persons with a disability have improved, persons with a disability continue to be marginalized and that differences continue to be accentuated in society.

However, such changes do not occur in a vacuum, nor do they occur without fundamental changes in social attitudes. In turn, such changes are catalysed by a number of key factors. We suggest that these factors include but are not restricted to: 1) the human rights movement, 2) the impact of human conflict, 3) humanitarian and advocacy organizations, 4) legislation, and 5) technological advances.

An Historical View

> **1** How has history influenced how we think and feel about disability and persons with disability?

Societal attitudes towards disability have varied significantly through history but, generally speaking, attitudes have been negative. Three perspectives of disability illustrate how attitudes and perceptions have changed, or alternatively how they have been perpetuated (Jansma and French 1994; Clapton and Fitzgerald 1997; Condeluci 1999). According to Jansma and French (1994), there are five distinct periods in the development of societal attitudes towards persons with a disability during which there is a demonstrable shift from negative to more positive attitudes. For the purposes of clarity we have labelled these periods but maintained the authenticity of the authors' descriptions. The **primitive era** (pre-history to 500 B.C.) was a period of fear, a period in which disability was considered the work of the gods and resulted in termination or abandonment. A period of **logical and natural explanation** (500 B.C. to 500 A.D.) followed in which the Greeks attempted to

understand emotional or mental disability, but it was a period in which the Greeks practiced infanticide and the Romans used people with disabilities for target practice. The **Middle Ages** (500 to 1500 A.D.) was a period of cruelty and confusion in which theological explanations and demonization of disability prevailed, and persons with a disability were treated cruelly. The **turning point** (1500 to 1900s A.D.) was a period in which there was increased recognition of human rights and a move to custodial and institutional care. The **landmark era** (1900s to the present day) is viewed as a time of de-institutionalization and increased community care and services.

Clapton and Fitzgerald (1997) acknowledge the pervasiveness of negative attitudes towards disability through history. They note that the story of persons with a disability has been one *of life on the margins*; those with a disability have traditionally been socially constructed as 'other'. They describe models of disability, all of which they argue have conferred, and arguably continue to confer, the concept of 'otherness' on the disabled. The three models are the *religious model*, the *medical/genetic model*, and the *rights-based model*. These models are outlined below.

In Western Judeo-Christian society, the roots of understanding physical and other bodily differences have been grounded in Biblical references. Disability was subsequently seen as a result of the work of evil spirits, the devil, witchcraft, or simply as God's displeasure. People with a disability were fundamentally different from able-bodied people. Society demonized and victimized persons with a disability, often with purging, exorcisms, and prayer for curative purposes. Alternatively, persons with a disability were cared for and given mercy and shelter by religious institutions.

With advances in medicine and technology, *"the doctor and the scientist replaced the priest as custodian(s) of societal values and curing processes"* (p. 2). Medical labels began to define individuals with disabilities; often the future of the affected individual was dictated and determined by medical diagnosis and prognosis, and there was a requirement of removal of 'other' from the normative realm. Institutionalization resulted in the marginalization of the individual and perpetuated the concepts of tragedy, burden, charity, dependency, and failure that were often attributed to disability.

Clapton and Fitzgerald (1997) suggest that,

> in more recent times, the notion of disability has come to be conceptualized as a socio-political construct within a rights based discourse. The emphasis has shifted from dependence to independence as people with a disability have sought a political voice. (p. 3)

However, they observe that the rights-based discourse still has become a way of constructing disability by locking people with a disability into an identity based on membership in a minority group. In this model, entitlement depends on being able to identify oneself as disabled, with the conceptual barrier between 'normal' and 'abnormal' remaining unchallenged.

Although rights-based movements have, at the strategic level, brought some additional entitlement to people with a disability, *"it has not significantly altered the way in which disability is constructed, and so, despite legislative changes, some people's lives have not necessarily changed"* (p. 3). Clapton and Fitzgerald (1997) suggest that new advances in medicine, advances such as genetic testing, threaten to further marginalize persons with a disability. They note that the rights-based discourse fails to address this issue and that it relies upon a medically constructed model of disability to support claims for rights and entitlements.

According to the authors, each model perpetuates the concept of 'otherness.' They call for a philosophy of universalism, where disability is actually a fluid and continuous condition, which has no boundaries but which is, in fact, the essence of the human condition. They conclude aptly with,

> At the level of our physical existence, diversity is a natural condition and the need is for us to welcome and embrace diversity outside of the hierarchical classification of difference...we are all interconnected and have flowing through each of us the same life force. (p. 4)

Like Clapton and Fitzgerald (1997), Condeluci (1996) notes that human and domestic services that advocate on behalf of persons with disabilities serve to perpetuate 'difference' and therefore maintain our societal views which often limit the potential of those living with disabling conditions. According to Condeluci, most formal or structured approaches to difference in the industrialized nations either 1) *fix the difference*–the person must make the adjustment in programmes designed to bring the person to normal; 2) *maintain the different person*– focusses on disability as something that cannot be resolved; or 3) *change the broader understanding about the difference*–through attempts made by organizations and advocacy groups to increase social understanding, often by overemphasizing or sensationalizing 'difference' in the interests of increasing financial donations. Like Clapton and Fitzgerald, Condeluci suggests that the common thread in all three approaches continues to contribute towards stigmatization and perpetuation of difference. These include common identification (e.g., labelling), a negative or deficit perspective (i.e., person is less than, has less than, is needy), congregation (i.e., people are served better in a group), and the role of helper or expert (i.e., an expert on 'them') is present and guiding. The result is "business as usual with agencies and organizations that surround people who have some type of difference" (Condeluci 1996, p. 46). This perpetuation of difference results in a cascade of impacts that include misunderstanding, avoidance, being unwelcome, exclusion, banishment, and finally destruction. Condeluci advocates for true inclusion of persons with a disability in society. This means:

> being at the table; being part of the discourse; being respected for who you are, not held accountable for what others might expect you to be. Inclusion acknowledges that people may be different and pushes us

to respect this diversity. It is a term that implies a welcoming to all. (Condeluci 1999, p. 4)

Condeluci therefore proposes and emphasizes that *interdependence* is the route to community, not the perpetuation of difference. Interdependence is about relationships, capacities, partnerships, and belonging. Interdependence suggests that we look at what is right and connectable about people and not what is wrong with them. We must build relationships from the commonalities we have and not from the differences. We must go beyond the admission of persons with a disability into our realm, to being concerned about being admitted into the realities of life for a person with a disability (Condeluci 1995). It is clear that for true attitudinal change to take place, inclusion and/or interdependence needs to occur, and we must deconstruct the 'difference', 'otherness', and 'dependency' perspectives.

2 Although we have made progress in our views regarding disability and persons with a disability, it could be argued that religious, medical, and rights-based advocacy 'scripts' serve to perpetuate a concept of 'difference' regarding persons with disability. Are persons with a disability 'different' than the so-called able-bodied, and what are the ramifications of treating persons as 'no different than' when it comes to issues of support, services, entitlement, etc?

At this juncture, let us consider important influences that have shaped and changed our views of disability and of persons with disabilities; that have changed the ways in which persons with a disability are treated in society; and, in particular, how this has influenced opportunities for physical activity in the community, school, and sport environments.

Advances in Human Rights

The historical shift with regard to respecting the human rights of individuals was an important factor in the development of a social environment that allowed persons with a disability to begin to partake on an equitable basis. The shift towards more humanistic views and an appreciation of the rights of persons can perhaps be traced to the early eighteenth century. One of the great figures of the French Enlightenment, and probably one of the most significant figures influencing nineteenth century Romanticism, was Jean Jacques Rousseau (1712–1778). Rousseau's most celebrated theory was that of the "natural man," and in his discourse on the inequalities of men (1754) and social contract (1762), he maintained that human beings were essentially good and equal in the state of nature. People entered into a social contract, establishing governments and educational systems to correct the inequalities brought about by the rise of civilization– a contract in which people are born free and equal and surrender none of that freedom to the state but rather agree to a protection of these rights. Rousseau's work had a profound influence on other eighteenth century philosophers such as Immanuel Kant (1724–1804). Like Rousseau, Kant emphasized the rights of persons as ends in and of themselves, rather than persons simply being a means to an end. Kant was key in the development of deontological, or non-consequentialist, ethics in which the focus is on the rights of persons and our duties to others. His focus on moral universalism is expressed in his "categorical imperative"–"act only according to the maxim by which you can, at the same time will that it should become a universal law." Rousseau and Kant established the early groundwork for the humanism movement and future human rights legislation, including society's treatment of persons with a disability.

Sherrill observes that the humanism movement of the 1950s marked a shift towards the concept of full actualization of the individual. Rooted in the self-actualization theory of Abraham Maslow and the philosophy of Carl Rogers, this movement marked a rebellion against Freudian theories of human development and the sickness and disease approach to disability that preceded this period (Sherrill 1996).

The Universal Declaration of Human Rights (United Nations 1948) (Web site 3) and the

Charter of Rights and Freedoms (Canada 1982) (Web site 3) are also based on this shift towards humanistic ideology in society in relation to disability.

War and Human Conflict

Disability–and death–have always been the tragic results of human conflict. Jansma and French (1994) describe periods of attitudinal development toward disability during which the world experienced wars between the Greeks and Romans, the brutal battles of the Middle Ages including Crecy and Agincourt, the horrendous conflicts of the Crimean War, the American Civil War, and more recently the "war to end all wars," World War I. These wars brought about massive loss of life and parallel increase in killing and maiming efficiency. However, prior to World War II, persons with serious injuries often died soon after their wounds from sepsis or shock. The discovery and use of effective antibiotics such as penicillin were major factors in relation to survival of persons with a variety of war-induced disabilities and changes in attitudes towards persons with disability. In 1928, Sir Alexander Fleming discovered penicillin by accident, although it would not be purified and concentrated for medical use for another decade. Penicillin became available for use at the end of the Second World War, and it had a remarkable impact on the survival rate of men and civilians suffering from a variety of traumatic wounds. In particular, it was important in the treatment of infection, tetanus, and septicemia, previously common causes of post-trauma death. The net effect of such advances as the discovery of penicillin, in conjunction with success of agencies such as the Red Cross, was that there were suddenly many more persons with a disability surviving. It is therefore not surprising that the end of the Second World War coincided with the development of a number of agencies that focussed on improving life for persons with a disability. The survival of spinal-injured individuals after the war served as one of the catalysts for the development of disability sports.

Humanitarian Agencies and Organizations

There is little doubt that changes in attitudes towards persons with disabilities are intimately linked to the development of agencies and advocacy organizations for the promotion of rights and services for persons with disabilities. However, one should not forget that, as Clapton and Fitzgerald (1997) and Condeluci (1996) point out, agencies and organizations also have inadvertently contributed to the perpetuation of the difference concept.

The UN and several other associated specialized agencies have directly influenced the quality of life of persons with a disability and have indirectly influenced the development of physical activity and sporting opportunities for people with disabilities. These specialized agencies include the International Labour Organization (ILO). The ILO is primarily responsible for improving access to labour markets and increasing economic integration through international labour standards and technical cooperation projects; the United Nations Educational, Scientific and Cultural Organization (UNESCO) is responsible for providing and improving special education; the United Nations International Children's Fund (UNICEF) is responsible for supporting childhood disability programmes and technical support in collaboration with Rehabilitation International (a nongovernmental organization); and the World Health Organization (WHO) is responsible for providing technical assistance in health and prevention (Web site 1). The UN's commitment to assisting the disabled has been evolving since it began to address the needs of individuals injured in World War II.

The UN's concern for the rights and well-being of persons with disabilities is rooted in its founding principles, which are based on human rights, equality of all human beings, and fundamental freedoms. The Charter of the United Nations (1945) (Web site 2), the Universal Declaration of Human Rights (1948) (Web site 3), the Declaration of the Rights of the Child (1959) (Web site 4), the two International Covenants on Human Rights (1966) (Web sites 5 and 6), and the Declaration on Social

Progress and Development (1969) (Web site 7) all attempt to ensure that persons with disabilities are entitled to exercise, on an equal basis, their political, civil, cultural, and social rights with persons who are nondisabled.

During the first decade of work in disability (1945–1955), the UN promoted a "welfare perspective of disability." Concern for individuals with a disability was expressed through the establishment of programmes to deal with disability issues, beginning with the promotion of the rights of people with physical disabilities. Initially, efforts were concentrated on rehabilitation and the prevention of disability. In the late 1950s, the focus on disability issues shifted from a welfare perspective to one of "social welfare." In 1958, the UN adopted the Discrimination (Employment and Occupation) Convention (Web site 8) The 1960s were characterized by fundamental re-evaluation of policy and the establishment of a foundation for the full participation of persons with a disability in society. The UN provided assistance to governments through advisory missions, personnel training workshops, and the creation or improvement of rehabilitation centres. It was not until the late 1960s that the UN recognized that societal attitudes were major obstacles in reaching its goals of equality. Attitudes began to shift towards a new social model for dealing with disability. This new social model resulted in the 1969 adoption of the UN's Declaration on Social Progress and Development (Web site 9).

The 1970s marked a new approach to disability. The UN's initiatives embraced the growing international concept of human rights for persons with disabilities and the equalization of opportunities for them. In 1971, the UN General Assembly adopted the Declaration on the Rights of Mentally Retarded Persons (Web site 10) and in 1975, the assembly adopted the Declaration on the Rights of Disabled Persons (Web site 11). In 1976, in recognition of the further need to promote the full participation of individuals with disabilities in the development and social life of their societies, the UN General Assembly proclaimed the year 1981 as the International Year of Disabled Persons (IYDP) (Web site 12) with the theme Full Participation and Equality. Furthermore, in 1977 the World Health Assembly at its general meeting decided that by the year 2000 the major social goal of governments and the WHO should be the attainment of a level of health that would permit all people of the world to lead a socially and economically productive life. In IYDP, the UN's General Assembly adopted a global strategy called Health for All by the Year 2000. This global strategy urged other concerned international organizations to collaborate with the WHO in achieving this goal (Web site 13).

The 1980s and 1990s represent a time of significant activity in the improvement of the status of persons with disabilities. Part of the shift in attitude and movement towards increased opportunity has been facilitated by changes in how disability was defined and classified. For example, in 1980, the WHO adopted the International Classification of Impairments, Disabilities and Handicaps (ICIDH), which made a clear distinction between 'impairment', 'disability', and 'handicap' (Web site 14). However, definitions of impairment, disability, and handicap were fundamentally based on the consequences of disease, and the loci of difficulties in full participation in society resided within the individual. In recognition of the focus on a disease approach to disability, the ICIDH has undergone a number of changes since 1997 including ICIDH-2 Beta 1 trials (1997), ICIDH-2 Beta 2 trials, (2000) and finally has been reformulated as the International Classification of Functioning, Disability and Health, or ICF (Web site 14b). In this classification, the focus is on how people live with their health condition and, in particular, the context and the environment in which people live. Therefore there has been a shift in focus from disease to function and health, and from the notion of disability as nested within the individual, to societal and contextual factors as determinants of health and participation.

The IYDP was celebrated in many countries with policy innovations, various research projects, and national and international conferences. On December 3, 1982, the UN General Assembly took a major step towards ensuring effective follow-up to the IYDP by adopting the World Program of Action (WPA) Concerning Disabled Persons (Web site 15). The WPA was a global strategy to enhance disability prevention, equalization of opportunities, and rehabilitation. This programme pertained to the full participation of persons with disabilities in life and it emphasized the need to approach disability from a human rights perspective. The Equalization of Opportunities was its guiding philosophy for the achievement of full participation of persons with disabilities in all aspects of economic and social life. An important principle underlying this theme was that persons with disabilities should not be treated in isolation, but rather within the context of normal community services.

In order to facilitate implementation of the various activities recommended in the WPA, the General Assembly declared 1983–1992 as the United Nations Decade of Disabled Persons (Web site 16). Emphasis was placed on improving education and employment opportunities for disabled people, raising new financial resources, and increasing their participation in the life of their communities and country. In 1987, at the mid-point of the UN-sponsored Decade of Disabled Persons, a review of the WPA and its effectiveness was undertaken. The review revealed that social progress had been slower than anticipated. Due to the slower-than-anticipated pace of progress during the first five years of the WPA, there was agreement that disability issues should be further addressed within a wider interdisciplinary setting. This approach took the form of a coordinated information and evaluation campaign combined with the creation of a technical cooperation programme. This strategy was supported through the establishment of a database on disability. Publication of the 1989 *Tallinn Guidelines for Action on Human Resources Development in the Field of Disability* encouraged recognition of disabled persons as agents of their own destiny rather than dependent objects of governments (Web

site 17). The *Tallinn Guidelines* provided a framework for participation. The framework focussed on the training and employment of disabled persons within all government ministries and at all levels of national policy-making in order to equalize opportunities. Moreover, the *Tallinn Guidelines* suggested that the training of disabled people should include independent socialization and self-help skills to prepare individuals for independent living. The same year (1989) marked the UN approval of the Convention on the Rights of the Child (Web site 18), which prohibits discrimination on the basis of disability and requires special measures to ensure the rights of children with disabilities.

In 1991, the UN General Assembly adopted the Principles for the Protection of Persons with Mental Illness and for the Improvement of Mental Health Care (Web site 19). The principles outlined fundamental freedoms and basic rights of persons with mental illness. Marking the end of the UN's Decade of Disabled Persons, the General Assembly proclaimed December 3 as the International Day of Disabled Persons (Web site 20). The day was initially established to commemorate the anniversary of the General Assembly's adoption of the WPA. In addition, in 1992 the General Assembly directed the secretary general to move from a role of consciousness-raising to an active role pertaining to disability. This placed the UN in a catalytic leadership position with the responsibility to place disability issues on the agenda of future world conferences. Also during 1992, the Economic and Social Commission of Asia and the Pacific proclaimed 1993–2002 as the Asian and Pacific Decade of Disabled Persons in order to implement the WPA in the Asian and Pacific region effectively (Web site 21).

The UN General Assembly decided in 1992 to change the objectives of the Trust Fund that was originally established for the IYDP, and that later became known as the Voluntary Fund for the UN's Decade of Disabled Persons. This Trust Fund would take on a new role as the fund to support practical action in achieving the target of a Society for All by 2010 (Web site 22). The intent of this decision was to use the resources of the fund to strengthen cooperation and technical activities in the disability field by cofinancing field-based action related to the strategies of the WPA, with a special emphasis directed to disadvantaged groups of society and developing countries.

One of the major outcomes of the UN Decade of Disabled Persons was the 1993 adoption of the Standard Rules on the Equalization of Opportunities for Persons with Disabilities (Web site 23). The Standard Rules consist of twenty-two rules essentially built on the concepts of the WPA concerning disabled persons (refer to Web site 23). There are three main areas that distinguish the Standard Rules from the WPA. These areas are: i) the rules are more concentrated and concrete in form; ii) they directly address the issue of member states' responsibility; and iii) they include an independent and active monitoring mechanism. Although not a legally binding instrument, the Standard Rules represent a strong moral and political commitment of governments to take action to attain equalization of opportunities for persons with disabilities. The Standard Rules were designed as an instrument for policy-making, and were intended to provide a basis for economic and technical cooperation within and among states, and between international organizations and governmental agencies.

In 1994 the UN secretary general appointed a special rapporteur on disability as part of the Commission for Social Development. The special rapporteur was given the task of monitoring and reporting on the implementation progress of the Standard Rules (Web site 23).

In 1994, at the World Conference on Special Needs Education in Salamanca, Spain, UNESCO adopted the Salamanca Statement and Framework for Action on Special Needs Education (Web site 24), with its framework stemming from the messages of the 1990 Jomtien World Conference on Education for All that was held in Thailand (Web site 25). The Salamanca Statement builds upon, and further develops, the ideas formulated in the Standard Rules (specifically rule 6) and makes

them more precise, thereby providing guidance for educational policies in the disability field. It is a powerful instrument that proclaims inclusive education as the leading principle in special needs education. However, it is also clear that neither the Standard Rules nor recommendations for special needs education (Jomtien World Conference) have been fully implemented.

In 1996, the special rapporteur prepared a report on the implementation, the Standard Rules on the Equalization of Opportunities for Persons with Disabilities, by members of the UN. The report was based on a survey sent to member nations of the UN to a) assess the level of implementation; b) identify the main changes and accomplishments in the field of disability, and c) identify major problems encountered in the implementation process of the Standard Rules of Equalization. One hundred and twenty-six countries were surveyed with a 45 percent response rate recorded from governments, and a 27 percent response rate from nongovernment organizations (NGOs). The response rate by question was quite varied (Web site 26) and it exposed many of the challenges that still remain in the field of disability and policy for governments in both the developed and developing countries.

For example, on disability policy, seventy governments stated that there was existing policy and eleven (ten of which were from developing countries) indicated that there was no policy. The special rapporteur's report exposed many concerns and issues including the right to vote, the right to marry, the right to education and employment, and the right to own property. In fourteen responding countries, persons with disabilities had no political rights (Web site 26).

The special rapporteur also reviewed UNESCO's 1993–1994 Review of the Present Situation of Special Education based on information collected through a questionnaire sent to ninety countries. Out of sixty-three countries responding, thirty-four reported that children with severe disabilities were excluded from education, and among these, eighteen of the countries excluded those children by law from the public education system. Regarding the rights of parents in decision-making for their child, twenty-four countries out of sixty-five that responded on special education questions reported that parents' involvement in decision-making and their rights to determining educational placement for their child was severely limited (Web site 26).

Another important area for action in disability policy pertains to the creation of equal job opportunities, since the overall goal of full participation is not possible without success in this area. The adoption of the Standard Rules on employment (rule 7)–along with the ILO Convention No. 159 on Vocational Rehabilitation and Employment (Disabled Persons) (Web site 27) and the related 1983 Recommendation No. 168 (Web site 28)–provided guidance on how to create job opportunities for those who are disabled. However in 1996, the special rapporteur indicated that only fifty-six countries had ratified the ILO Convention No. 159. Moreover, many governments that had ratified the convention failed to comply with important parts of the ILO Convention No. 159 requirements (Web site 26).

In 1993 at the World Conference on Human Rights in Vienna, 171 countries reiterated the importance of universality, indivisibility, and interdependence of human rights. They reaffirmed their commitment to the Universal Declaration of Human Rights by adopting the Vienna Declaration and Program of Action, which provided a new framework for planning, dialogue, and cooperation (Web site 29). This framework was meant to enable a holistic approach to promoting human rights that would involve actors at the local, national, and international levels. With regards to the rights of persons with a disability, the declaration states:

> The place of disabled persons is everywhere. Persons with disabilities should be guaranteed equal opportunity through the elimination of all socially determined barriers, be they physical, financial, social or psychological, which exclude or restrict full participation in society. (Web site 29)

In 1995, at the UN's World Summit for Social Development Conference in Copenhagen, Denmark, the summit delegates adopted the Copenhagen Declaration (Web site 30) on Social Development and the Program of Action (Web site 31) of the World Summit for Social Development. The declaration tries to respond to the spiritual and material needs of individuals, their families and communities, by stipulating that economic development, social development, and environmental protection are interdependent and mutually reinforcing components of sustainable development. Furthermore, the declaration noted that disadvantaged groups such as disabled persons were in need of special attention.

In 1998 the UN celebrated its fiftieth anniversary of the adoption of the Universal Declaration of Human Rights. The fiftieth anniversary theme was All Human Rights for All, which reinforced the idea that human rights–civil, cultural, economic, political, and social–should be taken in their totality and not disassociated one from the other (Web site 32).

Recent initiatives from the United Nations include the World Disability Report (1999) (Web site 33), the International Year of Older Persons (1999) (Web site 34), International Year for the Culture of Peace (2000) (Web site 35), and the Decade of Human Rights Education (1995–2004) (Web site 36).

3 How has the human rights movement and development and initiatives of humanitarian organizations influenced cultural attitudes towards disability and towards persons with disability?

Legislation and Government Action

The majority of legislation designed to protect the rights of persons with a disability through ensuring access to opportunity and resources has been passed in the last half of the twentieth century. Much of this legislation is a direct or indirect response to the UN's Decade of Disabled Persons (1983–1992) and the Standard Rules of Equalization of Opportunity for Persons with a Disability (1993). However, in some countries specific legislative provision for persons with disabilities either does not exist, or at best, is incorporated into general law and human rights legislation.

CANADA

In Canada, the major influence on the rights and opportunities for persons with disabilities is the Canadian Charter of Rights and Freedoms, adopted on April 17, 1982 (Web site 37). The supreme law of Canada, the Charter is a set of laws containing the basic rules about how Canada operates. It is universal in that it applies to all persons living in Canada and addresses the guarantee of rights, freedoms, mobility, legal, and equality rights. All other laws must be consistent with the rules set out in the Constitution. Since the Charter is part of Canada's Constitution, it supersedes any other law that may limit Charter rights. Disability is specifically mentioned under the domain of equality rights in section 15, subsections 1 and 2.

This section came into effect on April 17, 1985, and it states that:

15 (1) *Every individual is equal before and under the law and has the right to the equal protection and equal benefit of the law without discrimination and, in particular, without discrimination based on race, national or ethnic origin, colour, religion, sex, age, or mental or physical disability.*

15 (2) *Subsection (1) does not preclude any law, programme or activity that has as its object the amelioration of conditions of disadvantaged individuals or groups including those who are disadvantaged because of race, national or ethnic origin, colour, religion, sex, age, or mental or physical disability.*

The Supreme Court of Canada has stated that the purpose of section 15 is to protect those groups who suffer social, political, and legal disadvantages in society. At the same time, the purpose is to protect equality. Therefore, the Charter allows for certain laws

or programmes that may favour disadvantaged individuals or groups.

Section 24, subsections 1 and 2, outline the enforcement aspect of the Charter and state that anyone whose rights or freedoms are guaranteed by the Charter may apply to a court of competent jurisdiction to *"obtain such remedy as the court considers appropriate and just in the circumstances."* On the basis of the Canadian Charter of Rights and Freedoms, each province and territory has made provisions in legislation regarding services for persons with a disability, i.e., access to education.

Over the years, the Government of Canada has said that 'disability issues' were a Canadian priority. Examples are the development of the National Integration Strategy (1991), and the 1996 pronouncement by the prime minister and provincial premiers that disability issues had been identified as a Canadian priority. This was again reaffirmed in 1999 through the proposed strategy entitled, Federal Disability Strategy: Working in Partnership for Full Citizenship. In 1998, the federal, provincial, and territorial ministers responsible for social services and representing all Canadian jurisdictions (with the exception of Quebec) produced *In Unison: A Canadian Approach to Disability Issues. In Unison,* subtitled *A Vision Paper,* was intended to provide a blueprint for promoting the integration of persons with disabilities in Canada and became part of the Social Union initiative in Canada (HRDC, October 1998). It is based on the values of equality, inclusion, and independence, which together provide a "vision of full citizenship" (*In Unison,* p. 8, 1998).

Even though these initiatives are not always implemented as intended through policy changes, they do contain recognition of the denial of rights, lack of basic supports, and exclusion that are part of the day-to-day lives of far too many Canadians with disabilities. These strategy documents support the principles of equality, inclusion, and independence. They also acknowledge Canada's fundamental commitment to the equality of rights for persons with a disability and provide a basis on which the disability community can work with governments to address issues and concerns.

At the time of this writing there is no single piece of legislation aimed solely at disability, such as a Canadians with Disabilities Act (CDA), to parallel legislation that exists elsewhere in the world. While some advocates believe a CDA is necessary, others do not. Those against a CDA cite the current legal protection provided by the Charter of Rights and Freedoms and the Human Rights Act, as being sufficient, and/or that a CDA would not have the capacity to achieve the goals in Canada that the *Americans with Disabilities Act (ADA)* represents in the United States. This same perspective suggests that the true challenge is not to enact a USA-type of *ADA* equivalent, but rather to effect a change in the way that existing laws are being used and administered in Canada.

The Charter of Rights and Freedoms has influenced provincial and territorial governmental policies and encouraged governments to provide a 'universal' educational environment for children. In spite of this, exceptions have occurred. For example, the regulations that accompany the Nova Scotia government's education policies limit the right to education to students *"who are capable of benefiting."* Such regulations may exclude students on the basis of their disability. Legislation governing education in Alberta and Newfoundland includes provisions that restrict the 'right' to education for students with severe disabilities who are not considered to be 'educable' as determined by those in positions of authority. New Brunswick and Quebec are the only provinces that provide a right to early and extended schooling for students with disabilities. Only seven provincial jurisdictions provide for barrier-free access in new schools as per the standards set forth in the *National Building Code of Canada*, section 3.7–Barrier-Free Design (National Research Council 1990; 1995).

In Canada, the Charter of Rights and Freedoms has been used in determining issues of segregation and inclusion in schools through the process of litigation in the highest courts. These precedent-setting cases have helped shape the environment for inclusion that currently exists in most Canadian schools. *Emily Eaton v Brant County Board of Education* (1995) and the *Saint-Jean sur-Richelieu v Marcil* (1991) are two examples.

In February 1995, the Ontario Court of Appeal held that nonconsensual placement of Emily Eaton in a segregated setting was discriminatory and a violation of her rights under the Canadian Charter. The decision by the Ontario Court of Appeal reversed a lower court ruling as well as the original decision of the Special Education Tribunal. This decision by the Ontario Court of Appeal created a new judicial standard for the placement of students with disabilities in school settings. It is worth noting that the decision of the court is equivalent to the provision of the *least restrictive environment* that is contained in USA legislation. The least restrictive environment clause was considered but rejected in Ontario when drafting special education legislation back in 1980. The implication of the *Eaton v Brant* court decision was tantamount to a reversal of this fifteen-year-old policy decision.

In 1991 the Quebec human rights commission, Commission des droits de la personne et les droits de la jeunesse, reached a similar decision in the *Saint-Jean v Marcil* case. In the case, the parents of David Marcil contested the school board's refusal to integrate their nine-year-old autistic child, with related disabling and communication difficulties, into a regular school environment. The complaint was based on the board's refusal to fund an aide and to live up to the promised partial integration for their son. The commission ruled that the board must integrate David Marcil. The commission also awarded the parents certain material and moral damages based on the child's right to educational equality under the premise, *"without discrimination based on his handicap."*

UNITED STATES OF AMERICA
Much of the progressive legislation affecting persons with a disability originated in the United States of America with the most

influential and important legislation having taken place within the last quartile of the twentieth century.

The first federal law in the USA to provide substantial aid to education was the *Elementary and Secondary Education Act* (1965), which provided funds for compensatory education for disadvantaged students and for exemplary programmes. *The Education of the Handicapped Act, Title VI* (Public Law 91–230) was passed in 1970, and in 1990 it passed as the *Individuals with Disabilities Education Act* (*IDEA* – PL. 101–476). The *Americans with Disabilities Act* was passed in 1990 (*ADA* – PL. 101–336). *IDEA* covers disabilities from birth to twenty-one years of age, while the *ADA* legislation is applicable to all ages and applies to issues of physical and attitudinal access as it relates to employment, transportation, buildings, facilities, etc. Table 1 outlines the most important USA legislation and the key elements that are contained therein (Auxter, Pfyfer, and Huertig 1997).

As with the Canadian Charter, the true test for most enacted legislation is its ability to protect, in the face of challenges, those for whom it was intended. Like the Canadian Charter, laws in the US associated with equality for persons with a disability have been challenged on numerous occasions between 1954–1996 in relation to issues of segregation and placement, individual rights and equal opportunity, accessibility, and the provision of aides and services (Auxter, Pfyer and Huertig 1997) and will continue to be challenged.

For example, in 2001 the US Supreme Court ruled in favour of Casey Martin, the golfer, who was discriminated against by the Professional Golfers Association (PGA). The reason for the high-profile court case was that Casey Martin needed to use a golf cart due to a rare blood disorder which resulted in a mobility disability (Klippel-Trenaunay-Weber syndrome). The PGA would not allow the use of a golf cart and presented the argument that it would give Mr. Martin an unfair advantage over other professional golfers who had to walk the course, according to the PGA rules.

Bobby Silverstein, the chief counsel for the US Senate committee that drafted the *ADA*, believes the Martin case is one of the most important *ADA* victories because, "The Supreme Court sustained and reaffirmed this prong of civil rights [Title III]." The Martin decision is expected to play a critical role in a wide range of Title III *ADA* cases. Title I, dealing with employment, and Title II, which covers governmental entities, may be considered the meat-and-potatoes of the *ADA*, but Title III is extremely important. This is because full participation in the broad sweep of American culture will not be possible until private businesses that cater to the public–called public accommodations–modify the many practices and policies that have historically excluded people with disabilities. (Byzek and Gilmer 2002)

LEGISLATION IN OTHER COUNTRIES

It would be difficult, if not impossible in a chapter of this length, to cite all of the legislation that exists in the world pertaining to persons with a disability. However, examples of certain legislation from other countries are provided in table 6.2.

---

4 Legislation has been an important element with regard to securing equal access to opportunity for persons with disability, although influence on societal attitudes is difficult to measure. However, Canada does not have an Individuals with Disabilities Education Act or an equivalent to the *American Disabilities Act*, for example, and relies on the Charter of Human Rights and Freedoms, section 15. Would you support the development of specific-disability legislation in countries such as Canada? If so, why? If not, why not?

The Role of Technology

Technology has had a major impact on the inclusion of persons with a disability in education and society. An example is provided through the following illustration. Lawyer and polio survivor, Mr. Robert J. Provan, delivered a speech to the delegates at the Eighth International Post-polio and Independent Living Conference in June 2000. In his speech Mr. Provan stated, "The U.S. federal government was taking the lead in promoting universal access with the adoption of Section 508 of the *Rehabilitation Act*." He further stated that, "Section 508 requires federal agencies to ensure that its office machinery, electronic, and information technology purchased after August 2000 conforms to the principles of universal access." In this same speech Mr. Provan quotes Tim Berners-Lee, the inventor of the World Wide Web, when he says, "The power of the Web is in its universality. Access by everyone regardless of disability is an essential aspect." (Provan 2000).

The *Technology-related Assistance for Individuals with Disabilities Act* of 1988 (and amended in 1994) is a good example of legislation that has made provision to ensure equitable access to new technology for persons with a disability (Web site 38). The purpose of this act is to provide assistance to the state to support systems change and advocacy initiatives. The act is designed to assist each state to develop and implement a consumer-responsive comprehensive programme of technology-related assistance for individuals of all ages. For example, it is designed to increase the availability of funding for, access to, and provision of technology assistance devices and services.

There is little doubt that technology will continue to play a major part in increasing access for persons with a disability. Technology has revolutionized the mobility and participation opportunities for persons with disabilities. Computers and the Internet have arguably rendered disability virtually invisible in the workplace. For example, it allows people to work from home and often eliminates the need for travel, because transportation can be an impediment to employment for some. Technology has revolutionized sporting opportunities for athletes with a disability. You will read more about the impact of technology throughout this textbook.

5 How might these factors have influenced opportunities for persons with disabilities to access opportunities for active living in the community, physical education in schools, or the sports environment generally?

6 How might technological advances in wheelchairs and sports prostheses, for example, result in an unintentional discrimination issue among athletes with disabilities?

Impact of Active Living Opportunities for Persons with Disabilities

The aforementioned influences provide a backdrop to better understand the developments that led to adaptive physical activity and sporting opportunities for persons with disability. These influences have ultimately culminated in a shift towards a philosophy of inclusion in community, physical education, and sports. Throughout this text, you will be able to relate the development of so-called inclusive physical activity for persons with a disability to many of the events and initiatives we have introduced.

INCLUSIVE ADAPTED PHYSICAL EDUCATION IN SCHOOLS

A combination of the Canadian Charter and the influence of American law may be credited with advancing inclusive adapted physical activity opportunities in Canadian schools. The provisions of the Canadian Charter of Rights and Freedoms (1982) (Web site 37) and particularly section 15 (equality rights) provided a climate for the development of opportunities for persons with a disability, including *inclusive adapted physical education* (APE). The *Fitness and Amateur Sport Act* (1961) (Web site 39) established the federal government's formal and long-term commitment to fitness and health for all Canadians. Although disability is not mentioned specifically, the responsibility for fitness is assigned to the minister of health and, in part, is fulfilled through the Fitness and Active Living Program unit of

Table 6.1 USA Legislation Pertaining to Persons with a Disability

Date and Title of Key USA Legislation	Key Features of Legislation
1958 PL 85–926	Authorization of grants to universities for training personnel in mental retardation. The beginning of a federal commitment to the rights of persons with disabilities.
1961 PL 87–276 *Special Education Act*	Aimed at the preparation of teachers of deaf children.
1963 PL 88–164 Amendment to PL 85–926	Encompasses all handicapped groups requiring special education.
1964 PL 88–352 Civil Rights Legislation	
1965 PL 89–10 *Elementary and Secondary Education Act* (ESEA)	Access of states and local school districts to federal monies to develop programmes for economically disadvantaged children.
1966 PL 89–750 Amendment to *Elementary and Secondary Education Act*	Resulted in the creation of the Bureau of Education for the Handicapped.
1967 PL 90–170 ESEA amendment	Amended to support training, research, and demonstration projects, particularly physical education and recreation.
1968 PL 90–480 Elimination of the Architectural Barriers to Physically Handicapped	First federal legislation pertaining to architectural barriers.
1970 PL 91–230 *Education of the Handicapped Act Title VI* (EHA)	First major legislation leading to the passage of PL 94–142.
1973 PL 93–112 Rehabilitation Amendments: (Section 504 of the *Rehabilitation Act*)	Declared that handicapped people cannot be excluded from any programme or activity receiving federal funding on the basis of being handicapped alone.
1974 PL 93–247 *Child Abuse and Prevention Act*	Developed systems to protect children from abuse. Also mandated that anyone suspecting abuse of a child must report it.
1975 PL 94–142 *Education for All Handicapped Children Act*	Created free appropriate education for all handicapped children between the ages of 3–21 years. Education for children must be provided in a least restrictive environment; individualized education plans must be written; a continuum of placement services must be provided; portability of resources and services were mandated; rationale for separation must be provided. This was the first law in which physical education was specifically mandated.
1977 PL 94–142 Implementation of the *Education for All Handicapped Children Act*	Regulations for implementation of PL 94–142 were developed.
1978 PL 95–602 Developmentally Disabled Assistance and *Bill of Rights*	Updating developmental disability legislation of 1970 and 1975.
1978 PL 95–606 *The Amateur Sports Act*	Recognition of sports organizations for athletes with a disability as part of the US Olympic structure and recognition of eligibility for funding.

Date and Title of Key USA Legislation	Key Features of Legislation
1979 PL 96–88 *Department of Education Organization Act*	Changes status of the US Office of Education within Dept. of Health, Education and Welfare to a Department of Education
1981 PL 97–35 *Education Consolidation and Improvement Act*	
1983 PL 98–199 Amendments to the *Education for All Handicapped Children Act*	States were now required to collect information to determine the anticipated service needs for children with disabilities. It provided incentives to the states to provide services to handicapped infants and preschool children.
1986 PL 99–72 *Handicapped Children's Protection Act*	Legislated support for legal services for parents in litigation regarding placement of their child and provision of appropriate educational services.
1986 PL 99–457 *Education for All Handicapped Children Act* Amendments	Mandated development of comprehensive interdisciplinary services for handicapped infants, toddlers, birth through age 2, and to expand services for preschoolers, 3–5 years.
1987 h.r. 3839 Reauthorization of the *Child Abuse Prevention and Treatment Act*	Mandated a study on incidence of child abuse and disability resulting from child abuse (National Centre on Child Abuse and Neglect).
1988 PL 100–407 and 103–218 *Technology-related Assistance for Individuals with Disabilities Act*	Amended the Education of the Handicapped Act PL 100–407 to develop technology related assistance for individuals with disabilities. Note: Amended in 1994: The Technology-related Assistance with Disabilities Act amendments of 1994. To provide assistance to the states to support systems change and advocacy initiatives designed to assist each state in developing and implementing a consumer-responsive comprehensive statewide programme of technology-related assistance for individuals of all ages.
1990 PL 101–476 *Individuals with Disabilities Education Act* (IDEA)	Term *handicapped* is replaced with *disability*, and types of services offered extended.
1990 PL 101–336 *Americans With Disabilities Act* (ADA)	A widening of civil rights protections for all persons with a disability. Also addressed private discrimination.
1996 (Amendments to 101–476) *Individuals with Disabilities Education Act* Amendment	Amended and re-authorized discretionary programming and strengthened services to children at risk.
1997 PL 105–17 Amendments to the *Individuals with Disabilities Education Act*	

SOURCE: Adapted from *Principles and Methods of Adapted Physical Education and Recreation* (8th ed.) (p. 14) by D. Auxter, J. Pfyfer, and C. Huertig. St. Louis: MO: Mosby. Adapted with permission.

Table 6.2 World Examples of Legislation Impacting on Persons with a Disability

Country	Legislation Title	Date	Specific Provisions
Europe			
Britain	*The Education Act*	1981	Children with special needs should be taught in an integrated setting.
South America			
Republic of Ecuador	*Law for the Protection of the Disabled*	1982	Prevention and care of handicaps and social integration of disabled citizens under an equalization of access to culture, education, health, work, housing, recreation, and sports.
	Law 180 on Disabilities	1992	Aspects of protection of persons with a disability in society.
Costa Rica	Law 7600—Law for equality of opportunities for people with a disability in Costa Rica	1996	Guideline set for guarantee equal opportunities for all citizens with a disability.
Eastern Europe			
Czech Republic	National plan* of actions for: • handicapped persons • measures to reduce the negative impact of disability • equalization of opportunities for persons with a disability	1992 1993 1998	* note: not formal legislation but measures taken to raise awareness, reduce impact of disability, and equalize opportunity for persons with a disability.
Georgia	*Law on Social Defence of Disabled Persons*	1995	Addresses social infrastructure, medical, vocational, social rehabilitation, education, professional preparation, work, social emergency, and development of sports for disabled persons.
	Law on Veterans of War and the Armed Forces	1995	Support of persons lost or injured during war and their families.
Uzbekistan	*Law on Social Protection of Disabled People in the Republic of Uzbekistan*	1991	Mandates development of programmes of rehabilitation as well as provisions for physical culture and sport.

Country	Legislation Title	Date	Specific Provisions
Hungary	*The Act on Public Education*	1998	Allows for education of disabled children in special pedagogical institutions and/or integrated educational settings—ensures that no child is barred from education regardless of severity of disability.
	The Rights of Persons Living with a Disability and their Equality of Opportunity	1998	Subsequently referred to as the Equal Opportunities Act—mandates equalization of opportunity for persons with a disability.
Asia			
Mauritius	*The Employment of Disabled Persons Act*	1998	To sensitize employers on the need to provide persons with a disability the opportunity to contribute to the development of the nation.
	The Trust Fund for Disabled Persons Act	1998	To provide funding for vocational training of adults and adolescents with disabilities.
	The Building Act (Amendment)	1999	Authorities may impose building accessibility upgrades where necessary.
Pakistan	Disabled Persons Employment and Rehabilitation Ordinance	1981	Enforces a 1 percent quota of employment for persons with a disability in the public and private sector.
Philippines	The Magna Carta for Disabled Persons	1992	Provides for rehabilitation, self-development, and self-reliance in persons with a disability for integration into the mainstream of society.
	Accessibility Law (Amendment)	1992	Requirements of infrastructure accessibility.

Health Canada. This programme assumes responsibility for ensuring equity and access for active living for Canadians, and it also supports the work of the Active Living Alliance for Canadians with a Disability (Web site 40). Historically, it was the Jasper Talks conference held in Jasper, Alberta, in 1986 that laid the groundwork for the development of the Active Living Alliance (1989) and the subsequent Moving to Inclusion series. This series was developed in 1994 to provide teachers with information on how to include children with a disability in regular physical education classes. It was created by educators, parents, and adaptive physical education specialists, and supported by ministries of education across Canada. Over twenty-five thousand manuals have been distributed on a complimentary basis to more than fifteen thousand Canadian schools. There are now over four hundred leaders in nine countries, including Canada, who have been trained to use these resources (Steadward et al. 1997).

In the United States, much progress in the development of inclusive APA/APE opportunities has been made possible by legislation. Public Law 93–112 (PL 93–112), the *Rehabilitation Amendment* (enacted in 1973; implemented in 1977), contained a nondiscrimination clause that made it illegal to exclude children with disability from programmes receiving federal assistance. Schools providing physical education and interscholastic athletic programmes were legally bound to provide qualified students with the same opportunities as nondisabled population. Public Law 94–142 (PL 94–142), the *Education for All Handicapped Children Act* (enacted in 1973; implemented in 1977), stated that all children must receive a free and appropriate public education regardless of the level or severity of their disability. This opportunity had to be provided in the *"least restrictive environment"* possible. PL 94–142 mandated five rights that changed the nature of public schooling for children and youth with disabilities. These rights were, 1) a free and appropriate education, 2) nondiscriminatory testing, 3) evaluation and placement procedures,

4) education in the least restrictive environment, and 5) the due process of law (Auxter, Pfyfer, and Huertig 1997).

An absolutely critical aspect of PL 94–142 was the provision for parental input in individualized education plans. This provision allowed parents to be involved in the planning of physical activity programmes and to be a strong advocate for programmes involving access and opportunity for their children. PL 94–142 has been described as a "momentous achievement" (Sherrill 1993). This law has since become known as the *Education for All Handicapped Children Act–B*, and since 1990 it has been called the *Individuals with Disabilities Education Act–part B* or sub-chapter II. This law is re-authorized every three years and assigned a new number. Together, IDEA (birth to twenty-one years) PL 94–142 (three to twenty-one years) and the *Americans with Disabilities Act* (1990) (lifespan) are important legislative pieces that provide adapted physical activity opportunities for persons with a disability.

In 1978 in Quebec City, the International Federation of Adapted Physical Activity (IFAPA) was formed and gave further legitimacy to adaptive physical activity as a true academic discipline. The federation provided an international forum for APA specialists and other interested parties to discuss and share ideas, programmes, and research. The International Symposium of Adapted Physical Activity (ISAPA) is now held every two years. The North American Federation of Adapted Physical Activity (NAFAPA) was formed in 1989 as a regional affiliate of IFAPA and holds its meetings in alternate years to the ISAPA. The *Adapted Physical Activity Quarterly* (APAQ) was founded in 1984 and is an international, multidisciplinary journal designed to stimulate and communicate scholarly inquiry related to sport and physical activity. The journal has provided an important outlet for much of the work presented at symposia associated with NAFAPA and IFAPA and has been an important source of information for educators. Other publications such as *Palaestra* and *Sports 'n Spokes* have become important resources with regards to adapted physical activity.

COMMUNITY RECREATIONAL OPPORTUNITIES

In Canada, the Charter of Rights and Freedoms impacts on the provision of community recreation services for persons with a disability. Its legislative muscle is complemented by the Canadian Building Code. The Building Code provides a framework of guidelines and rules that directly affects the retrofitting and new construction of recreational facilities.

In the United States, the *ADA* (PL 101–336) legislation is important in terms of the provision of recreational sports opportunities because it mandated that persons with a disability should be afforded an equal opportunity and access to programmes and facilities such as health centres, swimming pools, golf courses, etc.

Developments in Sports

In the USA, Public Law 95–606–*The Amateur Sports Act* (1978), mandated the provision of encouragement and assistance to amateur athletic programmes and competition for disabled individuals, including participation where possible of handicapped persons in able-bodied competition and programmes.

One of the most important documents regarding the rights of persons with a disability to participate in physical activities is the *European Charter for Sport for All* (Council of Europe 1987). The European Charter's roots are grounded in the early 1980s when the Committee of Sport commissioned a study on sport for the disabled as a contribution to the International Year of the Disabled (1981). At the same time, European ministers responsible for sport adopted a resolution outlining the main priorities for European and national policies that impacted on sport for disabled persons. Six years later the European Charter was approved. The Charter's thirteen recommendations cover all aspects of the provision of sports for persons with a disability (DePauw and Doll-Tepper 1989).

As a result of the UN initiatives (e.g., *Standard Rules of Equalization of Opportunity for Persons with Disabilities,* 1993), legislation in other countries has also made provision for the inclusion of recreational and competitive sports opportunities for persons with a disability. A number of examples are cited below. In Ecuador, Law #180 was passed in 1992 and mandated equalization of opportunities permitting access to culture, education, health, work, housing, recreation, and sports. In Eastern Europe there has also been significant progress in relation to provisions for recreational and competitive sports opportunities that have been supported through a variety of legislative measures. The *National Plan of Action* (1992) was passed in the Czech Republic, which put a focus on barrier-free living and improvements to leisure services; and in Georgia, the *Law of Social Defense of Disabled Persons* specifically addresses the development of sports opportunities for disabled persons. In Uzbekistan, the *Law on Social Protection of Disabled People* passed in 1991. It was enacted via the Government Programme for Rehabilitation of Disabled People (1995) that undertook to implement a number of measures, including culture and sports for the disabled and to initiate support for the Georgian Disabled Person's Sport Federation.

Perhaps the greatest advancement of disability sports has been the development of the International Paralympic Committee (IPC) (1989). Based on a philosophy of elite sport and the autonomous rights of persons to participate at the highest levels possible, the IPC now oversees all elite disability sports and is the governing body for the Paralympic Games. The Paralympic Games are held every four years in conjunction with, and immediately following, the Olympic games. In the fall of 1999, the IPC opened its new headquarters in Bonn, Germany. The Paralympics represent the pinnacle of athletic achievement of persons with a disability. These games can be attributed in part to a fundamental change in attitudes towards persons with a disability as well as to the enormous efforts of all those who have worked tirelessly to bring about societal change.

Of course, technological changes have also had a significant impact in advancing performance of athletes with disabilities. The development of lightweight materials for the construction of wheelchairs and developments in hi-tech computerized prosthetic technology have all advanced disability sports.

You will learn much more with regard to the concept of inclusion and developments in community, physical education, and sports opportunities for persons with disabilities as you work your way through this text.

Problems Remain

You must recognize that this text does not have all the answers, that we are still faced with discrimination with regard to disability, and that the inclusion movement itself is fraught with challenges. With regard to adapted physical education, Block (1994) perhaps sums up the issues in his observations.

> Inclusion is perhaps the most feared and emotionally charged educational reform since passage of PL 94–142. Whether in formal debates at processional meetings or informal gatherings in teacher's lounges, nothing can divide a room of educators into two camps like discussions on inclusion.

According to Block (1999) we may have jumped on the "wrong bandwagon." He notes that inclusion has become a moral imperative and "in their zest to promote inclusion, many inclusionists forgot about the child." One of the unintended negative outcomes for some children has been a move to place children in a regular classroom environment, including physical education classes, without due regard as to the provision of appropriate individual programmes and supports within the larger class setting.

In disability sport also, inclusion has also become a source of debate although the meaning of the concept is somewhat different in this context. One of the goals of certain factions within the Paralympic movement has been to achieve the inclusion of selected full-medal events for athletes with a disability into the Olympic Games. This objective has met with significant criticism by many in the world of elite disability sports as either being misguided or elitist. Some athletes, for example, believe that full inclusion of a few athletes in the Olympic Games relegates those in the Paralympic Games and the Paralympic Games themselves to a second-class status. Athletes with intellectual disability have faced numerous difficulties in becoming included in the Paralympic family. Women are under represented in Paralympic Games competition, another inclusion issue about which you will learn more later in this text.

Concluding Comments, Cautions, and a Future Based on Interdependence

As the politics of inclusion move forward, there is a need for caution. Arguably, the move to inclusion has focussed principally at the level of the individual while failing to acknowledge and recognize the interdependence within the individual's environment, professional, and informal support system. The danger of the focus on independence to the exclusion of interdependence leads to the potential for an atmosphere of immersion, invisibility, anonymity, and a return to abandonment. If taken to the extreme, the normalization process (see Chapter 5 (Shogan)) could lead to the abdication of financial and moral responsibility for some people with disabilities.

No person alive today is truly independent from the rest of his or her fellow citizens. It is through this recognition of interdependence that society will have to respond to the needs and requirements of its disabled citizens in the future. This will occur because of an increasing visibility, acceptance, appreciation, and understanding of people with disabilities. Also, the aging of the population will bring disability closer to home for all citizens. The increased visibility will magnify the strengths, weaknesses, and vulnerability of the many disabled people who contribute in many different ways to the quality of community life.

The mid- to late-1990s saw a devolving of financial responsibility to the lowest level of government across most of the provinces and territories that make up Canada. The programmes, services, and delivery mechanisms available to Canadians vary according to the province in which they live.

Increasingly, this means that disabled individuals are reliant on the spirit and sense of fairness of their friends, neighbours, and civic leaders who make the policies that support inclusionary practices in their home communities. It also means that without 'a sense of fairness' disabled individuals will continue to be vulnerable and that society could be at risk of reverting to the days of isolation of the disabled individual, through financial and moral abandonment. At this point the Charter of Rights and Freedoms becomes even more important for the protection of individuals with disabilities.

Finally, in June 1999 the Parliamentary Sub-committee on the Status of Persons with Disabilities, tabled its first report in the House of Commons titled, *Reflecting Interdependence; Disability, Parliament, Government and the Community*. The authors of this report investigated the mountains of documents that have flooded the country over the years and that now sit on shelves collecting dust, and have resulted in little action when compared to the political rhetoric that accompanied them on their original release. The report made several recommendations about what should be done to get all levels of government and the disability community working together toward concrete implementation of common objectives. The main focus of the report was on a "future of interdependence."

Study Questions

1. A number of major factors have influenced the history of adapted physical activity in Canada. Identify the three most important factors and briefly justify your selection of them.
2. Based on your own experience, how successful have we been in developing 'inclusive' communities that facilitate 'active living' by all Canadians?
3. Select one of the people referred to in this chapter and using Internet or library resources develop a more complete biographical sketch of their role in the development of adapted physical activity in Canada.

References

BOOKS, JOURNALS

Auxter, D., Pfyfer, J., and Huettig, C. (1997). *Principles and methods of adapted physical education and recreation* (8th ed). St. Louis, MO: Mosby.

Block, M.E. (1994, Spring). Why all students with disabilities should be included in regular physical education. *Palaestra*, 17–24.

Block, M.E. (1999, Summer). Did we jump on the wrong bandwagon? Problems with inclusion in physical education. *Palaestra*, 30–42.

Byzek, J., and Gilmer, T. (2002, January). Casey Martin: The accidental advocate. *New Mobility Magazine*, p. 29. Available on-line: http://www.newmobility.com/review_article.cfm?id=491&action=browse.

Clapton, J., and J. Fitzgerald. (1997, April). The history of disability: A history of 'otherness'. *New Renaissance: A Journal of Social and Spiritual Awakening (7)*1. Available on-line: http://www.ru.org/artother.html

Condeluci, A. (1995). Interdependence: The route to community. In A. Condeluci, *The interdependence paradigm* (pp. 85–130). Winter Park, FLA: G.R. Press.

Condeluci, A. (1996a). Inclusion: Human services and culture. In A. Condeluci, *Beyond difference* (Introduction). Delray Beach, FLA: St. Lucie Press.

Condeluci, A. (1996b) The dualistic society. In A. Condeluci, *Beyond difference* (pp. 33–56). Delray Beach, FLA: St. Lucie Press.

DePauw, K., and Doll-Tepper, G. (1989). European perspectives on adapted physical education. *Adapted Physical Activity Quarterly, 6*, 95–99.

Eaton v. Brant County Board of Education (1997), 1 S.C.R. [On-line]. Available: http://www.lexum.umontreal.CA/csc-scc/en/pub/1997/vol1/html/1997scr1_0241.html

Human Resources Development Canada: Author. Social Services. (1998, October). In *In unison: A Canadian approach to disability issues: A vision paper*. Hull, QC. [Available from 140 Promenade du Portage, Phase IV, Level O. Hull, Quebec, K1A 0J9]. Available on-line at http://socialunion.gc.CA/news/102798_e.html

Jansma, P., and French, R. (1994). *Special physical education: Physical activity, and sports, recreation*. Englewood Cliffs, NJ: Prentice-Hall.

Jasper Talks. (1988). *Proceedings of the Jasper talks: Strategies for change in adapted physical activity in Canada*. Ottawa: CAHPER.

Lanoue et Commission des droits de la personne du Quebec. (1991). Commission scolaire de Saint-Jean-sur-Richelieu. *CAQ 130* (Call # R.J.Q. p. 44).

National Research Council of Canada, Canadian Commission on Building and Fire Codes. (1990, 1995). *The national building code of Canada, section 3.7: Barrier free design*. Ottawa: Author.

Provan R.J. (2000, Summer). Celebrating the Americans with Disabilities Act: The unfinished revolution. *Rehabilitation Gazette* [On-line], *40*, 2. Available: http://www.post-polio.org/gini/rg40-2.html#cele

Sherrill, C. (1996). *Adapted physical activity, recreation and sport: Crossdisciplinary and lifespan* (5th ed.). Boston: McGraw-Hill.

Steadward, R., Legg, D.F.H., Bornemann, R., Weiss, J.Y., Jeon, J.Y., and Wheeler, G.D. (1997, Autumn). Active Living Alliance for Canadians with a Disability: A ten year retrospective analysis. CAHPERD *Journal, 63*(3), 10–15.

WEB SITES

Web site 1
Persons with Disabilities. *The UN and persons with disabilities.* [On-line]. Available: http://www.un.org/esa/socdev/enable/ (URL on October 6, 2002).

Web site 2
United Nations. *Charter of the United Nations.* (1945). [On-line]. Available: http://www.un.org/aboutun/charter/index.html_ (URL on October 6, 2002).

Web site 3
United Nations. (1948). *Universal declaration of human rights.* [On-line]. http://www.un.org/Overview/rights.html Available: (URL on October 6, 2002).

Web site 4
United Nations. (1959). *Declaration of the rights of the child.* [On-line]. Available: http://www1.umn.edu/humanrts/instree/k1drc.htm (URL on October 6, 2002).

Web site 5
United Nations. (1966). *International covenant on human rights #1: International covenant on economic, social and cultural rights.* [On-line]. Available: http://www.unhchr.ch/html/menu3/b/a_cescr.htm_ (URL on October 15, 2000).

Web site 6
United Nations. (1966). *International covenant on human rights #2: International covenant on civil and political rights.* [On-line]. Available: http://www.unhchr.ch/html/menu3/b/a_opt.htm_ (URL on October 15, 2000).

Web site 7
United Nations. (1969). *Declaration on social progress and development.* [On-line]. Available: http://www.unhchr.ch/html/menu3/b/m_progre.htm_ (URL on October 15, 2000).

Web site 8
United Nations. Discrimination [Employment and Occupation] Convention. [On-line]. Available: http://www.unhchr.ch/html/menu3/b/d_ilo111.htmb_ (URL on October 15, 2000).

Web site 9
United Nations. *The United Nations and disabled persons: The first 50 years.* [On-line]. Available: http://www.un.org/esa/socdev/enable/dis50y00.htm (URL on October 6, 2002).

Web site 10
United Nations. (1971). *Declaration on the rights of mentally retarded persons.* [On-line]. Available: http://www.unhchr.ch/html/menu3/b/m_mental.htm (URL on October 6, 2002).

Web site 11
United Nations. (1975). *Declaration on the rights of disabled persons.* Available: http://www.unhchr.ch/html/menu3/b/72.htm (URL on October 6, 2002).

Web site 12
United Nations (1981). *International year of disabled persons 1981.* [On-line]. Available: http://www.un.org/esa/socdev/enable/disiydp.htm (URL on October 6, 2002).

Web site 13
World Health Organization. (1998). *Health for all in the 21st century.* [On-line]. Available: http://www.who.int/archives/hfa/ (URL on October 6, 2002).

Web site 14
World Health Organization. (1980) *International classification of impairments, disabilities and handicaps (ICIDH-1).* [On-line]. Available: http://www.alternatives.com/wow/who-old.htm (URL on October 6, 2002).

Web site 14b
World Health Organization. (2001). *International classification of functioning, disability and health (ICFDH).* [On-line]. Available: http://www.who.int/gb/EB_WHA/PDF/WHA54/ea5418.pdf (URL on October 6, 2002).

Web site 15
Persons With Disabilities. (1982). *World programme of action concerning disabled persons.* [On-line]. Available: http://www.un.org/esa/socdev/enable/diswpa00.htm (URL on October 6, 2002).

Web site 16

Persons With Disabilities. *United Nations Decade of Disabled Persons 1983–1992.* [On-line]. Available: http://www.un.org/esa/socdev/enable/dis50y60.htm (URL on October 6, 2002).

Web site 17

United Nations. (1989). *Tallinn guidelines for action on human resources development in the field of disability.* [On-line]. Available: http://hadar.m.se/svensk/text/sh711E.htm_ (URL on October 16, 2000).

Web site 18

United Nations Children's Fund (UNICEF). (1989). Convention on the Rights of the Child. [On-line]. Available: http://www.unicef.org/crc/crc.htm (URL on October 6, 2002).

Web site 19

United Nations. (1991). *Principles for the protection of persons with mental illness and the improvement of mental health care.* [On-line]. Available: http://www1.umn.edu/humanrts/instree/t2pppmii.htm (URL on October 6, 2002).

Web site 20

United Nations. (1992). *International Day of Disabled Persons.* [On-line]. Available: http://www.independentliving.org/LibArt/UN/IntlDoD_.html (URL on October 16, 2000). See also: http://www1.umn.edu/humanrts/resolutions/47/3GA 1992.html (URL on October 6, 2002).

Web site 21

United Nations Economic and Social Commission for Asia and the Pacific (ESCAP). (1992). *Asian and Pacific Decade of Disabled Persons, 1993–2002.* http://www.un.org/Depts/escap/decade/index.htm_ (URL on October 6, 2002).

Web site 22

United Nations Division for Social Policy and Development Department of Economic and Social Affairs. (1991). *United Nations voluntary fund on disability.* [On-line]. Available: http://www.un.org/esa/socdev/enable/disunvf.htm_ (URL on October 6, 2002).

Web site 23

United Nations. (1993). *Standard rules on the equalization of opportunities for persons with disabilities.* [On-line]. Available: http://www.un.org/esa/socdev/enable/dissre00.htm_ (URL on October 6, 2002).

Web site 24

UNESCO. (1994). *The Salamanca statement and framework for action on special needs education: Access and quality: Salamanca, Spain, 7–10 June 1994.* [On-line]. Available: http://www.unesco.org/education/educprog/sne/salam_anc/covere.html (URL on October 6, 2002).

Web site 25

UNESCO. (1990). *World conference on Education for All 1990, Jomtien, Thailand, 5–9 March 1990.* [On-line]. Available: http://www2.unesco.org/wef/en-conf/Jomtien%20Decla_rationpercent20eng.shtm (URL on October 16, 2000). http://www.unesco.org/education/efa/ed_for_all/background/world_conference_jomtien.shtml (URL on October 6,2002).

Web site 26

United Nations Division for Social Policy and Development Department of Economic and Social Affairs. (1993). *Monitoring the implementation of the standard rules on the equalization of opportunities for persons with disabilities.* [On-line]. Available: http://www.un.org/esa/socdev/enable/dismsreo.htm (URL on October 6, 2002).

Web site 27

International Labour Organisation General Conference. *C159: Vocational Rehabilitation and Employment (Disabled Persons) Convention, 1983.* [On-line]. Available: http://www.independentliving.org/LibArt/UN/ILOconv_.html (URL on October 16, 2000) http://ilolex.ilo.ch:1567/scripts/convde.pl?C159 (URL on October 6, 2002).

Web site 28

International Labour Office. (1983). *R168: Vocational rehabilitation and employment (disabled persons) recommendation, 1983.* [On-line]. Available: http://www.ilo.org/public/english/employment/skills/recomm/instr/r_168.htm (URL on October 6, 2002).

Web site 29

United Nations World Conference on Human Rights. (1993, June). *Vienna declaration and programme of action.* [On-line]. Available: http://www.hri.ca/vienna+5/ (URL on October 6, 2002).

Web site 30

United Nations Division for Social Policy and Development. (1995). Copenhagen declaration on social development and programme of action of the World Summit for Social Development. In *Report of the World Summit for Social Development, Copenhagen, 6–12*

March 1995. [On-line]. Available: http://www.un.org/
esa/socdev/wssd/agreements/decpa_rti.htm (URL on
October 16, 2000).
http://www.un.org/esa/socdev/docs/summit.pdf
(URL on October 6, 2002).

Web site 31

United Nations Division for Social Policy and
Development. Programme of action of the World
Summit for Social Development. In *In Report of the
World Summit for Social Development, Copenhagen, 6–12
March 1995*. [On-line]. Available: http://www.un.org/
esa/socdev/wssd/agreements/poach_i.htm (URL on
October 6, 2002).

Web site 32

United Nations. (1948, December). *All human rights for all:
The universal declaration of human rights*. [On-line].
Available: http://www.un.org/Overview/ rights.html
(URL on October 6, 2002).

Web site 33

(World Disability Report). (URL on October 16, 2000).

Web site 34

United Nations International Year of Older Persons. (1999).
United Nations principles for older persons. [On-line].
Available: http://www.un.org/esa/socdev/iyop/
iyoppop.htm_ (URL on October 6, 2002).

Web site 35

UNESCO. *The United Nations and the culture of peace:
International Year for the Culture of Peace 2000*. [On-line].
Available: http://www.unac.org/peacecp/iycp/
index.html_ (URL on October 16, 2000).
http://www3.unesco.org/iycp/ (URL on
October 6, 2002).

Web site 36

United Nations High Commissioner for Human Rights.
*United Nations Decade for Human Rights Education,
1995–2004*. [On-line] Available:
http://www.unhchr.ch/html/menu6/1/edudec.htm_
(URL on October 16, 2000).

Web site 37

Constitution Act, 1982 [en. by the Canada Act 1982 (U.K.),
c.11,s.1], pt. I (Canadian Charter of Rights and
Freedoms). [On-line]. Available:
http://www.laurentia.com/ccrf/default.htm (URL on
October 6, 2002).

Web site 38

U.S. Public Laws 100–407 and 103–218. Technology-
related Assistance for Individuals with Disabilities Act
of 1988 as Amended in 1994. [On-line]. Available:
http://www.resna.org/taproject/library/laws/techact9
4.htm (URL on October 6, 2002).

Web site 39

Canada. (1961). Fitness and Amateur Sport Act R.S., c.
F-25, s. 1. [On-line]. Available: http://www.pch.gc.CA/
progs/sc/pubs/act_e.cfm (URL on October 6, 2002).

Web site 40

Health Canada. Fitness and Active Living Programme
Unit. [On-line]. Available: http://www.hc-sc.gc.CA/
hppb/fitness/aboutus.htm_ (URL on October 6, 2002).

CHAPTER 7

Policy Strategies to Foster Active Living

Renée F. Lyons
Bruce Taylor
Lynn L. Langille

Learning Objectives
- To understand what policy is and why it is important.
- To understand key policy issues in adapted physical activity and disability.
- To learn how policy is made and influenced.
- To practice the art and science of policy development.

The Creation

In the beginning there was the plan
And then came the assumptions
And the assumptions were without form
And the plan was completely without substance
And darkness was upon the faces
Of the workers, and they spake
Unto their group heads, saying
 " This is very bad. It stinketh."
And the group heads went unto their section
   heads, and sayeth:
   " It is a container of excrement, and it
     Is very strong,
     Such that none can abide its strength."
And the managers went to their director and
   sayeth:
   " It contains that which aids plant
     Growth, and it is very strong."
And the director went to the vice-president
   and sayeth unto him:
   " This powerful new plan will
     Promote the growth and efficiency of this
     department."
And the vice-president looked upon the
Plan and saw that it was good
And the plan became policy.
                                    —Author Unknown

Introduction

"Policy, policy...yawn, yawn." (Herchmer 1994, p. 32)

What comes to mind when you think about the word *policy*? The term usually conjures up several uncomplimentary adjectives such as *boring, bureaucratic, authoritarian, restrictive,* and *time-consuming.* In truth, sometimes policy deserves these adjectives. And as "The Creation" suggests, the policy development process can make you shake your head in bewilderment. There also may be substantial discrepancies between what is written in the name of policy and how people interpret or act upon policy. Nevertheless, evidence suggests that one of the strongest determinants of sustainability of programmes and services is policy (Milio 1986; Mullen et al. 1995). Also, there is good evidence to suggest that collective efforts of community members and consumers **can** influence the policy process in ways that will create positive change (Devon Dodd et al. 1997).

Most people who read this text will have already developed a strong commitment to the value of physical activity. By the time they reach this chapter, they will have acquired considerable evidence of its importance for people with a disability. They will also be committed to gaining the skills necessary to provide leadership in fostering opportunities to be active.

But what does leadership in adapted physical activity mean?

One important aspect of leadership development is gaining technical skills. However, the application of these skills in providing direction and guidance to positively influence the decision-making process that creates opportunities for persons with a disability is of equal importance.

In order to function well, the 'system' (i.e., services, programmes, facilities, budgets, etc.) needs a strong framework that guides decisions. Knowing about the policy framework that facilitates or undermines opportunities, and knowing how to influence such policies, are central to your education and to your job as a practitioner. A person committed to providing adapted physical activity must be skilled in the policy arena. Individuals with a disability and practitioners both have an important role to play in crafting and influencing the policy development process in schools, communities, and governments.

Development of good policy "is carried out by and with people, not on or to people. It improves both the ability of individuals to take action, and the capacity of groups, organizations or committees to influence [change]" (adaptation of an excerpt from The Jakarta Declaration, WHO 1997).

It is helpful to know about the history of policy development for people with a disability. The following section provides some background on the development of policies for persons with a disability in Canada.

A SAMPLING OF CANADIAN POLICY MILESTONES

Here are highlights of landmark reports or events that have directly impacted on policy development in Canada related to disability.

- *Obstacles* (1981), tabled by the Special Committee on the Disabled and the Handicapped, contained 130 recommendations pertaining to all aspects of disability issues (Special Committee of Parliament on the Disabled and the Handicapped 1981).
- United Nations declared 1981 as the International Year of Disabled Persons. This event provided the focus for numerous initiatives in Canada and other countries (United Nations 1976).
- Rights of persons with disabilities included in the Canadian Charter of Rights and Freedoms (1982). Canada was (and still is) the only nation in the world that enshrines constitutional protection for persons with disabilities.
- Jasper Talks symposium held in 1986, representing a gathering of experts, athletes, and leaders in the field of adapted physical activity in Canada; recommendations and strategies put forth

helped shape the future of physical activity and disability in Canada. (Fitness Canada 1988).

- The federal government announced the National Strategy for the Integration of Persons with Disabilities (1991–96). This five-year strategy included eleven federal departments and focussed on the three theme areas: equal access, economic integration, and effective participation (Department of the Secretary of State of Canada 1991).
- The Task Force on Disability Issues tabled *Equal Citizenship for Canadians with Disabilities: The Will To Act* (1996) an examination of the role of the federal government through a "disability lens," containing fifty-two recommendations. This report led to the development of a document specifically on policy for active living for people with a disability (Active Living Alliance for Canadians with a Disability 1997).
- The Canadian federal government appointed a special parliamentary committee (1998) to review all federal legislation from the perspective of disability (Guarnieri and Bennett 1999).
- All governments except Quebec signed *In Unison: A Canadian Approach to Disability Issues* (1998), a national agreement on disability which described a bold vision of persons with disabilities as full citizens in work, culture, school, recreation, and all aspects of community life (Human Resources Development Canada 1998).
- The federal minister of health (1998) endorsed *Active Living for Canadians with Disabilities: A Blueprint For Action*, a national framework and focal point of consensus designed by "the disability community" to provide direction for the advancement of physical activity opportunities for Canadians with disabilities (Active Living Alliance and Health Canada 1998).

These actions represent significant moments in the history of policy development in Canada.

They also represent an evolution of thinking about people with a disability from the 'warehouse' approach (up to 1960), which was characterized by segregation, to the 'greenhouse' approach (1960–1980), which was characterized by specialized services and support, to the 'open house' approach (1980 to the present), which is characterized by access to mainstream services and social integration (Department of Secretary of State Canada 1993). As thinking about the treatment of people with a disability has progressed, policy has played a strong role in influencing social attitudes and structures.

---

1 Can you note any landmark decisions that have affected persons with disabilities in your community?

Step One: Understanding What Policy Is and Why It Is Important

A policy is a declaration that defines the intention of a community, organization, or government's goals and priorities. Policies outline the roles, rules, and procedures. They create a framework within which the administration and staff can perform their assigned duties (Mayer and Thompson 1982). In other words, policies add clarity to the mission of an organization, enabling people to better understand their role in accomplishing that mission. Policy can also refer to the establishment of standard ways of doing things that influence decisions, direction, and actions (Herchmer 1994). Policy is an evolving process that considers an organization's "best thinking and acting."

The idea of healthy public policy is relatively new (O'Neill and Pederson 1992). The concept was developed to stimulate thinking about the factors that determine health and to identify policy that would be supportive of health and wellness in Canada (Hancock 1982). Public policy is typically thought of as government policy, but it may also be the policy of a particular service institution such as a school or a not-for-profit agency operating at a municipal or provincial level. In *Promoting Health Through Public Policy* (1986), Milio argues that public policies shape the everyday environment in which people live and business operates, thus forming the foundation for health.

Policies serve many valuable functions:

- They reflect an organization's ideology and values.
- They are the principles that guide action.
- They are planning tools for goal-setting and service delivery.
- They provide the terms of reference for setting programme priorities and guiding programme development.
- They help set roles and delimit or define areas within the organization's role.
- They house the rules and regulations, and provide guidance for routine, unique, or controversial decisions.
- They provide the justification for, and the sanctioning of, resource allocations (e.g., budget, staff time).
- They provide for fairness of access by members of a community.
- They provide a tool to assist in evaluating progress and in providing accountability to constituents, funding agencies, etc.

Milio (1988) states that it is the responsibility of the government to set conditions that enable people to make healthy choices in their lives the "easiest choices" and to live in a health-enhancing physical, social, and political environment.

The secret of helpful policies is that they are relevant and useful for day-to-day activities; they can be operationalized and evaluated; and they can be changed if needed. A good set of policies should aid, not stifle, organizations. They should help people understand if they are on track in terms of mission and activities, and they should help define whether goals are being attained.

Policies can be straightforward or complex and can vary from a simple one-page statement to lengthy, sophisticated two-thousand-page legislation. It is also important to recognize that sometimes unwritten policies drive the direction of government and community organizational activity (e.g., personal agendas, availability of financial resources).

2 Can you provide some examples of unwritten policy?

So how does the presence of healthy public policy affect people with a disability?

Without consideration for persons with disabilities enshrined within an organization's mandate, it is easy for services to be eliminated, ignored, or forgotten, especially with budget reviews, changes in trends, and changes in leadership. As such, policy can serve as a means of ensuring social justice, reducing inequities, and protecting civil rights and interests.

The following scenarios provide insight into how policy may affect you (positively or negatively) as a practitioner and how important it is in the lives of persons with disabilities. The first scenario shows that policy at the school board level directly influences budget decisions about active living programmes for people with a disability. The others demonstrate that policies (or the lack of) at the level of the community and institution can directly impact on the accessibility of opportunities for active living.

Scenario 1: Harry is an adapted physical education teacher. One of his roles is to report regularly to the school board about his programme. A few years ago, Harry nearly lost his job because the school board had to cut costs. Adapted physical education was on the chopping block. Through a well-developed case demonstrating the value and benefits of the adapted physical education programme, and with support from parents and students, the school board reversed its initial budget policy decision and his services were maintained.

Scenario 2: Andrew is twenty-five years of age and lives in a small community in northern Canada. His family is on a fixed income, which hardly provides more than the bare necessities of life. Andrew has diabetes and has lost a leg due to circulatory problems brought on by his health problem. He would like to become involved in skating but he cannot afford skates, transportation to the rink (which is five miles away), or the admission fee for public skating. He also needs lessons on amputee skating, but there doesn't seem to be an instructor in his community. When he approached the municipal recreation department to inquire about possible supports, he was told that no policies existed that could meet the needs of individuals like him.

Scenario 3: Ann, an avid swimmer and wheelchair user, was unable to access a neighbourhood pool in her home town of Stockville. The town council had decided that "access to all" was too costly and declined requests to make the pool physically accessible.

Scenario 4: Peter participates in the Special Olympics. A recent policy change in his community provided for an integrated Summer Games. He now trains and competes in the same facilities with his friends—and for the same audiences as other athletes in that community.

Scenario 5: Karla is a therapeutic recreation (TR) coordinator in a nursing home. With the increased demand on nursing homes, it was decided that her facility would focus on older adults who required moderate to heavy nursing care. The facility policy for therapeutic recreation in nursing homes in Karla's district stated that the TR specialist-to-patient ratio for this level of care was one specialist for every forty patients. Therefore, Karla was able to add three new TR positions.

Each of these examples provides clues about what policy is and why it is extremely important to adapted physical activity. Ask yourself the following questions:

- What are the policy issues in each scenario?
- What are the different kinds of policy described in each of these case studies (e.g., budget, transportation, programme, etc.)?
- Who are the people who are making key decisions in each of these cases?
- Who needs to influence whom within the policy process?
- How can the input of people who are directly affected impact the nature of the policies that support adapted physical activity?
- When do policy approaches to active living have a greater impact than individual approaches?

---

3 Can you provide other scenarios of policies that could affect you, your community, your organization, and people with disabilities, positively and negatively?

A variety of public settings provide the backdrop for adapted physical activity, e.g., schools, workplaces, community indoor and outdoor facilities, provincial and national parks and museums. Each setting has its own orientation to policy and how it is developed. However, in all settings, policy that drives programmes and the allocation of resources is being based increasingly on evidence-based decision-making, (i.e., what evidence exists that a particular approach will be effective?). Therefore, individuals and groups must supply solid arguments in support of their case or approach (Mullen et al. 1995) and, where possible, give examples where similar actions have resulted in positive outcomes.

Step Two: Understanding Key Policy Issues in Adapted Physical Activity and Disability

Why create policies that foster inclusion of persons with a disability? What policy options will make it easier for people with a disability to be involved in physical activity? How can these policies be made easier for policy-makers to choose? In 1997, Judge Rosalie Silberman Abella addressed the social and policy changes that have paralleled the new policy perspectives on active living for Canadians with a disability.

One hundred years ago, the role of women was almost exclusively domestic; 50 years ago, some visible minorities were deprived of citizenship; 25 years ago, native people lacked a policy voice; and 10 years ago, disabled persons were routinely kept dependent. Today, none of these exclusionary assumptions are acceptable. (Government of Canada 1984)

However, perhaps the following comment by a recreation practitioner sums up the necessity for attention to policy that increases opportunities for people with a disability: "All this should be done so that the individual with disabilities can have an OK day." (Aylman in Lyons 1991, p. 2)

The presence of exclusionary practices contradicts the Canadian values of fairness, equality and respect for individual rights, values that Canada has assumed a leadership role in promoting worldwide. Nevertheless, there is much work to be done to improve our own record of discrimination. For example, we do not need to look far to see examples of inequities and systemic discriminatory practices. Systemic discrimination refers to the exclusion of certain groups of people through the application of policies and practices. These policies and practices are not programme, activity, or service related, nor are they required for the safe operation of the programme, activity, or service. Systemic discrimination creates barriers. These barriers are embedded in an organization's ways of carrying out its business as stipulated in the organization's policies, procedures, standards, rules, regulations, and practices, written and unwritten (Active Living Alliance for Canadians with a Disability 1994).

The following are key reasons why we need policies that support the inclusion of people with a disability.

- Many persons with a disability have been restricted from participation in the past. Policies that encourage and support opportunities are required **to make amends for the inadequacies and the constraints of the past.**

- Persons with a disability should feel **comfortable and welcome to participate** in physical activity, and have supports in place to ensure a safe and enjoyable experience. Policies are required for the provision of these supports.
- Persons with a disability may need to access **services that provide adaptations** for participating in physical activity. Policies are required to sustain and safeguard access to these services.
- Persons with a disability have a **right to access high quality facilities,** equipment and leadership on an equitable basis. As such, policies are needed which will safeguard this right.
- A fair and equitable portion of **budgets** dedicated to fostering recreation and physical activity should be devoted to persons with disabilities. Policies are required that ensure such allocations.
- Sometimes unique issues of access require **organizational decisions** (e.g., fees, participation, and renovations). These opportunities must be incorporated into the general set of access policies of a facility or service.

Policy that is written to include disadvantaged groups must be based on a clear ideology, or set of beliefs. In the context of adapted physical activity, **inclusive policy** has several fundamental dimensions. Inclusive policy

- safeguards access and participation in active living as a right of all Canadians
- respects the needs of each participant
- addresses the question, "Who is not in our programme?" and asks, "How do we include people with a disability?"
- respects, values and celebrates differences
- develops in consultation with 'community members' and builds consensus
- provides for shared authority and decision making
- ensures a safe and supportive environment

(Adapted from Active Living Alliance for Canadians with a Disability 1994)

Where does disability policy fit into the big picture of service delivery?

The value of policy development for persons with a disability is in its strategic use as a planning tool for service delivery decisions. It draws attention to the constraints faced in accessing opportunities for persons with a disability and also family members. It lays out the supports that are to be provided by a department or agency. In short, policy creates an awareness and knowledge of how issues of access will be dealt with and can help clarify where disability fits into the 'big picture' of service delivery. It has become popular to espouse a long list of benefits of physical activity to entice funders and consumers (Coyle et al. 1991). However, accumulating evidence of the value of physical activity can be overwhelming for some organizations as they try to determine what specific benefits they will aim for and with whom (Lyons 1994). Creation of policy can provide structure to an organization that is carefully considering its priorities.

How does one provide for sustainability and growth in services?

Without the establishment of services to persons with disabilities as a clear mandate of schools, municipalities, and public and private sector services, the realities of fiscal restraint and the ever-changing socio-political climate make these services very vulnerable to budgetary cutbacks. Too often, adapted physical activity has been supported by short-term projects with little sustainability once the project funds run out. However, policy development or change must pay careful attention to the following questions:

1. **What target population are we addressing with respect to a policy recommendation?**
   When we say "people with a disability," whom are we referring to? Chronic health problems, the largest producers of disability, are the major

health issues in Canada today. Health problems such as cancer, heart disease, stroke, diabetes, and asthma create substantive disabilities for people. However, the general public does not often include these populations when they think about disability. Also, people fail to consider the impact of disability as a family issue. The prevalence of disabling conditions and the widespread impact of disability are the kinds of information that need to be made public in order help to position disability as a big policy issue in Canada, affecting a large portion of the population.

2. **What is the intrusiveness of illness and disability on quality of life? What are the costs of inaction?**
   There is considerable evidence of suicide ideation, depression, poverty, and low self-esteem in the population of people with a disability. These problems result in lost wages, dependence, caregiver burden and burnout, and health costs (Lyons 1994). Policy-makers perk up and pay attention when we talk about connecting the issue (disability) with the 'big picture' (e.g., health care costs).

3. **What are the activity constraints and disability adjustment processes that policies will address?**
   In order to enhance opportunities for inclusion, we have sometimes downplayed what it takes to involve people with a disability in meaningful, healthy physical activity. What may be considered leisure for a person without a disability may be work for a person with a disability, due to the amount of time and energy required. For instance, in research on active living and multiple sclerosis, physical and mental energy must be allocated very carefully. Many activities, due to location, time of day, or the work needed to prepare to attend them, become more work

than enjoyment (Lyons and Meade 1993). Policies that address the details that will make active living pleasurable (e.g., reduced fees, transportation, staff training) and those responsible for implementing them, are critical. Obviously, the social rules and roles regarding responsibility for active living and disability are often very unclear in our society. Policy can help determine roles and clarify them for staff members and consumers.

4. **How do you get beyond all talk, no action?**
   There is a vast array of possibilities to focus on when it comes to policy, and it is easy for staff members to get bogged down. Rather than think broadly, think basic and strategic. Focus on the things that will truly make a difference. From the authors' experience in this field, three critical areas include allocating staff, establishing committees that can support the work of staff and volunteers, and building linkages between different service delivery systems (schools, workplaces, hospitals, etc.), so that appropriate services are developed, and so that there is continuity of service (e.g., a referral system between rehabilitation hospitals and community recreation departments).

Step Two has outlined why it is important to develop policies and analyze policies related to disability and active living. It has included relevant policy milestones that underline current policy and methods to help design a rationale for building healthy public policy for persons with a disability.

4 Think back to a field placement associated with this or other courses. How would you answer the questions in Step Two as they relate to the population or issue that you are interested in?

Step Three: Learning How Policy Is Made and Influenced

As a practitioner, one of the key things you can do is to contribute policy-relevant information for policy-makers. Such information would help others to identify, within their own situations, points of entry into the policy-making process, sources of support, and strategies to enhance the feasibility of particular policy options. It is important to be knowledgeable about the elements of policy frameworks. Generally, policy frameworks have four major elements.

POLICY FRAMEWORK: FOUR MAJOR ELEMENTS

1. Policy determinants
   The forces that shape the policy agenda (changes in social norms and values, traditions, changes in social conditions, and the political system within which policy decisions are made). Through the interaction of these forces during the policy process, a determination of changing needs, values attached to active living, opportunities, and differences in conditions for active living will emerge.

2. Policy content
   The clear statements of objectives and issues to be resolved; the enunciation of goals (intentions, principles, directions); arguments and rationale supporting the direction (including the underlying value system, causal assumptions, factual assertions, and calculations); instruments of implementation (authority, networks, funds, organization); and, expected impact or standard of success (direct, political, economic, social).

3. Policy process
   Process normally covers the following areas (the extent of coverage will depend on the nature of the issue at hand): devising ways of addressing and defining the public problem; formulating the policy, including the forging of means and

assessment of the feasibility of implementation; adopting the policy (public debate, parliamentary review and legislation); and the monitoring of success and failure.

4. Political community
People who are involved in the active living movement (citizens, groups, organizations) who share in the active living vision and strategies. They are an integral part of the movement for the advancement of active living and complement each other in their actions. They determine (based on historical patterns, prevailing beliefs, and the accumulation of previous policy decisions in the sector) the pattern of policy making that prevails for the sector (Health Canada 1995).

Policies should

- be simple, understandable, and practical
- be operationally feasible and measurable
- be flexible
- direct change
- show consistency between ideology and practice
- be responsive to consumer needs
- be directly relevant to constraints on physical activity
- be responsive to cultural characteristics and community characteristics
- be cognizant of current events or situations
- have direct application to everyday operations
- define roles and responsibilities
- be fiscally reasonable and responsible
- incorporate direction regarding resource utilization
- be consistent with general organizational polices
- be known and supported by key community agencies

MAJOR STAGES TO POLICY DEVELOPMENT: HOW TO BUILD EFFECTIVE POLICIES

Decision-making is not a single event. There are various approaches, or stages, in the policy development process.

1. **Observation and description:** Describe the key facts about the policy issue, process issues, and policy context. What are the components and the context of this issue? What are people's experiences of this issue?

2. **Analysis:** Identify the major issues, interests, costs, and benefits. What has taken place to create this issue? What has taken place to address this issue? How successful were efforts to address the issue? What were the costs and benefits, and to whom? What does the 'best practice' literature suggest?

3. **Options identification:** Identify the most likely choices to satisfy key stakeholders and avoid their major fears. What are the time frames?

4. **Advice:** Recommendations should include policy choices as well as next steps. How can the case be made? How will this approach be evaluated? What provision exists to change the policy if it doesn't produce anticipated results?

How can these efforts be implemented? Together is better; establish a small policy committee. Members can include individuals with a disability, staff, parents, university faculty, community agencies, and so forth. Decide upon a plan of action with deadlines and decision-making processes. Draft policy statements and submit statements for feedback. Submit proposed policies. Ensure that policies are followed. Evaluate and revise as necessary.

Any multistage process, in reality, never works systematically from one stage to the next. Many stages occur simultaneously and there is often a forward and backward motion to these processes. Usually the evidence brought to bear in influencing the process is not one single study or report, but a summary and synthesis of knowledge related to the issue (Lomas 2000). There are three interrelated domains that are useful to understand in the problem of decision-making: the structure (formal and informal), the values (beliefs and ideologies), and the information (producers and purveyors). There are also a number of factors to keep in mind when thinking about policy development:

- the balance between the individual good and the collective good
- time frames and budget cycles–when are your efforts most likely to effect change (could be tied to government spending cycles)
- the power of intersectoral action (people from different areas acting together)
- the language that the policy community uses as compared with the language of other sectors, i.e., each sector has it own set of terms that are understood within the sector
- the impact of the economic climate on policy

Examples of methods of policy development include:

1. Causal model evaluation–e.g., an incident occurs necessitating the development of a policy to deal with the current situation and future such incidences.
2. Consultation method–e.g., a townhall meeting is held to gain insight and input from the community in order to develop a relevant policy to address a particular concern.
3. Evaluation method–e.g., a trial period is held, after which a policy is re-examined and adjustments made accordingly.

Rating the Feasibility of a New Policy

---

1. What is the issue or problem?
2. What is the approach? What evidence exists for its effectiveness?
3. Is there a clear target population?
4. What changes can be expected by using this approach?
5. Is the approach feasible within the finances available?
6. Is there evidence from an economic or cost benefit analysis of the value of this approach?
7. Does this approach increase the capacity of communities and groups?
8. Does this approach capitalize on existing resources?
9. Is this approach sustainable?

SOURCE: Adapted from *Policy Analysis in Government: A Policy Wonk's Travel Guide* by I. Potter, 1997, unpublished manuscript; "Influencing the Policy Process with Qualitative Research" by R. Rist, 1994, in N.K. Denzin and Y.S. Lincoln (Eds.), *Handbook of Qualitative Research* (pp. 545–57). London: Sage. Adapted with permission.

SAMPLE POLICY ANALYSIS

A Policy Checklist for Municipal Recreation Services and Disability

This handy checklist could be adapted for any number of settings. It provides a menu of key factors that influence active living and disability that could be addressed in an organization's policies. The checklist and sample policies are from the publication *Municipal Government Policy Guidelines: Recreation Services for Persons with a Disability* (Lyons 1991). The key questions are: Does the organization have policies related to each of the following items? What are they?

The following are samples of questions that can be developed for several of the policy checklist items and samples of policy statements about them. These samples are a combination of statements from various communities across Canada which were collected from a study of municipal policies related to disability (Lyons 1991).

Policy Checklist

1. Departmental Roles and Responsibilities
   Statement of Beliefs   0
   Goals   0
   Objectives   0
   Evaluation   0

2. Programmes and Services
   Needs Assessment   0
   Leisure Education/Counselling   0
   Leisure Programmes   0
   Advocacy   0
   Financial Assistance   0
   Transportation   0
   Physical Accessibility   0
   Consultation/Collaboration   0
   Human Resource Development   0
   Promotion   0

3. Resources
   Budget   0
   Human Resources   0
   Facilities   0
   Equipment   0

Sample Policy Questions and Statements Related to Beliefs

What are the overriding ideologies of the department with respect to access to recreation and leisure opportunities for persons with a disability? How do they relate to departmental roles?

- "We believe all people have the right to become educated about the concept of leisure and to participate in recreational programmes and services of their choice. The use of leisure time is recognized as being an important and integral part of the quality of life for all people."
- "We believe in the need for support such as volunteers, staff, finances, information, adaptations to equipment, facilities, and services to ensure participation of people with disabilities."

- "We believe in the creation of an atmosphere where positive attitudes toward leisure integration are fostered and developed through collaborative efforts within the department, the entire municipal operation and the community at large…. Full community input and support is essential if the leisure integration process is to become operational. This input will help ensure that a proactive stance towards participation is nurtured."

Sample Policy Questions and Statements Related to Goals

What does the department hope to accomplish?

- "To identify leisure needs of persons with disabilities and to facilitate their participation in the life of the community."
- "To enable persons with disabilities to participate in leisure and recreation."

Sample Policy Questions and Statements Related to Objectives

What are the specific target areas that the department wishes to pursue?

- "To find out the leisure needs of consumers and caregivers."
- "To address the feasibility of developing support services for people with disabilities/special needs."
- "To develop a staff training plan."
- "To develop a strategy to promote our mandate and services to and for disabled users."
- "To develop a programme plan detailing recreation and culture opportunities for persons with disabilities or special needs."

Sample Policy Statement Related to Resources

The true measure of commitment to persons with a disability is demonstrated when a department devotes a portion of its physical, fiscal, and human resources to this area. The commitment may be related to the proportion of the population or based on needs and priorities.

- "In a town of 113,000, integration services has 10 percent of the recreation section budget and 20 percent of the staff allocation. This is informal, unwritten policy, but supported by the department."

In Step Three, we have included information on the components of a policy framework, what good policies include, the major stages in policy development, and several tools to assist you in organizing a policy process and conducting policy analyses.

---

5 Can you design an exercise to test the policy process? What organization or agency might you choose? How would you approach the organization or agency? What elements of Step Three would you use in building the policy process?

Step Four: Practicing the Art and Science of Policy Development

POLICY IMPLICATIONS—WHAT CAN I DO?

The following case study illustrates concerns that have arisen because of a lack of policy to address the issue. The ensuing exercise outlines a process to fill this void. The process is adapted from *Advocacy, the Process* (Active Living Alliance for Canadians with a Disability 1990).

Read the case study and work through the steps. Remember, there are no right or wrong answers. While every situation requiring policy will be unique and require its own solutions, the process described below is generic and can be applied across many settings.

CASE STUDY

Brenda was a first-year physical educator in a high school in rural Manitoba. In addition to her teaching duties, Brenda also coached several interscholastic teams including the senior girls' cross-country team in the fall and track team in the spring. Josie, a student who was

blind and ran with a tether and a sighted guide, was on the cross-country team. During the cross-country regional finals, Brenda was disappointed that, despite Josie's success during lead-up competitions, the school 'policy' related to budget did not permit provisions to support sending Josie's sight guide to out-of-town competitions. This was especially disturbing because the boys' football team was supported to participate in several exhibition games, including an out-of-province weekend event at a cost substantially greater than that needed to send an additional person to the cross-country finals.

During the spring track season, Brenda decided to take action when Josie's participation in a competition was once again constrained by a lack of funds to support the travel of her guide to an out-of-town event.

WHAT COULD/DID SHE DO?

The following section will walk you through a process for creating policy change, provide you with some valuable tips, and prompt you to apply this knowledge to the case study.

Phase One—Issue Identification and Support

STEP 1—DEFINE THE KEY ISSUE

Remember to talk about issues rather than solutions. To do this, you need to identify the central problem or need. A long list of issues can be overwhelming. Try to focus on a single issue and the source of the problem.

Finding funding support for Josie's guide is a solution, not an issue. Perhaps the issue is that there is no policy to address access for students with disabilities. List the possible sources of this problem.

If several issues appear to be equally important, choose the one most likely to be successfully resolved. By achieving one success, you are paving the way for subsequent advocacy efforts.

---

6 What is the key issue? Is it a gender inequity issue? Is it a budgetary issue? Is it a disability issue? Who are the people affected by this issue and how are they affected?

STEP 2—GATHER INFORMATION

Once the key issue is identified, it is time to gather information related to the issue. The amount of information you gather will depend upon the issue, the amount of time you have to prepare your case, the resources (staff, budget, etc.), and the availability of information.

7 What, if any, existing policies address the problem? Who are the key people to approach for help in rectifying the problem?

STEP 3—IDENTIFY SUPPORTERS

Now that the information is gathered, it is time to begin identifying potential supporters. Try to attract support from the following:

- consumers (those affected by the issue)
- decision-makers (those who could resolve the issue)
- public (community advocacy groups, teachers, etc.)

Find 'legitimizers'–those that have a reputation for doing good things for the 'community'–and gain their endorsement; when they endorse your issue they help to legitimize it.

8 Who is affected by the issue (e.g., participants? classmates? other coaches? parents?). Whose decisions could resolve the issue? Whose 'stamp of approval' would be helpful? Which groups or individuals may have an interest in the issue?

Phase Two—Make A Plan

STEP 1—REVIEW THE ISSUE AND IDENTIFY PREFERRED SOLUTION(S)

Review your answers to the following questions: What is the key issue? Why is it a problem? Who does it affect? How does it affect them? Who can resolve the issue? Whose support would help?

Now identify the preferred solution. Be as specific as possible. For most issues, the ideal and the realistic solution may be the same.

For complex issues, you may need to set a short-term target.

Remember that the simple, straightforward solution is often the best. Be careful not to blow a problem out of proportion that can make people defensive rather than supportive.

9 What policy outcome might Brenda and Josie anticipate as a result of successful changes? What would these changes be? What are the policy implications for elsewhere 'in the system?' Who would be affected and how?

STEP 2—DECIDE ON THE ROUTE

Identify who is/are the key decision-makers and the process for policy decisions. Find out others' opposing views; know their arguments and develop a strategy to counter these arguments. Identify the process of policy change. Do you have to get on the agenda of a board or committee meeting? Will you be required to submit a letter or document outlining the issue and your recommended solution(s)?

Approaching the wrong person or organization wastes time and causes frustration. Do not expect someone to change something if they have no influence in that area. Be sure to identify and reach out to those who do have the authority to make policy changes.

10 Who are the potential decision-makers (e.g., school board, parent/teacher association, principal, interscholastic athletic association, others)? What are some of the possible arguments to your proposed policy? What might you do to counter these arguments?

STEP 3—DEVELOP AN ACTION PLAN

1. **Brainstorm every potential strategy** for gaining support. Possible strategies might include circulating a petition, attending a parent/teacher association meeting, talking to the media, writing to the school board.
2. **Select the best strategy.** Remember, it is often necessary to educate the various individuals/groups in order to achieve a

favourable resolution; prepare back-up strategies in case first efforts fail.

3. **Formalize the action plan and prepare to implement it.** Organize yourself to achieve your goal (e.g., develop a committee and assign specific tasks to committee members).

---

11 What are the possible strategies and actions that would support Brenda's efforts to change or implement new policy? Identify those strategies that you feel merit most attention and effort. Why did you select these? What are the key steps in an action plan to implement these strategies?

Phase Three—Act On Your Plan!

IMPLEMENT THE PLAN

1. **Create a positive image** by taking a positive approach and building on past successes.
2. **Involve supporters** by raising public awareness of existing supporters and involving these individuals in the process.
3. **Schedule action steps,** remembering that timing is critical (e.g., select opportune moments to present the issue). Continue to focus on the issue and make constructive suggestions for resolving it.
4. **Present the issue** by sending a formal letter to the appropriate authority explaining the issue and requesting action. Find out what process they use to deal with an issue. Prepare a written brief with copies for each member. Inform your supporters to ensure their attendance. Work to make them feel that it is their issue, too. During the presentation, be positive and professional. By offering to cooperate with the decision-makers, you open the door for a positive reception of your issue. Give them a chance to change their minds gracefully.

---

12 What needs to be done to rectify the situation? How is this issue impacting on others? Draft a written brief outlining Brenda's issue. Create a policy statement that might serve to meet this need.

Possible road blocks and potential remedies might include the following:

Denial that the issue is a problem.
- Present your facts and figures.
- Place the onus on those who are responsible to prove that the issue is not a problem.

The issue is a low priority.
- Rally your supporters—the more, the better.
- Arrange media coverage.

There is no money available to support the desired change.
- Present a list of supporters (be sure to include your 'legitimizers').
- Arrange media coverage.
- Suggest a viable compromise.

You are getting the run-around.
- If your approach is correct, don't back down.
- If another 'system' would be more appropriate, try it.
- Set reasonable deadlines for action and monitor progress.
- Arrange media coverage.

If all else fails, remember, many first-time efforts are not enough. Have patience…everything you do is cumulative.

Phase Four—Evaluate
Assess the results. It should be possible to note positive changes which have occurred, and to identify areas which still need improvement.

1. **Examine the process**—What was the process? What were the key milestones in the process? What worked and what didn't work? Why? Even efforts that appear at first glance to have failed may have planted seeds that will eventually lead to future successes.

2. **Examine outcomes and impacts**–They may include an increase in levels of awareness, or of participation, changes in programme focus or changes in the quality of service. These are changes which occur over a period of time. They may include overall participation rates, performance improvements, and other behavioural changes.

3. **Acknowledge help**–Publicly thank individuals and agencies that helped to bring about positive change. Such acknowledgment helps attract allies for similar issues and efforts in the future.

Summary
This chapter has provided an introduction to adapted physical activity and policy. The chapter organized around an introduction and four learning objectives: understanding policy and why it's important; examining the key policy issues in adapted physical activity and disability; learning about how policy is developed; and practicing policy development. The chapter included information on what makes a helpful policy, how policies impact people with disabilities, and the field of adapted physical activity.

Although we set out processes for policy development, in real life, the process is not very linear and, in some cases, not altogether logical. Since we are talking about a process shaped by many factors including politics, public interest, timing, and sometimes crises, the role of the advocate and professional is to inject the best evidence and strategy to shape final results, and to ensure that unhelpful policies that constrain opportunities do not occur. The key is to be flexible, creative, and determined.

The chapter provided templates, examples, the use of a case study to practice policy-making, as well as critical thinking questions within each section. However, in order to transfer your reading to real-life situations, it will be important to find opportunities to immerse yourself in real-life situations. Placements, applied health research papers, and contact with policy-makers are your best avenues.

Increasingly, every field of endeavour is discovering the important role that policy plays in its work. We need good research on best practices in adapted physical activity, and those practices must impact policy. Policies are the key decisions that influence service provision, resource allocation, and the sustainability of service. We must all share the responsibilities for these efforts. That is the path to becoming a policy guru.

Study Questions
There is no doubt that we require systematic examination of good models of policy development in adapted physical activity and how to influence the policy process. Evaluation of research is new for practitioners in this area. Some questions that could be researched include:

1. What strategies inspire organizations to develop policy on disability?
2. Does policy actually influence access to opportunities? What are the steps that lead from policy to action?
3. Which people seem to be assisted by policy and who remains untouched by this process?
4. Are there a core set of policy issues that are central and others that are peripheral?
5. What are service agencies prepared to commit to? Is there some consistency, or is it variable? What are the determinants?
6. What can be learned from experiences that address other problems among other disadvantaged groups that would be useful for disability-related policy (e.g., women's rights, aboriginal rights)?

Acknowledgment

Very sincere thanks are extended to Dawn Schmidt, office administrator, AHPRC, for her editorial and word-processing savvy.

References

Abella, Rosalie S. (1984). *Report of the Commission on Equality in Employment/Rosalie Silberman Abella, commissioner.* Ottawa: Supply and Services Canada.

Active Living Alliance for Canadians with a Disability (1990). *Advocacy, the process: A resource in support of Canadians with a disability.* Gloucester, ON: Author.

Active Living Alliance for Canadians with a Disability. (1994). *The inclusion action pack: Increasing active living opportunities for persons with a disability.* Ottawa: AIS Publishing Solutions.

Active Living Alliance for Canadians with a Disability, and Health Canada. (1998). *Active living for Canadians with a disability: A blueprint for action.* Ottawa: Author.

Canada. Federal Task Force on Disability Issues. (1996). *The will to act: Equal citizenship for Canadians with disabilities.* Hull, QC: Minister of Public Works and Government Services of Canada.

Canada. Federal Task Force on Disability Issues. (1997). *The will to act: Equal citizenship for Canadians with disabilities.* Hull, QC: Human Resources Development Canada.

Canada. Department of the Secretary of State. (1993). Pathway to integration: Final report, mainstream 1992. In *Federal/provincial/territorial review of services affecting Canadians with disabilities: Report to ministers of social services.* Ottawa: Health Canada, Social Service Programs Branch.

Canada. Department of Secretary of State. (1991). *The national strategy for the integration of persons with disabilities.* Ottawa: Disabled Persons Secretariat.

Canada. Parliament. House of Commons. Special Committee on the Disabled and the Handicapped. (1981). *Obstacles: Report of the special committee on the disabled and handicapped.* 32nd Parliament, 1st Session. 3rd report. Ottawa: Dept. of the Secretary of State.

Coyle, C.P., Kinney, W.B., Riley, B., and Shank, J.W. (1991). *Benefits of therapeutic recreation: A consensus view.* Philadelphia: Temple University.

Devon Dodd, J., Buchan, M., Chaperlin, M, Crossman, D., and Oram, J. (1997). *Moving beyond hope: Consumers and communities in policy development.* Ottawa: Health Canada. (Available from Health Canada, Health Promotion and Programmes Branch, Suite 1802, MTT Building, 1505 Barrington Street, Halifax, NS B3J 3Y6).

Fitness Canada. (1988). *An information and communications guide for leaders.* Ottawa: Author.

Guarnieri, A., and Bennett, C. (1999). *Reflecting interdependence: Disability, parliament, government and the community: Report of sub-committee on Status of Persons with*

Disabilities. Ottawa: Human Resources Development Canada.

Hancock, T. (1982, August). Beyond health care. *The Futurist,* 4–13.

Health Canada. (1995). *Fitness strategic directions (1995–96): The policy and planning function.* Ottawa: Author.

Herchmer, B. (1994). Policy: a four letter word?? A question of planning and community development. *Journal of Leisurability, 21*(3), 32–34.

Human Resources Development Canada/Office of Disability Issues. (1998). *In unison: A Canadian approach to disability issues: Federal/provincial/territorial ministers responsible for social services discussion paper.* Ottawa: Author.

Jasper Talks. (1988). *Proceedings of the Jasper talks: Strategies for change in adapted physical activity in Canada.* Ottawa: CAHPER.

Lomas, J. (2000). Connecting research and policy. *ISUMA 1* (Spring).

Lyons, R. (1991). *Municipal government policy guidelines: Recreation services for persons with a disability.* Ottawa: Canadian Parks and Recreation Association.

Lyons, R. (1994). Recreation policy and disability: Where to from here? *Journal of Leisurability, 21*(3), 3–11.

Lyons, R., and Meade, D. (1993). The energy crisis: Mothers with chronic illness. *Canadian Woman Studies, 13*(4), 34–37.

Mayer, D., and Thompson, M. (1982). A case study of policy: Process, development and implementation. *Journal of Leisurability, 9*(3), 13–19.

Milio, N. (1988). Making healthy public policy: Developing the science by learning the art: An ecological framework for policy studies. *Health Promotion: An International Journal, 2*(3), 263–74.

Milio, N. (1986). *Promoting health through public policy* (2nd. ed.). Ottawa: Canadian Public Health Association.

Mullen, P., Evans, D., Forster, J., Gottlieb, N., Kreuter, M., Moon, R., O'Rourke, T., and Strecher, V. (1995). Settings as an important dimension in health education/promotion policy, programmes and research. *Health Education Quarterly 22*(3), 329–41.

O'Neill, M. and Pederson, A. (1992). Building a methods bridge between public policy analysis and healthy public policy. *Canadian Journal of Public Health, 83* (Suppl. 1), S25–S30.

Potter, I. (1997). *Policy analysis in government: A policy wonk's travel guide.* Unpublished manuscript.

Rist, R. (1994). Influencing the policy process with qualitative research. In N.K. Denzin and Y.S. Lincoln (Eds.), *Handbook of qualitative research* (pp. 545–57). London: Sage.

United Nations. (1976). *Proclamation of 1981 as the international year of disabled persons: Resolution A/RES 31/123.*

World Health Organization. International Conference on Health Promotion. (1997). *Jakarta declaration on health promotion in the 21st century.*

CHAPTER 8

The Role of Canadian Organizations in the Development of Adapted Physical Activity

Case Studies of the Active Living Alliance for Canadians with a Disability and the Canadian Paralympic Committee

David F.H. Legg

Learning Objectives

- To appreciate the role of Canadian organizations on the development of adapted physical activity.
- To understand the roles and challenges facing specific organizations dedicated to facilitating physical activity, sport, and recreation programmes for persons with disabilities.

Introduction

Several organizations have played an integral role in Canada's development of adapted physical activity. Among these are organizations that focus on active living, sport, recreation, and inclusion. While a number of organizations have played a significant role in promoting adapted physical activity, two will be profiled in this chapter: the Active Living Alliance (ALA) for Canadians with a Disability and the Canadian Paralympic Committee (CPC). Within the CPC's profile a significant sector will be devoted to the evolution of the Canadian Wheelchair Sports Association (CWSA). The CPC and ALA were chosen because of the broad multidisability nature of their partners and, secondly, because of their focus on both sport and active living issues.

Organization Profiles

ACTIVE LIVING ORGANIZATIONS FOR PERSONS WITH DISABILITIES

The Active Living Alliance for Canadians with a Disability (www.ala.ca) is a consortium of national organizations with similar mandates to enable active lifestyles for persons with disabilities. Since 1989, partner organizations to the alliance have included:

- Aboriginal Sport Circle (ASC)
- Active Living Coalition for Older Adults (ALCOA)
- Canadian Amputee Sports Association (CASA)
- Canadian Association for Disabled Skiing (CADS)
- Canadian Association for Health, Physical Education, Recreation, and Dance (CAHPERD)
- Canadian Blind Sports Association (CBSA)
- Canadian Cerebral Palsy Sports Association (CCPSA)
- Canadian Council of the Blind (CCB)
- Canadian Deaf Sports Association (CDSA)
- Canadian Intramural Recreation Association (CIRA)
- Canadian National Institute for the Blind (CNIB)
- Canadian Paralympic Committee (CPC)
- Canadian Paraplegic Association (CPA)
- Canadian Parks and Recreation Association (CPRA)
- Canadian Recreational Canoeing Association (CRCA)
- Canadian Red Cross Society (CRCS)
- Canadian Therapeutic Recreation Association (CTRA)
- Canadian Wheelchair Sports Association (CWSA)
- Health Canada, Fitness and Active Living Unit
- Learning Disabilities Association of Canada
- National Network for Mental Health
- The Roeher Institute
- Special Olympics Canada (SOC)
- YMCA

The idea of an alliance began at the Jasper Talks, where Dr. Robert Steadward and Dr. Ted Wall of the University of Alberta created an opportunity for discussion among Canadian professionals in the field of programmes and initiatives for persons with disabilities. In 1989 the alliance was formally created and, for the first time, received financial assistance from the federal government to pursue seven goals, or roles, reflected in a *Blueprint for Action* which had been written by the Alliance Coordinating Committee (Steadward et al. 1997).

Goal 1

The first goal described in the *Blueprint for Action* (first written in 1987, with subsequent editions published in 1993 and 1997) was to facilitate the growth of self-empowered individuals through awareness, education, and support (Active Living Alliance for Canadians with a Disability 1998). The alliance has pursued this goal by facilitating the development of advocacy groups and producing an *Advocacy in Action* workshop and video. Three other resources, *Words with Dignity*, *Fit for All*, and *Positive Images*, all first published in 1990, promoted the appropriate use of terminology when referring to individuals with disabilities. In 1997, the alliance, in cooperation with the Canadian Parks and Recreation Association (CPRA), developed *Opening Doors: Keys to Inclusive Recreation Policy for Persons with Disabilities* (Steadward et al. 1997).

The goal of self-empowerment was also facilitated through the creation of the Moving to Inclusion programme. This initiative was part of the Canadian government's project Active Living Through Physical Education: Maximizing Opportunities for Students with a Disability. This programme facilitated the inclusion of persons with disabilities into society while operating under the premise that participation in physical education is an important benefit for all students, including those with disabilities. This project, funded by Health Canada Fitness Program, was coordinated by the alliance, along with ten participating national partners and twelve provincial and territorial ministers of education. Led by Dr. Donna Goodwin and Dr. Dave Fitzpatrick, it developed a series of manuals categorized by both specific disability and leadership development components. Each of the nine resources, in complete and condensed versions, were intended to assist teachers in planning and teaching physical education classes that included students with disabilities. The manuals included adaptations to curriculum activities and other considerations, such as adaptations to space, distance, equipment, rules, and instructional strategies, which could enable the effective inclusion of a person with a disability (Active Living Alliance for Canadians with a Disability 1994).

Self-empowerment was also pursued through a marketing campaign initiated in 1999 when the alliance underwent a comprehensive strategic planning process that resulted in a new vision, Viabilité. Viabilité foresaw a 20 percent decrease in physical inactivity of persons with disabilities. This vision reflected, in part, federal Minister of Health Allan Rock's goal of seeing a 10 percent decrease in physical inactivity of all Canadians (Rock 1999).

From a choice of five options, Viabilité was selected, in part, because it was derived from the English words *viable* and *viability*, and the French words *viable* and *viabilité*. All of these terms represent either the premise of being able to live and grow independently or a process leading to a productive end result. The root *via* also suggested that a person could achieve health benefits by way of active living, while *ability* was perceived to have a positive association, in comparison to what some considered a negative connotation with the term *disability*. Finally, Viabilité could be appropriately presented in both English and French, a major communications advantage in Canada (Legg 2001).

Following the selection of Viabilité, the alliance developed a nationwide social marketing campaign. It was hoped that this plan would ultimately have a similar impact on the public's consciousness that the brand names Imagine had for volunteerism and Particip-ACTION had for active living. While Viabilité's

impact has yet to be assessed at the community level, it has already received a tremendous amount of support from the alliance's political partners. In June 1999, the federal, provincial, and territorial ministers responsible for fitness and active living publicly supported Viabilité and its social marketing campaign. Their support reflected, in part, a growing concern that health care costs in Canada were skyrocketing and recognition that physical activity could address this dilemma (Legg 2001).

Goal 2

The second goal listed in the alliance's *Blueprint for Action* was to develop a series of systems and networks with clearly defined roles, responsibilities, and communication links at each level of society. Networks have been established through the recruitment of organizations, the formation of the coordinating committee, continuous interaction and liaison with the federal government though Fitness Canada, the development of Provincial and Territorial Initiatives (PTI), and the creation of resources for people in the community.

The PTI was a partnership approach designed to strengthen networks of provincially- and territorially-based communication links, with the hopes of furthering the goal of full and equitable access to active living opportunities for Canadians with disabilities. With the financial and administrative support of the Active Living Alliance for Canadians with a Disability, PTI representatives from across the country developed community driven strategies that reflect the unique needs and resources available to their particular province or territory (Bourne and Legg 1998; Lawrence and Legg 1998). In collaboration with a local, regional, provincial, or territorial organization, PTI volunteers took a community development approach. The results of these efforts were activities that benefitted different levels and various sectors within the community (Bourne and Legg 1998).

PTI evolved over a ten-year period that began with the Jasper Talks in 1986. Several years following the alliance's creation, it recognized that there was a need to address issues pertaining to 'grass-roots' communication. The alliance thus identified one individual from every province and territory who was connected with activities and programmes at the local level and asked them to form a "network of networks." This network of networks eventually became known as the Linkage Initiative and later as the Provincial/Territorial Initiative (Bourne and Legg 1998).

Despite a number of common values, similar activities, and coinciding organizations, each PTI representative showed a unique approach to facilitating physical activity for persons with disabilities. This variability was as a response to the different responsibilities assumed by each level of government, public and private sectors, and various organizations with a stake in the provision of active living opportunities. The resources available and priority given to active living and disability issues differ between the provinces and territories and this disparity has certainly made it challenging to develop a comprehensive national strategy (Bourne and Legg 1998).

As a response to this variability, it was determined that all representatives should identify their own priorities and establish committees to assist in carrying out these objectives. PTI representatives were also asked to identify an organization that might be able to support their activities and officially administer the seed funds allocated by the alliance. In some cases, this partner organization was a provincial or municipal parks and recreation department, while in others it was a disability-specific organization. Three examples of partnerships are the Alberta Recreation and Parks Association, L'Association québécoise pour le loisir des personnes handicapées (the Quebec Association for Recreation of Disabled Persons), and the Ontario March of Dimes (Bourne and Legg 1998).

Providing services for persons with disabilities has sometimes been difficult due to the diversity within what we classify as 'disability.' PTI representatives had therefore been encouraged to focus on activities that were generic enough to address a majority of persons, regardless of ability, and to reflect the guiding principles of the alliance. These principles centred on quality of life being a fundamental right, empowerment, equal access, and respect and dignity. The other option that PTI representatives pursued were activities or programmes pertaining to a specific disability in their geographic area (Bourne and Legg 1998).

A second concern for the PTI, and common to most not-for-profit organizations, was funding. The alliance provided funds to support core PTI activities, with continuing support from the Fitness and Active Living Unit of Health Canada officially secured in July 1998. Fiscal reliance on the federal government, however, is not ideal and the alliance has discussed several strategies that would allow them to become more financially independent. One significant hurdle in this pursuit, however, is that while being a separate entity, the alliance is also responsible to a number of national partners and their provincial counterparts. Fundraising, without competing directly with any of these stakeholders, is difficult. One way in which the PTI has attempted to remedy this situation is by focussing on the sales of alliance resources. PTI members sell these resources within their own communities and retain the majority of funds for continued provincial or territorial programmes. Only a minimal amount is returned to the alliance to cover production costs. PTI members also purchase these resources for a nominal fee from the alliance using seed monies provided to each representative. They are then distributed by them at no cost to the consumer (Bourne and Legg 1998).

A third concern for PTI members is the inability to reach persons with disabilities in small communities. The majority of PTI representatives have resided in either the largest populated city or political capital of their province or territory. Dissemination of information to the smaller communities is therefore a significant issue. Some members have tried to combat this concern by using the Internet (although its effectiveness in reaching those in lower socio-economic groups is debatable), while others reached out to more remote areas through a travelling workshop and slide show (Bourne and Legg 1998).

A fourth issue for the PTI focussed on volunteer recruitment. Many PTI representatives were involved in a number of volunteer commitments and, in many cases, may have worked professionally within the field of active living for persons with disabilities for a number of years. The subsequent PTI committees were reliant upon many of the same people who contributed for several years, and volunteer burnout was therefore of paramount concern. To address this issue, some PTI representatives tried to tap into previously overlooked groups and existing networks. One example of this was in Newfoundland where the PTI representative successfully partnered with the Red Cross to help promote the alliance mandate and resources through their already existing province-wide network of volunteers (Bourne and Legg 1998).

Goal 3

The third goal of the alliance was to enhance organizational planning and policy development. Here, considerable time and effort has been spent trying to formulate policies that encourage inclusion and appropriate portrayal of persons with disabilities.

Goal 4

The fourth goal includes the identification, development, and promotion of relevant opportunities and related services. Many national partners noted earlier have pursued this goal. Specific examples include programmes developed by the YMCA, the Royal Lifesaving Society, and the Canadian Red Cross Water Safety Services. In 2001, the alliance in partnership with the YMCA–Youth Exchanges Canada enabled one hundred young Canadians to attend the alliance's annual forum in St. Catharine's, Ontario.

Goal 5

The alliance's fifth goal was to develop and promote leadership that would facilitate participation in physical activity. A significant programme that addressed this goal was the Moving to Inclusion (MTI) initiative which was noted earlier. As part of this initiative, a nationwide training programme was developed where alliance representatives conducted professional development sessions for teachers. In 1991, the Leadership Development Model Package was created for organizations active in leadership development and, in 2001, a speaker's bureau called Activating Opportunities was instituted. The Inclusion Action Pack was also created to help organizations move from developing inclusive policies to implementing effective inclusive programmes.

Goals 6 and 7

The sixth goal of public awareness is being addressed primarily through the Viabilité campaign addressed earlier. Finally, the seventh goal was to identify, promote, and support research, and to communicate state of the art information. The alliance is a hub of information for the national partners, provincial and territorial network members, and other stakeholders primarily through e-mail and Web-based means. Specific to research, in 1997 the alliance began to award the Ted Wall Research Award to a graduate student completing research in the area of adapted physical activity (Steadward et al. 1997).

FUTURE CHALLENGES

The alliance will face a number of challenges while continuing to provide a significant and important voice within Canadian society. A significant variable will be the success of the Viabilité social marketing plan. One of their most significant challenges will be showing the government and other funding bodies that they were able to achieve the goals of a 20 percent reduction in physical inactivity among Canadians with disabilities. For these purposes the alliance has formed a research committee to address this issue, which has a number of inherent challenges, foremost being the lack of a baseline measurement of active living patterns for persons with disabilities. A second challenge will be broadening the association's resource base, as long-term funding from sponsors and those outside of the traditional government sectors will enable greater flexibility and security. To date, only Pfizer Canada, a pharmaceutical company, and Wintergreen, makers of adapted learning materials, are national nongovernmental partners.

SUMMARY

The Active Living Alliance for Canadians with a Disability has, since 1989, worked with a broad spectrum of partners to ensure and enhance active living opportunities for persons with disabilities. Based on six goals outlined in its *Blueprint for Action*, the alliance has pursued equity for active living opportunities. While having achieved a great deal over a relatively short period of time, the alliance continues to face many challenges in fulfilling its mission.

1 Can marketing such as the Viabilité campaign decrease levels of physical inactivity among Canadians with a disability by 20 percent? What is required for the Viabilité marketing campaign to be successful?

2 Which individuals are unlikely to be served by this alliance, and why would this be so?

3 What steps can the Active Living Alliance for Canadians with a Disability take to ensure that it reaches its goal of a decrease in physical inactivity by 20 percent of persons with disabilities?

4 How can the Provincial and Territorial Committee address the issues it faces?

5 Are the seven goals identified in the *Blueprint for Action* still necessary and appropriate today?

THE CANADIAN PARALYMPIC COMMITTEE

While the Active Living Alliance for Canadians with a Disability addressed the recreation and active living needs of persons with disabilities, several disability sport organizations have been responsible for the development of elite athletes with disabilities. Many of these organizations are listed in the chapter appendix. Traditionally there have been five disability groups represented by these disability sport organizations, including those with spinal cord injuries (and polio, particularly in the earlier days), visual impairments, amputations, cerebral palsy, and intellectual disabilities. Those persons who are deaf or hard of hearing are also represented by a national disability sport organization, but for the most part they remain distinct and separate from the other disability sport organizations. There are also now a number of disability sport-specific national organizations, including the Canadian Wheelchair Basketball Association (CWBA) (www.cwba.ca), Canadian Association for Disabled Skiing (CADS) (www.disabledskiing.ca), and Sledge Hockey of Canada (SHOC) (www.shoc.ca). Finally, many sport organizations that previously only provided competitive sport administration for able-bodied athletes are now responsible for athletes with disabilities. Some of these include Swimming/Natation Canada (www.swimming.ca/) and Athletics Canada (www.athleticscanada.com/).

At the highest competitive level, the Canadian Paralympic Committee (CPC) (www.paralympic.ca) represents many of these disability groups. The CPC is a private corporation recognized by the International Paralympic Committee (IPC) since 1993 as the national Paralympic committee in Canada. Its mandate is to promote the Paralympic movement to the fullest by providing the professional management of Canada's Paralympic teams, while its vision is a Paralympic movement in Canada built on excellence at the Paralympic Games.

The Canadian Paralympic Committee, previously called the Canadian Federation of Sport Organizations for the Disabled (CFSOD), emerged as an organization shortly following the 1976 Olympiad for the Physically Disabled held in Toronto (also referred to then as the Torontolympiad and now called the Paralympics). The 1976 games were significant in that they were the first Paralympic Games where athletes other than those with spinal cord injuries were invited to participate. The chairman of the organizing committee for the games was Dr. Robert Jackson, who was previously the founding president of the Canadian Wheelchair Sports Association (CWSA) (www.cwsa.ca). The development of these games, and subsequently of the CPC, was thus significantly influenced by the evolution of wheelchair sports, although this does not imply that other disability sport groups were insignificant in their contributions.

Case Study: How one person can change the nation!

While organizations have had a profound impact on the development of adapted physical activity in Canada, obviously the impetus comes from personal commitment and leadership. The Canadian Paralympic movement started arguably when Dr. Robert Jackson attended the 1964 Paralympic Games in Tokyo, Japan. Canada did not compete, but Jackson, a medical student working as an orthopedic consultant with the Canadian Olympic Team in Japan, witnessed the games first hand. He questioned why a Canadian team was not participating. Dr. Jackson was interested in viewing the games because of a prior opportunity to see them in England at the Stoke Mandeville Games in 1961 where he was completing his medical postgraduate work at the Royal National Orthopedic Hospital in London. Dr. Jackson had met Sir Ludwig Guttmann, organizer of these games, and decided to approach him again in Tokyo to note his disappointment with Canada's absence. Sir Guttmann responded by expressing his own feelings regarding the apparent ambivalence shown by the Canadian Paraplegic Association (CPA) towards sport and recreation. In Guttmann's view, the CPA was over-focussing on occupational

rehabilitation, while it completely ignored the benefits of other modalities. Sir Guttmann was very persuasive, and Dr. Jackson left the tent promising to organize a Canadian team for the 1968 Paralympic Games near Tel Aviv.

Dr. Jackson forgot about his promise to Guttmann until 1967 when, as a personal project to commemorate Canada's Centennial birthday, he and his wife Marilyn invited a few patients from a Toronto hospital to stage a race. A few months following this track event, a formal club was created called the Coasters Athletic Club. That same summer, several other wheelchair sport clubs in Winnipeg, Vancouver, Edmonton, Montréal, and Halifax were formally created, with many of the founding members associated with the CPA.

During this time, a few CPA members began experimenting with amateur (ham) radio and, through word-of-mouth, the various wheelchair sports clubs began communicating on a regular basis. Wheelchair sport enthusiasts now had a forum to discuss the creation of a national wheelchair sport association. The use of ham radio became more prevalent within the wheelchair sport community in 1968 during the Canadian Postal Service strike, as amateur radio was the only viable and inexpensive method of communication.

The international wheelchair sport scene continued to become more sophisticated. In 1962, in Perth, Australia, the Commonwealth Games Federation hosted a set of events for athletes with a spinal cord injury. In 1966, the second Commonwealth Paraplegic Games were held in Kingston, Jamaica, with Ben Reimer from Winnipeg representing Canada.

Reimer's success helped to motivate a number of other Winnipeggers to approach the organizing committee for the Winnipeg Pan American (Pan Am) Games, scheduled for the summer of 1967, to request the inclusion of a wheelchair basketball game. The Winnipeg group, led by Al Simpson, was turned down initially but not discouraged. They knew they were in for difficult negotiations, as the Stoke Mandeville Games were also trying to have a parallel set of games with the Olympics in Tokyo, Rome, and Tel Aviv.

(The 1968 Paralympic Games were not held in Mexico City, as Olympic officials were concerned that the high altitudes would adversely affect the wheelchair competitors.)

The majority of the Winnipeg advocates, under Simpson's leadership, met at the Manitoba Monday Night Club, a sports and recreation drop-in centre for persons with physical disabilities. This group began to communicate with their counterparts in the United States, Jamaica, Trinidad and Tobago, and Argentina about the possibility of hosting a separate but parallel Pan Am Games for the physically disabled. "The point to this gathering was not necessarily for the love of sport, but instead to build social acceptance and undo the myth that persons with disabilities were a burden to society" (Legg 2000).

For Simpson, this desire and energy led him to protest the Pan Am Games organizing committee in their Winnipeg hotel. Eventually, the Pan Am Games organizing committee agreed to recognize the creation of a Wheelchair Pan Am Games section.

Once given the mandate to host the games, the next problem was how to pay for them. Federal minister John Munro agreed to provide a grant, but regulations stipulated that the money be distributed to a national organization. The Canadian Wheelchair Sports Association (CWSA) did not officially exist at that point, so the CPA Board of Directors agreed to act as the temporary national association.

While the Manitoba group was preparing for the games, the CPA was linking with people using the aforementioned ham radio network. Hookup was at 11:00 A.M. on Saturday morning, Winnipeg time, on the 20-metre band at 14160 kcs. The ham radio hookups were illegal because they circumvented the Bell telephone system, but fortunately Bell Canada chose to overlook them. Through this network, the Manitoba organizers discovered Dr. Jackson, who was meeting with wheelchair athletes in Toronto on a regular basis.

In the winter of 1966, the organizing committee began arranging a series of trials to select a national team. Direct competition was impossible because of the vast distance and cost, so the organizers simply compared the best times or distances taken from local events. In reality, there were not that many qualified athletes, so every effort was made to bring anyone who was sincere in their efforts to compete (Legg 2000).

On August 8, 1967, the Wheelchair Pan Am Games were officially opened with athletes representing Argentina, Jamaica, Mexico, Trinidad and Tobago, and the United States of America. While the athletes were competing and training, numerous others were discussing the merits of a Canadian national wheelchair sport organization. On Thursday, August 10, 1967, a motion was presented "that a national wheelchair sports association in Canada be formally established." A draft constitution and by-laws would be circulated at a meeting held in conjunction with the Centennial Games in Montréal later that fall. (The Centennial Games were originally scheduled prior to the Winnipeg event but because of organizational difficulties were postponed.)

The Centennial Games included a number of wheelchair events and were held to celebrate Canada's Centennial. On September 9, 1967, at Montréal's Loyola College (now Concordia University), Dr. Jackson commented on the progress that he and the ad-hoc organizing committee had made.

> It is my pleasure to say a few words about the back room happenings of the past three days. As you now know, we are finally organized on a national scale with representation from 7 of the 10 provinces. We should note with some pride that although wheelchair sport may have started earlier in England and the USA, that the Canadian organization was started by paraplegics themselves, with full cognizance of the many benefits that they would receive. In fact 10 of the 14 board members were in a chair. Our new organization (if you'll excuse the medical analogy) was formally conceived at the Pan Am Games in Winnipeg and after a very short pregnancy with severe labour pains for the past three days was delivered into the world at noon today. The constitution has been drawn up and is now ready for

submission to the secretary of state for approval. (Jackson 1997)

Remembering his promise to Guttmann, Jackson set out, after CWSA's creation in 1967, to develop a national team to compete in the 1968 Paralympic Games. Athletes were invited to Edmonton for trials at the University of Alberta, and the first Canadian team travelled to Israel for the Paralympic Games.

In the 1970s, CWSA continued to focus on its national teams. One CWSA respondent recalled that, in preparation for the team to attend the 1972 Heidelberg Paralympic Games, "someone out in the west started a rumour that Heidelberg Beer, which was a Canadian brewery, would give one cent for every bottle cap that was collected to recognize that the games were being held in their namesake" (Jackson 1997). In pubs and bars, people started collecting Heidelberg beer caps. Eventually the brewery became aware of this mythical fundraising campaign when thirteen thousand beer caps were hand-delivered to its head office. The brewery contacted CWSA executives, embarrassed that they had not made the original offer to sponsor CWSA athletes. After several conversations, the brewery agreed to be the official sponsor for CWSA and donated $14,000 (Jackson 1997).

With Montréal hosting the Olympics in 1976, it was hoped that someone in Canada would correspondingly host the fourth Paralympic Games. In 1973, Dr. Robert W. Jackson resigned as president of CWSA in order to chair the organizing committee. Jackson was also elected vice-president of the International Stoke Mandeville Games Federation (ISMWGF) and, upon the death of Sir Ludwig Guttmann, was unanimously elected as its president. As chair of the Torontolympiad organizing committee, Jackson gave up his medical practice for six months and tackled everything, "from planning menus and working with foreign ambassadors, to arranging for the inoculation of the police horses that would be prancing in the opening day parade" (Jackson 1997).

A total of sixteen hundred athletes and nine hundred coaches from 44 countries participated in the fourth Paralympic Games.

Many of these athletes had a visual impairment or amputation. The addition of these two disability groups resulted, in part, from a chance meeting between Dr. Jackson and a friend who was working with the Swedish national team. This friend told Dr. Jackson that the Swedish team had already planned to include other disability groups based on an unfounded rumour. Dr. Jackson thought about this dilemma and decided that philosophically it made sense to include them (Legg 2000).

The addition of athletes with disabilities other than those that were spinal-cord-injury-related had an enormous impact on CWSA, on disability sport throughout Canada, and on disability sport internationally. The addition of these athletes forced organizers to change the name of the event from the Paralympics to the Olympiad for the Physically Disabled. "The term Paralympics was studiously avoided because it had the connotation of paraplegic games and so was objected to by the amputee and blind athletes" (Jackson 1997). Ironically, Paralympics would be chosen as the official term for the event with *Para* denoting in parallel to the Olympics and not a shortened version of paraplegic.

While a tremendous success, the Torontolympiad was not without its controversy or challenges. Funding from the federal government to host the games was withdrawn at the last minute because of the participation of a South African team. The federal government's decision to withdraw funds from the hosting organization was due to an international ban that disallowed South African athletes from competing in any international sporting events because of international condemnation of South Africa's apartheid policies. The South African wheelchair sports team, however, was racially mixed, and for this reason, ISMWGF had accepted their bid to join the International Wheelchair Sport Association. Dr. Jackson recognized that the South African team had a unique commitment to equality and thus felt that they deserved to be invited to the Torontolympiad (Jackson 1997). The federal government, meanwhile, was already feeling international pressures surrounding this issue due to a potential boycott from a number of African countries at the Montréal Summer Olympic Games because of the participation of New Zealand, which had competed against South Africa in an exhibition able-bodied rugby match.

Marc Lalonde, the Canadian minister of National Health and Welfare, expressed concern that South Africa was only attempting to propagate the impression of equality in South Africa by the registration of a racially integrated wheelchair team (Milner 1990). The official stance of the Canadian government was that it would not prevent the participation of the team, but as a government it could not associate itself with the South African team or the games through financial support. Ultimately, South Africa competed, with several countries boycotting including Jamaica, India, Hungary, Poland, Yugoslavia, Sudan, Uganda, and Kenya (Jackson 1997).

Financially, the Canadian government's opposition to South Africa's inclusion and its subsequent withdrawal of support had a dramatic impact. Dr. Jackson was hopeful that a fourth of the funds needed to host the games would come from the Ontario provincial government, a fourth from the federal government, and a fourth from ticket sales and sponsorship. The final fourth would come from the different countries and athletes themselves. Only two months prior to the games, however, the Canadian government made its decision to withdraw the agreed-upon support of $450,000 and asked to have a $50,000 advance reimbursed. The Ontario government, following the federal government's lead, also decided to follow suit and withdraw its funding (Jackson 1997).

This announcement was made only a few months prior to the game's opening ceremonies. The Torontolympiad organizing committee, in desperate need of funds, argued that the South African team had both black and white athletes and thus it deserved international support. The federal government appeared somewhat conciliatory and requested proof that the team was truly representative of racial integration. It was arranged that the Canadian ambassador in Cape Town would visit the selection camp of the South African team, but at the last minute the consulate said that the Canadian embassy could not verify the games as it had other more pressing matters. The embassy staff never witnessed the selection events and the Canadian government withdrew its support (Milner 1990).

The withdrawal of funds made it next to impossible to host the games, resulting in a public outcry of support for persons with disabilities. A political cartoon in the *Toronto Sun* newspaper reflected this mood by showing the provincial and federal ministers of health pushing a black African wheelchair athlete over a cliff (Jackson 1997). Eventually, the provincial government relented to public pressure and agreed to honour its commitment. The federal government, however, refused to budge.

The games went ahead with a massive debt looming. The presumed deficit from these games, however, never occurred as ticket sales and donations far surpassed expectations. The opening ceremonies, which were not supposed to generate much interest, attracted over twenty thousand people. *Toronto Sun* columnist George Gross noted that these games were "sport and not like something else on the back pages of the social pages" (Gross 1976, p. 36).

Three days before the games ended, the federal government relented to public pressure and reallocated its original commitment of $450,000. These funds, while not used for the games themselves, were designated to create and support a coordinating committee for all Canadian athletes with disabilities. The purpose of this newly formed coordinating committee was to establish one governance mechanism for the government and to ensure a proper disbursement of funds towards the disability sport movement.

This committee was comprised of representatives from the Canadian Association for Disabled Skiing (CADS), Canadian Amputee Sports Association (CASA), Canadian Wheelchair Sports Association (CWSA), and Canadian Blind Sports Association (CBSA). By 1979, with the federal government funding dispersed, many members of this group thought that the maintenance of a cooperative relationship, such as a coordinating committee, would be beneficial. As a result, in 1980 the coordinating committee was formalized to become the Canadian Federation of Sport Organizations for the Disabled (CFSOD). It was incorporated with the mandate to "coordinate those activities common to member sport organizations for the physically disabled on matters pertaining to promotion, rule integration, coaching integration, and participation in national and international competitions, and administration involving more than one disability group" (www.paralympic.ca/about/historye.html).

The Formation of the Canadian Federation of Sport Organizations for the Disabled

In CFSOD's early years, the focus of activities was on the establishment of the organization in terms of membership, governance, and coordinating role in major international events. At the same time, CFSOD was involved in coordinating national games with Brantford, Ontario, becoming the host of the Canadian Games for the Physically Disabled in the late 1980s. The host organizing committee then successfully negotiated a long-term sponsorship agreement with the Canadian Foresters, and in 1989 the games became known as the Canadian Foresters Games. This funding remained in place until 1993. Another activity of CFSOD included the lobbying effort for the integration of athletes with disabilities into major international competitions. The result of much of this work was the establishment of the International Committee on Integration (ICI) in 1990, later renamed as the Commission for the Inclusion of Athletes with Disabilities (CIAD) and supported by the International Paralympic Committee (IPC). Both the ICI and CIAD were due, in part, to Rick Hansen's Man in Motion world tour and Anne Merklinger's administrative leadership. CFSOD also coordinated the efforts of member national sport organizations in lobbying for the inclusion of athletes with disabilities in Canada Games.

This effort was successful, and since 1993 in Kamloops, BC, athletes with disabilities have been fully included (www.paralympic.ca/about/historye.html).

Throughout the 1980s, CFSOD continued to be the coordinating body for many multi-disability events and forums. By the early 1990s, the sport community for athletes with disabilities was changing. Following the success of the 1988 Seoul Paralympic Games, the games started growing in recognition and acceptance. Around the same time, a direct mail campaign was becoming less profitable. CFSOD was struggling to meet its current mandate, as it became more focussed on games (www.paralympic.ca/about/historye.html).

THE FORMATION OF THE CANADIAN PARALYMPIC COMMITTEE AND CHALLENGES FACING MEMBER ORGANIZATIONS

In 1992 and 1993, CFSOD undertook a strategic review of its mandate and objectives. The review resulted in changes to the structure of the organization and new objectives to better reflect its focus on the Paralympic Games. In April 1993, the CFSOD board of directors approved a name change to the Canadian Paralympic Committee (CPC). In addition to the name change, a new logo was adopted incorporating the IPC logo with the Canadian flag.

At the same time, a number of federal government decisions were made pertaining to funding and inclusion. In 1993, the federal government was close to circulating the *Core Sport Report*, a government document addressing ways to categorize sports and its financial contributions. While it was not officially released until the spring of 1994, the rumours of its ramifications had a direct impact on several national sport organizations. Rumours relating to the report included the possibility of several sports losing their funding. Many national sport organizations responded by becoming inwardly focussed and preparing for worst-case scenarios. This hurt disability sport organizations in that they were unable to implement many inclusion-based strategies. The process used to create the *Core Sport*

Report also affected disability sport organizations as they were assessed under a special target group category. While this segregation ensured that disability sport organizations would retain a higher level of funding, it also meant that other sports would perceive them as special. Disability sport organizations thus found themselves in a difficult position. They knew they had the expertise, resources, and mandate to serve as an essential partner in the evolution of an inclusive, equitable Canadian sport system, and they knew that they wanted to be judged on their own unique ability to facilitate a more inclusive and equitable sport system. The special priority designation given to disability sport organizations, however, opened them to the whims of changing government priorities, particularly in the area of entry-level criteria. The challenge, under Core Sport funding within the special priority category, therefore, was to have the criteria structured to meet the association's evolving needs, while not making the government appear to be overly generous.

In 1994, funding from the federal government also changed, in part, because of the new *Sport Funding Accountability Framework* (SFAF) for able-bodied sport organizations (Sport Canada 1994). The federal government endeavoured to reshape its contribution programme and focus on fewer sport organizations. Originally the fear of cuts was high, as the *Core Sport Report* suggested that disability sport organizations should be assessed under the same guidelines as able-bodied sport organizations (Sport Canada 1994). Ultimately, however, it was decided that there should be a modified assessment system for disability sport organizations (Sport Canada 1994). Regardless of this change, most disability sport organizations still received a significant funding cut.

In 1996, Sport Canada decided to pursue what was referred to as fast-tracked inclusion: an immediate transfer of athletes with disabilities into the able-bodied sport system. Financially, this meant that Sport Canada would be transferring most of the sport technical and administrative funding that was previously earmarked for disability sport organizations to various able-bodied sport organizations.

From Sport Canada's perspective, the funding cuts would eventually reflect feedback from the Funding and Accountability Framework for Athletes with Disabilities (FAFAD) (Ostry 1995). Scores from this assessment were based on three main categories including high performance, sport development, and management (Ostry 1995). The analysis included site visits to major international competitions, extensive reviews of NSO annual reports, and funding submissions. The federal government's assessment concluded that in disability sport, the technical competency was severely lacking. In particular, the government was disappointed with the complete lack of qualified and trained coaches and the poor relationship with the National Coaching Certification Programme (NCCP). Most disability sports, in the government's opinion, were not operating at a national calibre. Sport Canada believed that the best way to alleviate this was to fund one national sport system.

While encouraged by the government, significant challenges still face the inclusion process. One may be a perception that many Paralympic athletes are still competing at a developmental level. The CPC believes, however, that the Paralympic movement should be seen as having emerged from the rehabilitation and therapeutic recreation roots to a point where it is now seen as the highest testing ground of athletic excellence for athletes with a disability. This goal would mirror the same principles and values as their able-bodied, high-performance sport peers. One reason for the perception that Paralympic athletes are still in a developmental stage may be that some entry-level athletes have, in fact, advanced to the international arena too quickly. This rapid advancement may have resulted from not having enough competitors to challenge them, or from a lack of appropriate coaching and leadership. Regardless of whether or not this is true, it is still important to understand that it is a perception.

Assisting with the inclusion process, however, are partnerships that mirror the same sentiments at the international level. The International Paralympic Committee (IPC) and International Olympic Committee (IOC) signed a contract in November 2001 recognizing a new commitment to work together, while other examples of successful partnerships between the national Paralympic and Olympic partners also have been initiated in the United States, Great Britain, and Australia. Finally, it seems that the timing for inclusion between able-bodied and disabled athletes is particularly inviting because of how Canada proudly presents its heritage of promoting the inclusion of persons with disabilities into mainstream society. Government, labour, the private sector, and volunteer groups across the country have been working to remove the barriers to full participation. The sport system is an appropriate arena to continue promoting the removal of this barrier.

THE FUTURE

Disability sport organizations such as the Canadian Paralympic Committee will continue to face many challenges in the coming years. The most significant of these challenges will pertain to inclusion. It has never been clear whether disability sport organizations should work themselves out of business per se through the inclusion model, or just change responsibilities to one of developing and discovering athletes with disabilities, rather than duplicating elite programming opportunities. There has always been the need for development and discovery of athletes with disabilities because it is not always possible to emulate the able-bodied structure when it comes to these responsibilities. This means that in all probability there will continue to be a role for established organizations dealing with disability and sport.

Disability sport organizations and particularly the CPC also need to play an advocacy and watchdog role ensuring that elite opportunities for athletes with a disability continue far into the future and are not relegated only to those that are currently at the national level. While *Sport: The Way Ahead–The Report of the Minister's Task Force on Federal Sport Policy*

(Best 1992) and the sub-committee's report on the study of sport in Canada, *Sport: Leadership, Partnership and Accountability* (Lincoln and Mills 1998) suggested that further steps were needed to encourage the inclusion of persons with a disability into national sport-governing bodies, it is still questionable whether this is in fact occurring. For many people associated with disability sport, the commitment made by able-bodied sport organizations to provide continued opportunities for athletes with disabilities is tenuous. Some sport administrators perceive the fast-tracked inclusion mandate as a cost-cutting measure taken by the federal government, possibly without the support of the able-bodied sport organizations. Most of the national sport governing bodies had already dealt with massive funding cuts, and any further demands placed on stretched resources might not be welcomed.

For disability sport in general, future directions were outlined at COMPASS 2010, a national symposium on sports development for Canadian athletes with a disability, hosted by the CPC. This symposium helped identify key priorities for the disability sport community which included an increase in participation at all levels of competition, ensuring that a sport programme and competition continuum be in place, that coaches were appropriately educated and certified from the grassroots to high-performance levels, that there was an increased rate of participation at the elite level, that a national database of Paralympic sport research existed, and an evaluation of the inclusion process take place.

With these goals in place, COMPASS 2010 also was a time to reflect on how far the disability sport community had come in a relatively short period of time. In 2001, it can be argued that athletes with disabilities have more opportunities than any time previous. Elite athletes with disabilities are afforded similar if not equal status in many regards including access to government carding and programmes offered at national sport centres. Canadian athletes with disabilities are also achieving unparalleled success. In Sydney,

Canada tied with Spain for third place for gold medals and fifth overall, for total medals behind only Australia, Great Britain, Spain, and the United States, with thirty-eight gold, thirty-three silver, and twenty-five bronze medals. In Nagano, Canada placed tenth overall with fifteen medals: one gold, nine silver, and five bronze. Both are significant gains from previous competitions where in Atlanta 1996 Canada placed seventh and in Lillehammer 1994 placed fourteenth.

6 What should be the primary role of the Canadian Paralympic Committee?

7 What should be the focus for the Canadian Paralympic Committee as sport at the national level becomes more and more integrated?

8 What are the advantages and disadvantages of including athletes with disabilities into the able-bodied sport system?

9 What assumptions about disability underlie decisions to have separate organizations in a specific sport for those with and without disabilities?

Summary

From an organizational perspective, Canada has made significant contributions to adapted physical activity. With dedicated, passionate, and visionary leadership from countless volunteers, parents, coaches, officials, and staff, those organizations outlined in this chapter and several others noted in the appendix met numerous goals and in many respects surpassed expectations. These organizations developed comprehensive programmes, promoted wellness, and helped cultivate numerous national athletes and teams that consistently ranked among the world's best. These organizations also facilitated social change by influencing the public's perceptions and attitudes towards persons with disabilities and drove the inclusion process. Finally, these organizations continue to lead the evolution of sport for athletes with disabilities as advocates and promoters of athletic excellence.

Study Questions

1. Is there still a need for sport and recreation organizations specifically for athletes with disabilities?
2. Have the goals and objectives of the Active Living Alliance for Canadians with a Disability and the Canadian Paralympic Committee been achieved?
3. What will be the future challenges to organizations providing recreation and elite sport opportunities for persons with disabilities?

References

Active Living Alliance for Canadians with a Disability. (1994). *Active living through physical education: Maximizing opportunities for students with a disability.* Ottawa: Health Canada.

Active Living Alliance for Canadians with a Disability. (1998). *Active living for Canadians with a disability: A blueprint for action* (3rd ed.). Ottawa: Health Canada.

Best, J.C. (1992). *Sport: The way ahead: The report of the minister's task force on federal sport policy.* Ottawa: Minster of Supply and Services.

Bourne, C., and Legg, D. (1998). Linking to the community: The Active Living Alliance for Canadians with a Disability. *Journal of Leisureability, 25*(3), 11–16.

Canadian Paralympic Committee. (2001). Web site. Available: http://www.paralympic.ca (URL on October 7, 2002).

Gross, G. (1976, June 4). The Olympiad for the Physically Disabled. *Toronto Sun,* p. 36.

Jackson, R. (1997). Personal interview, Dallas, TX: David Legg.

Lawrence, L., and Legg, D. (1998). The linkage initiative: A cross Canada approach to creating opportunities for persons with disabilities. *Parks and Recreation Canada, 57*(4), 8–9.

Legg, D. (2000). *Strategy formation in the Canadian Wheelchair Sports Association (1967–1997).* Unpublished doctoral dissertation, University of Alberta.

Legg. D. (2001). Viabilité: A new initiative, a new identity. *Palaestra, 17*(2), 28–33.

Lincoln, C., and Mills, D. (1998). *Sport: Leadership, partnership and accountability.* Ottawa: House of Commons.

Milner, J. (1990). Wheelchair sports: Canada leading the way. *Rehabilitation Digest, 21*(2), 8–10.

Ostry, A. (1995) A. Personal correspondence to Clare Gillespie.

Rock, A. (1999). House of Commons Debate, March 17th. Ottawa: Hansard.

Sport Canada (1994). *Discussion paper on the sport Funding and accountability framework.* Ottawa: Author.

Steadward, R., Legg, D., Bornemann, R., Weiss, C., Jeon, J., and Wheeler, G. (1997). Active living for Canadians with a disability: A ten year retrospective analysis. *Canadian Association for Health, Physical Education, Recreation and Dance Journal, 63*(3), 10–15.

Appendix

ORGANIZATION ADDRESSES

Active Living Alliance for Canadians with a Disability, 720 Belfast Road, Suite 104, Ottawa, ON, K1G 0Z5, T: 1–800–771–0663 or (613) 244–0052, F: (613) 244–4857

Athletics Canada, 606–1185 Eglinton Ave East, North York, ON, M3C 3C6, T: (416) 426–7181, F: (416) 426–7182 Paralympic Sports: Athletics (amputee and wheelchair)

Canadian Amputee Sports Association, 217 Holmes Avenue, Willowdale, ON, M2N 4M0, T: (416) 229–9324, F: (416) 229–6547, Paralympic Sports: Powerlifting

Canadian Association for Athletes with an Intellectual Disability, 402–200 Main Street, Winnipeg, MB, R3C 4M2, T: (204) 925–5632, F: (204) 925–5635, Paralympic Sports: Athletics, Swimming

Canadian Association for Disabled Skiing, P.O. Box 307, Kimberly, BC, V1A 2Y9, T: (250) 427–7712, F: (250) 427–7715, Paralympic Sports: Alpine Skiing

Canadian Blind Sports Association, 7 Mills Street, Lower Level, Almonte, ON, K0A 1A0, T: (613) 256–7792, F: (613) 256–8759, Paralympic Sports: Athletics, Goalball

Canadian Cerebral Palsy Sports Association, 1010 Polytek St., Unit 14, Gloucester, ON, K1J 9H9, T: (613) 748–1430, F: (613) 748–1355, Paralympic Sports: Athletics, Boccia, Powerlifting

Canadian Cycling Association, 212A–1600 James Naismith Drive, Gloucester, ON, K1B 5N4, T: (613) 748–5629, F: (613) 748–5692, Paralympic Sports: Cycling (Athletes with C.P. or visual disability)

Canadian Fencing Federation, 305–1600 James Naismith Drive, Gloucester, ON, K1B 5N4, T: (613) 748–5633, F: (613) 748–5742, Paralympic Sports: Fencing

Canadian Table Tennis Association, CTTC Building, 2800–1125 Colonel By Drive, Ottawa, ON, K1S 5R1, T: (613) 733–6272, F: (613) 733–7279, Paralympic Sports: Table Tennis

Canadian Therapeutic Riding Association, 550 Imperial Road North, P.O. Box 24009, Guelph, ON, N1E 6V8, T: (519) 767–0700, F: (519) 767–0435, Paralympic Sports: Dressage

Canadian Wheelchair Sports Association, 200–2460 Lancaster Road, Ottawa, ON, K1B 4S5, T: (613) 523–0004, F: (613) 523–0149, Paralympic Sports: Rugby

Canadian Wheelchair Basketball Association, 402–2781 Lancaster Road, Ottawa, ON, K1B 1A7, T: (613) 260–1296, F: (613) 260–1456, Paralympic Sports: Wheelchair Basketball

Canadian Yachting Association, 504–1600 James Naismith Drive, Gloucester, ON, K1B 5N4, T: (613) 748–5687 ext: 2974, F: (613) 748–5688, Paralympic Sports: Sailing

Cross Country Canada, 100–1995 Olympic Way, Canmore, AB, T1W 2T2, T: (403) 678–6791, F: (403) 678–364, Paralympic Sports: Cross-Country Skiing, Biathlon

Federation of Canadian Archers, 200–2460 Lancaster Road, Ottawa, ON, K1B 4S5, T: (613) 260–2113, F: (613) 260–2114, Paralympic Sports: Archery

Judo Canada, 301A–1600 James Naismith Drive, Gloucester, ON, K1B 5N4, T: (613) 748–5640, F: (613) 748–5697, Paralympic Sport: Judo

Shooting Federation of Canada, P.O. Box 181, Station "A", Fredericton, NB, E3B 4Y9, T: (506) 444–4588, F: (506) 363–4610, Paralympic Sports: Shooting

Sledge Hockey of Canada, P.O. Box 20063, Ottawa, ON, K1N 5W0, T: (613) 723–5799 or 1–888–857–8555, F: (613) 995–2520, Paralympic Sports: Sledge Hockey, Ice Racing

Special Olympics Canada, 60 St. Clair Avenue East, Suite 700, Toronto, ON, M4T 2N5, T: (416) 927–9050, F: (416) 927–8475

Swimming/Natation Canada, 503–1600 James Naismith Drive, Gloucester, ON, K1B 5N4, T: (613) 748–5673, F: (613) 748–5715, Paralympic Sports: Swimming

Tennis Canada, 175 Salisbury Avenue, Cambridge, ON, N1S 1K3, T: (519) 624–6399, F: (519) 624–6401, Paralympic Sports: Wheelchair Tennis

Volleyball Canada, 197 Sylvan Avenue, Scarborough, ON, M1E 1A4, T: 1–800–363–4067, F: (416) 297–2650, Paralympic Sports: Volleyball

IV ■ DELIVERING ADAPTED PHYSICAL ACTIVITY SERVICES

CHAPTER 9

Moving Toward Inclusion

Greg Reid

Learning Objectives

- To write an essay describing the positive aspects of including individuals with a disability in physical activity programmes with their nondisabled peers.
- To describe the historical factors that led to mainstreaming, including the concept of normalization.
- To describe the differences and similarities among the terms *mainstreaming*, *least restrictive environment*, and *inclusion*.
- To describe the criticisms of *mainstreaming*, *least restrictive environment*, and *inclusion*.
- To write an essay describing their own philosophical perspective on including students with a disability in physical activity programmes with their nondisabled peers.

Introduction

When *adapted physical education* was defined by our American neighbours in 1952 (Committee on Adapted Physical Education; see Chapter 2 (Reid)), a setting other than regular physical education was assumed. After all, it was defined as a programme for those who could not keep up in the vigorous physical education programme. Thus, students with disabilities in regular school classrooms were removed and possibly taught individually or in small groups. More frequently, they were simply excused from physical education. At that time, however, the majority of students with a disability in both Canada and the United States were not enrolled in regular classrooms. They were in segregated settings: special classes within regular schools, special schools, institutions, or hospitals. The interaction between people with and without a disability was almost nonexistent. In fact, the public school system could prevent a student with a disability from attending a local school, and it was the parents' responsibility to find alternative education, often at their own expense. This educational landscape mirrored that of society in which people with disabilities were largely excluded from job opportunities, public transportation, leisure, and private living accommodations. Many parents were even advised to place their child with a disability in an institution soon after birth. Thus, exclusion and segregation of people with a disability guided many practices in education and society.

Adapted physical activity has developed in the past fifty years, in terms of what it is, and in terms of where it occurs. In fact, probably more has been written and debated about where it occurs, than about what it is. Where it occurs refers to the degree of interaction between people with and without disabilities. Words and concepts about placement and interaction of people with and without disabilities have emerged. These include *integration*, *mainstreaming*, *normalization*, *least restricted environment*, and *inclusion*. Many authors have noted that these terms have been used in different ways, thus confusing the debate about the process and extent of including people with disabilities along side those without disabilities, in society and education. The purpose of this chapter is to describe these terms, why they emerged, what they originally meant, and how and why meanings changed. The term *integration* will be used to refer to the most general sense of having people with disabilities learn, work, and recreate among peers without disabilities. *Mainstreaming*, *normalization*, *least restricted environment*, and *inclusion* are consistent with *integration*, but each has a distinct meaning, history, and implications, which will unfold in the ensuing pages.

---

1 Does integration occur at the expense of individuals without a disability? Is it not better for the people with a disability to be excluded for their own good? Do not people with disabilities have different needs, and therefore special settings might be best for them?

Mainstreaming and Normalization

Mainstreaming was the first concept associated with the education of children with a disability in the same class as their age peers without a disability. The term *mainstreaming* originated in the context of racial integration, but by the 1960s became associated with integration of children with a disability into regular classrooms. However, its roots are deep. Howe observed in 1851 that it was desirable for blind children to "associate with the seeing" (Connor 1976). There were a number of arguments put forth by proponents of mainstreaming (table 9.1). In a landmark paper, Dunn (1968) argued that much of special education for students with mild mental retardation was not justified because they were not more academically successful in special classes than they were in regular classes (see also efficacy studies by Guskin and Spiker 1968; Kirk 1964). Also, these special education classes were composed of an inordinate number of youngsters from cultural minority and otherwise disadvantaged groups. Special education was not considered to be very special, according to Dunn. One reaction to the challenge issued by Dunn might have been to improve the education received in segregated special schools and classes. But other factors pushed toward a solution via mainstreaming.

For example, normalization was a concept that became important for people with a disability. Normalization was a societal concept, with implications much beyond the education system (Wolfensberger 1972). Normalization originated in the Scandinavian countries and meant valuing people with a disability and having them experience the same daily rhythm of life as people without a disability. Most adults live in apartments or homes independently or in small groups (families or roommates). They leave their residence in the morning to go to work or school. Throughout the day they make a number of decisions such as where to eat lunch, whether to go to the bank, and what to do after work or school. Thus, it was not normalizing to live in a large

Table 9.1 Reasons for Mainstreaming

• Effectiveness of special classroom instruction was questioned	

• Normalization	• Undesirable effects of a label which accompanies special education placement
• Parental pressure	• Advances in special education which could accommodate wider range of student in regular classrooms
• Inappropriate placement in special classroom	• Changing educational philosophies toward greater acceptance education of minority children of individual diversity

SOURCE: From "Mainstreaming: Implications for Physical Educators" by G. Reid, 1979, *McGill Journal of Education, 14,* pp. 367–77.

institution on a ward without privacy, to never leave the grounds, and to engage in 'therapy' or 'rehabilitation' during the day, while having all decisions made for you. Such a life is not typical of the daily rhythm of most people without a disability. Normalization did not advocate that people with a disability should be 'normal,' rather that they should be provided opportunities to experience a fuller, self-determined, and empowered life.

2 Think about people with a disability whom you know and list some of their activities that reflect normalization. Can you find instances that do not reflect normalization?

Normalization had an enormous impact on social services for people with a disability, including the closing or downsizing of many institutions, providing public transportation for people with a physical disability, having adults live independently or with support in communities, and having recreation facilities accept their role in providing opportunities for all citizens. Normalization is clearly supportive of children with a disability attending their neighbourhood schools.

Therefore, for a number of reasons, mainstreaming was supported as an educational alternative to ineffective special education that isolated and segregated children (Reid 1979).

3 Do you think those reasons are as valid today as they were in the 1960s and 1970s? But what exactly was intended by mainstreaming?

Many definitions were offered (e.g., Bundschuh 1976; DiRocco 1976: Dunn 1976; Dunn and Craft 1985), but Birch (1974) was quite comprehensive when he stated that mainstreaming referred to enrolling and teaching exceptional children in regular classes for the majority of the school day, but at the same time assuring that the children received high quality special education. In other words, mainstreaming was about regular class placement, but maintaining special education services. A student could be placed in a regular class, but removed for part of the day if that was deemed educationally necessary. Special educators would work with the child if removed from the class, but would also provide support for the regular teacher.

Dunn's (1968) pivotal paper about the quality of segregated special education dealt only with children who had a mild intellectual disability. Thus, early discussions of mainstreaming clearly indicated that it was designed for children with mild disabilities, and not the whole range of disabilities (Block and Krebs 1992; Reid 1979). Mainstreaming did not refer to the wholesale transfer of all special education students to regular classes.

Moreover, it was also designed to occur on an individual basis. For example, segregated programming was largely based on labels (if the label was 'blind,' then the child should be placed in the blind programme). Mainstreaming was supposed to occur only after assessment deemed it an appropriate placement for that specific *individual*. It is fair to say that mainstreaming meant that children had to gain entrance into the mainstream by demonstrating certain skills in the assessment process. In other words, educational authorities had to believe the individual's needs could be met in the mainstream.

Thus, the concept of mainstreaming included much more than a physical placement of a student; it involved maintaining special education services, and it occurred on an individual basis. As noted, it was not designed for all people with a disability. Mainstreaming resulted in many children with disabilities being taught in regular physical education classes in the 1970s and 1980s. As we will see however, mainstreaming became criticized from two distinct viewpoints: some people believed it went too far and too fast, with insufficient planning, and others believed it did not go far enough, nor quickly enough!

A number of problems in physical education mainstreaming were identified (see DePaepe 1984; Grosse 1991; Lavay and DePaepe 1987; Sherman 1996; Stein 1976; Watkinson 1991). Many of the difficulties are summarized in table 9.2. If one looks at the list in table 9.2, it becomes immediately clear that some of the problems were direct contradictions of the meaning of mainstreaming.

4 Can you identify these?
Read the first two under the topic Student. It is stated that mainstreaming is not the best place if the student has not been fully assessed and is placed on the basis of the whole special education class, not the individual.

5 Did the concept of mainstreaming imply that whole special education classes were supposed to be disbanded and that all the children were placed in a regular class without assessment?
Mainstreaming was not supposed to happen this way. It was supposed to be an individual placement decision based on assessment.

6 What went wrong?

It seems that mainstreaming was often implemented inappropriately. First, it occurred without a great deal of planning (Lavay and DePaepe 1987) and before physical educators were ready. Many did not even have a preliminary course in adapted physical activity. This writer remembers a teacher telling him that the school administration decided on a Thursday afternoon that the special education class in the school would be dismantled on Monday morning. A member of the physical education staff who had an interest in special education had taught these students as a group. But on Monday all physical educators would find the special education students in their regular gym classes. There was no time to prepare, to learn from their experienced colleague, and no assessment to determine if the students should be in the regular class. A second problem with implementation was lack of adequate staff. If a special educator retired or resigned, he or she was often not replaced, since the students were mainstreamed. Hence, the support for regular teachers that was part of the original concept of mainstreaming, designed to assist in the instruction for the children, was reduced or eliminated. Mainstreaming became a way of saving money in some school boards. If this scenario produced larger class sizes, it is no wonder teachers complained that they were not doing enough for the children with a disability, and that their time was diverted from the children without a disability.

Table 9.2 Mainstreaming Is Not Always the Better Place When...

Student	Teacher	Environment
The mainstream is not always a better place to be when... ... a full physical evaluation, including movement patterns, skills, knowledge, and fitness, is not performed prior to placement decisions; ... a student is placed based on a decision about an entire exceptional special education class group rather than on individual needs; ... a student is placed there even though that student does not have direction following, focusing, and on task behaviours necessary for participation; ... a student is placed there without necessary auxiliary support needed to involve that student in the education process; ... a student does not have prior experience or acquired skills necessary to participate on level with the rest of the class; ... a student is subject to ridicule by other classmates; the health and safety of the student would be compromised; and, ... a student is incapable of participating in or benefiting from the class in a manner consistent with goals of the physical education program.	The mainstream is not always a better place to be when the teacher... ... is not receptive to having that special needs student in class ... is neither trained in adapting equipment, curriculum, and teaching techniques to meet individual needs, nor is able to receive supportive assistance from a qualified adapted physical education specialist; and, ... has sound reasons for a student not being mainstreamed.	The mainstream is not always a better place to be when... ... no possibility exists for adaptive equipment and/or facilities; ... class is overcrowded or overloaded with students; ... participation in the mainstream hinders development in other educational areas; ... particular activities or curriculum of the mainstream group would not contribute to optimum development of the individual, consistent with goals of the physical education program; and ... placement decision is based on mainstream being the only available instructional opportunity.

SOURCE: From "Is Mainstreaming Always a Better Place to Be?" by S. Grosse, 1991, *Palaestra, 7*(2), 40–49. Reproduced with permission from Challenge Publications, Macomb, IL 61455.

Mainstreaming was never conceptualized or defined as a means to reduce services or staff. Yet, this seems to have occurred. Third, the original idea that only children with mild disabilities should be mainstreamed became blurred as students with a severe disability, and having distinct and unique needs, were also included in the mainstreaming movement.

Mainstreaming as a 'dumping ground' became a significant and comprehensive criticism. This phrase meant that the original meaning of individual placement on the basis of need was lost. And once in the mainstream, education was not appropriate. It was simply a physical placement of children with disabilities in settings with their age peers without disabilities, with minimal interaction. Mainstreaming became the brunt of criticisms, not because it was a poor ideology, but because it was often implemented incorrectly.

Despite the difficulties with mainstreaming, it was effective in some places with some children (sidebar). Unfortunately, we do not know the exact reasons for the successes.

7 Was mainstreaming implemented correctly? Was it a matter of teacher skill and attitude?

The term *mainstreaming* is not used a great deal today in education. In part, this is because poor planning and implementation (too far, too quickly) resulted in a 'bad name.' Broadhead (1985) stated that the term become distorted and misused, and it was therefore unceremoniously retired as a concept. Before we move on, it must also be stated that mainstreaming was also criticized because it was the only alternative to segregation. New models of placement were being described, which had several options (e.g., Reynolds 1962). These models depicted the *least restrictive environment* philosophy. We turn to this discussion next. Also, it should be noted that the inclusion movement (which will be described later) argued for *all* children to be integrated into regular classrooms, and its proponents disagreed with the original mainstreaming restriction to students with mild disabilities. Thus, for some people, mainstreaming did not go far enough.

Figure 9.1 Least Restrictive Environment Model

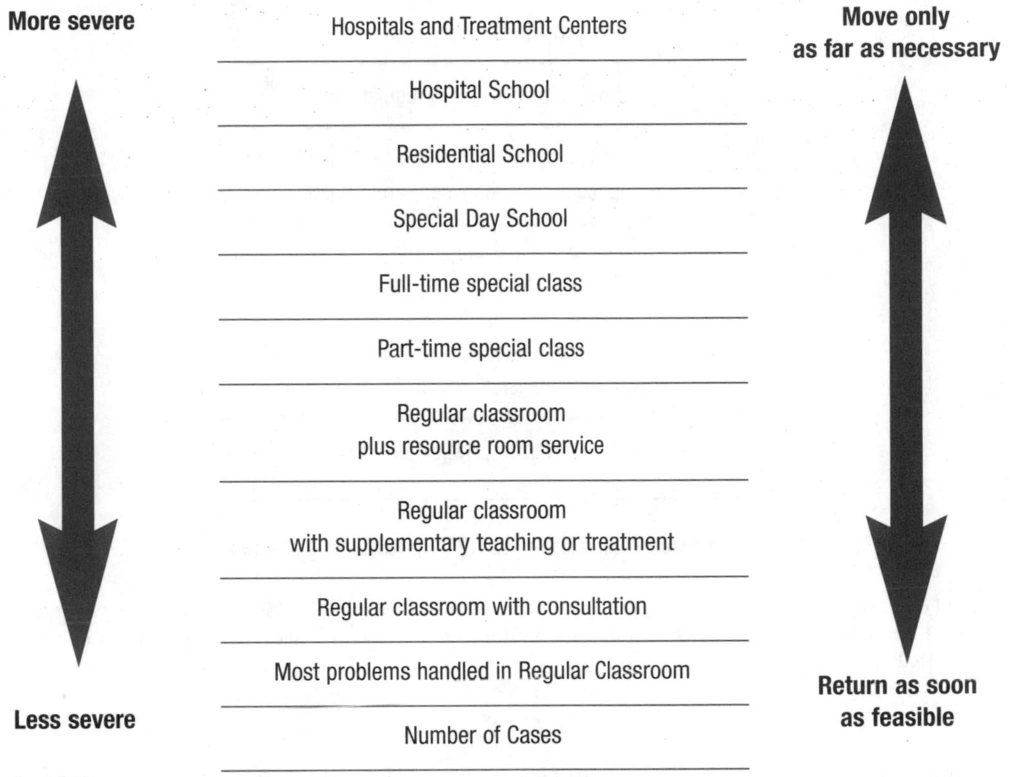

More severe		Move only as far as necessary
	Hospitals and Treatment Centers	
	Hospital School	
	Residential School	
	Special Day School	
	Full-time special class	
	Part-time special class	
	Regular classroom plus resource room service	
	Regular classroom with supplementary teaching or treatment	
	Regular classroom with consultation	
	Most problems handled in Regular Classroom	Return as soon as feasible
Less severe	Number of Cases	

SOURCE: From "A Framework for Considering Some Issues in Special Education" by M. Reynolds, 1962, *Exceptional Children, 29*, pp. 367–70. Copyright 1962 by the Council for Exceptional Children. Reprinted with permission.

Least Restrictive Environment Philosophy

The least restrictive environment (LRE) philosophy is based upon a model of special education (figure 9.1) put forth by Reynolds (1962). In part, this model was developed to deal with alternatives to segregation of students in special classes and schools, although mainstreaming was not mentioned as a term in the original 1962 paper. LRE is based on a multiple number of placement options that were called "the cascade of services" by Deno (1970). Some environments such as hospitals included twenty-four-hour residential care and, therefore, were deemed more restrictive than a special school, which in turn was more restrictive than a regular school. Theoretically, children could move up and down the cascade as needed, but the intent was to move them in one direction, to less restrictive placements as

academic and social skills were acquired. It was assumed that by adopting this line of thinking individuals would move to less restrictive settings over time.

For example, a child might be receiving education in a special day school (see figure 9.1) for students with an intellectual disability. A special bus owned by the school transports the child, many kilometres from home. A meeting is held at which his or her progress and skills are reviewed, and an analysis is presented to the local community school. It is determined that this student knows how to use public transportation, has reasonable social skills, enjoys reading in the library, and is generally well behaved. The school has a special education class and there is the possibility of integration in social studies, art, and physical education. The decision is

Figure 9.2 A Least Restrictive Environment Model in Adapted Physical Education

Adapted P.E. in a Special School

Full time adapted P.E. in a regular school

Adapted P.E. with regular P.E.
for specific activities where appropriate

Part time regular P.E.,
part time adapted P.E.

Regular P.E. with consultation
from the adapted physical education specialization

Full time regular physical education

Modified Cascade System of Continuum Services

SOURCE: From "Adapted Physical Education: A Look Back, A Look Ahead" by P.M. Aufsesser, 1981, *Journal of Physical Education and Recreation, 52*(6), pp. 28–31. Copyright 1981 by the American Alliance for Health, Physical Education, and Recreation. Reprinted with permission.

made that the local school can accommodate his or her educational needs, and it is less restrictive because the student remains in his or her local community. Therefore the student is moved two steps down in the model in figure 9.1. These models became quite popular and some were adapted for physical education (Aufsesser 1981; 1991; Sherrill 1993) (figure 9.2).

LRE became a popular term in the United States because it was entrenched in their federal special education laws as early as 1975. Legally, our American counterparts are bound by a law that states children with disabilities should be educated in regular settings to the extent possible, but that they can be removed if the nature and severity of the disability makes education in regular classes unsatisfactory (Aufsesser 1991; Sherrill 1994). The law requires that school officials articulate a continuum of alternative placements, which is some form of the LRE options. There are no Canadian laws that specify the LRE, but the concept remains legitimate.

Thus, the LRE included mainstreaming as one of the placement options, but also included several other potential placements. It was designed for all children, not only those with mild disabilities. Placement along the continuum was based on an individual education plan (Sherrill 1994). Beyond requirements of the United States law, some authors have argued that LRE is the most sensible and comprehensive philosophy of placements available (Grosse 1991; Sherrill 1994). Sherrill (1994) stated that 93 percent of children with a disability in the United States are now being educated in regular schools and, therefore, the LRE philosophy is facilitating integration.

8 While the LRE may enjoy wide support as a sensible concept, it has been criticized for a number of reasons. Can you think of some negative aspects or drawbacks to the LRE?

Some problems of the LRE have been highlighted (Block and Krebs 1992; Grineski 1994; Stainback, Stainback, and Forest 1989; Taylor

1988). Most of the criticisms have come from individuals who adhere to an inclusion philosophy and therefore believe that the rightful place of *all* children with a disability is in the regular school classroom. It has been argued that the LRE legitimizes restrictive environments such as residential facilities, and despite the intention of the LRE model, there is little chance of movement to less restrictive placements, in particular for those with more severe disabilities. Second, the focus of LRE is physical settings and concepts of integration and segregation, rather than more appropriately on services and supports that are required by people. Third, the LRE is a 'readiness' model in which people must earn the right to move to another level, but little is specifically stated about how segregation prepares the individual for a less restricted level. Fourth, many believe integration is a moral issue and not a decision that can be left in the hands of professionals (which occurs with the LRE). Everyone has the right to be included, according to advocates of inclusion. Fifth, it has been argued that the LRE is a basic infringement of rights, because it deals with the extent of restriction, not whether or not such restriction should occur.

Inclusion

Inclusion is essentially a term of the 1990s. As Block (1994b, p. 17) remarked, "inclusion is perhaps the most feared and emotionally charged educational reform since the passage of PL 94–142 [the United States law for children with disabilities that included the least restrictive environment]. Whether in formal debates at processional meetings or informal gatherings in teacher's lounges nothing can divide a group of educators into two camps like discussions of inclusion" (information in brackets added).

9 What is this concept? How is it different from mainstreaming or the LRE?

"An inclusive school is a place where everyone belongs, is accepted, supports, and is supported by his or her peers and other members of the school community in the course of having his or her educational needs met" (Stainback and Stainback 1990, p. 3). Thus, inclusion is more than a placement; it is an attitude of acceptance (DePauw and Doll-Tepper 2000; Kozub, Sherblom and Perry 1999). Inclusion involves teaching all students with a disability in their local community schools, in age-appropriate classrooms, with supplementary aids and services, and support personnel (Block 1992, 1994a, 1994b, 1996). An inclusive physical education environment is "one which provides the opportunity for students of all abilities and interests to participate in physical education (Active Living Alliance for Canadians with a Disability 1994, p. 2). While inclusion will be described primarily from an educational viewpoint in this section, readers should realize that inclusive communities are ones in which all people are fully functioning citizens. Regardless of disability label, there are ample opportunities for friendship and support, transportation, housing, recreation, and employment. However, there is more than just the opportunity 'to do,' because inclusive 'doing' occurs in a context that accepts diversity as a natural dimension of humanity, which accentuates our similarities rather than differences and relegates disability to, largely, differences that make no difference. Therefore, inclusion can be conceptualized as a broad societal idea, a philosophy in which "all people are valued as unique contributing members of society and included" (DePauw and Doll-Tepper 2000, p. 139). These ideas are similar to Condeluci's (1995) ideas of interdependence (see Chapter 6 (McPherson, Wheeler, and Foster) for further details).

There are some important educational implications in the concept, which have been articulated by those writing extensively about inclusion. First, *all* students are included, not just those with mild disabilities, as was the case with mainstreaming. Some writers may use terms such as *full* and *partial inclusion* to allow for some children to be excluded, but original definitions from its most strident advocates refer to *all* children. Second, the regular

Table 9.3 Benefits of Inclusion

Benefits for Children with Disabilities	Benefits for Children without Disabilities	Benefits of Inclusion to Teachers
• More stimulating environments • Role models who facilitate communication, social and adaptive behaviors • Improved competence in IEP objectives • Opportunities to make new friends and share new experiences • Greater acceptance by peers • Membership in a class and in the school	• More accepting of individual differences • More comfortable with students with disabilities • Become more helpful in general • Acquire leadership skills • Improved self-esteem	• Awareness/appreciation of individual differences in all children • Access to specialists/resources that can help all children • Learn new teaching techniques that can help all children

SOURCE: From "Did We Jump on the Wrong Bandwagon? Problems with Inclusion in Physical Education" by M. Block, 1999, *Palaestra, 15*(3), pp. 30–36, 55. Copyright 1999 Challenge Publications. Reproduced with permission.

classroom is the starting point for instruction, not a reward for good performance elsewhere. Proponents of inclusion reject the notion of LRE, and any other form of segregation, for the reasons noted in the section on LRE. Thus, all students with a disability begin kindergarten in the local school. Also, students with a disability are included in a given classroom to reflect natural proportions and age. If 10 percent of the school-aged population is believed to have a disability, then the natural proportion of a thirty-member class would be three students with a disability. Inclusion is not placing the nine children with a disability in grade four into one class with students who do not have a disability. Third, inclusion supports the merger of regular education and special education (in some school boards, special education is a separate department) since it is recognized that students must continue to receive support services and, by extension, the regular teacher will need assistance with some children. This will occur most efficiently if the two systems are merged. Fourth, inclusion accepts the fact that some students with a disability may be outside the classroom if required by their educational needs. For example, students with intellectual disabilities sometimes have difficulty with generalizing their learning. Therefore, an appropriate place to learn about money and change is while shopping or at a restaurant. It would also be sensible to use weight rooms and fitness facilities at the actual site in the community rather than in the school gym. While the student may be outside for some time, he or she is still considered to be part of the group of students in the classroom. Inclusion is more than simply placing students in classrooms; it is creating a learning environment in which all feel accepted as an integral part of the whole. Fifth, supplementary services and aides assist successful inclusion. Thus, instructional adaptations and special equipment are brought to the student, rather than the student being placed in a hospital or special rehabilitation centre because of 'special' equipment. Also, the programme must be appropriate and individualized. The child may practice wheelchair basketball techniques during a basketball unit but engage in a separate activity such as wheelchair racing during the outdoor rugby unit, which has been deemed inappropriate for that individual.

10 Can you see how inclusion is more a concept about accepting and belonging than it is about placement? You may also wish to reread the sections on the supports-based and empowerment/self-determination paradigms in Chapter 2 (Reid) since these parallel inclusion. Mainstreaming and LRE emphasized placement, or where education (and recreation) of a student with a disability would occur. But if inclusion does not acknowledge any placement but regular classrooms or gyms, can it accept sport programmes such as Special Olympics and Paralympics? Are not these programmes designed essentially for individuals with a disability?

Table 9.4 Problems and Challenges to Inclusion in Physical Education

It became a 'cause' or moral imperative

In reality, the needs of some children were ignored

Parental preferences were ignored

Lack of individualized physical education programmes

Teachers feel they are ill-prepared and not supported

Many elementary school physical education programmes are taught by classroom teachers

SOURCE: From "Did We Jump on the Wrong Bandwagon? Problems with Inclusion in Physical Education" by M. Block, 1999, *Palaestra, 15*(3), pp. 30–36, 55. Copyright 1999 Challenge Publications.

Inclusion has been advocated for many reasons (Stainback, Stainback, and Forest 1989). All things being equal, Block (1994a) suggested that inclusion is better than segregation since inclusive programmes can lead to better instruction for all students, because good physical education is good adapted physical education. Also, many parents wish to have their children be part of the larger community so that potential friendships might develop. But much of the rationale for inclusion is a philosophical one: it is simply argued to be the best place for all children, and those with a disability have a moral right to be in the regular class. Potential benefits from inclusion have been outlined in more detail by Block (1999) and are seen in table 9.3.

Inclusion was an integral part of the dialogue at the Jasper Talks (see Chapter 3 (Wall)). The Active Living Alliance for Canadians with a Disability (1994), created from the Jasper Talks, sponsored the Moving to Inclusion project to support the inclusion of children in regular physical education programmes. There are several chapters in this book that deal with inclusion in addition to this one. Therefore, inclusion is a prominent issue in Canada. However, the Supreme Court of Canada ruled in 1997 that a child with a disability could be removed from the regular classroom if it were deemed necessary by

educators. Thus, inclusion remains a goal and process for many schools and school boards, but it is not a requirement by law. Also, special schools still exist in many parts of Canada, which, of course, is inconsistent with inclusion. Therefore, university students graduating in the early years of the twenty-first century will find that some school boards have adopted inclusion as a policy, or are actively working toward it, while others support segregated classes.

Inclusion, like mainstreaming and the LRE, has come under attack (table 9.4).

11 Can you imagine some of the criticisms of inclusion? As you read on, see if any of the perceived problems of inclusion are similar to those of mainstreaming or LRE.

Block (1999) has described some of the problems from an American perspective, but many are relevant to Canada as well. However, we must introduce this discussion by noting that many children with disabilities are included in regular schools and classrooms across Canada and are functioning quite well. Strong advocates of the concept of inclusion argue that everyone should be included.

One of the problems articulated by Block (1999) was that inclusion became a cause, a moral imperative, that did not have to be supported by research, according to its proponents. Thus, there was little systematic study of inclusion, for example, or the education needed by the teachers, or specific inclusion techniques that were effective. Second, zealots of inclusion forgot about the needs of individual children, since they were more concerned with placement of children in regular classes. Thus, there was little consideration that some children who were medically fragile, or with very serious emotional problems, might actually benefit from some form of alternative placement and education outside regular classes and schools. Third, the preferences of parents were often ignored. Some parents believed their children flourished in settings other than the regular schools. Fourth, many regular physical education programmes were not particularly individualized and therefore could not accommodate many youngsters with a disability. Often, physical education classes had such large numbers that class management was difficult and quality instruction impossible. Block suggested that many physical educators did not take ownership of children with a disability, believing these children were outside their responsibilities. Even when the teachers were highly skilled and experienced, they still expressed frustration at not being able to deal simultaneously with all the children in their class (Lienert, Sherrill, and Myers 2001; LaMaster, Gall, Kinchin, and Siedentop 1998). These teachers wanted to do more but did not believe they had adequate preparation and time. Fifth, lack of personnel support was noted as a significant problem, and it was claimed that children were simply 'dumped' into large physical education classes without teaching assistants or adapted physical activity consultants. This is particularly a problem at the elementary level, since classroom teachers are often responsible for instruction in physical education in many parts of Canada. Therefore, including children with a disability was an added challenge to someone who might be uncomfortable teaching physical education in the first place (Karper 1995).

12 Are some of these difficulties with inclusion similar to those mentioned with mainstreaming or LRE? Which ones?

The attentive reader will note considerable similarity between the problems of inclusion and mainstreaming. Both have been charged with being poorly implemented as intended (e.g., lack of support personnel) and becoming a 'dumping ground.' It was claimed that physical educators were not ready to accept children with disabilities and that their programmes were so inflexible that there was little opportunity to accept even a modest range of individual differences. Finally, each has been criticized for forgetting about the individual in the rush to implement the concept. Has mainstreaming just been repeated under the guise of inclusion? It is hoped that this is not the case. There may have been more progress than seems evident. Possibly the individuals now being 'included' have more severe disabilities than those integrated into the 'mainstream.' It is possible, for example, that physical education programmes can now accommodate those with disabilities who were candidates for mainstreaming fifteen to twenty years ago, but current difficulties remain with the support of those with more challenging disabilities. Also, there are many reports of successful inclusion in physical education (e.g., Block, Zeman, and Henning 1997; Heikinaro-Johansson, Sherrill, French, and Huuhka 1995; Houston-Wilson, Dunn, van der Mars, and McCubbin 1997; Lieberman, Dunn, van der Mars, and McCubbin 2000). Nonetheless, there seems much to be done.

So Tell Me What To Do!

We have waded through the concepts of mainstreaming, normalization, LRE, and inclusion. Let us remember that each was a response to the unacceptable segregation of most children and adults with a disability that characterized Canadian society until the 1970s. Despite the weakness or challenges described above, the beginning of the twenty-first century finds many children with a disability successfully receiving education in community-based schools and more adults with a disability in the workforce, at community recreation facilities, and enjoying a meal at a restaurant. Many things are proceeding very well, and there have been positive changes in the past thirty years.

Yet how do we deal with the difficulties in physical activity settings? After reading all the benefits of and problems with mainstreaming, normalization, LRE, and inclusion, the reader may be asking the following question,

13 "Tell me what to do as a young professional in physical activity with regard to inclusion." You will have to reflect on the contents of this complete book, including the chapters dealing with the 'how' of inclusion, and build a working philosophy on these important issues by yourself.

However, some points in the following paragraphs may assist you, and they begin to describe this author's viewpoint.

Jane Watkinson, a University of Alberta professor, published a paper in 1991 titled "The Mainstreaming Bandwagon: A Need for Reassessment." More recently, Block (1999) produced a paper titled "Did We Jump On the Wrong Bandwagon? Problems With Inclusion in Physical Education." Finally, DePauw and Doll-Tepper (2000) produced a piece titled "Toward Progressive Inclusion and Acceptance: Myth or Reality? The Inclusion Debate and Bandwagon Discourse." Each of these scholars used the term *bandwagon* to describe some of the difficulties with mainstreaming and inclusion.

14 What does "jumping on a bandwagon" imply to you?

To jump on a bandwagon suggests quick acceptance of an idea without considering the issue fully. A bandwagon often has the appearance of being contemporary and enjoying such wide support that opposing it seems almost heresy. Bandwagons tend to say, "This approach is great for everyone and other alternatives are wrong"; "Get on board, or you will be left behind."

In reality, bandwagons constrain rather than liberate thinking and practice. For example, when mainstreaming and normalization were developed, it became common to criticize programmes such as the Special Olympics because they were largely segregated. Some suggested that these programmes be discontinued. But as Watkinson (1991) noted, thousands of individuals with an intellectual disability learned to skate, ski, and/or swim because of Special Olympics. They learned social skills through Special Olympics, and many travelled to competitions throughout their province and some across Canada. Jumping on the bandwagon of mainstreaming, if it meant eliminating Special Olympics, may have prevented meaningful athletic practice for some individuals. Mainstreaming and inclusion are not poor ideologies, but in some instances they were implemented poorly and too quickly, often forgetting about the individual person who was thrown on the bandwagon and found the trip to be unrewarding. Therefore, it is likely wise to avoid bandwagon thinking in the future.

15 How do we avoid "jumping on a bandwagon"?

The easiest way is to resist absolute statements, such as, this is wonderful for everyone. Such comments deny individual choice, decision making, empowerment, and self-determination. Diversity is a key to physical activity programming today. There are hockey programmes for children of all ages and abilities, including older adults over sixty, and range from recreation to highly competitive. People bring different interests and competencies to the rink. One programme can not fit all. Another way to avoid bandwagon thinking is to allow people to choose. Therefore, participants should have access to a host of programme opportunities. If a programme that is largely segregated (e.g., a Special Olympic swim team) does not fulfill a need, it will eventually cease to operate. An individual who uses a wheelchair likely has a wide range of friends and will want access to the local fitness facility to socialize and exercise with those without a disability. But this same person may choose to participate in wheelchair sport and aspire to the Paralympics, a programme that is restricted to people with a disability (Yilli 1994). We should support individuals who wish to move in and out of inclusive and segregated settings as required and articulated by them. Another way to prevent bandwagon discourse is to redefine inclusion as a more flexible and accepting philosophy, more accommodating to true individual needs, and be more willing to include alternative views that aim for similar goals. Of course, strong advocates of inclusion for all will disagree with this posture and argue that it justifies segregated thinking. Yet, by redefining inclusion it may remain an excellent goal to guide many of our practices in the future.

We also need to conduct research on the impact of inclusion on students with and without disabilities (Block and Vogler 1994; see Goodwin and Watkinson 2000; Vogler, Koranda, and Romance 2000, as examples). Recently, Goodwin and Watkinson (2000) reported that students with physical disabilities experience good and bad days in inclusive physical education. Good days were associated with a sense of belonging, sharing the benefits of physical education, and sense of skillful participation. The bad days occurred when they became socially isolated, their competence was questioned, and their participation was restricted. We must know more about how to maximize the good days and minimize the bad.

Summary

This chapter has described the very powerful concepts of mainstreaming, normalization, LRE, and inclusion. They have had a profound influence on how we view disability, education, and leisure, as well as housing, transportation, and employment. Normalization challenged us to ensure that experiences for those with a disability reflected our own daily, weekly, and yearly rhythms and activities. Institutional living, attending special schools at great distance from local schools, lack of choice or responsibility, and low expectations were not 'normalizing.' Mainstreaming was a response by schools to normalization and other factors, and it promoted the integration of students with mild disabilities into regular school programmes. The LRE was a continuum of educational placements, which varied by degree of restriction and freedom offered the person with a disability. It was intended to promote progressive movement toward less restrictive settings, the least restrictive being the mainstream. Inclusion supported the placement of *all* people with a disability into regular classrooms, with supports being brought to the individuals, rather than having the children leave the class or school to receive the supports. Inclusion was more than just a placement, it was an attitude of belonging and acceptance of diversity. Mainstreaming, normalization, LRE, and inclusion have been criticized by some, and professionals should be aware of this commentary. Much of the dialogue is critical of how integration of individuals with a disability has been implemented, rather than the concepts themselves.

Surely, no thoughtful argument would suggest a return to the segregated settings and neglect for people with a disability that typified the early twentieth century. Without question, our society has moved to greater acceptance and concern for people with a disability. In fact, our Canadian society has made remarkable strides toward acceptance of other aspects of diversity such as racial background and sexual orientation. We need to continue to move toward integration at every available opportunity in education and recreation settings. But inclusion for all, as desirable as it is, will require positive attitudes on the part of teachers, additional preparation for them, and more money for appropriate supports (Karper 1995). In one published account of successful inclusion in physical education (Block et al. 1997), there was a physical education specialist as the regular physical education teacher, a full-time one-to-one teaching assistant for the student who had a disability, and a specialist in adapted physical education who functioned as consultant. Unfortunately, not many schools in Canada enjoy this luxury of support. This should not be an excuse to avoid inclusion, however. Going backward is not a solution.

Innovative thinking can overcome some of the obstacles. In Finland, for example, Heikinaro-Johansson et al. (1995) demonstrated the considerable success of a consultant model, which assisted elementary school classroom teachers to deal with integration as they taught physical education. In Canada, we have access to the excellent Moving to Inclusion series, which can assist. But we must determine if teachers are aware of this resource, is it being used, is it helpful? What is the perception of teachers to inclusion? What factors positively influence inclusion? What are the barriers? We also have Canadian scholars who have made significant contributions to re-thinking the role of leisure in the life of the individual with a disability (e.g., Hutchison and McGill 1992 and the journal *Leisurability*). Therefore, we should move forward toward inclusion as a desirable philosophical goal of acceptance, but with concern, intelligence, and openness, ever vigilant for arguments that "one size must fit all."

Study Questions

1. You are a parent of young child with a disability who has been denied access to the Saturday morning gym/swim programme in your local community. Develop an essay of why your child should be allowed to participate.
2. For the first half of the twentieth century, people with a disability were largely excluded from society. What factors led to more integrated concepts, specifically mainstreaming?
3. What are the similarities and differences among mainstreaming, LRE, and inclusion?
4. List the criticisms of mainstreaming, LRE, and inclusion.
5. You have been asked to address the school or recreation advisory board on integration with physical activity programmes. Prepare an essay that describes your personal philosophy, being careful to be explicit and to offer support for your stance.

References

Active Living Alliance for Canadians with a Disability. (1994). *Moving to Inclusion*. Ottawa: Author.

Aufsesser, P.M. (1981). Adapted physical education: A look back, a look ahead. *Journal of Health, Physical Education and Recreation, 52*(6), 28–31.

Aufsesser, P.M. (1991). Mainstreaming and the least restrictive environment: How do they differ? *Palaestra, 7*(2), 31–34.

Birch, J.W. (1974). *Mainstreaming educable mentally retarded children in regular classes*. Minneapolis: Leadership Training Institute, University of Minnesota.

Block, M. (1992). What is appropriate physical education for students with profound disabilities? *Adapted Physical Activity Quarterly, 9*, 197–213.

Block, M. (1994a). *A teacher's guide to including students with disabilities in regular physical education*. Baltimore: Paul H. Brookes.

Block, M. (1994b) Why all students with disabilities should be included in regular physical education. *Palaestra, 10*(3), 17–24.

Block, M. (1996). When can I remove a child with disabilities from regular physical education? *Palaestra, 12*(2), 45–50.

Block, M. (1999). Did we jump on the wrong bandwagon? Problems with inclusion in physical education. *Palaestra, 15*(3), 30–36, 55.

Block, M., and Vogler, E.W. (1994). Inclusion in regular physical education: The research base. *Journal of Physical Education, Recreation, and Dance,* 40–44.

Block, M.E., and Krebs, P.L. (1992). An alternative to least restrictive environments: A continuum of support to regular physical education. *Adapted Physical Activity Quarterly, 9,* 97–113.

Block, M.E., Zeman, R., and Henning, G. (1997). "Pass the ball to Jimmy": A success story in inclusive physical education. *Palaestra, 13*(3), 37–41.

Broadhead, G.D. (1985). Placement of mildly handicapped children in mainstream physical education. *Adapted Physical Activity Quarterly, 2,* 307–13.

Bundschuh, E.L. (1976). Preparation of undergraduate physical education majors for mainstreaming. In *Mainstreaming physical education.* The National Association for Physical Education of College Women and the National Association College Physical Education Association for Men.

Committee on Adapted Physical Education. (1952). Guiding principles for adapted physical education. *Journal of Health, Physical Education, and Recreation, 23,* 15, 28.

Connor, F.L. (1976). The past is prologue: Teacher preparation in special education. *Exceptional Children, 42,* 336–78.

Deno, E. (1970). Special education as development capital. *Exceptional Children, 37,* 229–37.

DePaepe, J. (1984). Mainstreaming malpractice. *Physical Educator, 41* (1), 51–56.

DePauw, K.P., and Doll-Tepper, G. (2000). Toward progressive inclusion and acceptance: Myth or reality? The inclusion debate and bandwagon discourse. *Adapted Physical Activity Quarterly, 17,* 135–43.

DiRocco, P. (1976). Political and economic implications of mainstreaming. In *Mainstreaming physical education.* The National Association for Physical Education of College Women and the National Association College Physical Education Association for Men.

Dunn, L.M. (1968). Special education for the mildly retarded: Is much of it justifiable? *Exceptional Children, 35*(1), 5–22.

Dunn, J. (1976). Mainstreaming: Definition, rationale and implications for physical education. In *Mainstreaming physical education.* The National Association for Physical Education of College Women and the National Association College Physical Education Association for Men.

Dunn, J.M., and Craft, D.H. (1985). Mainstreaming theory and practice. *Adapted Physical Activity Quarterly, 2,* 273–76.

Goodwin, D., and Watkinson, E.J. (2000). Inclusive physical education from the perspective of students with disabilities. *Adapted Physical Activity Quarterly, 17,* 144–60.

Grineski, S. (1994). Dilemma of educational placement for students with severe disabilities. *Palaestra, 10*(3), 21–22.

Grosse, S. (1991). Is the mainstream always a better place to be? *Palaestra, 7*(2), 40–49.

Guskin, S.L., and Spiker, H.H. (1968). Educational research in mental retardation. In N.R. Ellis (Ed.), *International review of research in mental retardation: Vol. 3.* New York: Academic Press.

Heikinaro-Johansson, P., Sherrill, C., French, R., and Huuhka, H. (1995). Adapted physical education consultant service model to facilitate integration. *Adapted Physical Activity Quarterly, 12,* 12–23.

Houston-Wilson, C., Dunn, J.M., van der Mars, H., and McCubbin, J. (1997). The effect of peer tutors on motor performance in integrated physical education classes. *Adapted Physical Activity Quarterly, 14,* 298–313.

Hutchison, P., and McGill, J. (1992). *Leisure, integration and community.* Concord, ON: Leisurability Publications.

Karper, W.B. (1995). Problems with inclusive elementary school physical education. *Palaestra, 11*(2), 32–35.

Kirk, S.A. (1964). Research in education. In H.A. Stevens and R. Heber (Eds.), *Mental retardation.* Chicago: University of Chicago Press.

Kozub, F.M., Sherblom, P.R., and Perry, T.L. (1999). Inclusion paradigms and perspectives. A stepping stone to accepting learner diversity in physical education. *Quest, 51,* 346–54.

LaMaster, K., Gall, K., Kinchin, G., and Seidentop, D. (1998). Inclusion practices of effective elementary specialists. *Adapted Physical Activity Quarterly, 15,* 64–81.

Lavay, B., and DePaepe, J. (1987). The harbinger helper: Why mainstreaming in physical education doesn't always work. *Journal of Physical Education, Recreation, and Dance, 58*(7), 98–103.

Lieberman, L.J., Dunn, J.M., van der Mars, H., and McCubbin, J. (2000). Peer tutors' effects on activity levels of deaf students in inclusive elementary physical education. *Adapted Physical Activity Quarterly, 17,* 20–39.

Lienert, C., Sherrill, C., and Myers, B. (2001). Physical educators' concerns about integrating children with disabilities: A cross-cultural comparison. *Adapted Physical Activity Quarterly, 18,* 1–17.

Reid, G. (1979). Mainstreaming: Implications for physical educators. *McGill Journal of Education, 14,* 367–77.

Reynolds, M. (1962). A framework for considering some issues in special education. *Exceptional Children, 29,* 367–70.

Sherrill, C. (1993). *Adapted physical activity, recreation, and sport: Crossdisciplinary and lifespan* (4th ed.). Madison, WI: Brown and Benchmark.

Sherrill, C. (1994). Least restrictive environment and total inclusion philosophies: Critical analysis. *Palaestra, 10*(2), 25–35, 52–54.

Sherman, A. (1996). Mainstreaming: Where did we fail? *Palaestra, 12*(2), 25–27.

Stainback, S., and Stainback, W. (1990). Inclusive schooling. In W. Stainback and S. Stainback (Eds.), *Support networks for inclusive schooling* (pp. 3–24). Baltimore: Paul H. Brookes.

Stainback, S., Stainback, W., and Forest, M. (1989). *Educating all students in the mainstream of regular education.* Baltimore: Paul H. Brookes.

Stein, J. (1976). Sense and nonsense about mainstreaming. *Journal of Physical Education and Recreation, 47*(1), 43.

Taylor, S. (1988). Caught in the continuum: A critical analysis of the principles of the least restrictive environment. *Journal of the Association for Persons with Severe Handicaps, 13*(1), 41–53.

Vogler, E.W., Koranda, P., and Romance, T. (2000). Including a child with severe cerebral palsy in physical education: A case study. *Adapted Physical Activity Quarterly, 17,* 161–75.

Watkinson, E.J. (1991). The mainstreaming bandwagon: A need for reassessment. *Canadian Association of Physical Education and Recreation Journal, 57*(1), 39–42.

Wolfensberger, W. (1972). *The principle of normalization in human services.* Toronto: National Institute of Mental Retardation.

Yilli, A.B. (1994). Full inclusion: A philosophical statement. *Palaestra, 10*(4), 18.

CHAPTER 10

Professional Preparation

Claudia G. Emes

Learning Objectives

- To describe the key factors that influence an abilities-based approach to adapted physical activity.
- To discuss APA in relation to service delivery.
- To define the components of an abilities-based service delivery process.
- To relate the APA practicum to an abilities-based service delivery process.

Introduction

As we begin the twenty-first century, preparing for a professional future that includes working with people who have a disability includes almost everyone who will receive professional credentials, whether in the fields of fitness, sport, dance, physical education, or recreation. The opportunities are endless for people with a disability to participate in physical activity. Whether it is first-time entry to a swim lesson or training for an elite competition, the experience the participant has will be directly affected by the encounter she or he has with the professional who is delivering the programme. This encounter is part of a larger concept called *service delivery*.

The purpose of this chapter is to present professional preparation in adapted physical activity using an *abilities-based service delivery model*.

Abilities-based Practice

Application of an abilities-based approach is fundamental to the undergraduate preparation, education, and training of future adapted physical activity (APA) professionals. Professional preparation in APA is based on the delivery of service that is:

- person-centred
- enquiry-based
- focussed on abilities
- inclusive

PERSON-CENTRED

Person-centred planning helps the professional move from the superior role of **expert** to the more humble role of **partner**, someone who is interested in supporting and negotiating the learning needs of a person. It begins with listening. In fact, the first planning step is to listen to the person with whom you will work. It requires active listening that faithfully demonstrates to that person that he or she has been heard and understood. It employs the use of the following simple techniques:

- Position yourself physically so you are close and at eye level with this person.
- Repeat while conversing what you think you heard him or her say.
- Summarize your conversation and ask if you got it right.
- Share your feelings.

This component of planning is exciting because it is based on a process of discovery. Frequently, the interests, capacities, and aspirations of a person with a disability are buried under labels and the lack of or limited information. It is empowering for the person to convey information she or he wants you to know. It will likely increase motivation toward activity to be part of the decision making about the type of activity and the goals and objectives associated with a programme.

1 Think of someone in your life whom you consider a good listener. What attributes, in your opinion, do you see in him or her that makes a good listener? Write down the attributes and check off those that you have and those that you would like to practice. Is there any evidence that good listening helps to get to know someone better if you listen well? What do you see as the key differences in what you learn about people using good listening skills compared to not listening well?

ENQUIRY-BASED

To enquire is to seek to learn by asking. Posing good questions is critical to successful enquiry. A product of posing good questions is valuable information and, in order to provide the best service possible in APA, you will want the best information available to you. Posing good questions also affords the opportunity to challenge the status quo. It is important not to get too comfortable with the way things have been done in the past, as learning to be a professional includes seeking new solutions to old challenges. The concept of individualization is fundamental to working in a model that relies on abilities-based and person-centred planning. In order to make an individual plan that considers both the needs and potential of a person, you must seek to learn by asking.

2 Compare the questions you ask a friend and those you ask a stranger to learn more about that person? What are the differences? What types of questions are most revealing? How do these questions compare to those that you ask when you are questioning about things?

FOCUS ON ABILITIES

Focussing on capabilities and competencies is the basic tenet of an abilities-based approach to service delivery in APA. It compares the functional abilities of a person with the demands of specific activities and measures the 'compatibility overlap'. If the person's abilities match or exceed the functions required by the activity, then there exists a strong likelihood that participation in that activity will be successful. Therefore, in order to focus on abilities, it is important to determine what abilities a person has in relation to those that will be required of him or her to participate in an activity. This can be accomplished effectively by making simple comparisons. Generally, those comparisons are instructed by the specific activity, but they include skills in the cognitive, communicative, social, fitness, motor, and object manipulation areas.

3 Select two activities or sports that you currently enjoy doing and two that you would like to learn. Compare your abilities with those demanded by the activities that you have selected in the following categories: What are the minimal, relevant demands of the activities in communication skills, social skills, fitness levels, motor skills, and object manipulation skills? What are your skills in these areas? What is your 'compatibility overlap' in these activities? How does understanding 'compatibility overlap' affect your interest in and attitude toward learning these new activities?

INCLUSIVE

Inclusion is an imperative that promotes the creation of communities that support all of their members and ensures they share equitably in its contributions and resources regardless of their differences (Jeffreys and Gall 1996). It is often used interchangeably with the word *integration*, but they are not the same in that integration usually addresses efforts to manage the reversal or reduction of segregation. Integration ensures the physical presence of people with disability among those without disability, it does not ensure social, emotional and intellectual participation. Inclusion, on the other hand, results from valuing all members of society in the same way. This philosophy emerged from an earlier theory of normalization that originated in Scandinavia. It did not suggest that people with disability become normal through treatment, but that their patterns and conditions can be normalized to resemble those of the mainstream of society. *Social role valorization* is central to this understanding. That is, valued social status is important for all members of our society (Galambos and Whetstone 1989). It has become evident over time that both an inclusive attitude and an inclusive environment are the outcomes of valuing people regardless of their differences.

4 Think about your own social role. What are the factors that influence your social role? Have you ever been in a position where you feel your opinion is not valued? Why do you think it was not valued? How did that experience affect your feelings at the time? How do you think your opinion may have been better valued? How do you like to be valued?

Professional Preparation

Preparation to enter into a career where one works with people with a disability includes expanding one's knowledge base, participating in a practicum (experiential learning) where knowledge, understanding and skills can be tested within the safety of a well-defined environment, and developing critical thinking and analytical skills that continuously challenge traditional attitudes and assumptions in APA.

EXPANDING ONE'S KNOWLEDGE

Adapted physical activity is defined as a cross disciplinary body of knowledge directed toward the identification and solution of individual differences in the psychomotor domain. It is a service delivery profession and an academic field of study which supports an attitude of acceptance of individual differences, advocates to enhance access to active lifestyles and sport, and promotes innovation and cooperative service delivery and empowerment systems. Adapted physical activity includes but is not limited to physical education, sport, recreation, dance and creative arts, nutrition, medicine and rehabilitation. (Sherrill 1993, p. 5)

The delivery of services that meet the needs of people with disability is the cornerstone of the APA profession. Service delivery is a complex process that relies a variety of professional activities and behaviours. Studying the components of service delivery provides an effective guide to the generic preparation of professionals who service people with disability in a physical activity setting.

UNDERSTANDING SERVICE DELIVERY
Service delivery accounts for the quality and the manner in which people receive information, instructions, directions, and services such as therapy, programmes of activity, and social support. It accounts for the way services are delivered, what type of services, and the quality and the timeliness of the services. Service delivery is determined by both the people and the materials or equipment that are part of a service. In APA, service delivery is defined by the programmes we offer: school-based adapted physical activity, adapted fitness and recreational community-based programmes, and elite sport such as Paralympics and Special Olympics.

UNDERSTANDING ABILITIES-BASED SERVICE DELIVERY
In abilities-based service delivery, the person receiving the service is placed in the centre of the system of delivery. Abilities-based service serves this person by directing attention away from asking "What's wrong with this client and how can professionals fix it?" toward such questions as "What are this person's capacities and abilities and what supports are needed to express them?" and "What works well for this person?" Person-centred planning does not ignore disability; it simply shifts the emphasis to a search for capacity in the person. A person's difficulties are not relevant to the process until his or her goals and visions are clear. At that point, it may be appropriate to ask, "What particular assistance do you need because of your specific limitations (not labels)?" Service delivery has shifted from a focus on accurate diagnosis, therapeutic

interventions, and developing skills in small steps, to listening respectfully and imaginatively to the person (parents or guardians) and standing with them to thoughtfully consider how to work together (O'Brien and O'Brien 1998). Rarely is a prescription or a ready-made remedy available; each person requires unique attention. Finding what works best often includes using techniques that have been previously successful, but an established formula is not a starting point. The starting point is recognizing the unique needs, feelings, and capabilities of a person and acknowledging the growth and learning potential of this person.

COMPONENTS OF APA SERVICE DELIVERY
Depending on the purpose of providing an APA service (e.g., training for an international competition versus delivery of a school-based sport programme), good service delivery may or may not require all the components or factors generally associated with APA service delivery. However, a comprehensive programme of service delivery will include the following components:

5 What is advocacy? Why is it the overarching concept that is part of every aspect of service delivery?

1. Advocacy
Advocacy means "promoting or pleading a case or a cause in a convincing way," while an *advocate* is "someone who uses advocacy tools in his or her own interest or on behalf of another." In APA, advocacy is an integral part of all aspects of service delivery, and as a professional, you should consider carefully when it is important for you to be an advocate and, more importantly, when can you support the person with whom you work to be a self-advocate.

Advocacy is empowering because its success depends on the articulation of a solid argument or cause. During preparation and presentation of the argument we learn about the issues around it. We are also reminded that advocacy does not occur in isolation, but is part of all aspects of service delivery. It is an imperative in planning, assessing individual abilities, taking different professional roles, creating connections for APA participants, and evaluating programmes.

We can use our voice to advocate and support advocacy in many ways. Writing letters, making presentations and speeches, creating position papers, and role modelling are standard examples of advocacy. Depending on your role, whether it be a coach, counsellor, or teacher, the way in which you use advocacy may vary. For example, Steve, a practicum student, started working with a young person who is visually impaired. Steve's passion is cycling, so he introduced her to this sport. Soon she was cycling successfully and Steve was seeking opportunities for her to compete. As there were no programmes specifically for cyclists with visual impairment, Steve became an advocate to include her in existing programmes. He promoted support for cycling competition from a provincial organization for athletes with visual impairment and, as a result, this cyclist was financially sponsored to compete in an event out-of-province. He now has a successful programme in operation with two more cyclists and support for programme development from the national cycling body. What were the tools he used as an advocate? First, he advertised his interest in coaching cycling in a provincial newsletter for people with visual impairment. Although he received just one response, he saw this as an opportunity to launch a programme of cycling for people with visual impairment. His next step as an advocate was a letter-writing campaign to get financial support for his participant as an athlete. He then encouraged her involvement as an advocate and they both spoke to various organizations, not only for support, but to encourage new members to join them. One year later, their sights were set on international competition. Eventually, Steve will support the cyclist to be a self-advocate whenever possible.

6 Assuming that you are participating in a practicum, consider the people whom you work with in your practicum. If you are not in a practicum, consider one of your personal experiences. How could you use advocacy to improve or change the programme? What tools would you use? Who would be the advocate?

2. Assessment
Deciding where to begin.

When you are placed in a situation of responsibility, regardless of context or activity there are certain understandings that will assist you in determining where to begin and what to do. Whether you are planning an inclusive games unit in physical education or a work-out routine in a private gym, you can gather generic information that will guide decisions which you and the learner with whom you are working will make together. What information do you need? Start by asking the following questions.

A. WHO IS THIS PERSON?

Learn as much as you can about him or her: likes and dislikes, interests, preferences, recreational pursuits, significant accomplishments. If necessary, speak to family members and friends. A person whom others find extremely difficult to understand may have no one close enough to interpret and speak up for his or her personal interests. This will result in little or no information about this person's strengths and uniqueness. Unfortunately, lack of personal information may be justified by devaluing, self-defeating statements such as, "She's too low-functioning to have any interests," or, "His behaviour is so severe no one can get near him." In challenging cases such as these, the highest priority of quality service delivery is to start building a relationship (O'Brien and O'Brien 1998, p. 46). Building a relationship can occur without using verbal communication. Pictures, objects, and technologically-driven communication can be used as an alternative.

Table 10.1 Statements of Observation

Needs Work	Better Examples
1. Is hard of hearing	Constantly needs repetition of instruction
2. Needs more social interaction	Has a tendency to play alone and does not share toys
3. Can not throw a ball very well	Demonstrated an immature throwing pattern—no opposition or weight transfer
4. Seems lazy	Low activity level—does not initiate activities, always sits down to listen to instructions

7 Think about how you can establish a relationship with a person who has disability without using verbal communication. How could you begin to establish a relationship using an object?

B. WHAT ARE THIS PERSON'S OBSERVABLE ABILITIES?

Observe skills and abilities in the environment in which you will be working together. This can be done by conducting authentic assessments wherein performance in specific skills is assessed when they are demonstrated in an authentic situation (i.e., observing a forward pass during a soccer game rather than as an isolated skill). Alternatively, you may merely record personal observations when the two of you happen to be in the same place. Regardless, learn to make good observational statements. Try not to interpret the behaviour you see. Concentrate on what you are observing, not what you think is going on. The following chart compares statements that record observations versus those that record interpretations.

8 How do the incomplete statements differ from the better examples provided above? What characterizes a good observational statement?

Depending on the person and the place in a learning experience, the focus of an observation may differ. General guidelines for points of observation are:

- Overall movement, posture, gait, balance, and eye-hand coordination
- Movement planning–evidence that the person find solutions to movement problems; evidence of willingness to attempt difficult tasks
- Interaction with peers–how others interact with one another and with this person; evidence of communication
- Response to instruction–evidence of attention span, understanding instruction (Gavron 1996)

Enhance your observations by complementing them with information acquired from the following assessments (see Chapter 21 (Longmuir)): communications skills, mobility, object manipulation, cognitive skills, and behaviour and social skills.

C. WHAT DOES THIS PERSON HOPE TO ACHIEVE?

Learning more about this person's aspirations will significantly influence the goals and objectives that you set for a programme. Setting goals and objectives are shared activities that include the person with whom you are working.

3. Planning for learning in APA

You may be planning to coach an elite athlete, provide personal fitness training, guide a rock-climbing activity, or teach a dance class. Regardless of how you are involved in the APA experience, it is important to think very carefully about the purpose, objectives, and possible outcomes before you prepare the learning or practice episode. Successful planning is usually reflected in how well the expected outcomes of a programme are achieved. Although we may have our sights on the outcomes, it's what we do, how and where we do it, and with whom that gets us there. In other words, we must help create the right circumstances to achieve our intended outcomes.

Programme planning, as a part of service delivery, is like creating a banquet. You must consider who will be dining, what will be served, who will serve and where it will be served, and not necessarily in that order. Are you considering fast food for children served in a community hall by parents, or gourmet dining, adults only, at an elegant restaurant with experienced waiters? How will these different factors affect the service at the banquet? Planning a programme should be viewed from the same perspective. Schwab (1966) suggests that we should plan for a total learning experience that includes the interaction of the four places of learning: milieu, student (learner), instructor, and content.

MILIEU

Clustered in the milieu are the needs, demands, and conditions that social structures place on the learner. To return to our metaphor, if the banquet hall is constructed well it should be able to serve different people at different times and with a variety of menus. A good hall can be set for 400 or reconfigured to host 30 intimately. It welcomes all with an inviting atmosphere that suits people from age eighty to age eight. It accommodates those who use wheelchairs alongside those who use strollers and those who have limited vision. The hall is a structure that cannot discriminate who will access it according to age,

disability, or any other factor. The doors and windows, however, can be opened and closed by those who plan the banquet. The doors and windows represent the social structures that determine who will enter and who will leave, how the world sees the banquet, and how those at the banquet see the world. Social structures influence our attitudes and affect policy. They are political (governments, schools, health care organizations), religious (churches, schools, charities), gender-based (schools, organized sports), ethnic (communities, schools, churches), socio-economic (housing, schools, health care, organized sports), and disability-based (housing, schools, health care access, organized sports). The frequency with which the "doors and windows" remain open to the banquet hall has changed over time. Within APA we are reminded of the historical norm of institutionalizing people with developmental disability. Over time that norm has all but disappeared in North America. When the doors and windows of the banquet hall are permanently open, then the *milieu* for learning will account for all participants, including those with diability.

> **9** Besides deinstitutionalization, is there other evidence that the social norm for serving people with disabilities has changed? What influence do social structures have on how people with disabilities participate in physical activity and learn in physical education classes? How does social norm influence the milieu? Consider the milieu of your university education. How can you describe the milieu of your total learning experience in a first-year class?

STUDENT

The student represents a cluster of abilities, past experiences, and current and future needs in a constellation unique to every individual. She or he is at the banquet to have a feast of learning. Therefore, we must identify the most important considerations for choosing an individual menu. We must determine from which table at the banquet buffet it is best for that individual to choose items for his or her plate. We must also make sure that the other tables hold enough options for everyone else to fill their plates equally well.

INSTRUCTOR

Schwab considers the instructor, or teacher, and the teaching process together and advocates professional preparation and practices that encourage learner independence. The instructor is the chef who has the skills to prepare the feast. Often they have prepared this kind of feast in the past, but something always has to be adapted to meet the unique needs of today's guests, who will participate in decisions about the food and in its preparation. This is consistent with the type of service delivery presented here, as the learner (person) is in the centre of the process. Each aspect of the process nourishes greater independence, or less dependency, by the learner. The learner is encouraged to take responsibility. This also affords the opportunity to risk failure as well as success.

10 Think about the learning experiences you have enjoyed the most. What characterized those experiences? If you were learning from a teacher, what behaviours did you observe? What are the professional practices that teachers engage in that encourage greater independence?

CONTENT

The fourth determinant of the total learning experience is the content, or subject-matter. Without food there is no feast. Food, not just any food, must be chosen on the basis of colour, consistency, and nutritional contribution to the feast. The outcome is variety, interest, and balance. We make learning interesting by varying the content and the way in which it is delivered. It should also reflect planning and preparation that considers age-appropriateness, cultural appropriateness, and relevance to proposed outcomes. Proposed learning should be made clear in the stated objectives of any programme plan.

Together, these four determining factors continuously interact in an environment that supports enquiry and creativity. The four places of learning are also the framework within which planning for a programme occurs. It is the ideal environment in which to modify standard protocol and adapt to situations that depart to a greater or lesser extent from the norm.

4. Implementing an APA programme

Given that the milieu, student, instructor, and content are well understood, different support skills emerge as prerequisites for planning to move into implementation. Working in a physical activity setting requires different knowledge and skills at different times, and it further requires that you understand when and how to execute those skills effectively. During professional preparation, you should learn the basics of using the following tools. Depending on the outcome of the assessment phase of the APA service delivery process, there are a variety of ways you can support and contribute to learning. These include:

- teaching
- brokering
- facilitating
- consulting
- coaching
- leading
- co-learning
- advocating

11 Expand your definition of each of the above actions by describing the common critical skills that all of these actions require and what skills distinguish these actions. For example, each requires good communication skills, but in teaching, you may be required to create explicit lesson plans, whereas consulting might require that you file a site evaluation report. How can the above list of actions be further compared and contrasted? Can you create examples of how these might be used in the same physical activity learning environment?

Regardless of the part you take during learning, as a professional you should be prepared to create documents that demonstrate knowledge and skills associated with explicit planning. The ability to create goals, objectives, timelines, and programme evaluations is fundamental to this skills set.

GOAL-SETTING

Whenever possible, goals should be created with the person who is trying to attain those goals. Some might argue that, when setting goals together with the person(s) with whom you are working, expectations could easily become unrealistic. Is this true? Does it matter? What is another way of viewing the inclusion of this person in goal-setting? Research has shown (Fuchs, Fuchs, and Deno 1985) that learners are motivated by the ambitiousness of their goals, even if they fail to achieve them, whereas mastery of less ambitious goals is not as motivating as one might expect.

Goals are person-centred statements of programme outcomes that describe in general terms how things will be in the person's future. Usually, goals are created annually and therefore become predictors of what one might expect a year from now. They describe results rather than the methods to be used. Have you ever heard someone say as they usher in the New Year, "This year my goal is to lose ten pounds and keep it off"? Is this statement person-centred? Is it in general terms? Does it speak to results or method?

12 What are your personal goals for your APA class? Analyze them in terms of being predictors. What factors will influence how well they will predict for you the future outcome of the course?

Goals also guide the implementation of a programme. They should reflect values in the programme and relate to the person in more than one way; that is, they should cover several dimensions, such as, physical, intellectual, social, emotional, and cultural.

WRITING OBJECTIVES

The method by which goals are achieved is made explicit through specific behavioural objectives. Objectives will be addressed further in Chapter 16 (Goodwin), but by way of introduction, objectives will be examined here in terms of how they translate the methods of achieving goals. Standard guidelines for writing objectives include the following: *person* (by name), behaviour or *action*, *criterion*, *elements*, and *date*. They follow a simple to remember acronym: PACED. Objectives are person-centred so they begin by stating the person's name, followed by the behaviour or action she or he will demonstrate, including at what level or standard (criterion), all of the elements that will characterize the behaviour, and the date by which all of this will be achieved. For example, an objective that reflects the goal to become a competitive tandem cyclist might be stated as follows: Tanya will tandem cycle at least 10 km on flat terrain in 30 minutes by May 15 (4 weeks). Identifying Tanya by name personalizes the activity (cycling) while identifying a specific distance (10 km), the elements (flat terrain), and the speed (criteria) clarifies how the action will take place. The date provides a time target to work toward.

Objectives can guide long-range activities, intermediate range, short range or 'just-in-time' activities. If you are in a practicum placement where you work with someone different every time you meet, you may be called upon continually to create just-in-time objectives. The PACED guideline works in all cases, but a just-in-time objective is made on the basis of a situation as it presents itself at the moment. For example, your placement may involve a weekly swimming programme but you rarely work with the same person in consecutive weeks. To bring focus to your time in the pool, assess your situation from a person-centred perspective and create a just-in-time objective that will guide your experience together and provide a common outcome toward which you both are working. The result could be, "Today Jason will practice the survival role, without a floatation device, at

Goal: To Become a Competitive Tandem Cyclist

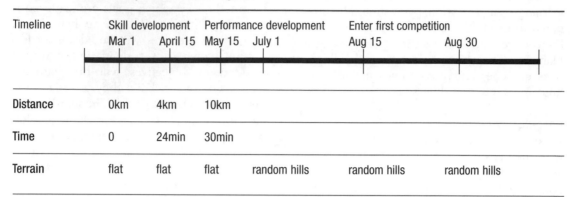

Timeline	Skill development		Performance development		Enter first competition		
	Mar 1	April 15	May 15	July 1	Aug 15	Aug 30	
Distance	0km	4km	10km				
Time	0	24min	30min				
Terrain	flat	flat	flat	random hills	random hills	random hills	

least six times before we leave the pool." This objective could guide the entire time in the pool or it could be integrated with other activities. Further information about objectives in relation to programme planning is provided in Chapter 16 (Goodwin).

CREATING TIMELINES

Timelines provide points of reference that not only indicate a start and a finish point to a programme, but they also indicate milestones when various outcomes should be achieved and how quickly you expect to advance toward your goals.

EVALUATION

Programme evaluation provides important feedback about the impact it is having on the person(s) for whom it's designed. First, evaluation can be a measure of how well programme goals were met and how many objectives were achieved. This is usually a quantitative assessment that can be made using objective measures. More importantly evaluations can also be an opportunity for the person to whom the service is provided, to comment on their own satisfaction with the outcomes of their total learning experience. These are usually qualitative measures that rely on personal perceptions, opinions, and judgements. Both types of evaluation offer valuable insight about the impact of a programme.

5. Creating Connections

"Facilitating community inclusion is an art form" (Uditsky 1999) that requires practitioners who are committed to learning the values, understandings, and talents that will make a qualitative difference to the lives of people with disabilities. APA service delivery goes beyond schools and specialized programmes to building bridges with the community. Participating in APA should be a fluid event that includes the possibility of a transition from a physical education class to community recreation, or from lessons in a sport to a competitive programme; or from standardized school-based curriculum content to lessons in an activity that requires a unique environment or specialized equipment. Participation in activity is a life-long skill and therefore successful service delivery sets the stage for seamless *transition* into the community.

Consider your practicum and ask how well prepared those you work with are to move between different types of programmes.

13 What would the person with whom you are working do if the programme that you are currently working in no longer existed?

6. Evaluation

Evaluation provides valuable information that can be gained through both qualitative and quantitative procedures. During the assessment stage, information regarding "what is" was accumulated by asking questions of and about the person. It uses tools of listening, asking, critical observing, and testing to determine strengths and abilities. By comparison, evaluation focusses on outcomes. It should reflect the extent to which goals are being achieved. Evaluation answers the question, "What worked?" It can be used at critical times throughout a programme to determine if any modifications are necessary and at the conclusion to determine the extent to which goals and objectives have been successfully achieved. If a goal is not achieved, the evaluation continues on to re-examine aspects of programme preparation and implementation that may have affected the outcome. Examples include accurateness of information provided by the initial assessment, appropriateness of the goal, and availability of appropriate support and resources.

Consistent with a person-centred approach, the evaluation process should include the person. After all, this person was part of planning, goal setting, and implementation; therefore he or she likely will want to be involved in evaluation. Negative feelings about evaluations can be diffused by person-centred involvement, and they will be seen as useful, instructive activities.

INCORPORATING EXPERIENTIAL LEARNING

Experiential learning refers to engaging in practical learning beyond the normal instructional setting, and, because it leads to broader and more enduring learning outcomes, it should be an integral part of professional preparation. An essential component of experiential learning is that the learner is guided towards reflective observation so that the relevance of the experience can be assessed and placed into context. In APA, experiential learning is usually achieved through a practicum placement, working with a person who has a disability in a physical activity setting. During this experience the learner has the opportunity to apply newly acquired knowledge, to challenge some existing assumptions, and to test developing professional skills. The formal and informal reflection that is part of journal writing about such an experience is essential. Reflective activity is synonymous with doing research on oneself, making the obvious dubious, making the hidden obvious—and it relies on self-honesty (Connelly 1994).

THE APA PRACTICUM

Practicum means "a context for practice." It is an essential part of learning in APA because it offers an opportunity to experience, first-hand, the effect of utilizing professional skills in service delivery while working with a person(s). A practicum may vary in terms of the activities or roles undertaken by students and supervisors. Generally, it offers the opportunity to observe other professionals working in the field and, ultimately, you will assume some level of responsibility for the activities of the person(s) with whom you are working. However, minimal level of responsibility within a programme does not mean minimal responsibility for your own learning. Practicum learning is a process, not a body of knowledge to be mastered as in a theory course. In other words, a practicum placement has to do with the journey, not just the destination. (Reimer, Thomlison, and Bradshaw 1999).

Each practicum should be viewed according to the beginning, middle, and end. The beginning includes all the activities associated with determining your placement, doing the appropriate *pre-practicum preparation*, and actually getting started. The next phase, while the practicum is underway, is one of on-going *formative evaluation* and adjustment. The final phase is a time of reflection and *summative evaluation*.

Pre-practicum preparation

Take advantage of all orientation meetings and opportunities. Ask other students who have completed this particular practicum about their experiences. Learn as much as you can about the agency or organization that is sponsoring the programme. Be clear about its expectations of you and its responsibility to you as a practicum student. Be sure you understand the objectives of your particular practicum. Prepare yourself by:

- thinking about your attitude and expectations for this practicum
- thinking about your personal learning plan in the practicum
- formulating questions that you have for your instructor and your supervisor

FORMATIVE EVALUATION

During this phase, it will help you to seek regular feedback on the progress you and the person with whom you are working are making toward the goals and objectives of the programme. A formative evaluation seeks information that will form and develop the delivery of the programme as it transpires. This information might cause you to correct your course within the programme, perhaps by increasing intensity or decreasing the number of objectives you hope to achieve. It also serves to inform your personal skills and abilities as a leader, instructor, or coach. To get this kind of feedback you often have to ask for it. Start with the person you are working with and ask him or her how you might have done things differently. Similarly, request feedback from your immediate supervisor. Ask your peers or colleagues who might be working at the same placement.

SUMMATIVE EVALUATION

It is here that you reflect on the experience and consider those things that have changed, for both you and the person(s) with whom you were placed. Now is the time to think about the new things you have learned, as well as those things that you now realize you would like to learn. Consider the high-level success of the practicum and what contributed to each success. When things didn't go as well as you wanted, how might you have done things differently? What would you like your next practicum to be?

JOURNAL WRITING

One of the most effective ways to focus on learning during a practicum is to record what happened in each session. This is an opportunity to chronicle significant and meaningful events, but what is more important is the process of writing. Writing about your practicum forces you to be reflective and critical of the experience, and through this process you will improve your learning.

Your journal should include:

- a record of facts, events, and process
- a record of observations and experiences
- an appraisal of the personal impact of these events on you

Journal writing can begin with an observation, a question, a feeling, but the most important part of writing is to get started. The purpose of creating a journal is self-assessment and, therefore, the end product must be meaningful to you. Some helpful guidelines that you should consider are:

- Develop a routine of writing in your journal immediately after or close to the time of your weekly practicum experience.
- Be brief but make sure you get a point across.
- Use language that won't embarrass you when others read your journal.
- Balance entries by thinking in terms of opposites (e.g., strengths and weaknesses).
- Identify recurring patterns of interaction.
- Reflect on the language you use and the thinking it reflects.
- Recognize changes in your behaviour, thinking, and self-awareness.

The words *reflect* and *reflective* have been used in this section to describe an important process used in journal writing. Reflecting is a cognitive process that promotes self-assessment and self-awareness. To reflect on your experience ask yourself what your thoughts are about your personal contribution, i.e., what you perceived to be your strengths and weaknesses. Focus on your understanding of meaning, values, and interrelationships that are unfolding for you through this experience.

The journal also provides the opportunity to identify how much you have integrated your learning in courses that deal directly with APA, as well as those that support your understandings in APA. You may wish to compare how things in the field are done differently, how reality may or may not reflect theory. Remember, this is a personal journey, and learning on this journey and writing about that learning should not be the same for any two individuals.

Challenging Traditional Assumptions

Given that the abilities-based service delivery process works well in a variety of settings where professionals are working with people who have disability, can we just adopt it without questioning its use? Yes, of course we can use it, but it is important to remember that it has evolved just as our understanding of APA in today's society has evolved. We should continually seek to improve the delivery of professional service. Consider the progress in service delivery for people with disability that has been made in the past fifty years. That progress has occurred in response to those who have questioned existing practice. Progress depends on a willingness to question or challenge the status quo.

The learning experience you undertake during professional preparation in APA should prepare you to go beyond merely functioning well in the field. Professional preparation means developing disciplined thinking within the entire area of APA. It means giving up preconceived notions about what is good or bad, what is possible or impossible. As a critical thinker, you will develop new insights, and questions will emerge during your day-to-day practice. By analyzing your work, new ideas will evolve that will lead to creative approaches to planning, and new ways of offering service delivery will surface. Approach your work strategically. Focus on on-going learning, continue to seek alternative ways of doing things, differentiate facts from opinions, look for themes or clusters of related information that will inform your professional understanding. Question your lived experience in relation to current professional practice and search for new ways to improve professional practice.

Summary

This chapter focussed on professional preparation based on an abilities-based service delivery procedures. Referencing this process, numerous skills and competencies required of the APA professional were identified and discussed. As these are mastered, an outcome of professional preparation is a wide knowledge-base and a strong sense of self or self-knowledge. Learning does not stop here; the journey continues. You must be willing to participate in other learning experiences such as workshops, other courses, perhaps other degree programmes. You must know yourself, know your strengths and your limitations in order to distinguish between personal preferences and those that are best for the person(s) whom you are serving. Constantly compare the world of theory to the world of reality and evaluate your interpretation of theoretical constructs. Always look for a better way of doing things.

14 Ask yourself, "Are you willing to read regularly in the area of APA?" "Do you read regularly outside the area to expand your scope and perspective?"

Study Questions

1. Using your practicum as an example, explain what you have done or could do to ensure that a person-centred approach is used in your delivery of the programme.
2. What types of information can you accumulate about a person with disability when you focus on their abilities?
3. What is APA service delivery?
4. Describe each of the points at which a person with disability should be involved in the decisions that are part of the planning and implementation of an APA programme.
5. What is the purpose of journalling a practicum experience?

References

Connelly, M. (1994). Practicum experiences and journal writing in adapted physical education: Implications for teacher education. *Adapted Physical Activity Quarterly, 11*, 306–28.

Fuchs, L.S., Fuchs, D., and Deno, S.L. (1985). Importance of goal ambitiousness and goal mastery to student achievement. *Exceptional Children, 52*(1), 63–71.

Jeffreys, M., and Gall, R. (1996). *The learning journey.* Calgary, AB. Detselig.

Galambos, D., and Whetstone, W. (1989). *Individual programme planning.* Oakville, ON: Sheridan College of Applied Arts and Technology.

Gavron, S. (1996). Personal communication.

O'Brien, J., and O'Brien, C.L. (1998). *A little book about person centered planning.* Toronto: Inclusion Press.

Reimer, M., Thomlison, B., and Bradshaw, C. (1999). *The clinical rotation handbook: A practicum guide for nurses.* Albany, NY: Delmar.

Schwab, J. (1966). The teaching of science as enquiry. In P.F. Brandwein, *Elements in a strategy for teaching science in the elementary school.* Cambridge, MS: Harvard University Press.

Sherrill, C. (1993). *Adapted physical activity recreation and sport* (4th ed.). Madison, WI: WCB/McGraw-Hill.

Uditsky, B. (1999). The erosion of individualized funding in Alberta. *Connections, 6*(1), 1–7.

CHAPTER 11

Foundations of Assessment

Marcel Bouffard

Learning Objectives

- To define assessment and state key reasons for assessing people.
- To define reliability and state why, as a test user, you should be concerned about the reliability of a measurement procedure.
- To state the difference between the modern definition of validity provided by Messick and the older conception of validity accepted during the middle of the twentieth century.
- To state at least five ethical issues related to assessment.

The delivery of services to people is at the core of adapted physical activity. The services are typically related to the development of movement skills, games, and sports, fitness and health as well as leisure counselling. Adapted physical educators typically acknowledge that they want to offer the best services possible given the financial, physical, and social constraints they have. In addition, as noted by Sherrill (1993), adapted physical activity encompasses "*attitudes* supportive of individual differences and adaptation" (p. 6).

To offer services implies that *decisions* have to be made about what services to offer and how to offer them. Assessment is used to guide these decisions. In fact, although there are different viewpoints about what constitutes assessment, it could be defined as the process of collecting data for the purpose of making decisions about people (Salvia and Ysseldyke 1995). According to this viewpoint, we never talk about assessment, but instead we talk about "*assessment for the purpose of...*" (Salvia and Ysseldyke 1995, p. 5). In addition,

I personally endorse the viewpoint stating that the participant should be involved, to the largest extent possible, in the decision-making process. This is in opposition to assessment models where the expert decides what to do, and the participant is expected to follow the recommendations.

Although tests can be used for assessment purposes, 'test' and 'assessment' are not synonymous. A test refers to an examination or a standardized procedure conducted for examining some characteristics of people (or sometimes a group). A test is an instrument which when administered often yields a measure. Assessment involves more than the use of a test. As noted by Cronbach (1960), assessment "involves the use of a variety of techniques, has a primary reliance on observation [of performance], and involves an integration of [diverse sources of] information in a summary judgment" (p. 582). Assessment often begins with observations and attempts to explain observations. Sometimes these observations are made through testing.

In this chapter, a brief review of assessment purposes is undertaken. Although test and assessment are not synonymous, tests are frequently used for assessment purposes and an introduction to fundamental testing ideas is made. Reliability and validity will be covered in this section. Problems with testing and assessment will be outlined, and alternative, emerging views briefly sketched. A summary of the material covered, and not covered, will conclude this chapter.

Some Comments About the Jargon

Understanding the literature on assessment can be a complex venture. It is often similar to learning another language. The meanings of key expressions need to be learned to understand the literature. In addition, although there is general consensus about the meaning of key words or expressions used, careful reading often reveals slightly different word usages. Most concepts have 'fuzzy boundaries'. Personally, I became acutely aware of the fuzziness of language while taking a course in genetics during the mid-1980s. Before that course, I had rather tacitly assumed that it was easy to define what the word *sex* meant and how to use this concept to identify the sex of a person. Dr. Claude Bouchard, our instructor, revealed that twenty-two different genetic markers could be used to identify the sex of a person and that a different answer could be obtained by using different markers. This awareness made it clear to me that if an apparently simple concept such as sex could have fuzzy boundaries, then many other concepts could also be fuzzy. In fact, I would argue that most of the concepts we use in our language have fuzzy boundaries and are, therefore, imprecise.

Definitions are human creations. They often stipulate what is or is not part of a concept. If you keep reading about this field, you will soon realize that some expressions such as *assessment, measurement, test, evaluation,* etc., are used differently by different people. One may be inclined to lament this situation. However, the lack of unanimous agreement about the meaning of key concepts often reveals fundamental differences in viewpoints and assumptions made by people. It is beyond the scope of this chapter to review these differences. The essential point for you to remember is that you should not assume that the same word means exactly the same thing for different people. To understand the meaning of a document, you must spend time understanding the meaning of key concepts as used by the author you are reading. This chapter is an introduction to some key assessment ideas and issues. You should not assume that the language will be used in exactly the same way when you read other papers about assessment.

Purposes of Assessment

The reasons for assessing vary considerably across many groups within the adapted physical activity community. Policy makers, administrators, adapted physical educators, and parents may want to know different 'things' before making decisions. Frequently-listed reasons for conducting assessment are to screen, to diagnose, to place people into groups, to know the person, to determine progress, to compare with others, to compare against a norm, etc. Although it is possible to assess programmes, facilities, or the environment, this chapter will be limited to the assessment of people.

SCREENING

When assessment is used for screening purposes, fast and efficient data collection procedures are used to decide whether more comprehensive assessment is necessary. The notion that difficulties may go unnoticed if we do not carefully study this possibility (Salvia and Ysseldyke 1995) is implicit in screening. For example, a checklist may be completed by a school teacher to identify children who may have movement difficulties (i.e., children who have movement coordination problems and perform culturally normative skills significantly below the level expected for their age). In this case, the checklist is used as a screening instrument, and a person who meets the screening criteria should be referred for diagnostic assessment. Screening does not imply that someone necessarily needs special services.

DIAGNOSTIC

Diagnostic assessment is usually an intensive, in-depth, systematic collection of information that covers a specific area. The purpose of this process is to determine as accurately as possible capabilities and limitations of a person as well as the specific needs of the individual. Recommendations about how the specific needs could be met are usually included in this process. A diagnosis need not be medical. It does not necessarily lead to a label that describes a syndrome.

PLACEMENT

In educational settings, people are often placed into relatively homogeneous groups. The results of assessment are frequently used to form these groups.

KNOW THE LEARNER

To foster human development, one must first know the characteristics of the learner before one can determine which developmental activities should take place. Oftentimes, when people enroll in a programme the teacher knows little about the participant. Spending time getting to know each person is a prerequisite to good decision-making. In addition, knowing the participant is a continuous process which can occur before, during, and after the delivery of a programme. For example, when a teacher asks Peter to throw a ball to Mary, he can directly observe Peter's throwing pattern and discover that Peter does not step forward with his left foot while throwing with his right arm. Consequently, Peter cannot throw the ball for a long distance. This assessment may immediately lead to a teaching recommendation. In addition, assessing the learner can occur at the end of the programme. If good data are available about each participant before and after the programme, assessment of progress can be made.

DETERMINE PROGRESS

To justify a programme, one must show that it is functioning effectively. From an administrative viewpoint, stakeholders want to know whether it is appropriate to invest time, facilities, and money into a programme. Without evidence of beneficial effects, stakeholders are likely to be reluctant to invest in a programme of uncertain quality. Furthermore, we have a moral obligation to determine the effects of our programmes. We live in a democratic society in which it is assumed that fostering personal development is a legitimate goal. Under this assumption, the demonstration of positive beneficial effects is essential. Why should we spend time offering a programme without positive consequences? Time might be better spent doing other things.

TO COMPARE AGAINST OTHERS

Assessment is sometimes conducted to compare a person's performance against norms. The expression *norm-referenced measurement* is often used to refer to this type of assessment. Norms are statistical descriptions of the performance of a reference group which often include descriptive statistics such as the mean, the mode, percentile, etc. Although norms are obtained from a particular group, a selection process is used to ensure that the sample of participants is likely to be representative of the population of interest. When norms are available, the performance of a person can be compared to the norms. For example, the results of the Test of Gross Motor Development (TGMD) (Ulrich 1985) administered to Peter indicate that his performance level on the object control subscale is at the 10th percentile. This indicates that, given his age and gender, 90 percent of children in the population have a score higher than his. From a normative viewpoint, Peter's performance is different from the typical, average performance. In brief, when norm-referenced measurement is used, the meaning of a score is derived by comparing a score to a norm.

TO COMPARE AGAINST A CRITERION

Assessment can also be conducted to compare actual performance to a desired level of mastery. The expression *criterion-referenced measurement* is often used to refer to this type of assessment. Contrary to norm-referenced measurement, criterion-reference measurement does not indicate a person's relative standing; it measures a person's performance in relation to a desired standard of mastery. For example, an adapted physical educator using the TGMD could compare a child's movement execution to a standard of mastery. For each skill in the TGMD, the standard of mastery is defined as a mature movement pattern (e.g., see Wickstrom 1977).

QUALITY OF A MEASUREMENT PROCEDURE

To conduct an assessment, adapted physical educators may use already available tests. Some of these tests have been well standardized, while for others standardization has been minimal or absent. A standardized test is an instrument which is administered under controlled conditions. In addition, the test has been developed following a careful standardization procedure, including the selection of items, their initial administration and

analysis, reliability studies, validity studies, the development of norms, and the like.

A large number of testing instruments are presently available to assist you to conduct an assessment. However, the availability of an instrument does not imply that you can obtain good information by using it. It is essential to understand that there is no multi-purpose instrument available: instruments have been developed with a specific purpose in mind. For example, you will not find an instrument to assess the level of movement competency of a child, his or her intrinsic motivation towards physical activity, as well as the same child's attitude towards persons with a disability. On the other hand, you can find instruments to assess the level of movement competency of a person (e.g., Ulrich 1985), or the person's degree of intrinsic leisure motivation (e.g., Beard and Ragheb 1983), or a person's attitude towards persons with a disability (e.g., Yuker, Block, and Young 1966).

Although instruments are developed for a rather specific purpose, it does not imply that the procedure will yield data that are of sufficient quality for your work. People attempting to summarize information using logic and numbers (often called quantitative researchers), often refer to the *reliability* and *validity* of a measurement procedure to convince others that the procedure, if properly applied, produces data that can be relied upon to make decisions. An introduction to these key measurement concepts is presented next.

Reliability

People interested in measurement issues have developed a number of measurement theories. Classical true-score theory (CTT), generalizability theory, and item-response theory are the most frequently used ones. It is beyond the scope of this chapter to introduce the last two theories; the discussion will be limited to classical true-score theory. It is probably correct to assert that this theory, although the oldest, has been used more frequently than the other two theories to develop assessment tools.

A basis assumption of CTT is that when we measure an attribute (e.g., height, weight,

Figure 11.1 Observed scores obtained using a more reliable measurement procedure (left panel) and less reliable one (right panel)

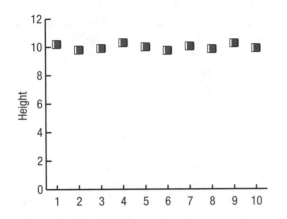 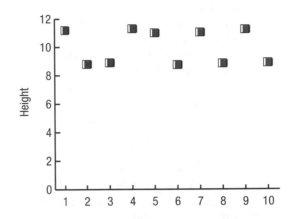

attitude towards inclusion), the observation or score we get may not really correspond to what is. More specifically, CTT states that an observed score (X) is the algebraic sum of two components: a true-score (T) and an error-score (E). In brief, **X = T + E**. To explain the thinking behind this equation, assume that we know the true height (i.e., true-score) of Mary, which is 150 cm. Someone measuring Mary's height might obtain an observed score of 149 cm. In this case, the observed score is 1 cm below Mary's true-score (149 cm = 150 cm - 1 cm) and the measurement error is -1 cm. Repeating the same measurement procedure may lead to another observed-score. For example, if the observed-score on the second occasion is 150.5 cm, then the measurement error is + 0.5 cm.

Stated differently, CTT makes a basic assumption about the nature of reality. What is real is the true-score and an observed-score in itself cannot be trusted. According to the thinking behind CTT, observations contain errors and these errors should be minimized to inform us well about what is real. If these errors are relatively small, we can safely state that we can rely on the observed-score to make an inference about the true-score. If this is the case, then the measurement procedure is declared reliable. Conversely, if there is a large measurement error, the observed-score

cannot be trusted as an adequate representation of the true-score, and the measurement instrument is declared unreliable.

Assume that you have measured Mary's height ten times within a period of five minutes. During such a short time period, it is plausible to assume that Mary's height did not change and, therefore, any difference in observed-scores is due to measurement error as opposed to a change is Mary's height. On the left panel of figure 11.1, you can observe that there are small differences between the observed-scores while there are larger differences on the right panel. In this case, the observed scores on the left panel suggest that the measures are more reliable than the observed scores on the right panel. In summary, reliability refers to the consistency or stability of the results of a measurement procedure from one use to the next. When repeated measurements of the same thing give identical or very similar results, the measurement instrument is said to be reliable. A measure is reliable to the extent that it is free of random error (Vogt 1993). When random errors are small, observed-scores can be trusted as good indicators of true-scores.

To explain the foundations of CTT, I have assumed that we know the true-score. However, the true-score, although postulated to be "the real thing," cannot be observed directly. It is only through observed-scores that we can know the true-score. To define the true-score, measurement specialists rely on a well known fact of statistics which states that if you randomly sample multiple observations from a population, then the long-run average of all these observations will equal the mean of the population. Stated differently, if you randomly select an infinite number of observations from a population, the mean of your observations will correspond to the mean of the population. Consequently, in CTT, the true-score is defined as the long run average of all the observed-scores.

You may ask, why bother about all this stuff? Why should I spend time to learn the foundations of CTT? Please, take time to ponder over these questions. A fundamental answer is that you need good information, that is, information which you can rely upon to make adequate professional decisions. Let us illustrate this point with an example. Assume that you offer a movement skill acquisition programme to John who has difficulty learning the movement skills required for ball skills (e.g., throwing, catching, kicking, batting, etc.). To determine John's entry level, you elect to administer the TGMD (Ulrich 1985). Briefly, when using this test, you can obtain a score that represents a child's level of movement competency on object control skills and locomotor skills. On the basis of these scores, you decide to administer a remedial intervention programme to John.

Now, let us assume that when you administer the TGMD you obtain unreliable results. This means that if you were re-administering the test to John, within a short-time span, John's results are likely to be quite different. Sometimes, these differences could be very important. The lesson here is that with an unreliable test you may recommend a remedial intervention programme if the results are below typical expectations. In this case, you may be wasting John's time, your time, and booking facilities that are not required for remedial intervention. Conversely, if a test is unreliable, you may not detect a child who needs special assistance. In addition, if you offer

a programme, you may be unable to determine whether John really improved his level of movement competency or if the 'observed change' is simply the result of measurement error. In summary, unreliable data may lead to faulty decisions and the impossibility to determine clearly whether real progress occurred.

The basic lesson to be learned here is that when you plan to use a standardized instrument, read the documentation accompanying the instrument. You need to know whether (and how) reliability was established. During your acquaintance with instruments you may encounter expressions such as *test-retest reliability*, *equivalent-form reliability*, *split-half reliability*, *internal consistency reliability*, and the like. It is beyond the purpose of this chapter to clarify the meaning of these expressions. An attempt to estimate the extent to which the data obtained from a measurement procedure contain random error is common to all of them.

Validity

The meaning of *validity* has changed over time during the twentieth century. You may have heard or read something like "a test is valid if it measures what it is supposed to measure." Although this definition was accepted during the middle of the twentieth century, the above definition of validity has been abandoned, for two major reasons. First, assessment specialists nowadays prefer to refer to a measurement procedure instead of a test per se. A test is usually administered by people to people living in a physical and a social context. Second, assessment specialists gradually realized that they were validating statements, not tests. Nowadays, it is commonly accepted that we are validating the inferences from a test, not the test itself. It is the *use* of the test (the inference made from the test) that is the thing to be validated; not just the test itself (Rubin 1988).

Messick (1989) offered a commonly accepted definition of validity. He states that

> validity is an integrated evaluative judgment of the degree to which empirical evidence and theoretical rationales support

the *adequacy* and *appropriateness* of *inferences* and *actions* based on test scores or other modes of assessment…. It is important to note that validity is a matter of degree, not all or none." (p. 13)

A number of important points are made in Messick's definition. First, the word *integrated* means that many sources of information are used to document the appropriateness of inferences. Second, questions of validity are questions about the soundness of interpretation of a measure. We should never forget that the interpretation of a measure is made by humans. Third, validity issues are studied by using two major modes of thinking: empiricism and rationalism. That is, validity evidences are obtained by obtaining both qualitative and quantitative data about people. These data are used in combination with what is assumed to be sound and reasonable to provide a rationale supporting the interpretation of test scores. Stated differently, the validation process relies heavily on human judgement. Fourth, as noted earlier, inferences are what are validated, not tests. Fifth, in his definition, Messick refers to the appropriateness of actions. Here, Messick raises questions and issues about the consequences of test use. Although Messick includes consequences of test use in his definition of validity, this is still a controversial issue in the field. People who object to the inclusion of the "appropriateness of actions" within the definition of validity are not opposed to the study of consequences of test use. They object to the inclusion of this component within the definition of validity (Maguire, Hattie, and Haig 1994). Sixth, validity is not an all or none property, it is a matter of degree. The results of a test may have "many interpretations which differ in their degree of validity and in the type of evidence required for the validation process" (Linn 1979, p. 109). This viewpoint implies that expressions such as "this test is valid" or "this test is not valid" are incorrect. We do not validate a test, and validity is a matter of degree, not 'black or white.' In addition, although not noted in Messick's definition, validation is a never-ending process. As noted by Cronbach (1988):

As psychological science generates new concepts, test interpretations will have to be reconsidered. Also, because psychological and educational tests influence who gets what in society, fresh challenges follow shifts in social power or social philosophy. So validation is never finished. (pp. 4–5)

Like a scientist who often questions the interpretation of her results, interpretations of test scores are open to reinterpretations.

It is a common practice to break down validity issues into three major types: content validity, criterion-related validity, and construct validity. A brief introduction to each type of validity issue is presented next.

CONTENT VALIDITY

The administration of a bowling test is unlikely to inform you about people's basketball abilities. If you have taken a motor learning course, you may have learned that the general motor ability hypothesis has not been supported. Simply stated, the general motor ability hypothesis would imply that if you are a very good basketball player, you are also a very good bowler. In fact, the specificity hypothesis has received more support. This means that even if you are a very good basketball player, it does not imply that you are a very good bowler. In addition, you know that bowling and basketball are different types of activities. A key difference is that in bowling the environment is stable and does not change prior to or during movement skill execution, while in basketball the environment is unstable, changing. Stated differently, to be successful at basketball requires that you anticipate the state of the environment in the future, while bowling does not require anticipation. The essential point here is that the task demands of bowling and basketball are different. Consequently, a bowling test will not include items measuring anticipatory capabilities required in basketball, while anticipation items included in a basketball will be irrelevant to bowling.

A test is developed for a specific purpose. In addition, a test typically contains a number of items. Which items should be included and which items excluded is a central issue. An instrument has content validity if the items accurately represent the 'things' we would like to know something about. In the above example, a bowling test does not include items representing anticipatory capabilities and, hence, lacks content validity in regard to basketball. On the other hand, the inclusion of items representing anticipatory capabilities would be irrelevant to bowling.

Usually, test developers provide an argument supporting the content validity of an instrument. It is assumed that test developers know something about a domain of interest and that this knowledge could be used to justify the inclusion of certain items and the rejection of others. The content validity process essentially relies on human judgment. A typical content validation strategy is to ask experts whether the content of the instrument is representative of the domain of interest. Content validity evidence tends to be nonstatistical in nature.

CRITERION-RELATED VALIDITY

Another question frequently asked is whether the results of a test can be used to make predictions. Can the results from one variable be used to predict the results on another variable? Based on the timespan between two tests, it is customary to differentiate between *concurrent* and *predictive validity*. Ideally, concurrent validity concerns the extent to which the results of a test can be used to predict the results of another test administered at the same time. Obviously, strictly speaking, two tests cannot be administered at the same time. The expression 'at the same time' refers to tests taken 'nearly at the same time.' As you may already have anticipated, predictive validity concerns the extent to which the results of one test can predict the results of another test administered at another time.

Criterion-related validity evidence is used to validate inferences the following way: in criterion-related validity, inferences based on the results of an assessment instrument are compared to inferences based on a criterion measurement that is accepted as a standard indicator of the target construct, or trait. Stated differently, it is assumed that the interpretation of the results of an assessment instrument is correct and, then, the results of another instrument are compared to it. For example, a few decades ago, estimation of percentage of body fat using skinfold callipers was validated against the results of hydrostatic weighing. At that time, hydrostatic weighting was viewed as the 'gold standard.' Nowadays, due to the availability of better technology, hydrostatic weighing has been gradually replaced by magnetic resonance imagery (MRI). Irrespective of the emerging trends, the results of a skinfold calliper could be compared to the results of an accepted gold standard to provide criterion-related validity evidence. An obvious limitation of this validation strategy is that the accepted gold standard could be inadequate. Criterion-related validity evidence is usually statistical in nature. That is, the argument supporting criterion-related validity evidence often relies on measures of association or correlation. It is commonly accepted that the test developer must provide relevant criterion-related validity evidences.

CONSTRUCT VALIDITY

Questions of construct validity are a consequence of fundamental assumptions made by researchers. Construct validity issues are mainly the result of the adoption of a realist philosophy (Maguire, Hattie, and Haig 1994). It is assumed that there is a reality that exists which is independent of people, and some of this reality cannot be directly observed. According to a realist philosophy, a construct is something that exists but is not directly observable. Since Newton's work, people have used gravity as a construct to explain the movement of objects in the universe. In psychology, constructs such as emotion, motivation, or attitude are frequently used to explain human behaviour. If there is a reality we cannot directly observe, how can we know something about this reality? This is the fundamental issue of construct validity. When issues of construct validity emerge, there is no obvious gold standard, or criterion, against which to validate a test. All we can do is to find indicators of the construct, none of which is perfect.

According to a realist philosophy, it is sensible for humans to search for hidden causes. This viewpoint has not always been accepted. At the beginning of the twentieth century, when a philosophical movement called *logical positivism* was dominant, issues of construct validity were deemed nonsensical. Logical positivists developed a theory of meaning that declared that statements about non-observables were meaningless. Behaviourism in psychology, particularly represented by the work of Watson and Skinner, was strongly influenced by logical positivism.

Logical positivism is no longer a dominant philosophy. Signs of this rejection appeared in a classic paper published in 1955 by Cronbach and Meehl. In this paper they affirmed that a language referring to non-directly observable entities could be meaningful. They defined a construct as "some postulated attribute of people, assumed to be reflected in test performance" (p. 115). Hence, the fundamental construct validity issue is the extent to which the test performance reflects the postulated attribute (sometimes called trait) of a person. Stated differently, how can we make appropriate inferences to the non-observable on the basis of what we can observe? The search for an answer to this question is still ongoing and it is beyond the purpose of this chapter to review the work completed in this regard. It could be an interesting exercise for you to ask how you can use what you can see, hear, smell, and so forth to make a plausible inference about the nonobservable. By going through this exercise, you can develop a feel for what is at stake in construct validation.

Validity issues are essentially issues about knowing. The bottom line is that assessment specialists ask whether we really know people with whom we are working. Do we really have information that we can trust to make appropriate decisions? Earlier, assessment was defined as the process of collecting data for decision-making purposes. Obviously, from the viewpoint outlined above, not all kinds of 'data' are adequate. You need good data. This is what assessment specialists say when they refer to the need for high reliability and validity.

Some measurement specialists may object to the treatment of construct validity as presented in this chapter. To them, issues of content-validity and criterion-related validity are all subsumed under constuct validity. It is beyond the scope of this chapter to highlight the nature of the present debate amongst specialists. For pedagogical reasons, I find it is easier to clarify validity issues by dividing them into smaller ones.

Ethics and Assessment

Assessment raises a number of questions about how we ought to behave (i.e., ethics). Assessment implies that information is collected about people and, hence, when you assess you invade a person's privacy. This obviously raises a number of ethical questions about the right people have to collect information about other people and use it to make decisions likely to affect people's lives. In the past, some tests have been inappropriately used to label people as imbeciles or morons. It has been argued that some standardized tests may favour the glib and penalize the thoughtful (Lyman 1998). You may already have criticized one of your teachers for test unfairness, that is for administering a test that was too difficult or a test that did not cover the material studied in class (i.e., a test that did not have sufficient content validity). Furthermore, due to cultural differences, tests can be biased and unfair to some groups. Tests can also give changing results even if the time delay between two administrations is, to the best of our knowledge, too short to lead to a significant change in a person's characteristic. In addition, tests and test results can be misused, misinterpreted, and so forth (for elaboration see Lyman 1998).

The above paragraph raises a number of issues about assessment and test use. Some of these issues are discussed at greater length by Shogan (1998) (also Chapter 5 (Shogan)) and

I invite you to ponder carefully over her papers. The available assessment technology shows what might be done. It says little about what ought to be done. Your work as a professional in adapted physical activity cannot be divorced from ethics. The use of assessment tools often makes ethical issues salient and I invite you to reflect on these questions and issues. As noted in Chapter 1 (Bouffard and Strean), critical thinking cannot be divorced from ethics. Moral principles ultimately guide our actions.

Emerging Trends

This chapter is a general introduction to some key assessment ideas and issues. However, the 'assessment territory' is much broader and complex than this presentation might suggest. To use a metaphor, together we only scratched the surface of the visible part of an iceberg in this chapter. Comments about some parts of the uncharted territory are presented next.

Although most of the material included in this chapter refers to standardized tests, this should not be viewed as a recommendation to use only standardized tests for assessment purposes. The main intent was to introduce you to issues (decision-making, reliability, validity, ethics) you are likely to be concerned with when you assess people. Like most instruments, standardized tests have both strengths and limitations which could be viewed as both sides of a coin. Although standardized tests often increase the plausibility of inferences, they are quite often narrow in scope and cannot capture what really happens in people's lives. Instead of obtaining precise information about only a few dimensions of a person, many assessment specialists argue for the inclusion of a rich and broad base of information to make decisions.

The work on qualitative assessment is not discussed in the present chapter. Attempts to summarize information using numbers has been severely criticized during the last two decades of the twentieth century. A number of qualitative researchers argue that not all data are quantifiable. Important information is lost when attempting to quantify. For example, proponents of qualitative methods argue that a much better ('thick') description of people's attitudes toward inclusion could be obtained by speaking to people and using their own (nonquantified) words to understand their attitude. A good introduction to qualitative assessment was published by Cook and Reichardt (1979) as well as other qualitative research textbooks (e.g., Patton 1990).

Tests are usually administered under standardized conditions. This implies that the environment in which the test is administered is somewhat artificial. The use of assessment tools in contrived situations lacking ecological validity has been severely criticized by some. Nowadays, many recommend conducting assessment in natural settings. One assessment strategy frequently used is to use direct observation of behaviour (e.g., see Martin and Bateson 1993; Pellegrini 1996). Another related line of investigation is the work of Watkinson and Causgrove Dunn on ecological task analysis described in Chapter 15.

Concluding Comments

When assessing, what you intend to do comes first. That is, you must clarify your objectives. You cannot spend all your time assessing; you must clarify what you want to know. Given the time and the resources you have, assessment must be of the highest quality possible. A large number of assessment tools are available for your work. For a brief description of some of them see Burton and Miller (1998) and Burlingame and Blaschko (1990). It is essential to remember, however, that instruments presently available may not be adequate for your work. They may not correspond to what you want to do, be too costly, or too time-consuming. In addition, although some instruments are published with a clearly stated purpose, the argument supporting the plausibility of inferences made from test scores is often tenuous. In addition, some instruments are available on the market but the purposes for using them is not stated. With the knowledge you presently have after reading this chapter, you should be able to ask questions about the value of these instruments. In brief, availability does not ensure quality. When you assess you collect information about people to make decisions. The collection and use of information about people raises a number of ethical questions. Finally, some recent trends in assessment highlight the benefits of assessing people in ecologically valid settings and of using qualitative data.

Study Questions

1. What is assessment? In your professional work, why would you assess persons with a disability?

2. What is reliability? Is it ethical to make placement decision (for example, place a child in a special classroom), on the basis of a 'test' that is unreliable?

3. One of your professional colleagues states that an assessment instrument, for example, a document called *Attitude Towards Inclusion,* is not valid. In your own words, state what your colleague is implicitly saying. Outline what you can do to determine whether you agree with your colleague's assertion.

4. List at least five ethical issues you may face when assessing people. Say why you consider them to be ethical issues.

References

Beard, J.G., and Ragheb, M.G. (1983). The leisure motivation scale. *Journal of Leisure Research, 15,* 219–28.

Burlingame, J., and Blaschko, T.M. (1990). *Assessment tools for recreational therapy.* Ravensdale, WA: Idyll Arbor.

Burton, A.W., and Miller, D.E. (1998). *Movement skill assessment.* Champaign, IL: Human Kinetics.

Cook, T.D., and Reichardt, C.S. (Eds.). (1979). *Qualitative and quantitative methods in evaluation research.* Beverly Hills, CA: Sage.

Cronbach, L.J. (1960). *Essentials of psychological testing* (2nd ed.). New York: HarperCollins.

Cronbach, L.J. (1988). Five perspectives on validity argument. In H. Wainer and H.I. Braun (Eds.), *Test validity.* Hillsdale, NJ: Erlbaum.

Cronbach, L.J., and Meehl, P.E. (1955). Construct validity in psychological tests. *Psychological Bulletin, 52,* 281–302.

Linn, R.L. (1979). Issues of validity in measurement for competency-based programmes. In M.A. Bunda and J.R. Sanders (Eds.), *Practices and problems in competency-based measurement* (pp. 108–23). Princeton, NJ: Educational Testing Service.

Lyman, H.B. (1998). *Test scores and what they mean* (6th ed.). Boston: Allyn and Bacon.

Maguire, T., Hattie, J., and Haig, B. (1994). Construct validity and achievement assessment. *The Alberta Journal of Educational Research, 49,* 109–26.

Martin, P., and Bateson, P. (1993). *Measuring behaviour: An introductory guide* (2nd ed.). New York: Cambridge University Press.

Messick, S. (1989). Validity. In R.L. Linn (Ed.), *Educational measurement* (3rd ed., pp. 13–103). New York: American Council of Education.

Patton, M.Q. (1990). *Qualitative evaluation and research methods* (2nd ed.). Newbury Park, CA: Sage.

Pellegrini, A.D. (1996). *Observing children in their natural world.* Mahwah, NJ: Erlbaum.

Rubin, D.B. (1988). Discussion. In H. Wainer and H.I. Braun (Eds.), *Test validity* (pp. 241–56). Hillsdale, NJ: Erlbaum.

Salvia, J., and Ysseldyke, J.E. (1995). *Assessment* (6th ed.). Boston: Houghton Mifflin.

Sherrill, C. (1993). *Adapted physical activity, recreation and sport: Crossdisciplinary and lifespan* (4th ed.). Madison, WI: Brown and Benchmark.

Shogan, D. (1998). The social construction of disability: The impact of statistics and technology. *Adapted Physical Activity Quarterly, 15,* 269–77.

Ulrich, D.A. (1985). *Test of gross motor development.* Austin, TX: Pro-Ed.

Vogt, W.P. (1993). *Dictionary of statistics and methodology.* Newbury Park, CA: Sage.

Wickstrom, R.L. (1977). *Fundamental motor patterns* (2nd ed.). Philadelphia: Lea and Febiger.

Yuker, H., Block, J., and Young, J. (1966). *The measurement of attitudes toward disabled persons.* Albertson, NY: Human Resources Center.

CHAPTER 12

Physical Activity as Rehabilitation

David F.H. Legg

Learning Objectives

- To understand the benefits of physical activity within the rehabilitation process for persons with disabilities.
- To understand the allied professionals involved in providing physical activity for persons with disabilities during the rehabilitation process.
- To understand the challenges inherent within physical activity programmes during the rehabilitation process for persons with disabilities.

Introduction

The realm of adapted physical activity has, in many respects, evolved from the field of rehabilitation. Today, there is still a significant relationship between the two. The purpose of this chapter is to emphasize the nature of the relationship between physical activity and rehabilitation by focussing on interventions for persons with disabilities. This will be accomplished by reviewing the history of physical activity used within rehabilitation programmes and settings, clarifying the definition of rehabilitation and how physical activity is incorporated into it, outlining the benefits of including physical activity into a rehabilitation programme, and identifying the challenges to implementation.

When reading this chapter, it is important to remember that, while best practices are noted, they are just that—the current best practices. The use of physical activity within the rehabilitative process is continually expanding and redefining itself. It is also important to regard rehabilitation beyond its traditional confines, which have been viewed as occurring only in hospitals and rehabilitation centres. The rehabilitative process, however, is not restricted to any specific environment and is addressed in this chapter with examples from clinical, educational, and other settings.

History

The use of physical activity as a form of rehabilitation evolved from the Greek, Roman, and Chinese empires. The Chinese (3000 B.C.) used physical activity as a means of rehabilitation to divert a patient's attention away from the primary treatments of bodily ailments (Jansma and French 1994). Hippocrates in 460 B.C. used physical activity to strengthen muscles and aid rehabilitation (Auxter and Pyfer 1985) and to treat mental disorders, by combining music with gymnastics and dancing. The Romans from 500 B.C. until 1500 A.D., heralded the virtues of diet and exercise as a tonic for the body. Physical activity was also identified as a form of rehabilitation in the late 1700s when Phillippe Pinel (1745–1826), a French physician, treated persons with a mental illness. Pinel's techniques became known as moral treatment (Carter, Van Andel, and Robb 1995), and were later applied by Jean Itard (1775–1838). Itard, another French physician, was an early teacher of the deaf and persons with developmental disabilities. He also used games and physical activity for rehabilitative purposes.

In the early 1900s, segregated schools for children with developmental disabilities also used physical activity as a form of rehabilitation. Here, the activities were designed not for play, but for specific goals related to coordination, control, and attention (Avedon 1974; Frye and Peters 1972). The underlying rationale was that physical activity reduced tension and anxiety, believed to result from the unconscious conflict among inner motives and desires.

In the 1920s, the use of physical activity as therapy in health care settings proliferated in Red Cross programmes initiated in the United States following World War I. Based on their success, recreation and physical activity programmes appeared in mental health settings in the 1930s. This pattern was further reflected in England at the Stoke Mandeville Rehabilitation Hospital following World War II. The large influx of returning war veterans with disabilities facilitated the development of new innovative methods for treatment and rehabilitation, with particular emphasis given to physical and spiritual elements. Sir Ludwig Guttmann, the hospital's director, pioneered the use of physical activity as a form of rehabilitation, although it was presented to patients as sport (see Chapter 26 (Steadward and Foster) for additional information). These forays into wheelchair sport then evolved into an annual international competition known as the Stoke Mandeville Wheelchair Games, the first of which was held in 1948 (Legg 2000).

In Canada, the first organized use of physical activity took place in 1946 as a form of rehabilitation for persons with spinal cord injuries on the front lawns of the Deer Lodge Rehabilitation Hospital in Winnipeg, Manitoba. Some of the events included archery, milk bottle pitching, basketball throwing, ring tossing, croquet, and golf putting. Competitions were held on an inter-ward basis with nine teams consisting of eight patients each. Similar competitions were then held at a number of other rehabilitation hospitals across Canada, spurring on the growth and development of disability sport in Canada and organizations such as the Canadian Wheelchair Sports Association (CWSA) (formed in 1967) (http://www.cwsa.ca/) (Legg 2000). (See Chapter 8 (Legg) for further information on the Canadian Wheelchair Sports Association).

The large rehabilitation hospitals established in major urban centres in Canada shortly after World War II eventually gave way to the development of community-based rehabilitation programmes in the 1970s. Community-based rehabilitation, also referred to as independent-living, differed from traditional rehabilitation models by placing a greater emphasis on consumer and community participation and decision-making. This change emerged from criticisms of the traditional rehabilitation model, with its dependence on highly trained health professionals and a commitment to top-down, paternalistic models of decision-making (Lysack and Kaufert 1994). Economics also influenced this change towards a more community-directed approach, as politicians recognized that it was less expensive to facilitate the rehabilitation process for persons with disabilities in their own homes instead of hospitals. The independent-living movement thus reflected a broadening of rehabilitation goals with the emphasis placed on individual needs (Pollock and Stewart 1990).

In the late 1990s, both traditional and community-focussed approaches of rehabilitation were recognized as necessary and valuable with each representing different ends of an important treatment continuum. This continuum allowed a person with disability to enter rehabilitation in a hospital, but quickly transfer from that setting to a community-based, independent-living scenario when it was appropriate. The use of physical activity as part of the rehabilitation programme thus took its cues from the programme delivery sites, as well as the client's ability and the situational context. One example of this is the Steadward Centre (http://www.steadward-centre.org) at the University of Alberta which provides segregated and inclusive physical training opportunities for individuals based on their specific rehabilitative needs.

What Is Rehabilitation?

Throughout its historical evolution, rehabilitation was based upon the notion that improved physical and psychosocial functioning led to a more meaningful life. As the understanding of what constituted a meaningful life underwent significant changes, so did the definition of rehabilitation and the role that physical activity played within it.

Traditionally, a meaningful life was based for many on the concept of wealth and employment. Therefore, access to work opportunities or retraining for immediate employment received the focus in early rehabilitation programmes. Slowly, other areas of a person's life were recognized as equally important. Wright (1980) addressed this change in his text, *Total*

Rehabilitation, where the goal of rehabilitation services was to facilitate rewarding, useful, and satisfying activity—not just for finding employment. From this perspective, physical activity was seen as a primary mechanism for rehabilitation, as persons with disabilities relied on sport as a means of social reintegration, a positive use of leisure time, and a means for self-actualization. The definition of rehabilitation thus evolved toward a more dynamic process with the purpose of restoring an individual's physical, mental, and emotional functioning to a valued status and role within society. This holistic perspective included a focus not only on the physical realm, but also on the vocational, social, and psychological elements. The centre of attention, however, was still on restoring what was lost because of the disability.

Rehabilitation was operationalized by the International Classification of Impairments, Disabilities, and Handicaps (ICIDH) developed by the World Health Organization (WHO) (1980). Their model emphasized the importance of social, attitudinal, and environmental influences on individuals with impairments (Fuhrer 1987). This suggested that, instead of restoring what was lost, the focus should be on accentuating what remained.

While these varied definitions presented a number of unique interpretations of the rehabilitation process, they espoused one common element: the need to focus on rehabilitating the whole person. Therefore, physical activity was viewed as an excellent medium for rehabilitation as it simultaneously addressed the person's physical, mental, emotional, social, and spiritual components. With this recognition, there followed a new-found respect for physical activity, which subsequently gave it a more prominent role within the rehabilitation setting. This was followed by growth, eventually giving way to specialization and the emergence of numerous professionals claiming expertise for its delivery. These included therapeutic recreation specialists, occupational therapists, physical therapists, and physiatrists, each of which will now be reviewed separately. Adapted physical activity specialists can be involved in the rehabilitation process but are not recognized by an official governing body. For this reason their involvement as a professional group in providing physical activity programmes during the rehabilitation process will not be addressed in this chapter.

THERAPEUTIC RECREATION SPECIALISTS

Therapeutic recreation (TR) specialists work within the health and human service sector in both community and institutional settings. They are sometimes referred to as recreation therapists, although some would regard this as technically incorrect. Nevertheless, in Canada the distinction between the two terms has rarely been made (Alberta Therapeutic Recreation Association 1998).

The evolution of therapeutic recreation as a profession began in the United States, with early terms that included *hospital recreation* and *medical recreation*. In 1967, the National Therapeutic Recreation Society (NTRS) (http://www.nrpa.org/branches/ntrs.htm) of the United States was founded as a branch of the National Recreation and Park Association (NRPA) (http://www.activeparks.org/) (Howe-Murphy and Charboneau 1987). In 1984, the American Therapeutic Recreation Association (ATRA) (http://www.atra-tr.org/atra.htm) was formed in response to needs expressed by professionals working in health and human care facilities who believed that the NTRS was too focussed on recreation-driven facilities. Independent of other therapeutic recreation or leisure service organizations, ATRA emphasized the treatment and educational functions of therapeutic recreation (Howe-Murphy and Charboneau 1987). ATRA chose as its guiding philosophy Petersen and Gunn's (1984) theoretical model (later updated by Peterson and Stumbo 2000), which was developed in the mid-1970s, and based on a synthesis of existing literature. Petersen and Gunn's (1984) Leisure Ability model clustered TR into three major areas: rehabilitation, leisure education and counselling, and recreation participation. The leisure ability model was adaptable to a variety of clinical and community settings with a focus on the facilitation of the development,

maintenance, and expression of an appropriate and satisfying leisure lifestyle.

In Canada, the profession of therapeutic recreation was formalized in 1985 with the creation of the Alberta Therapeutic Recreation Association (http://www.alberta-tr.org/index.htm). Eventually, a number of other provinces formed associations, which then led to the need for a national governing body. In 1995, the Canadian Therapeutic Recreation Association (CTRA) (http://www.canadian-tr.org/), was established to act as an advocacy group and central governing body. Similar to its predecessor in the United States, CTRA accepted Petersen and Gunn's (1984) Leisure Ability model as its theoretical foundation.

The main reason that TR used Petersen and Gunn's (1984) model was to provide treatment for those identified as needing it. The second purpose was to provide recreation opportunities for those needing special programme adaptations. This facilitated participation irrespective of the setting in which the service was provided. Choosing the programme delivery mechanism, meanwhile, depended on the degree of freedom in participation exhibited by the client and the degree of control exhibited by the specialist. The leisure-based philosophy was consistent with a revised therapeutic recreation service outcome model developed by Carter, Van Andel, and Robb (1995). Another model utilized by TR professionals was treatment-centred recreation. This model was closely linked to the medical-clinical model identified by O'Morrow and Reynolds (1995). This approach, also referred to as prescriptive therapeutic recreation, had as its primary emphasis the use of recreation as a tool to accomplish important treatment or rehabilitative goals. To achieve the goals of these models, a few modalities used physical activity to help restore, enhance, or maintain levels of health and functional ability. Modalities are referred to under several general headings that include music, art, pets, horticulture, play, and dance therapy. Some of these then incorporate various levels of physical activity in order to address therapeutic goals.

OCCUPATIONAL THERAPISTS

Founded 1926, the Canadian Association of Occupational Therapists describes its field as that which helps people to lead a more productive, satisfying, and independent life by assisting them to manage daily living functions (e.g., dressing, eating, and shopping) and those activities that enable work or the enjoyment of free time (http://www.caot.ca/). Consistent with this description was the identification of recreation as being within the occupational therapist's (OT) scope of practice. This resulted in a number of conflicts with TR practitioners who also claimed leisure as their professional domain (Smith, Perry, Neumayer, Potter, and Smeal 1992).

Occupational therapy has also been defined as "the therapeutic use of self-care, work, and play activities to increase independent function, enhance development, and prevent disability" (Hopkins and Smith 1993, p. 4). Occupational therapy thus uses goal-directed activities, appropriate to each person's age and social role, to restore, develop, or maintain the ability for independent and satisfying lives. More specifically, occupational therapists evaluate, treat, and consult with individuals whose abilities to cope with the tasks of everyday living are threatened or impaired by physical illness or injury, psychosocial disability, or developmental deficits. These activities can take place in hospitals, schools, rehabilitation agencies, long-term care facilities, and other health care organizations.

PHYSICAL THERAPISTS

Physical therapy (also known as physiotherapy) is defined as treatment that uses heat, cold, light, water, electricity, massage, ultrasound, exercise, and functional training for the purposes of relieving pain, preventing deformity and further disability, developing or improving muscle strength or motor skills, and restoring or maintaining maximal functional capacities (Sherrill 1996). Founded in 1920, the Canadian Physiotherapy Association defines their field as a health care profession concerned with the assessment, maintenance, and restoration of the physical function and performance of the body (http://www.physio therapy.ca).

Physical therapists utilize physical activity to maintain motor functions by planning and implementing strategies for evaluation through tests and measures of neuromuscular, musculo-skeletal, cardiovascular, respiratory, and sensory-motor functions (Litton, Veron, and Griffin 1990). They are concerned with the restoration of physical functioning and prevention of disability following disease, injury, or loss of body parts and thus utilize physical activity as a therapeutic exercise for functional training procedures.

PHYSIATRISTS

Physiatrists are physicians who specialize in rehabilitation, a medical specialty that deals with the evaluation and treatment of those whose functional abilities are impaired. The inaugural meeting of the Canadian Association of Physical Medicine and Rehabilitation was held on May 30, 1952, with the association incorporating on October 15, 1962. The Association of Academic Physiatrists suggests that their members help improve a person's functional capabilities by medical treatment and organizing and integrating a programme of rehabilitation (http://capmr.medical.org/index.html). Therefore, the physiatrist is not directly involved in the actual implementation of physical activity programmes for the purposes of rehabilitation, but is more concerned with the assessment, overview, and management of the programme delivery and, in some cases, may prescribe a physical activity programme.

ALLIED PROFESSIONS OVERVIEW

There appears to be a great deal of overlap among the four professions that have been reviewed in this section, although there may be sufficient diversity for each to be regarded as unique. Therapeutic recreation appears to deal more with the psychosocial domain while physical therapy and occupational therapy address the physical domain. Recreation therapy thus tends to focus on the meaning of activity and self-actualization, otherwise known as 'the little things that make life worth living', while physical and occupational therapists deal with the daily living skills. Finally, physiatrists coordinate these activities focussing on the person's well-being. Theoretically, these four professions can work together with the goal of delivering a high standard of care tailored to the client's needs. Although teamwork is popular with most health professionals, its effectiveness has not yet been conclusively established in rehabilitation (Bakheit 1996).

---

1 There appears to be a great deal of overlap among the professions that use physical activity within the rehabilitation process. Do you think that there is sufficient diversity among them? What would be the risk of making them into only one profession? What are the potential problems of having so many professions think that physical activity is at the heart of their 'treatments'?

---

2 What would be the consequence if any of these professions moved away from the medical model?

---

3 What role can adapted physical activity specialists play during the rehabilitation process? What impact do these various professions have on the adapted physical activity specialist?

The Benefits of Physical Activity During Rehabilitation

The multiplicity of professions that deliver physical activity programmes throughout the rehabilitation process is a reflection of the many benefits that participation provides for the client. The benefits of physical activity are well documented for many different special populations, whether they are related to physical fitness, social networking, spirituality, or psychological well-being (Balmer and Clarke 1997; Canadian Parks/Recreation Association 1997; Coderre 1999; Godbey, Graefe, and James 1992; Koop 1999; Lincoln and Mills

1998; Bouchard, Shephard, and Stephens 1994; Sport Ontario 1992). In addition, benefits have also been quantified economically.

Alan Rock, the federal minister responsible for Health Canada in 1999, pointed to the importance of physical activity in terms of financial costs. Rock reported to the House of Commons that "the connection between physical activity and health is both direct and dramatic and if over the next five years Canadians could reduce their levels of inactivity by 10 percent, Health Canada would save about $10 billion" (Cleary 1999). In the early 1990s, it was also revealed that 50 percent of Ontario's provincial budget was spent in the health and social services sectors. The rate at which these expenditures were growing was a concern and more money was not necessarily an appropriate answer. Instead, there was a need for better management of the health care system with a renewed focus on physical activity (Symington 1994).

The financial independence of the individual with a disability is another economic benefit to the health care system. A 1995 study conducted by the Canadian Paraplegic Association (CPA) reported that 33 percent of people who had spinal cord injuries had not held a job since their injury, and an additional 17 percent were not even looking (Fawcett 1996). This issue was an impetus for the development of wheelchair sport. Dr. Robert Jackson, CWSA's first president, suggested that employers who saw a person with a disability bench press four hundred pounds, or wheel around a track at a blazing pace, were likely to perceive that person as being able to work a forty-hour week and make a significant contribution (Jackson 1974). More recently, this association between physical activity and employment has also been noted with McCleary and Chesteen (1990) who suggested that participation in a wilderness trip that included those with disabilities and those who were able-bodied would encourage those who were able-bodied to hire a person with disabilities in their own business.

Play therapy for children with disabilities was also recognized as an excellent medium for addressing long-term economic issues pertaining to employability. Children with disabilities may have limited play experiences because of physical limitations and social isolation. As a result, they might not have opportunities for exploration or experimentation within a variety of roles and mediums. By not experiencing through trial and error, children with a disability may not develop an accurate appraisal of personal capabilities. A third deterrent to future employment is that children with a disability may not be encouraged to think about having jobs, as those around them may feel that it is unrealistic. Finally, there may be limitations placed on the child's development of occupational choice based on a lack of information about what services or adaptations are available. Through play, children with a disability can address many of these concerns by learning to cope with their own capacities, experiment with different roles, practice leadership and organizational skills, and explore their own creative potentials (Pollock and Stewart 1990).

In addition to the practical benefits of helping a person with a disability find gainful employment, there are other more generic benefits. They are divided into two main categories: psychological and physical. Of these there are special populations where the benefits are clearly identified. Examples include spinal cord injuries, stroke, and cardiovascular disease. There are also groups, such as mental illness and youth at risk groups, where there remains a good deal of speculation about the benefits of physical activity, because it is difficult to identify the exact parameters of interventions that actually provide the benefit. There are also conditions such as AIDS about which we have conflicting information concerning the rehabilitative effects of physical activity. Finally, there are some conditions where activity has to be provided in a certain well-planned way to avoid unpleasant or harmful effects such as diabetes. Recognizing this variability in knowledge as it pertains to the understanding of physical activity during rehabilitation, it is important to consider the suggestion of Bouffard and Strean in Chapter 1

that adapted physical educators must continuously confirm with other experts the benefits of intervening with physical activity prescriptions.

PSYCHOLOGICAL BENEFITS

Humans are not content just to survive. Instead, we seek to thrive and build lifestyles filled with meaningful and valued activities. This is captured in Maslow's Hierarchy of Needs (1954) and is described as the desire for belonging and the pursuit of self-actualization.

Physical activity during the rehabilitation process addresses these needs by enabling participation in what many would consider to be mundane tasks, also referred to as *microflow activities* (Csikszentmihalyi 1975). Microflow activities have been defined as everyday activities that have nonfunctional significance; they are not essential for carrying out the tasks of our daily lives. Csikszentmihalyi (1975), while focussing specifically on the older adult, discovered that these microflow activities fulfilled an essential function of maintaining involvement in other more important activities. They provided stimulation in a nonstimulating environment and thus helped maintain arousal and reduce tension by involving social interaction, body movement, imagination, attention, or creativity. Csikszentmihalyi (1975) claimed that individuals who were deprived of these activities for one or two days tended to complain about fatigue, increased concerns about health, and increased tension. Normal activities thus became more stressful, and people were more irritable. Participation in physical activity, meanwhile, can allow people to partake in many of these microflow activities directly while also enabling them to participate in others indirectly through improved mobility and independence.

Participation in meaningful physical activity programmes during the rehabilitation process also encourages better long-term use of personal leisure time. Day (1990) noted that a great deal of leisure time for persons with disabilities is spent in ways considered to be of poor quality or of having low value. The leisure activities typically selected by those leaving a rehabilitation programme are passive, unplanned, solitary, and require no financial investment. Conversely, society tends to value leisure activities that are active, preplanned, done in groups, and require organization, equipment, rules and a financial investment. Day (1990) further suggested that part of this dichotomy stemmed from an over-focus during rehabilitation on vocational training for employment purposes and not enough on leisure education such as identifying accessible recreation facilities. This suspicion was confirmed as 28 percent of those leaving rehabilitation programmes received training in leisure education, while 92 percent received training in vocational skills (Day 1990). Appropriate use of leisure time would also promote the inclusion of these persons into the community by enabling new friendships and facilitating the break from an institutionalized setting or overprotected home environments (Hale et al. 1979).

PSYCHOLOGICAL BENEFITS
FOR YOUNG CHILDREN

The independence gained from family members is a benefit often overlooked in physical activity programmes during rehabilitation. The extent to which adolescents with disabilities are granted independence and autonomy from the family is often related to the parents' perception of their children's physical and emotional strength (Voll and Poustka 1994). Participation in physical activity and sport, meanwhile, may be a medium that allows parents to view their children as strong and independent.

Young children can also utilize physical activity through play to help develop motor and socialization skills. Williams and Lair (1991) noted that lack of mobility, overprotective parental attitudes, preoccupation with medical treatments, authoritarian treatment climates, limited personal responsibility, and lack of decision-making experiences result in children with a disability who perceive themselves as less than competent. Play therapy in a nonevaluative environment provides opportunities for children with a disability to address these concerns and gain self-confidence, take

advantage of their abilities, and accept or overcome limitations associated with their disabilities (Carmichael 1994). An Alberta-based, nonprofit organization, GRIT (Getting Ready for Inclusion Today), incorporates many of these principles within their programmes for preschool-age children with a disability. Developmental specialists are assigned to children on a one-to-one basis and design programmes based on the principles of play therapy. One example is using games that require sounds to form the foundation for further feeding skills or linguistic abilities.

PSYCHOLOGICAL BENEFITS
FOR YOUTH AT RISK

Physical activity helps address psychological issues in rehabilitation programmes for youth at risk, by being both diversionary and therapeutic (McCall 1996). Diversionary programmes are designed to allow youth at risk a chance to 'burn off' excess energy and hostility in a controlled environment, which allows them to attend to other learning situations. One example is Enviro's, a non-profit organization in Alberta, Canada, that uses a high-ropes course to teach youth at risk the importance of relying on others, the significance of cooperation, and the need to handle stress and anger in a safe and effective manner.

Youth at risk may also benefit from physical activity programmes that address concerns related to substance abuse. This is achieved by showing clients how to achieve a natural high through physical performance. Physical activity can also be used to release excess energy and negative feelings such as anger, frustration, and emotional distress in a more socially appropriate and healthy manner (Kunstler 1996).

PHYSICAL BENEFITS

While providing a number of social and psychological benefits throughout the rehabilitation process, participation in physical activity can also address a number of disability specific issues. For the purposes of this chapter, a few specific examples will be presented, by no means implying that this is an exhaustive list.

Physical Benefits for Persons with a Spinal Cord Injury

Lack of physical activity for persons with a spinal cord injury following trauma is correlated to a number of diverse medical complications, including loss of bone integrity in the paralyzed limbs (osteoporosis), bladder infection, and pressure sores. The adoption of an active lifestyle and incorporation of physical activity during the rehabilitation process can help avoid these obstacles while also offering the prospect of protection against further health complications such as arthritis, heart disease, type II diabetes, and obesity (Jeon, Weiss, and Steadward 1997; Kaprielian 1994). These benefits are particularly important for those with spinal cord injuries, as mobility is already a concern and issues such as obesity further complicate transportation challenges. Finally, participation in physical activity enhances existing physical capacities including improved cardio-respiratory function and muscular strength. As these elements improve, so does the person's overall health, mobility, life-satisfaction, and sense of well-being (Noreau, Shephard, Simard, Pare, and Pomerleau 1993).

Physical Benefits for Persons with Cardiovascular Disease

Physical activity programmes provide tremendous benefit for persons with cardiovascular disease (CVD). CVD is recognized as a leading cause of mortality in North America, however, a number of people are now surviving open-heart surgery and myocardial infarction. These people require the assistance of cardiac rehabilitation programmes that incorporate a significant component of physical activity to reduce the risk of having a heart attack. This is accomplished through risk factor modifications that incorporate physical activity to help lower blood cholesterol levels and maintain ideal body weight (McGuire, Young, and Goodwin 1996).

Stroke rehabilitation, which is often associated with CVD, also utilizes physical activity as a therapeutic technique. Here, physical activity is used to assist with impaired mobility as the effects of the attack on the brain may require relearning or redefining participation in daily activities. Rehabilitation, and particularly the use of physical activity, would not reverse the effects of the stroke, but it can help develop strength to enable adaptations that facilitate continued involvement.

Physical Benefits for a Person with a Mental Illness

A third group where participation in physical activity programmes is speculated as being beneficial is those with a mental illness. Skrinar, Ungar, Hutchinson, and Faigenbaum (1992) suggested that voluntary participation in supervised exercise training improved the fitness profile of people with mental illness who were frequently overweight, had excessive body fat, were cardiovascularly unfit, and displayed physical and lifestyle profiles similar to people with heart disease. People with mental illness also tended to exhibit sluggishness, low energy, poor body image, and low self-concept. These important secondary characteristics represented serious barriers to their rehabilitation (Skrinar et al, 1992).

A second advantage of aerobic exercise for persons with mental illness, and particularly those with schizophrenia, is the possibility of decreasing reliance upon psychotropic medication. Aerobic exercise provides an alternative technique and possible reduction of the drug's detrimental side effects, while also being far more cost-effective for the consumer and the health care system (Pelham and Campagna 1991).

Physical Benefits for Persons with HIV and AIDS

A final group that may benefit from participation in physical activity (although not necessarily in a rehabilitation programme) include persons with AIDS. AIDS was first reported in the United States in 1981 and since that time the number of people dying from it and those being infected with the human immunodeficiency virus (HIV) causing AIDS have escalated. Research regarding the value of exercise for persons with HIV and or AIDS, however, has been inconclusive. In their chapter addressing therapeutic recreation and AIDS,

Grossman and Caroleo (1996) cited two references (Goleman 1992; Schlenzig et al. 1989) suggesting that exercise programmes increased one's T4 cell count, helping to fight infections. Grossman and Caroleo (1996) then further suggest that prolonged aerobic physical activity may actually be detrimental to the individual's overall level of health.

4 Can you think of other people with disabilities or disabling conditions that may (or may not) benefit from physical activity during rehabilitation? Why might they benefit? Why not?

Challenges

Although persons with disabilities are often those who can benefit the most from physical activity, they are also the least involved. The Active Living Alliance for Canadians with a Disability's *Blueprint for Action* (1999) referred to a national population health survey, noting that 16.4 percent of persons with a disability had not participated regularly in physical activity programmes in the previous three months, compared to 7.9 percent of other Canadians (Industry Canada 1995). Ironically, the same survey and others suggested that Canadians with disabilities wished they were more physically active (Industry Canada 1995; Statistics Canada 1991).

Three barriers may stop persons with disabilities from participation. These include a perceived incompetence to participation, inaccessible programmes or facilities (Calloway 1993; Triemstra and Murdock 1995; Witt 1988), and high cost, which became particularly relevant with the elevated levels of unemployment noted earlier (Fawcett 1996).

The implication for adapted physical activity professionals involved in the rehabilitation setting is, therefore, to address these three barriers. Physical activities should be promoted that require little cost and can be easily accessed. Activities should also be promoted that accentuate existing skills. Finally, it is important to involve the client in deciding which activities they want to pursue, which will hopefully lead to continued participation after they leave the rehabilitation continuum (Active Living Alliance for Canadians with a Disability 1999; Itzhaky and Schwartz 1998; Kosciulek 1999).

A final challenge is the inconclusive nature regarding the benefits of physical activity during the rehabilitation process for all persons with disabilities and disabling conditions. There are many areas where we still lack knowledge about the role of physical activity during rehabilitation. As noted earlier in this chapter, we must be careful to not make assumptions that physical activity is always beneficial.

5 Can you state with confidence that physical activity during rehabilitation will benefit people with various types of disabling conditions (e.g., cancer, diabetes, etc.)?

6 Does having activity used by the professionals outlined in this chapter and coordinated by a physiatrist in a hospital setting contribute to the perpetuation of the medical model of dealing with disability?

Summary

This chapter addressed the importance of including physical activity into a rehabilitation process for persons with disabilities. The professionals involved in providing these services throughout the rehabilitation continuum were reviewed, as were the assumed benefits associated with participation. The chapter concluded with a review of three barriers to participation for persons with disabilities in physical activity programmes, which mirrors many of the comments made by Dr. Longmuir in Chapter 21. It is hoped that recognizing the numerous benefits of physical activity and the challenges to accessing them will enable practitioners to acquire the necessary resources to enable greater participation.

Study Questions

1. Compare and contrast the various allied professionals involved in providing physical activity programmes for persons with disabilities during their rehabilitation process.
2. What are the benefits of incorporating physical activity into the rehabilitation process for two special populations?

References

Active Living Alliance for Canadians with a Disability. (1999). *A blueprint for action* (3rd ed.). Ottawa: Health Canada.

Alberta Therapeutic Recreation Association. (1998). Is recreation therapy the same thing as therapeutic recreation? *ATRAbute, 58*: 10.

Alberta Therapeutic Recreation Association. (2001). atraWeb. [Home page] Available http://www.alberta-tr.org/index.htm (URL on October 20, 2002).

American Therapeutic Recreation Association. (2001). American Therapeutic Recreation Association. [Home page] Available: http://www.atra-tr.org/atra.htm (URL on October 20, 2002).

Austin, D., and Crawford, M. (1996). *Therapeutic recreation: An introduction* (2nd ed.). Needham Heights, MA: Simon and Schuster.

Auxter, D., and Pyfer, J. (1985). *Adapted physical education and recreation.* Toronto: Times Mirror/Mosby College Publishing.

Avedon, E. (1974). *Therapeutic recreation service: An applied behavioural science approach.* Englewood Cliffs, NJ: Prentice Hall.

Bakheit, A. (1996). Effective teamwork in rehabilitation. *International Journal of Rehabilitation Research, 19*: 301–6.

Balmer, K., and Clarke, B. (1997). *Benefit indicators: Measuring progress towards effective delivery of the benefits of parks and recreation.* Calgary, AB: Author.

Balmer, K., and Clarke, B. (1997). *The benefits catalogue: Summarizing why recreation, sports, fitness, arts, culture and parks are essential to personal, social, economic and environmental well-being.* Ottawa: Canadian Parks and Recreation Association.

Bouchard, C., Shephard, R., and Stephens, T. (1994). *Physical Activity Fitness and Health: International Proceedings and Consensus Statement.* Champaign, IL: Human Kinetics.

Calloway, J. (1993). Future challenges for therapeutic recreation services. *Leisure Watch Canada, 2*(2): 1–2.

Canadian Association of Occupational Therapists. (2001). [Home page] Available http://www.caot.CA (URL on October 20, 2002).

Canadian Association of Physical Medicine and Rehabilitation. (2001). [Home page] Available: http://www.capmr.medical.org/index.html (URL on October 20, 2002).

Canadian Physiotherapy Association. (2001). [Home page] Available: http://www.physiotherapy.CA (URL on October 20, 2002).

Canadian Therapeutic Recreation Association. (2001). [Home page] Available: http://www.canadian-tr.org (URL on October 20, 2002).

Carmichael, K. (1994). Play therapy for children with physical disabilities. *Journal of Rehabilitation, 60*(3): 51–53.

Carter, M., Van Andel, G., and Robb, G. (1995). *Therapeutic recreation: A practical approach.* Prospect Heights, IL: Waveland.

Cleary, M. (1999, June 11). Campaign urges disabled to get active. *Ottawa Citizen,* p. 42.

Coderre, D. (1999, October). *Speaking notes for the Honourable Denis Coderre, P.C., M.P., Secretary of State (Amateur Sport) on the occasion of the Athletes Can Forum.* Alliston, ON: Author.

Csikszentmihalyi, D. (1975). Beyond boredom and anxiety. In E. Crepeau (Ed.), *Activity planning for the elderly.* Boston: Little, Brown and Company.

Day, H. (1990). A study of quality of life and leisure. In M. Nagler (Ed.), *Perspectives on disability.* Palo Alto, CA: Health Markets Research.

Fawcett, G. (1996). *Living with a disability in Canada: An economic portrait.* Ottawa: Office for Disability Issues.

Frye, V., and Peters, M. (1972). *Therapeutic recreation: Its theory, philosophy, and practice.* Harrisburg, PA: Stackpole Books.

Fuhrer, M. (1987). Overview of outcome analysis in rehabilitation. In M. Fuhrer (Ed.), *Rehabilitation outcomes: Analysis and measurement* (p. 1–15). Baltimore: Paul Brooks.

Godbey, G., Graefe, A., and James, S. (1992). *The benefits of local recreation and parks services.* Washington: National Recreation Foundation.

Goleman, D. (1992, February 12). Relaxation and exercise plan may slow pace of AIDS virus. *The New York Times,* p. C12.

Grossman, A., and Caroleo, C. (1996). Acquired immunodeficiency syndrome (AIDS). In D. Austin and M. Crawford (Eds.), *Therapeutic recreation* (2nd ed., p. 285–301). Needham Heights, MA: Allyn and Bacon.

Hale, G., Barr, P., Buckman, G., Goodman, S., Jimenez, H., Naylor, V., and Seddon, G. (1979). *The source book for the disabled.* New York: Paddington.

Hopkins, H., and Smith, H. (1993). Willard and Spackman's occupational therapy. (8th ed.). In C. Sherrill (Ed.), *Adapted physical activity, recreation and sport: Crossdisciplinary and lifespan* (5th ed.). Boston: McGraw-Hill.

Howe-Murphy, R., and Charboneau, B. (1987). *Therapeutic recreation intervention: An ecological perspective.* Englewood Cliffs, NJ: Prentice Hall.

Industry Canada. (1995). *National population health survey.* Ottawa: Author.

Itzhaky, H., and Schwartz, C. (1998). Empowering the disabled: A multidimensional approach. *International Journal of Rehabilitation Research, 21*: 301–10.

Jackson, R. (1974). Editorial. In *Official programme: 6th national wheelchair games.* Ottawa: Canadian Wheelchair Sports Association.

Jansma, P., and French, R. (1994). *Special physical education: Physical activity, sports and recreation.* Englewood Cliffs, NJ: Prentice Hall.

Jeon, J., Weiss, C., and Steadward, R. (1997). Reducing the risk: Why you may be at risk of developing diabetes and cardiovascular disease and what you can do to prevent them. *Caliper, LII*(3): 8–14.

Kaprielian, R. (1994). Why work out? The benefits of exercise for people with paraplegia. *Rehabilitation Digest, 25*(3): 3–5.

Koop, C. (1999). *Results and recommendations of the World Summit on Physical Education.* Berlin: International Council on Sport Science and Physical Education.

Kosciulek, J. (1999). Consumer direction in disability policy formulation and rehabilitation service delivery. *Rehabilitation Digest, 65*(2): 4–9.

Kunstler, R. (1996). Substance abuse. In D. Austin and M. Crawford (Eds.), *Therapeutic recreation* (2nd ed., p. 95–111). Needham Heights, MA: Allyn and Bacon.

Legg, D. (2000). *Organizational strategy formation in the Canadian Wheelchair Sports Association (1967–1997): A comparison to Leavy and Wilsom (1994).* Doctoral dissertation, Edmonton: University of Alberta.

Lincoln, C., and Mills, D. (1998). *Sport leadership, partnership and accountability, Standing Committee on Canadian Heritage, Sub-committee on the Study of Sport in Canada.* Ottawa: House of Commons.

Litton, F., Veron, L., and Griffin, H. (1990). Occupational therapists and physical therapists: Vital members in the rehabilitation and educational processes of disabled students. In M. Nagler (Ed.), *Perspectives on disability.* Palo Alto, CA: Health Markets Research.

Lysack, C., and Kaufert, J. (1994). Comparing the origins and ideologies of the independent living movement and community based rehabilitation. *International Journal of Rehabilitation Research, 17*: 231–40.

Maslow, A. (1954). *Motivation and personality.* New York: Harper and Row.

McCall, G. (1996). Corrections and social deviance. In D. Austin and M. Crawford (Eds.), *Therapeutic recreation* (2nd ed., p. 78–94). Needham Heights, MA: Allyn and Bacon.

McCleary, I., and Chesteen, S. (1990). Changing attitudes of disabled persons through outdoor adventure pro-grammes. *International Journal of Rehabilitation Research, 13*: 321–24.

McGuire, F., Young, J., and Goodwin, L. (1996). Cardiac rehabilitation. In D. Austin and M. Crawford (Eds.), *Therapeutic recreation* (2nd ed., p. 258–68). Needham Heights, MA: Allyn and Bacon.

National Recreation and Parks Association (2001). [Home page] Available http://www.activeparks.org/ (URL on October 20, 2002).

National Therapeutic Recreation Society (2001). [Home page] Available http://www.nrpa.org/branches/ntrs.htm (URL on October 20, 2002).

Noreau, L., Shephard, R., Simard, C., Pare, G., and Pomerleau, P. (1993). Relationship of impairment and functional ability to habitual activity and fitness following spinal cord injury. *International Journal of Rehabilitation Research, 16*: 265–75.

O'Morrow, G., and Reynolds, R. (1995). *Problems, issues and concepts in therapeutic recreation.* Englewood Cliffs, NJ: Prentice Hall.

Pelham, T., and Campagna, P. (1991). Benefits of exercise in psychiatric rehabilitation of persons with schizophrenia. *Canadian Journal of Rehabilitation, 4*(3): 159–68.

Petersen, C., and Gunn, S. (1984). *Therapeutic recreation programme design: Principles and procedures* (2nd ed.). Englewood Cliffs, NJ: Prentice Hall.

Peterson, C., and Stumbo, N. (2000). *Therapeutic recreation program design: Principles and procedures* (3rd ed.). Boston: Allyn and Bacon.

Pollock, N., and Stewart, D. (1990). A survey of activity patterns and vocational readiness of young adults with physical disabilities. *Canadian Journal of Rehabilitation, 4*(1): 17–26.

Schlengzig, C. et al. (1989). Supervised physical exercise leads to psychological and immunological involvement in pre-AIDS patients. *Proceedings of the V International Conference on AIDS, Montreal, Canada.*

Sherrill, C. (1996). *Adapted physical activity, recreation and sport: Crossdisciplinary and lifespan* (5th ed.). Boston: McGraw-Hill.

Skrinar, G., Ungar, K., Hutchinson, D., and Faigenbaum, A. (1992). Effects of exercise training in young adults with psychiatric disabilities. *Canadian Journal of Rehabilitation, 5*(3): 151–57.

Smith, R., Perry, T., Neumayer, R., Potter, J., and Smeal, T. (1992). Inter-professional perceptions between therapeutic recreation and occupational therapy practitioners: Barriers to effective interdisciplinary team functioning. *Therapeutic Recreation Journal, 4*: 31–42.

Sport Ontario. (1992). *For the love of sport: A resource kit for sport leaders in Ontario.* Toronto: Ministry of Tourism and Recreation.

Statistics Canada. (1991). *Health and activity limitation survey.* Ottawa: Author.

Symington, D. (1994). Megatrends in rehabilitation: A Canadian perspective. *International Journal of Rehabilitation Research, 17*: 1–14.

The Steadward Centre For Personal and Physical Achievement (2001) [Home page] Available www.steadwardcentre.org (URL on October 20, 2002).

Triemstra, C., and Murdock, W. (1995). Therapeutic recreation: A decade of change. *Leisureability, 2*(4): 1–12.

Voll, R., and Poustka, F. (1994). Coping with illness and coping with handicap during the vocational rehabilitation of physically handicapped adolescents and young adults. *International Journal of Rehabilitation Research, 17*: 305–18.

Williams, W., and Lair, G. (1991). Using a person-centered approach with children who have a disability. *Elementary School Guidance and Counseling, 25*(3): 194–203.

Witt, P. (1988). Therapeutic recreation research: Past, present and future. *Therapeutic Recreation Journal, 22*(1): 14–23.

World Health Organization. (1980). *International classification of impairments, disabilities, and handicaps: A manual of classification relating to the consequences of disease.* Geneva: Author.

Wright, B. (1980). Total rehabilitation. In R. Lyons (Ed.) (1993). Meaningful activity and disability: Capitalizing upon the potential of outreach recreation networks in Canada. *Canadian Journal of Rehabilitation, 6*(4): 256–65.

V ■ THE SCHOOL ENVIRONMENT

CHAPTER 13

Inclusive Physical Education

A Conceptual Framework

Donna L. Goodwin
E. Jane Watkinson
David A. Fitzpatrick

Learning Objectives

- To define *inclusion* within the instructional context of physical education.
- To identify and describe the components of an inclusive physical education programme.
- To discuss and illustrate the appropriateness of the goals of the physical education programme for students with disabilities.
- To illustrate how the conceptual framework can be used to plan, implement, or evaluate the effectiveness of inclusive physical education programmes.
- To identify areas in need of further investigation to advance our understanding of the process of inclusive physical education.

Introduction

The provision of appropriate educational experiences for all students within the regular classroom and mainstream of school life reflects the current educational ideology of inclusive education. Within the inclusive setting, students with physical or learning disabilities, those at risk of educational failure, and those who surpass age-equivalent educational expectations and are considered gifted receive their education from general education teachers in the regular classroom (Stainback and Stainback 1990; York, Vandercook, MacDonald, Heise-Neff, and Caughey 1992). The ideology of inclusive education emanated from dissatisfaction with the earlier educational perspective of integration.

Integration within the school system was based upon a service-based model that labelled, grouped, and placed students according to their abilities into special education classrooms (Polloway, Smith, Patton, and Smith 1996). By grouping students, specialized on-site services, such as teachers with special education backgrounds, consultant expertise, technical support, and specially designed classrooms could be efficiently and effectively delivered and managed. A dual system of education emerged, one for students who participated in regular or mainstream educational programmes, and another for students who participated in special education programmes.

Integration was founded on the assumption that special programmes, delivered within protected environments, would be followed by successful placement in regular settings. Advocates for inclusive education rejected the notion of protected environments, however, stating that students with disabilities learn more in the regular classroom than they do in segregated settings, and that inclusive educational experiences better prepare students with disabilities for community living. They also contended that the general school population learned to interact and communicate with others according to individual strengths rather than stereotypic generalizations (Stainback and Stainback 1992; Kerzner Lipsky and Gartner 1992).

The purpose of this chapter is to explore the complex phenomenon of inclusive physical education. A conceptual framework, identifying the variables that contribute to the planning, implementation, and evaluation of inclusive physical education will be presented. The relationship of the variables to each other will be discussed within the context of professional practice and the need for ongoing empirical study. A definition of inclusive physical education will also be put forward.

---

1 What value conflicts resulted in a dual system of education being rejected by advocates of inclusive education?

---

2 What were the premises underlying integrated education?

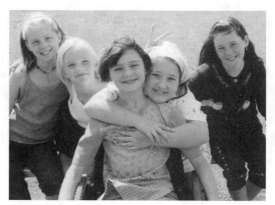

School Friends

Inclusive Physical Education

Inclusive education reflects a commitment to a support-based model of education that places students with disabilities in a regular educational setting immediately upon school entry. The model presumes that necessary technical and educational supports will be provided on an ongoing basis, thereby ensuring success and continuation in the inclusive setting. An unfortunate paradox of inclusive education, however, is that the supports necessary for success are not always known, provided, or empirically evaluated (Block 1999a; LaMaster, Gall, Kinchin, and Siedentop 1998; Watkinson and Bentz 1986).

The interpretation and day-to-day implementation of inclusive physical education has been left largely to regular classroom teachers, with the outcome that it has different meanings for different people (Decker and Jansma 1995; Kauffman 1995; Sherrill 1994). This has resulted in differing interpretations of programme goals, instructional context, relevant and ecologically valid content, and needed support structures across school districts and even individual schools (Davis 1989; Davis and Burton 1991; Karper and Martinek 1985; Sherrill and Montelione 1990). Block (1999a) argues that, among the problems faced by practicing teachers of physical education, inclusion is not being carried out properly. Decisions about placement in regular physical education classes have been made based on philosophy and not student need, parental preferences have been ignored, and the

Figure 13.1 The Cascade System of Educational Placement

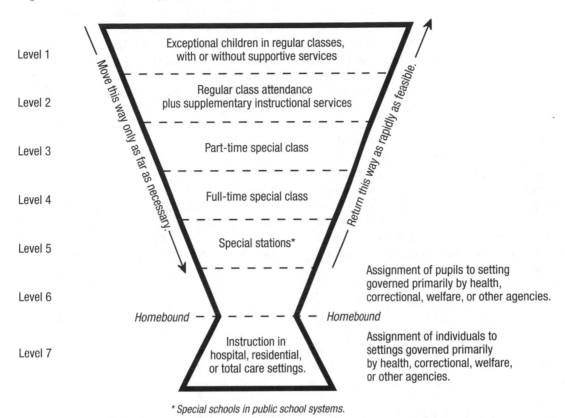

Level 1 — Exceptional children in regular classes, with or without supportive services

Level 2 — Regular class attendance plus supplementary instructional services

Level 3 — Part-time special class

Level 4 — Full-time special class

Level 5 — Special stations*

Level 6 — Assignment of pupils to setting governed primarily by health, correctional, welfare, or other agencies.

Homebound — Homebound

Level 7 — Instruction in hospital, residential, or total care settings.

Assignment of individuals to settings governed primarily by health, correctional, welfare, or other agencies.

Move this way only as far as necessary.

Return this way as rapidly as feasible.

* Special schools in public school systems.

SOURCE: From "Special Education as Developmental Capital," by E. Deno, 1970, *Exceptional Children, 37*(3), pp. 229–37. Copyright 1970 by the Council for Exceptional Children. Reprinted with permission.

support for adapted physical education specialists has been lacking. The need to clarify the educational experiences, expectations, and supports required for successful inclusion appears to be overwhelming (Hamre-Nietupski 1993; Sherrill and Williams 1996).

The dynamic and complex nature of inclusive physical education has been evident in the conceptual writings of many adapted physical activity leaders. Such writers have addressed adaptations to the curriculum (Block and Vogler 1994), as well as strategies for individualizing assessment and instruction (Davis and Burton 1991). They have investigated the social acceptance of individual differences through frequent, long-term, positive, and mutually respectful peer interactions (Tripp and Sherrill 1991; Sherrill, Heikinaro-Johansson, and

Slininger 1994) and acknowledged the importance of sharing the responsibility of participation with peers, parents, instructional assistants, and professionals through collaborative working relationships (Block 1994; Maguire 1994).

LEAST RESTRICTIVE ENVIRONMENT

The philosophy of inclusive education, or what has been termed special education reform, was precipitated by a lack of satisfaction with the principle of least restrictive environments (LRE). The principle was most commonly represented by the cascade system (figure 13.1) and referred to the right of students to be successfully educated in the setting that was most like the educational setting of students without disabilities (Friend, Bursuck, and Hutchinson

1998). LRE was resulted in the development of a continuum of placements that led to the development of placement options that were ranked hierarchically from most restrictive to least restrictive (Wehman, Sherron, and West 1997). To some, LRE was interpreted to mean the degree to which students with disabilities were separated from students without disabilities (Block and Krebs 1992).

The principle of LRE was supported by adapted physical educators and modified for physical education settings (Aufsesser 1991). The intent was to provide support services for students with disabilities with the aim of moving students through the continuum of options toward the ultimate goal of regular physical educational placement alongside their peers without disabilities.

The principle of LRE came under criticism, however (see Block and Krebs 1992 for an in-depth discussion of LRE) for perpetuating the labelling of students by characteristics at the macro level (e.g., learning disability, emotional disturbance). These generalized characteristics were then broadly applied to instructional planning (Kauffman 1995; Wang 1996). Further, LRE supported the primacy of professional decision making as students had to demonstrate to the satisfaction of teachers and administrators that they were eligible to progress through the continuum (Gartner and Kerzner Lipsky 1996). In essence, students were asked to 'earn their way' out of special education classrooms to join their peers in regular or classrooms.

For a more in-depth discussion of the philosophy of least restrictive environment as it has been applied to physical education, the reader is directed to Chapter 9 (Reid) titled "Moving Toward Inclusion." An illustration of the cascade system as it has been adapted for use in physical education settings can be found there.

WHERE, WHAT, AND HOW

It is apparent that one of the themes that runs through our current understanding of inclusive physical education is *where* students with disabilities should receive their education, in regular classrooms or in special education classrooms? Current ideology promotes the educational and social merits of the regular classrooms for all students, from early childhood programmes, during elementary grades, and through secondary school (Friend et al. 1998). Inclusive classrooms are promoted over other settings because all children are valued, can learn, and belong in the mainstream of school and community life. Diversity is a valued and celebrated reflection of the human condition, which strengthens classrooms and provides greater learning opportunities for everyone (Jacobsen and Sawatsky 1993; Stainback and Stainback 1996). As many students with disabilities are already involved in regular physical education programmes (Decker and Jansma 1995) the prominence of the *where* debate has faded from recent literature (Block and Vogler 1994; Sherrill 1994).

A second theme that runs through our discussion of inclusive physical education is *what*. What do we teach students with disabilities? Is the regular curriculum appropriate, or is something different desired or needed? Closely associated with the *what* theme is the *how* theme. Once the appropriateness of the curriculum has been determined, *how* is it best implemented? Are some instructional strategies better suited to the needs of students with disabilities than others? Are support services and aides needed, and if so, what and who are they, and to what extent are they needed? These questions have yet to be fully answered. Although the *where* question appears to have reached resolution, the *whats* and the *hows* of inclusive physical education appear to be operating at a conceptual level of understanding and knowledge (Block 1999b).

A DEFINITION

Reid (1992) reminds us that language is a dynamic and evolving system and we must expect changes in its interpretation as societal values and beliefs evolve and change. As such, our understanding of inclusive physical education is maturing over time. We no longer focus only on *where* students receive their physical education programme. Nor do we focus on how well students with disabilities 'fit into' the regular physical education programme.

Our pedagogical focus has shifted to a more ecological view of the larger instructional setting. We acknowledge the complex roles of classmates, teachers, and administrators, while also recognizing the importance of support systems such as families, instructional assistants, physical education consultants, and adapted equipment or specially designed environments (Sherrill 1994). We also acknowledge the appropriateness of the goals of the regular physical education programme within this supported environment and how students experience them (Goodwin and Watkinson 2000; Goodwin 2001). As such, *inclusive physical education means providing all students with disabilities the opportunity to participate in regular physical education with their peers, with supplementary aides and support services as needed to take full advantage of the goals of motor skill acquisition, fitness, knowledge of movement, and psycho-social well-being, toward the outcome of preparing all students for an active lifestyle appropriate to their abilities and interests.*

GOALS OF INCLUSIVE PHYSICAL EDUCATION

The appropriateness of the standard curriculum is fundamental to the discussion of inclusive physical education. Endorsing the *where* (i.e., regular physical education programme) as one of the delineating features of inclusive physical education presupposed the appropriateness of the goals and objectives of the regular programme for students with disabilities. To suggest otherwise presents a contradiction between the *where* and the *what* that cannot be easily resolved. Recommending placement in the regular physical education programme while advocating for alternate programme content may in essence be promoting the creation of a programme within an existing one, thereby bringing us full circle in the inclusion debate. Separate programme content could result in removing students with disabilities from interaction with classmates and an increased workload for teachers (Fuchs and Fuchs 1994).

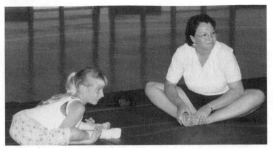
In the Gym

There are four generally agreed upon goals of physical education: (a) knowledge acquisition and application, (b) motor skill acquisition, (c) health related fitness, and (d) psycho-social well-being (Arnold 1991; Graham 1987). The goal of knowledge in physical education can be viewed in a number of ways. Knowledge about action that is stored in memory and can influence the development and execution of skilled action has been referred to as *declarative knowledge* (Wall 1986; Wall, McClements, Bouffard, Findlay, and Taylor 1985). Depending on the learner, it can include knowledge of biomechanics, motor-learning principles, and activity-specific information such as timing, stance, swing, and follow-through.

Knowledge about how to perform or use the information to control and execute skilled movement is *procedural knowledge* (Ennis 1994). Procedural knowledge is used when a performer visually identifies relevant performance information, deploys attentional strategies, or selects a response to meet the task demands (Wall et al. 1985). Both declarative and procedural knowledge are crucial to skill acquisition and thus are basic to participation in physical education irrespective of the presence or absence of a disability. Fundamentally, Grosse (1978) reminds us, "Whether the individual is to become a sports announcer or a television football fan, he/she still needs a basic knowledge of how the game is played" (p. 1).

The practical application of declarative and procedural knowledge occurs during the process of motor skill acquisition. Whereas the motor domain is central to physical education, motor skill acquisition is fundamental to the curriculum (Arnold 1991; Davis 1989;

Sherrill and Montelione 1990). Students are expected to participate in a range of activities and to do so requires a minimal level of skill proficiency that can only be achieved with appropriate opportunities for practice (Wall 1982). The question then remains, is the goal of motor skill acquisition attainable by students with disabilities? The authors join others in replying, "yes" (Block 1992; Sherrill 1998; Stein 1987). However, the context of assessment and instruction must be conceptualized from a functional outcome perspective and not from a normative developmental sequence perspective (Davis and Burton 1991).

As early as 1978, there was a call to individualize instruction by allowing the student to perform standard skills in the most functional manner possible (Grosse 1978). Interpreting the curriculum from a traditional motor development perspective, which defines performance attributes solely by the achievement of hierarchical stages of skill proficiency, may mean that the goal of motor skill acquisition becomes unattainable by and inappropriate for some students.

An alternative approach to motor skill acquisition has been proposed. Ecological task analysis (Davis and Burton 1991) links the requirements of the task to environmental conditions and performer capacities. In this approach, curriculum activities are categorized by function and intention (i.e., moving from one point to another, propelling a stationary or moving object or person, receiving a stationary or moving object or person, and changing position relative to an object, person, terrain, or event). Achieving the outcome of the task (e.g., getting the volleyball into the opponent's court) takes precedence over achieving the 'correct' movement form for an overhand volleyball serve, for example. Students, with the support of the teacher, are freed to discover the movement form that best meets the movement outcome, as dictated by the task. The solutions are collaboratively determined through exploration and self-discovery by the student and direct instruction by the teacher (Burton and Davis 1996). An ecological task analysis approach

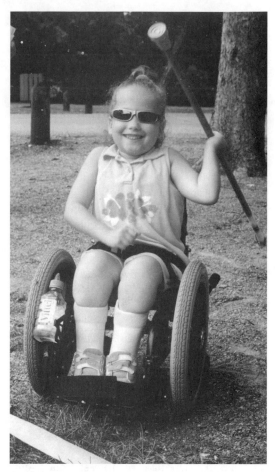

Javelin

to assessment and instruction removes the onerous responsibility of having to know, or presume to know, the best movement form for students with disabilities. This approach is consistent with the goal of skill acquisition and hence well suited to inclusive physical education programmes.

Endorsing the goals of motor skill acquisition also removes us, one more step, from previous models of disability that emphasized individual weakness and physical rehabilitation to ameliorate problems. Our current understanding validates the capabilities of persons with disabilities and their capacity for development and self-determination. Instructional accountability in inclusive physical education rests with the recognition that the goals of the regular physical education programme are purposeful and meaningful for all students

(Davis 1989). The degree to which specific activities with programme dimensions of the curriculum (e.g., dance, gymnastics, aquatics, individual and team activities) are suited for all students remains open for discussion, however.

The goal of fitness is promoted in physical education curricula. Only insofar as fitness can be shown to assist functional participation in the activities of the curriculum can it be regarded as serving an educational objective for any student (Arnold 1991). Furthermore, if circuit training, aerobic exercises, or calisthenics are used to meet the curricular goal of fitness, the educational component is lost to simple physical conditioning. The students must be simultaneously developing an understanding of what they are doing and why they are doing it. It is the educational worth of fitness that makes this goal appropriate for students with disabilities. Ultimately, fitness is an individual matter that requires personal commitment to daily activities that will address cardiovascular efficiency, strength, muscular endurance, and flexibility (Arnold 1991).

Students with disabilities were frequently placed in regular physical education on the belief that it would contribute to a wider degree of social acceptance of disability. The social context (peers, teachers, environment), through personal contact with persons with disabilities, would move toward an atmosphere of increased acceptance of, and appreciation for, human diversity. The goal of psycho-social well-being implies that social development is not necessarily consistent with social acceptance by others, but rather that the larger social context must be one that allows for individual expression. An increased tolerance of individuality promotes a social context in which students with disabilities experience a sense of belonging and acceptance because of who they are and not how much they conform to their peer groups (Block 1999a; Sherrill and Montelione 1990).

3 What modifications were made to the cascade system as it was applied to physical education?

4 What issues surrounded the ability of students to move from one LRE to another?

5 What assumption underlies a commitment to inclusive physical education programming?

6 What is the distinction between instruction that is functionally based and that which is based on normative developmental sequences?

A Conceptual Framework

A conceptual framework that provides both structure and boundaries for the discussion and investigation of inclusive physical education is provided in figure 13.2. It provides a visual conceptualization of the context, consequences, and interrelationships among the variables (Ennis 1999). Undoubtedly, new components will be added over time as our knowledge and understanding of teaching and learning in inclusive physical education increases.

WHY A CONCEPTUAL FRAMEWORK?

The need for consultation in inclusive physical education programmes has become increasingly important (Block and Conatser 1999). The consultant's role is extremely diverse and very challenging. Consultants are asked to address problems as diverse as a mismatch between a teacher's value system and the school district's commitment to a support-based or inclusionary model of education, fears about the safety of the students in the class, a lack of general preparation in the teaching of physical education, inadequacy of facilities or equipment, paucity of supports to implement the programme, overprotective parents, and students with limited motor skill repertoires (Heikinaro-Johansson, Sherrill, French, and Huuhka 1995).

A framework that identifies the interacting variables in the inclusive physical education environment would be valuable during the first step of the consultation process, the needs assessment. During a needs assessment the consultant assists the teacher to identify,

Figure 13.2 A Conceptual Framework for the Study and Practice of Inclusive Physical Education

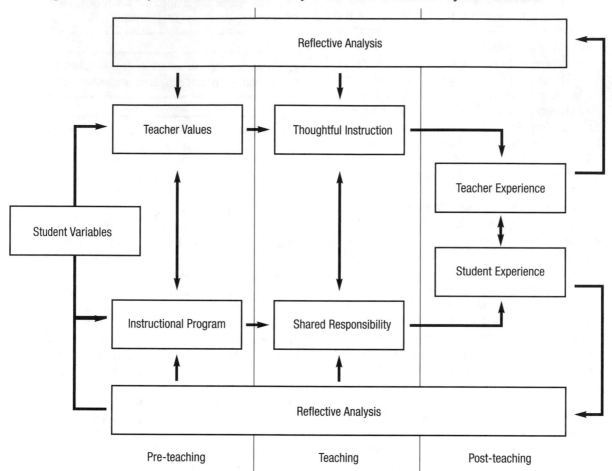

SOURCE: Adapted from *The Study of Teaching* by M.J. Dunkin and B.J. Biddle, 1974, New York: Holt, Rinehart, & Winston. Adapted by permission.

clarify, and prioritize concerns. Even though the teacher often initiates the consultation process (Block and Conatser 1999), there are times when the exact nature of the concern cannot be articulated beyond a sense that things are not going well. The conceptual framework would provide a systematic way of identifying the nature of the concerns and thereby facilitate problem-solving. Concerns over a school administrator's relegation of instructional assistance support within the school and the need for a volunteer to assist with the upcoming aquatics programme, although related, may require very different action plans. Similarly, a teacher who does not

see the benefits of the physical education programme for students with disabilities will not be responsive to programme modifications, no matter how innovative or appropriate they may be designed to increase the student's participation in the programme.

The conceptual framework also provides a template from which to begin planning for a student with a disability who may be joining a class in the upcoming year. It becomes apparent that there is much to consider beyond getting to know the student better. Attention needs to be given to teacher expectations, curriculum adaptations, support systems, and instructional strategies. The framework can also be used to evaluate how well things are going in an existing inclusive physical education setting. The experiences of the students and teacher will provide a context from which to reflect on how well resources were allocated, the responsibility was shared, or teacher and student expectations were in line with the curriculum.

In summary, if 'best practices' in inclusive physical education are to be built upon more than personal insight and positive intentions, applied research must play a prominent role in guiding practice. Although a conceptual framework is useful for visualizing and revealing patterns of relationships among interacting instructional variables, it can also be useful in providing structure and boundaries for empirical study (Miles and Huberman 1994; Snow 1973). Karper and Martinek (1985) contend that the believability, replicability, and generalizability of school-based research can only be enhanced with a clearer understanding of the content and context of inclusive physical education. Nonetheless, neither the framework, nor its testing, would question the assumptions upon which a framework is built (Slife and Williams 1995). That is to say, not only are the variables identified within the framework and their relationships open to investigation, but also so are the ideas upon which the framework was developed. Given these cautionary notes, the conceptual framework may provide a useful heuristic representation for the discussion and study of inclusive physical education is proposed.

DEVELOPMENT OF THE CONCEPTUAL FRAMEWORK

The conceptual framework was adapted from a model for classroom teaching by Dunkin and Biddle (1974). The model distinguished between four regions: presage, context, process, and product variables. The *presage* variables were concerned with the characteristics of teachers and the effects of these characteristics on the teaching process. For example, an inexperienced teacher's formative background (e.g., social class, age), or a veteran teacher's experiences (e.g., repeated years of single-grade teaching) may influence the teaching process. Similarly, the experiences gained at university during teacher preparation, practice teaching, through in-service development, or post-graduate education may also influence classroom instruction. Teacher properties such as attitudes, beliefs, motives, and abilities may also have a potential effect on teaching.

Context variables included those characteristics of the environment to which the teacher must adjust. It may include the physical building, budget constraints, or the influences of the parent association. Students are also included within the context region. Like teachers, students can influence the instructional setting.

Process variables were concerned with the actual activities and behaviours of teachers and students in the classroom. Only those behaviours that were overt and could be measured were deemed to be process variables according to Dunkin and Biddle (1974). Teacher behaviours have been the primary focus of research on the teaching process.

Product variables concerned change in students, or the outcome of teaching that resulted from participation in classroom activities with the teacher and other students. Within this model, student growth, as measured by subject-matter learning, was presumed to be an indicator of teaching effectiveness.

The strength of the Dunkin and Biddle model of teaching over earlier models was its explicit recognition of student behaviour as a process variable, and the influence of context variables as something with which teachers must contend. Previous models defined research on teaching as that which placed the behaviour or characteristics of the teacher as the central variable (Gage 1963a, 1963c). Research on teaching was aimed at the identification and measurement of teacher behaviour and revealing their consequences on student growth. The three central categories of this early research on teaching involved teaching methods (e.g., lecturing, project model), instruments of teaching (e.g., textbooks, films), and teacher personality and characteristics (e.g., subject knowledge, intelligence) (Gage 1963c). Although other relevant variables, such as social interaction and the social background provided by the school, home, and community at large were noted to be part of the larger landscape, "they are neither necessary nor sufficient to characterize a piece of research as research on teaching" (Gage 1963c p. vii).

Gage set the stage for the "criteria for effectiveness paradigm" or what has come to be known as the "process-product" paradigm of educational research (Gage 1963b; Garrison and Macmillan 1984). Research on teaching (e.g., teaching styles, teaching methods) became synonymous with the identification of criterion, or set of criteria, teachers might implement to bring about effectiveness (the product) as reflected by student change (e.g., achievement and attitude). The assumption of causality in this paradigm is evident as the causes or teacher behaviours that bring about student change are sought. Doyle (1975) suggests, "two factor causal analyses–i.e., where teacher behaviour and student achievement are the only two factors considered–overlook the importance of the mediating processes of student activities and of the classroom ecology" (p. 62). The activities of the student, according to Doyle, were skipped over in the search for a causal relationship between the teacher's activities and the students' achievement.

According to Dewey (1938), "Perhaps the greatest of all pedagogical fallacies is that a person learns only the particular thing he is studying at the time" (p. 48). What might students learn or not learn because of the way learning was experienced? Dewey contemplates the quality of the educational experience and advocates that the business of the school is more than the transmission of bodies of information to the new generation. Relating to students as a 'class' rather than a 'social group' contributes to teachers acting largely from the outside. Relating to students as a social group changes the compulsion of control to that of facilitating exchange.

Dewey's (1938) theory of experience is based on two principles: continuity and interaction. Experiences can be judged as educational only to the degree with which they are agreeable and they have an influence upon later experiences; "the principle of continuity of experience means that every experience both takes up something from those which have gone before and modifies in some way the quality of those which come after" (p. 35). Secondly, the educational experience should be interpreted as an interaction, with equal weighting being given to the objective conditions of the environment as well as internal conditions of the learning. The violation of this principle brings the largest criticism of process-product models of teaching, including that of Dunkin and Biddle (1974). Educational research has taken a one-sided view of teaching and sought to identify, measure, and correlate teacher and context variables to student achievement (Garrison and Macmillan 1984). The experience of the student had been all but ignored in our quest to advance our understanding of teaching and, in particular, the phenomenon of inclusive physical education.

To address this major shortcoming, researchers in the area of adapted physical activity have adapted the Dunkin and Biddle (1974) model. DePauw and Goc Karp (1992) incorporated the four regions of presage, context, process, and product within a socio-historical and socio-cultural framework for pedagogic research for diverse learners (see figure 13.3). Heikinaro-Johansson's (1995) studies on including students with special needs in physical education were also based on a framework adapted from Dunkin and Biddle (1974). She however, expanded the outcome region to explicitly include both teacher and student experiences as outcomes of the inclusive physical education programme, although this region of the framework is not directly addressed in her studies.

The conceptual framework presented in figure 13.2 adapts the Dunkin and Biddle (1974) and DePauw and Goc Karp (1992) models further. It incorporates the presage (teacher values), context (student variables), process (thoughtful instruction, shared responsibility),

Figure 13.3 Framework for Conducting Pedagogical Research for Diverse Learners

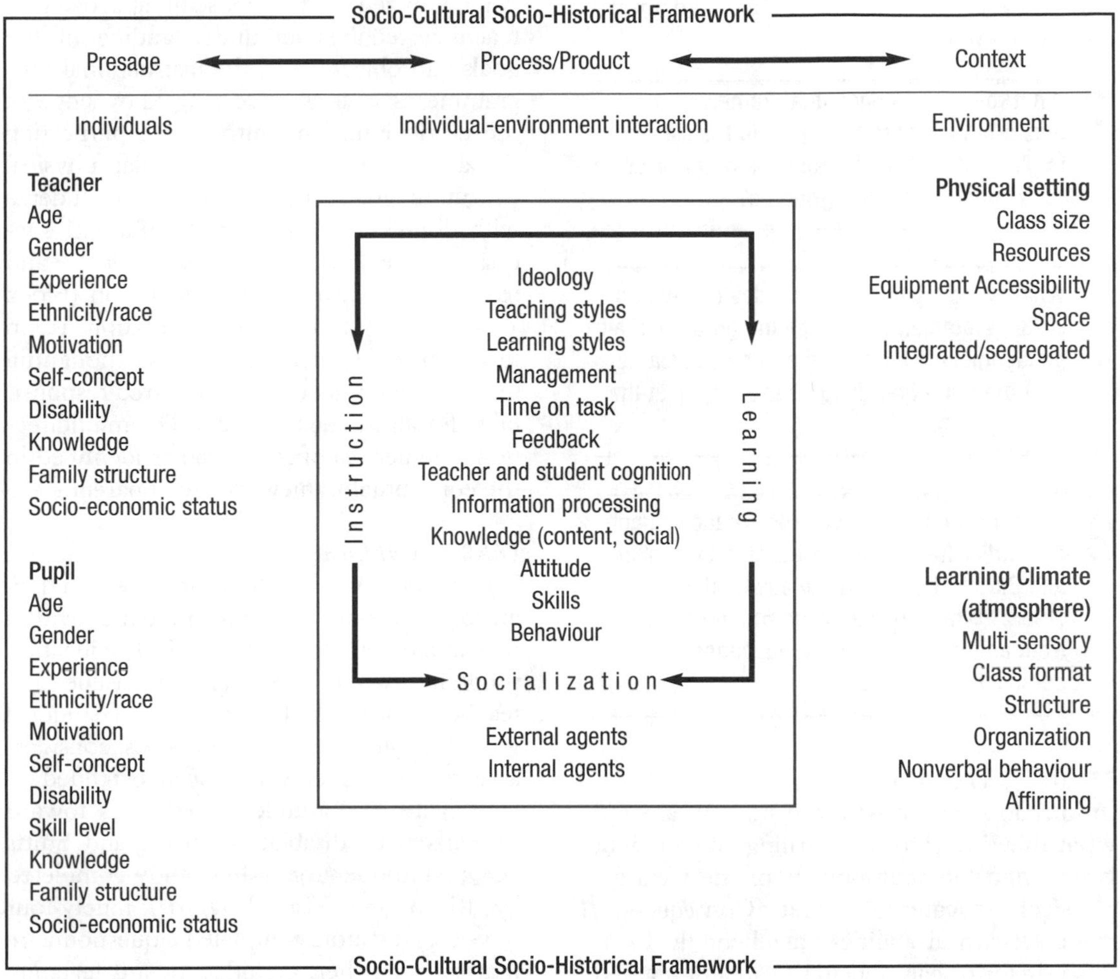

─── Socio-Cultural Socio-Historical Framework ───

| Presage | ⟷ | Process/Product | ⟷ | Context |

| Individuals | Individual-environment interaction | Environment |

Teacher
Age
Gender
Experience
Ethnicity/race
Motivation
Self-concept
Disability
Knowledge
Family structure
Socio-economic status

Pupil
Age
Gender
Experience
Ethnicity/race
Motivation
Self-concept
Disability
Skill level
Knowledge
Family structure
Socio-economic status

Instruction

Ideology
Teaching styles
Learning styles
Management
Time on task
Feedback
Teacher and student cognition
Information processing
Knowledge (content, social)
Attitude
Skills
Behaviour

Learning

S o c i a l i z a t i o n

External agents
Internal agents

Physical setting
Class size
Resources
Equipment Accessibility
Space
Integrated/segregated

Learning Climate (atmosphere)
Multi-sensory
Class format
Structure
Organization
Nonverbal behaviour
Affirming

─── Socio-Cultural Socio-Historical Framework ───

SOURCE: From "Framework for Conducting Pedagogical Research in Teaching Physical Education to Include Diverse Populations" by K.P. DePauw and G. Goc Karp, 1992, in *Sport and Physical Activity: Moving Toward Excellence* (pp. 243–48) by W.L. Almond and A. Sparkes (Eds.). London: E and FN Spon. Reprinted with permission.

and product (teacher and student experiences) regions of the model, but the focus on the teacher effectiveness alone, as measured by student achievement (process-product paradigm) has been expanded. The notion of shared *responsibility* within the instructional process, and student and teacher *experience* as an outcome of the instructional process have been incorporated.

The phases of implementation of an inclusive physical education programme include information gathering and synthesis, programme execution, student and teacher change, and evaluation (Dunkin and Biddle 1974). These temporally-sequenced activities have been referred to as pre-teaching, teaching, and post-teaching responsibilities and are represented on figure 13.2 by the vertical lines that dissect the framework (Kysela, French, and Brenton-Haden 1993). The constituent elements within each phase will be briefly explained. The intent is not to present a review of the related literature in each area, but to describe their interactive and multidirectional nature.

7 What role can a conceptual framework, as illustrated in figure 13.1, play in the planning, implementation, and evaluation of an inclusive physical education programme?

8 What is the significance to today of Dewey's (1938) statement, "Perhaps the greatest of all pedagogical fallacies is that a person learns only the particular thing he is studying at the time" (p. 48)?

9 What reasons were given for expanding upon the earlier frameworks presented by Dunkin and Biddle (1974) and DePauw and Goc Karp (1992)? Why was the expansion important from an inclusive physical education perspective?

STUDENT VARIABLES

Information about who the students are and what they bring to the learning environment is an important component of the inclusive physical education context. Consequently, students with disabilities have been the focus of study for researchers in the area of adapted physical activity for some time. A considerable early research legacy has resulted in an abundant accumulation of knowledge in such areas as fitness, motor learning, motor skill acquisition, and attitudes toward physical activity (Broadhead 1986; Pyfer 1986). Research in the biological, social psychological, behavioural, and cognitive domains of persons with disabilities and physical activity continues to be represented in the current literature (Broadhead and Burton 1996).

INSTRUCTIONAL PROGRAMME

An organized and purposeful approach to teaching requires an understanding of the goals and objectives of the instructional programme as well as a working knowledge of the curriculum. The authors are purporting the appropriateness of the regular physical education goals and objectives for students with disabilities. However, the ultimate success of the programme for students and teachers lies with its implementation (Block 1999b). Programme implementation is, in turn, linked to teacher values, thoughtful instructional practices, and a shared responsibility for all students' success. The multidirectional influences of the variables identified in the conceptual framework are apparent.

TEACHER VALUES

The teachers' value systems or the worth they attribute to something* are embedded within the implementation of physical education programmes. To understand the value that teachers place on the presence of students with disabilities in their classrooms, considerable research energy has been extended to investigate the attitudes of teachers toward students with disabilities (Rowe and Stutts 1987; Santomier 1985). In a study completed by Rizzo and Vispoel (1991), ninety-four physical educators completed a questionnaire that assessed their attitudes toward teaching students who were classified as having developmental disabilities, behaviour disorders, or learning disabilities. The results indicated that there was a significant positive correlation between favourable teacher attitudes and years of teaching students with disabilities and a negative correlation with years of overall teaching. It was concluded that fostering positive attitudes toward the teaching of students with disabilities required more than teaching experience. Hands-on experience teaching

---

* Values can be intrinsic, instrumental, inherent, or contributory in nature. *Intrinsic value* refers to the inherent value that something possessed by virtue of its own sake. *Instrumental value* is present when a contribution is made to something. *Inherent value*, in turn, refers to an experience, awareness, or contemplation that, in and of itself, has intrinsic value. Finally, *contributory value* exists when a contribution has been made to the value of the whole. (Audi 1995)

ADAPTED PHYSICAL ACTIVITY

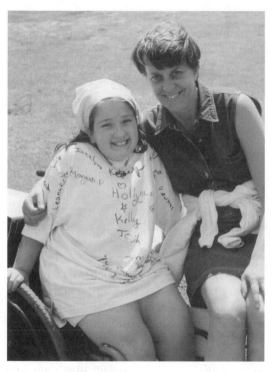

Instructional Assistant

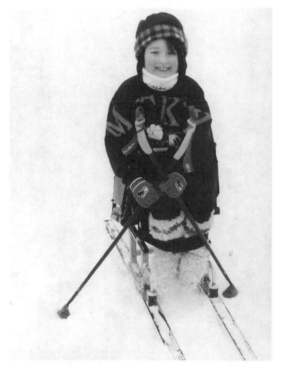

Cross-country Skiing

students with disabilities was needed to foster positive attitudes.

It was further noted that the teachers held more favourable attitudes toward teaching students with learning disabilities than toward students who had developmental disabilities or behaviour disorders. In contrast, a later study with undergraduate physical education majors it was found that they had more favourable attitudes toward teaching students who had developmental disabilities (Rizzo and Vispoel 1992). In both studies, students with behavioural disorders were perceived less favourably than students who had learning disabilities or developmental disabilities.

It was also noted in the former study (Rizzo and Vispoel 1991) that perceived competence was strongly related to positive attitudes. Teachers who perceived themselves as competent in their teaching had more favourable attitudes toward teaching students with disabilities over those who perceived themselves to be less competent. This finding was consistent with an earlier study (Rizzo and Wright

1988). Although this research is of extreme value, alone it leads to the assumption that beliefs and moral commitments about what is 'good' and 'should work' is enough to sustain and guide inclusive physical education practices (LaMaster et al. 1998). A broader understanding of the dynamic process of inclusive physical education is needed.

Teacher competence is a reflection of pedagogical tactfulness, or what van Manen (1986) calls a special kind of knowledge, that which is obtained through a certain kind of seeing, listening, and responding. He suggested that teacher competence is more than professional or clinical knowledge; it is the knowledge that comes from the thoughtfulness that results from asking the question, "How is the child experiencing this situation" (p. 8)? It is this underlying ethic of caring that guides our interactions and responses to children (Clandinin 1993). Seeking to meet the needs of students by modifying and manipulating activities may be of little consequence if we are not mindful of how the students are experiencing the

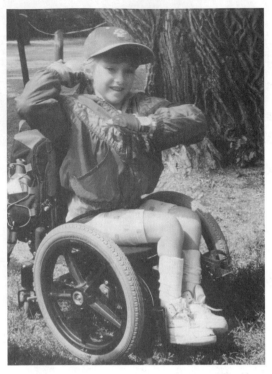

Shot-put

activity. Research on teachers' values is but one piece of a very complex phenomenon.

Providing opportunities for attitude change toward teaching students with disabilities in physical education settings over the course of undergraduate professional preparation programmes remains a concern for university and college personnel across North America (Rizzo, Broadhead, and Kowalski 1997). Tools such as the Physical Educators' Attitude Toward Teaching the Handicapped Measure-II (PEATH-II) (Rizzo and Vispoel 1991) and the Teacher Integration Attitudes Questionnaire (TIAQ) (Sideridis and Chandler 1997) have been developed to assess empirically the efficacy of hands-on experiences in bringing about attitude change. Evidence such as this, combined with efforts to infuse knowledge about disability throughout undergraduate physical education curriculum, may encourage students to think differently about human diversity as they acquire knowledge and construct new understandings (DePauw and Goc Karp 1994; Rizzo et al. 1997).

THOUGHTFUL INSTRUCTION

Teaching tasks are those that facilitate 'on the floor' student success. The effective use of available resources and ongoing adjustment to the lesson are characteristic of thoughtful and effective instruction. Although many adapted physical education specialists advocate individualizing instruction by adapting equipment, modifying activities, and providing instructional support (e.g., peer tutors), there has been little empirical evidence supporting these premises (Davis and Burton 1991).

Proponents of inclusion often advocate on behalf of all children, but when carefully questioned, they may actually be advocating on behalf of children with very specific needs and abilities, (e.g., students with multiple disabilities or those with developmental disabilities). The extent to which instructional strategies that are applicable to one disability can be generalized to another is uncertain. Is it possible some instructional approaches can be broadly applied, or are all students to be viewed as individuals (Sherrill and Williams 1996)? Further investigation is needed into the pedagogic strategies and instructional techniques that can best accommodate the educational needs of diverse groups of students within the physical education classroom. Chapter 16 (Goodwin) discusses further the instructional approaches that have been used in adapted physical education settings.

SHARED RESPONSIBILITY

The current conceptual framework expands upon the previous frameworks by including the notion of shared responsibility (Jacobsen and Sawatsky 1993; Sherrill 1994). Classmates and instructional assistants, as well as teachers, students, and administrators are fundamental to the inclusion process (Block 1994). By placing inclusive physical education within a social context, the accountability for its success immediately moves beyond that of the student with a disability.

A genuine commitment to quality programmes for students with disabilities requires a school and system-wide commitment (Stainback and Stainback 1996). The range of student abilities and needs in inclusive class-rooms may surpass the resources available to one teacher. Group problem-solving and the sharing of programme responsibilities can bring diversity to instructional methodology and an expanded interpretation of the curriculum (Kysela et al. 1993). From a pragmatic point of view, partnerships among students, parents, paraprofessionals, administrators, and other professionals may be a necessary corequisite of inclusive physical education.

Sharing responsibility for inclusive physical education assumes there is agreement among those who may have input into the students' programmes (e.g., teacher, physical therapist, parents, classmates). In addition to agreement among the partners, there must also be a commitment to equal access of information and participation in problem identification, discussions, and decision making (Stein 1994; Wang 1996). Bringing about successful collaboration remains an ongoing challenge as the support systems most needed by teachers and students, the extent of the support, and systems for its delivery continue to be identified (Block 1999b; Jacobsen and Sawatsky 1993).

In acknowledging the need for a team approach to including students with disabilities in physical education, students without disabilities are often overlooked (Block 1994). Although numerous benefits are purported for the classmates of students with disabilities in inclusive education settings (e.g., more accepting of individual differences, more comfortable with students with disabilities, more helpful, increasing leadership skills, and improving self-esteem) (Block 1999b), little empirical research specific to physical education has been conducted (Slininger, Sherrill, and Jankowski 2000).

To measure the impact of including students with disabilities on the students of a regular physical education class, twenty students from a grade six physical education class that included three students with severe disabilities were compared to twenty students from another grade six physical education class, none of whom were known to have any disabilities (Block and Zeman 1996). Prior to and upon completion of a three-and-a-half-week basketball unit, the students participated in sport skill tests and completed the Children's Attitudes Toward Integrated Physical Education–Revised (CAIPE-R) Survey.

The results indicated that including students with severe disabilities did not negatively impact on skill improvement. Similar gains in passing and shooting were observed for both classes. In addition, there was no reported difference between the two groups in general attitude toward students without disabilities. "Including students with disabilities in physical education did not result in unfavorable attitudes for children without disabilities" (Block and Zeman 1996, p. 47).

Block and Zeman's (1996) findings support an earlier study that compared the attitudes of elementary school students, nine to twelve years of age, who participated in physical education classes that included students with disabilities (119 girls and 107 boys) and classes that did not (122 girls and 107 boys) (Tripp, French, and Sherrill 1995). The students completed the Peer Attitudes Toward the Handicapped Scale (PATHS), and the analysis of the findings indicated that there were no differences in overall attitudes toward students with disabilities by the students who did or did not participate in physical education that included students with disabilities.

TEACHER AND STUDENT EXPERIENCES
Post-teaching involves comparing the planning and implementation phases of the process to the outcomes and experiences of the students and teachers. Whereas research has addressed such outcomes as fitness and skill acquisition (e.g., Harvey and Reid 1997; Jansma, Decker, Ersing, McCubbin and Combs 1988; Winnick 1985) little attention has been given to the post-teaching experiences of teachers or students with disabilities.

Insights into the views of students have only recently been addressed in the physical education literature. In 1995, a special edition of the *Journal of Teaching in Physical Education* was dedicated to physical education through students' eyes and in students' voices. The purpose of the monograph was to describe and analyze what students think, feel, and know about various aspects of their physical education programmes. The contributors to the special edition revisited the assumption that teachers know and understand the needs and interests of the students they teach.

Portman (1995), a contributor to the monograph, looked at the experience of low-skilled sixth grade students using the theoretical construct of learned helplessness. Teacher judgement and skills tests were used to identify thirteen low-skilled students (eleven girls and two boys) from four sixth-grade classes. Interviews and field observations revealed four themes: (a) I like PE when I am successful, (b) I can't because I can't, (c) mostly nobody helps, and (d) mostly everyone yells at me. Portman suggested that the thirteen low-skilled students exhibited symptoms of learning helplessness and believed themselves to be fatalistically doomed to failure. The pattern of failure was attributed to lack of ability, and the students were largely unwilling to expend and sustain efforts to learn skills.

Other contributors addressed specific aspects of physical education, such as student responses to formative grading in physical education, physical fitness testing, and keeping score in children's games. In a study of responses to grading practices (Nugent and Faucette 1995), two sixth-grade students, one classified as academically gifted by the education system and another as having a learning disability, were interviewed. These students also completed two written questionnaires. The students were initially selected for the study based on teacher referral. The teacher was asked to identify one female who was predicted to achieve a high mark in physical education and one who was predicted to achieve a low mark. Although these students were later classified as gifted and possessing a learning disability, based on performance on the Stanford-Binet and three tests of learning achievement respectively, their classifications were not known to the researchers at the time of the study. The analysis of the data revealed that both students experienced frustration and disappointment over their grades. The student classified as gifted displayed creativity in her suggestions for how the grading process could be better implemented and the student classified as having a learning disability discussed her vulnerability to lower grades due to problematic behaviours.

In a further study, Hopple and Graham (1995) presented what children think, feel, and know about physical fitness testing, particularly when the mile-run test was administered each fall and spring. The participants were fifty-two grade four and five students from two different schools. Analysis of the interview, written quiz, and teacher-supplied physical education artifact data revealed three main themes: students' understanding, test dodging, and options for change. The authors indicated that most students did not understand why they were taking part in the mile-run physical fitness test. Although the link to cardiovascular fitness was demonstrated by the responses of some students, their understanding appeared to be incomplete.

Students who tended to perform poorly on the test commented that the mile-run test was 'the' test to be avoided. Some of the methods used to avoid the test were faking illness or injury, staying away from school on test administration day, or producing a written note from home. Physical pain and discomfort were reasons cited for dodging the test. If provided the opportunity, some students would have changed the mile-run to make it more fun. Fun was equated with easier (shorten the distance), not keeping track of the score (recording times), and adding equipment to make it more game like (jumping over cones, kicking a ball). Overall, the authors concluded that for many students of this study, the mile-run test was not a meaningful or positive experience, but rather a painful, negative one that was to be avoided.

The meaning of score-keeping in children's games was investigated in yet another area of physical education (Wessinger 1994). The pervasiveness of games in our elementary curriculum and the controversy surrounding the potential outcomes of competition in children's play led Wessinger to seek an understanding of the meaning of score-keeping from the children's perspective. Students from two fourth-grade classes were interviewed. By keeping track of the score, individual students believed they could help the team to win. Scoring against the odds, with finesse, or spectacularly was particularly valued. The public glory bestowed on students for scoring contributed to good feelings about physical education. The implication resulting from these students' experiences was that small teams (one-on-one, two-on-two), which matched the participants' skills to the game challenges, were desirable because they increased the opportunity for scoring and hence the enjoyment of physical education.

In a further study, Carlson (1995) investigated the actions and feelings of students who have become alienated from physical education. In-depth phenomenological* interviews with 2 junior high students and four teachers, a survey of 105 students in six different grade levels, and interviews with a further 6 students identified from the survey results, resulted in the construction of a model to help explain the alienation process associated with physical education. Extrinsic and intrinsic factors were advanced to explain why some students 'hate gym' (p. 475). Factors contributing to alienation included a lack of personal importance and identification with physical education, feelings of lack of control brought on by competitiveness and 'being on display', and a sense of isolation associated with perceptions of poor skill development. The students of this study responded to their adverse experiences in physical education by attempting to hide their displeasure from others, being spectators by withdrawing from participation and bench-sitting, becoming wallflowers by participating minimally, faking illness or injury, or self-banishment through non-attendance.

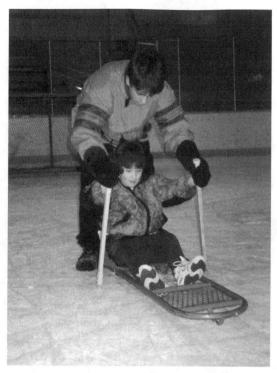

Sledge Hockey

In one of the few studies of physical education experiences for students with physical disabilities, Blinde and McCallister (1998) interviewed twenty students (seventeen boys and three girls) with an average age of thirteen. The disabilities represented were cerebral palsy, spina bifida, birth defects, head injury, paraplegia, and polysonic fibrous dysplasia. A content analysis of the interview data revealed that, although some students expressed happiness or satisfaction with physical education, these comments were activity- or class-period-specific. More typical responses were represented by the themes of limited participation and negative emotional responses. The authors concluded that students offer a unique vantage point from which to view the physical education environment and resulted in a number of teacher recommendations.

---

* Phenomenological interviews are conversations to obtain descriptions about what people know, the manner in which they experience what they know, and what it means (Kvale 1996).

The perspectives of persons with developmental disabilities have also been sought. Quality of life studies have been conducted to obtain the values, views, and preferences of persons with developmental disabilities with regard to such areas as home, work, leisure, and relationships, as institutional or facility-based service delivery systems gave way to community-based support systems (Hoge and Dattilo 1995; Neumayer and Bleasdale 1996; Wheeler 1996). Only recently has interviewing been promoted as a viable method for collecting research data about the lives of persons with developmental disabilities (Malik, Ashton-Shaeffer, and Kleiber 1991). The use of interviews is not without its challenges, however. Acquiescence, or the inclination to answer "yes," regardless of the question asked, threatens the validity of the responses of persons with developmental disabilities (Heal and Sigelman 1995; Matikka and Vesala 1997; Sigelman, Budd, Spanhel, and Schoenrock 1981).

Other aspects of verbal communication have also been raised. Speech defects may make recorded interviews difficult to transcribe. Also, a tendency for a higher incidence of hearing disorders in persons with developmental disabilities over the general population may also influence the ability to hear the interviewer correctly. The interpersonal dynamics between the interviewer and the interviewee may also contribute to the degree in which active and full involvement of both parties is achieved (Atkinson 1989). Perhaps most significantly, the question of the linguistic abilities of persons with developmental disabilities has been raised (Owens 1989). How well can they understand words, concepts, and questions? The Research and Training Center in Mental Retardation at Texas Tech University addresses this complex question in a series of studies (e.g., Sigelman and Budd 1986; Sigelman, Budd, Spanhel, and Schoenrock 1981). In reviewing the research to that time, Sigelman et al. (1981) concluded that persons with developmental disabilities

appear to be able to understand and use semantic information in much the same

way as non-retarded persons of the same mental age do....Therefore, the semantic system of mentally retarded children develops normally, although they tend to lag behind in their rate of acquisition.... Consequently, in developing interview questions for mentally retarded consumers with low mental ages, one should, to the extent possible, use very simple sentence constructions which draw on concrete and commonly used words. (p. 216)

To overcome the tendency to discount the opinions and information provided by persons with developmental disabilities, techniques for improving their ability to talk for themselves have been sought. Drawings and pictures have been used to increase the reliability and validity of self-report, as well as posing questions in multiple and triangulated formats, (e.g., open-ended questions to compliment close-ended questions, and supplementing participant information with other data-collection techniques) (Sigelman and Budd 1986; Wadsworth and Harper 1991).

In a study by Dattilo, Hoge, and Malley (1996), one hundred persons with developmental disabilities and their parents or caregivers were interviewed about their current and past recreational activities, the quality of their participation, and constraints to leisure participation. The researchers documented their actions to enhance the validity and reliability of the responses. The procedures they implemented included avoiding temporal and numerical concepts, including concrete visual cues, and using different types of questions. Systematic interviewer training was also undertaken.

In a study completed by Wyngaarden and associates (1981) with 440 persons with developmental disabilities, he concluded, "One of the most important findings of the study was that mentally retarded people can and are eager to provide complex and moving accounts of their experiences in returning to community life" (p. 113). He remarked that the decision to interview persons with developmental disabilities was guided by two assumptions: persons with developmental disabilities are valid sources of information, and for some aspects of their lives they are the only appropriate source for information. Ongoing dialogue and continued investigation into the phenomenon of inclusive physical education is required if student and teacher experiences are to be meaningful and positive in nature.

10 What reasons are given for including *shared responsibility* in the conceptual framework?

11 Why would teachers who perceive they are competent teachers have more favourable attitudes toward teaching students with disabilities?

12 What value conflicts may exist among those who share the responsibility of success in a regular physical education programme for a disability?

13 What contribution does an understanding of the experiences of students bring to the planning, implementation, and evaluation of an inclusive physical education programme?

Summary

Inclusive physical education evolved from a system of educational placement that grouped students with similar educational needs into intact classrooms with specialist teachers. Today, priority is given to the merits of the regular classroom. The definition of inclusive physical education reflects this ideology as it acknowledges the intrinsic worth of the goals of regular physical education for students with disabilities. To benefit from the goals of motor skill acquisition, fitness, knowledge of movement, and social well-being toward the development of an active lifestyle appropriate to the students' abilities and interests, however, there may be a need for supplementary aide or support services.

To plan, implement, and evaluate an inclusive physical education programme, attention must be paid to the dynamic and complex interactions of the students, the teachers, the instructional programme, and the supports available. A conceptual framework was offered that identified three broad areas or phases of instruction, associated with the teaching of an inclusive physical education programme pre-teaching, teaching, and post-teaching.

Pre-teaching tasks included student variables, teacher values, the instructional programme itself and the manner in which they interact in planning for instruction. Teaching tasks included thoughtful instructional strategies and the idea of sharing the responsibility for a successful programme among school personnel, fellow students, and parents. Finally, the post-teaching phase acknowledged the importance of student and teacher experiences resulting from participation in the programme and the meaning given to those experiences. The process of reflective analysis highlighted the continuous and cyclical nature of planning for improvement physical education programming.

Future Study

The conceptual framework is useful in identifying areas of inclusive physical education that are in need of further consideration. Although the goals of the regular physical education programme, identified as the *instructional programme* within the conceptual framework (figure 2), appear to have merit (Goodwin and Watkinson 2000), the degree to which specific activities within the curriculum programme dimensions (e.g., dance, gymnastics, aquatics, individual and team activities) are relevant and appropriate to students with disabilities is open to further discussion and investigation. What programme modifications are best suited to which activities, and to what degree should they be implemented? Who is the best source of information when activity modifications are required? What role should the teacher, the student in question, or classmates play? When should modifications be implemented and when should one activity be abandoned for another? What theoretical framework provides the needed backdrop from which to address these questions?

We often *share the responsibility* of programme success and task completion by soliciting the support of others. Inclusive educational settings utilize the instructional strategy of tutoring to meet the diversity of learning needs (Block and Krebs 1992). Does peer tutoring enhance learning or does it remove the opportunity for students to exercise independence and interfere with their ability to develop and exercise their own strategies? What is the impact of ongoing support on the self-esteem and self-efficacy of students with disabilities during physical education? These questions remain to be answered.

Our understanding of how students take advantage of the affording qualities of their instructional environments is not well understood. How prepared are students to perceive, attend to, or actively seek out affording qualities of their instructional environment? What processes are needed to facilitate the identification and manipulation of the affording qualities of the equipment or play area, for example? What *student variables*, or individual qualities, are most reflective of potential success in inclusive physical education? Under what circumstances are students active decision-makers in the form their involvement takes? How do we assist students to take advantage of their instructional environment? Preparing students to take an active role in how their programme is experienced may be useful in promoting self-help and self-regulatory behaviours.

Questions pertaining to the affording qualities of the instructional environment can also be asked of teachers. Are teachers cognizant of, or can they make use of, the environmental affordances that can constrain students' experiences? Introducing the notion of affordances to teachers may support the operationalization of what van Manen (1993) referred to as "tactful teaching," or what has been referred to within the conceptual framework as *thoughtful instruction.*

The *teachers' values* can be an important contributor to what they and their students ultimately experience within the instructional setting. A value system that defines disability in terms of personal weakness, loss of function, or need for remediation may logically assume that nonparticipatory or restrictive roles are to the students' benefits. Alternately, a value system that accepts diversity as a natural expression of the human family may set about creating an environment that enables people to respond to the best of their abilities and in ways that are meaningful to them. By giving voice to persons with disabilities and their teachers, the complexity of inclusive ideology can be better understood.

Study Questions

1. What variables need to be taken into consideration when planning for an inclusive physical education programme and how to these variables relate to one another?
2. What problems were associated with early models of integrated education?
3. What distinctions exist between the principle of LRE and the definition of inclusive physical education that was presented?
4. What does *shared responsibility* mean within the context of inclusive physical education?
5. What is the significance of including the *teacher's and student's experiences* in the conceptual framework of inclusive physical education?
6. What is the impact of the *teacher value system* on the planning, implementation, and evaluation of inclusive physical education?
7. Comment on the appropriateness of the goals of the regular physical education programme for students with disabilities.

References

Arnold, P.J. (1991). The preeminence of skill as an educational value in the movement curriculum. *Quest, 43*, 66–77.

Atkinson, D. (1989). Research interviews with people with mental handicaps. In A. Brechin and J. Walmsley (Eds.), *Making connections: Reflecting on the lives and experiences of people with learning difficulties* (pp. 63–73). London: Hodder and Stoughton.

Audi, R. (Ed.). (1995). *The Cambridge dictionary of philosophy*. Cambridge, UK: Cambridge University Press.

Aufsesser, P.M. (1991). Mainstreaming and the least restrictive environment: How do they differ? *Palaestra, 7*(2), 31–34.

Blinde, E.M., and McCallister, S.G. (1998). Listening to the voices of students with physical disabilities. *Journal of Physical Education, Recreation, and Dance, 69*(6), 64–68.

Block, M.E. (1992). What is appropriate physical education for students with profound disabilities? *Adapted Physical Activity Quarterly, 9*, 197–213.

Block, M.E. (1994). *A teacher's guide to including students with disabilities in regular physical education*. Baltimore: Paul H. Brookes.

Block, M.E. (1999a). Problems with inclusive physical education. *Palaestra, 15*(3), 30–36, 55–56.

Block, M.E. (1999b). Did we jump on the wrong bandwagon? Making general physical education placement work. *Palaestra, 15*(4), 34–42.

Block, M.E., and Conatser, P. (1999). Consulting in adapted physical education. *Adapted Physical Activity Quarterly, 16*, 9–26.

Block, M.E., and Krebs, P.L. (1992). An alternative to least restrictive environments: A continuum of support to regular physical education. *Adapted Physical Activity Quarterly, 9*(2), 97–113.

Block, M.E., and Vogler, W. (1994). Inclusion in regular physical education: The research base. *Journal of Physical Education, Recreation, and Dance, 65*(1), 40–44.

Block, M.E., and Zeman, R. (1996). Including students with disabilities in regular physical education: Effects on nondisabled children. *Adapted Physical Activity Quarterly, 13*(1), 38–49.

Broadhead, G.D. (1986). Adapted physical education research trends: 1970–1990. *Adapted Physical Activity Quarterly, 3*(2), 104–11.

Broadhead, G.D., and Burton, A.W. (1996). The legacy of adapted physical activity research. *Adapted Physical Activity Quarterly, 13*(2), 116–26.

Burton, A.W., and Davis, W.E. (1996). Ecological task analysis: Utilizing intrinsic measures in research and practice. *Human Movement Science, 15*, 285–314.

Carlson, T.B. (1995). We hate gym: Student alienation from physical education. *Journal of Teaching in Physical Education, 14*, 467–77.

Clandinin, D.J. (1993). Teacher education as narrative inquiry. In D.J. Clandinin, A. Davies, P. Hogan, and B. Kennard (Eds.), *Learning to teach, teaching to learn: Stories of collaboration in teacher education* (pp. 1–15). New York: Teachers College Press.

Dattilo, J., Hoge, G., and Malley, S.M. (1996). Interviewing people with mental retardation: Validity and reliability strategies. *Therapeutic Recreation Journal, 30*(3), 163–78.

Davis, W.E. (1989). Utilizing goals in adapted physical education. *Adapted Physical Activity Quarterly, 6*, 205–16.

Davis, W.E., and Burton, A.W. (1991). Ecological task analysis: Translating movement behaviour theory into practice. *Adapted Physical Activity Quarterly, 8*, 154–77.

Decker, J., and Jansma, P. (1995). Physical education: Least restrictive environment continua in the United States. *Adapted Physical Activity Quarterly, 12*(2), 124–38.

Deno, E. (1970). Special education as developmental capital. *Exceptional Children, 37*(3), 229–37.

DePauw, K.P., and Goc Karp, G. (1992). Framework for conducting pedagogical research in teaching physical education to include diverse populations. In W.L. Almond and A. Sparkes (Eds.), *Sport and physical activity: Moving toward excellence* (pp. 243–48). London: E and FN Spon.

DePauw, K.P., and Goc Karp, G. (1994). Integrating knowledge of disability throughout the physical education curriculum: An infusion approach. *Adapted Physical Activity Quarterly, 11*(11), 3–13.

Dewey, J. (1938). *Experience and education*. London: Collier Books.

Doyle, V. (1975, April). *Paradigms in teacher effectiveness research*. Paper presented at the annual meeting of the American Education Research Association, Washington, DC.

Dunkin, M.J., and Biddle, B.J. (1974). *The study of teaching*. New York: Holt, Rinehart, and Winston.

Ennis, C.D. (1994). Knowledge and beliefs underlying curricular expertise. *Quest, 6*, 164–75.

Ennis, C.D. (1999). A theoretical framework: The central piece of a research plan. *Journal of Teaching in Physical Education, 18*, 129–40.

Friend, M., Bursuck, W., and Hutchinson, N. (1998). *Including exceptional children: A practical guide for classroom teachers*. Scarborough, ON: Allyn and Bacon.

Fuchs, D., and Fuchs, L. (1994). Inclusive schools movement and the radicalization of special education reform. *Exceptional Children, 60*, 294–309.

Gage, N.L. (Ed.). (1963a). *Handbook of research on teaching*. Chicago, IL: Rand McNally.

Gage, N.L. (1963b). Paradigms for research on teaching. In N.L. Gage (Ed.), *Handbook of research on teaching* (pp. 94–141). Chicago, IL: Rand McNally.

Gage, N.L. (1963c). Preface. In N.L. Gage (Ed.), *Handbook of research on teaching* (pp. v–ix). Chicago, IL: Rand McNally.

Garrison, J.W., and Macmillan, C.J.B. (1984). A philosophical critique of process-product research on teaching. *Educational Theory, 34*(3), 255–74.

Gartner, A., and Kerzner Lipsky, D. (1996). Serving all students in inclusive schools: Contrasts in Canadian and U.S. experience. In J. Lupart, A. McKeough, and C. Yewchuck (Eds.), *Schools in transition: Rethinking regular and special education* (pp. 60–78). Toronto: Nelson.

Goodwin, D.L. (2001). The meaning of help in PE: Perceptions of students with physical disabilities. *Adapted Physical Activity Quarterly, 18*(3), 289–303.

Goodwin, D.L., and Watkinson, E.J. (2000). Inclusive physical education from the perspective of students with physical disabilities. *Adapted Physical Activity Quarterly, 17*(2), 144–60.

Graham, G. (1987). Motor skill acquisition: An essential goal of physical education programmes. *Journal of Physical Education, Recreation, and Dance, 59*(8), 44–48.

Grosse, S.J. (1978). Mainstreaming the physical handicapped student for team sports. *Practical Pointers, 1*(8), 1–8.

Hamre-Nietupski, S. (1993). How much time should be spent on skill instruction and friendship development? Preferences of parents of students with moderate and severe/profound disabilities. *Education and Training in Mental Retardation, 28*, 220–31.

Harvey, W.J., and Reid, G. (1997). Motor performance of children with attention-deficit hyperactivity disorder: A preliminary investigation. *Adapted Physical Activity Quarterly, 14*(3), 189–202.

Heal, L.W., and Sigelman, C.K. (1995). Response biases in interviews of individuals with limited mental ability. *Journal of Intellectual Disability Research, 39*(4), 331–40.

Heikinaro-Johansson, P. (1995). *Including students with special needs in physical education.* Jyvaskyla, Finland: University of Jyvaskyla.

Heikinaro-Johansson, P., Sherrill, C., French, R., and Huuhka, H. (1995). Adapted physical consultant service model to facilitate inclusion. *Adapted Physical Activity Quarterly, 12*(1), 12–33.

Hoge, G., and Dattilo, J. (1995). Recreation participation patterns of adults with and without mental retardation. *Education and Training in Mental Retardation and Development, 30*(4), 283–98.

Hopple, C., and Graham, G. (1995). What children think, feel, and know about physical fitness testing. *Journal of Teaching in Physical Education, 14*(4), 408–17.

Jacobsen, S.S., and Sawatsky, D.C. (1993). Meeting the challenge of integrating students with special needs: Understanding, building and implementing integration as inclusion. *Canadian Journal of Special Education, 9*(1), 60–66.

Jansma, P., Decker, J., Ersing, W., McCubbin, J., and Combs, S. (1988). A fitness assessment system for individuals with severe mental retardation. *Adapted Physical Activity Quarterly, 5*(3), 223–32.

Karper, W.B., and Martinek, T.J. (1985). Problems in mainstreaming research: Some personal observations. *Adapted Physical Activity Quarterly, 2*(4), 347–50.

Kauffman, J.M. (1995). How we might achieve the radical reform of special education. In J.M. Kauffman and D.P. Hallahan (Eds.), *The illusion of full inclusion: A comprehensive critique of a current special education bandwagon* (pp. 193–211). Austin, TX: Pro-ed.

Kerzner Lipsky, D., and Gartner, A. (1992). Achieving full inclusion: Placing the student at the center of education reform. In W. Stainback and S. Stainback (Eds.), *Controversial issues confronting special education: Divergent perspectives* (pp. 3–12). Neeham Heights, MA: Allyn and Bacon.

Kvale, S. (1996). *Interviews: An introduction to qualitative research interviewing.* Thousand Oaks, CA: Sage.

Kysela, G. M., French, F., and Brenton-Haden, S. (1993). Legislation and policy involving children with special needs. In L.L. Stewin and S.J.H. McCann (Eds.), *Contemporary education issues: The Canadian mosaic* (pp. 279–99). Mississauga, ON: Copp Clark Pitman.

LaMaster, K., Gall, K., Kinchin, G., and Siedentop, D. (1998). Inclusion practices of effective elementary specialists. *Adapted Physical Activity Quarterly, 15*(1), 64–81.

Maguire, P. (1994). Developing successful collaborative relationships. *Journal of Physical Education, Recreation, and Dance, 65*(1), 32–36, 44.

Malik, P.B., Ashton-Shaeffer, C., and Kleiber, D.A. (1991). Interviewing young adults with mental retardation: A seldom used research method. *Therapeutic Recreation Journal, 25*(1), 60–73.

Matikka, L.M., and Vesala, H.T. (1997). Acquiescence in quality-of-life interviews with adults who have mental retardation. *Mental Retardation, 35*(2), 75–82.

Miles, M.B., and Huberman, A.M. (1994). *Qualitative data analysis.* Thousand Oaks, CA: Sage.

Neumayer, R., and Bleasdale, M. (1996). Personal lifestyle preferences of people with an intellectual disability. *Journal of Intellectual and Developmental Disability, 21*(2), 91–114.

Nugent, P., and Faucette, N. (1995). Marginalized voices: Constructions of and responses to physical education and grading practices by students categorized as gifted or learning disabled. *Journal of Teaching in Physical Education, 14*, 418–30.

Owens, R. (1989). Cognition and language in the mentally retarded population. In M. Beveridge, G. Conti-Ramsden, and I. Leudar (Eds.), *Language and communication in mentally handicapped people* (pp. 112–42). New York: Chapman and Hall.

Polloway, E.A., Smith, J.D., Patton, J.R., and Smith, T.E.C. (1996). Historic changes in mental retardation and developmental disabilities. *Education and Training in Mental Retardation and Developmental Disabilities, 31*, 3–12.

Portman, P.A. (1995). Who is having fun in physical education classes? Experiences of sixth grade students in elementary and middle schools. *Journal of Teaching in Physical Education, 14,* 445–53.

Pyfer, J.L. (1986). Early research concerns in adapted physical education 1930–1969. *Adapted Physical Activity Quarterly, 3*(2), 95–103.

Reid, G. (1992). Editorial. *Adapted Physical Activity Quarterly, 9*(1), 1–4.

Rizzo, T.L., Broadhead, G.D., and Kowalski, E. (1997). Changing kinesiology and physical education by infusing information about individuals with disabilities. *Quest, 49*(2), 229–37.

Rizzo, T.L., and Vispoel, W.P. (1991). Physical educators' attributes and attitudes toward teaching students with handicaps. *Adapted Physical Activity Quarterly, 8,* 4–11.

Rizzo, T.L., and Vispoel, W.P. (1992). Changing attitudes about teaching students with handicaps. *Adapted Physical Activity Quarterly, 9,* 54–63.

Rizzo, T.L., and Wright, R.G. (1988). Secondary school physical educators' attitudes toward teaching students with handicaps. *American Corrective Therapy Journal, 41*(2), 52–55.

Rowe, J., and Stutts, R.M. (1987). Effects of practica type, experience, and gender on attitudes of undergraduate physical education majors toward disabled persons. *Adapted Physical Activity Quarterly, 4*(4), 266–77.

Santomier, J. (1985). Physical education, attitudes and the mainstream: Suggestions for teacher trainers. *Adapted Physical Activity Quarterly, 2*(4), 328–37.

Sherrill, C. (1994). Least restrictive environments and total inclusive philosophies: Critical analysis. *Palaestra, 10*(3), 25–35.

Sherrill, C. (1998). *Adapted physical activity, recreation, and sport: Crossdisciplinary and lifespan* (5th ed.). Dubuque, IA: Brown and Benchmark.

Sherrill, C., Heikinaro-Johansson, P., and Slininger, D. (1994). Equal-status relationships in the gym. *Journal of Physical Education, Recreation, and Dance, 65*(1), 27–31, 56.

Sherrill, C., and Montelione, T. (1990). Priorizing adapted physical education goals: A pilot study. *Adapted Physical Activity Quarterly, 7*(4), 355–69.

Sherrill, C., and Williams, T. (1996). Disability and sport: Psycho-social perspectives on inclusion, integration, and participation. *Sport Science Review, 5*(1), 42–64.

Sideridis, G.D., and Chandler, J.P. (1997). Assessment of teacher attitudes toward inclusion of students with disabilities: A confirmatory factor analysis. *Adapted Physical Activity Quarterly, 14*(1), 51–64.

Sigelman, C.K., and Budd, E.C. (1986). Pictures as an aid in questioning mentally retarded persons. *Rehabilitation Counseling Bulletin, 29*(3), 173–81.

Sigelman, C.K., Budd, E.C., Spanhel, C.L., and Schoenrock, C.J. (1981). When in doubt, say yes: Acquiescence in interviews with mentally retarded persons. *Mental Retardation, 19,* 53–58.

Sigelman, C.K., Schoenrock, C.J., Winer, J.L., Spanhel, C.L., Hromas, S.G., Martin, P.W., Budd, E.C., and Bensberg, G.J. (1981). *Communicating with mentally retarded persons: Asking questions and getting answers.* Lubbock: Texas Tech University.

Slife, B.D., and Williams, R.N. (1995). *What's behind the research: Discovering hidden assumptions in the behavioural sciences.* Thousand Oaks, CA: Sage.

Slininger, D., Sherrill, C., and Jankowski, C.M. (2000). Children's attitudes toward peers with severe disabilities: Revisiting contact theory. *Adapted Physical Activity Quarterly, 17*(2), 176–96.

Snow, R.E. (1973). Theory construction for research on teaching. In R.M.W. Travers (Ed.), *Second handbook of research on teaching* (pp. 77–112). Chicago, IL: Rand McNally.

Stainback, S., and Stainback, W. (1990). Inclusive schooling. In W. Stainback and S. Stainback (Eds.), *Support networks for inclusive schooling: Interdependent integrated education* (pp. 3–23). Baltimore: Paul H. Brooks.

Stainback, S., and Stainback, W. (1992). Schools as inclusive communities. In W. Stainback and S. Stainback (Eds.), *Controversial issues confronting special education: Divergent perspectives* (pp. 29–43). Needham Heights, MA: Allyn and Bacon.

Stainback, S., and Stainback, W. (1996). Merging regular and special education: Turning classrooms into inclusive communities. In J. Lupart, A. McKeough, and C. Yewchuck (Eds.), *Schools in transition: Rethinking regular and special education* (pp. 43–59). Toronto: Nelson.

Stein, J. (1987). The myth of the adapted physical education curriculum. *Palaestra, 4*(1), 34–37.

Stein, J. (1994). Inclusion articles questioned. *Journal of Physical Education, Recreation, and Dance, 65* (2), 11.

Tripp, A., French, R., and Sherrill, C. (1995). Contact theory and attitudes of children in physical education programme toward peers with disabilities. *Adapted Physical Activity Quarterly, 12*(4), 323–32.

Tripp, A., and Sherrill, C. (1991). Attitude theories of relevance to adapted physical education. *Adapted Physical Activity Quarterly, 8*(1), 12–27.

van Manen, M. (1986). *The tone of teaching.* Richmond Hill, ON: Scholastic.

van Manen, M. (1993). *The tact of teaching: The meaning of pedagogical thoughtfulness.* London, ON: Althouse Press.

Wadsworth, J.S., and Harper, D.C. (1991). Increasing the reliability of self-report by adults with moderate mental retardation. *Journal of the Association for Persons With Severe Handicaps, 16*(4), 228–32.

Wall, A.E. (1982). Physically awkward children: A motor development perspective. In J.P. Das, R.F. Mulcahy, and A.E. Wall (Eds.), *Theory and research in learning disability* (pp. 253–67). New York: Plenum Press.

Wall, A.E. (1986). A knowledge-based approach to motor skill acquisition. In M.G. Wade and H.T.A. Whiting

(Eds.), *Motor development in children: Aspects of coordination and control* (pp. 33–49). Boston: Martinus Nijhoff.

Wall, A.E., McClements, J., Bouffard, M., Findlay, H., and Taylor, M.J. (1985). A knowledge-based approach to motor development: Implications for the physically awkward. *Adapted Physical Activity Quarterly, 2*(1), 21–42.

Wang, M. (1996). Serving students with special needs through inclusive education approaches. In J. Lupart, A. McKeough, and C. Yewchuck (Eds.), *Schools in transition: Rethinking regular and special education* (pp. 143–63). Toronto: Nelson.

Watkinson, E.J., and Bentz, L. (1986). *Cross Canada survey on mainstreaming students with physical disabilities into physical education in elementary and secondary schools: Final report.* Gloucester, ON: CAHPER.

Wehman, P., Sherron, P., and West, M.D. (1997). Education for individuals with disabilities. In P. Wehman (Ed.), *Exceptional individuals* (pp. 3–56). Austin, TX: Pro-ed.

Wessinger, N.P. (1994). "I hit a home run!" The lived meaning of scoring in games in physical education. *Quest, 46,* 425–39.

Wheeler, J.J. (1996). The use of interactive focus groups to aid in the identification of perceived service and support delivery needs of persons with developmental disabilities and their families. *Education and Training in Mental Retardation and Developmental Disabilities, 31*(4), 294–303.

Winnick, J.P. (1985). The performance of visually impaired youngsters in physical education activities: Implications for mainstreaming. *Adapted Physical Activity Quarterly, 2*(4), 292–99.

Wyngaarden, M., and Abt Associates. (1981). Interviewing mentally retarded persons: Issues and strategies. In R.J. Bruininks, C.E. Meyers, B.B. Sigford, and K.C. Lakin (Eds.), *Deinstitutionalization and community adjustment of mentally retarded people* (pp. 107–13). Minneapolis, MN: American Association on Mental Deficiency.

York, J., Vandercook, T., MacDonald, D., Heise-Neff, C., and Caughey, E. (1992). Feedback about integrating middle-school students with severe disabilities in general education classes. *Exceptional Children, 58*(3), 244–58.

CHAPTER 14

Facilitating Independence

Implications for the Learner and the Instructor

Karen Calzonetti

Learning Objectives

- To understand the terminology related to independence, including the constructs of self-determination, autonomy, self-regulation, and empowerment.
- To become familiar with contemporary literature related to independence and related constructs, including Wehmeyer's model of self-determination.
- To learn the value of promoting independence and related constructs for both the learner and the instructor in adapted physical activity.
- To understand instructional considerations for the learner and the instructor when facilitating independence in a physical activity/learning environment.

Introduction

From a theoretical and practical perspective, researchers often speak of the person-centred approach and of the importance of recognizing the individual separately from his or her disability. As adapted physical activity practitioners, how much of a person-centred approach do we *really* take? Consider, for example, the number of choices you make in a single day. Now try to imagine another person limiting the number of choices you make to one a day, or perhaps removing any personal power to make choices all together. Consider a situation in which you are denied access to a physical activity or recreational pursuit because you are presumed to be incapable of making your own decisions, or identifying your own goals, or because an instructor assumes that you simply do not have the skills required to participate. In other words, imagine feeling disempowered in a way that not only makes you dependent on others, and undermines your decision-making capabilities, but also leads to feelings of diminished self-worth and incompetence. Clearly, this is not a picture consistent with the educational ideal of facilitating independence for *any* learner, with or without a disability.

The purpose of this chapter is to explore the notion of independence, and related constructs such as self-determination, self-regulation, and psychological empowerment, in relation to instructional practices within adapted physical activity. History tells us that people who are disabled have often been excluded from any personal control over their own learning. This chapter will reinforce the value of facilitating independent behaviours and self-determined actions for all individuals, including the individual with a disability.

Supporting independence means that people with disabilities have a right to participate in decisions about their lives in a meaningful way, to the greatest degree possible, and should be provided the skills and opportunities to make choices about their lives (Bosner and Belfiore 2001; Watkinson 1994; Wehmeyer 1992; Wehmeyer and Schwartz 1998). This requires a strong commitment by researchers and practitioners to the development of instructional methods that encourage the learner's independence, personal control, and growing sense of empowerment. Guided by Wehmeyer's model of self-determination (1992, 1997), part one of this chapter will explore the notion of independence and self-determination for individuals who are disabled and for their instructors. Part two briefly discusses supporting evidence for instructional programmes concerned with independence and self-determination. Part three highlights some theoretical and practical implications underlying independence and self-determination within the instructional setting. Finally, case studies that illustrate examples of instructional strategies an instructor may incorporate into the physical activity setting to encourage the development of independent behaviours for the learner are provided in part four.

Part One: The Language of Independence

Contrary to popular opinion, independence, or the act of being independent, does not mean the ability to do things without help or assistance. Cited as a Western notion of independence (Oliver 1990), voices within the disability movement suggest that independence is not a simple measure of performance in skills related to self-care, or other activities taught by professionals in traditional rehabilitative settings. Rather, independence may be more accurately defined as the ability to be in control of, and make decisions about, one's own life despite the presence of assistance (Reindal 1999). Based upon the "choice of acceptable options that minimize reliance on others in making decisions and in performing everyday activities" (Nosek 1992, p. 103), being independent means an individual has control over his or her own life.

A term known as *self-determination* is directly related to this view of independence. While not a new concept (Bowman 1999), self-determination is a particularly dominant theme in disability literature today (Brotherson, Cook, Cunconan-Lahr, and Wehmeyer 1995; DePauw and Sherrill 1994; Reid 2000). Often defined in dictionaries at a collective or political level, self-determination may also be viewed at the individual or personal level (Wehmeyer and Bolding 1999). As a personal construct, self-determination has been defined in the context of human rights advocacy (Nirje 1972), as an issue of empowerment (Rappaport 1981), as a motivational construct (Deci and Ryan 1985), and as an educational outcome (Wehmeyer 1992, 1996a). Self-determined people know what they want and how to get it; they make choices in their lives, and have control over decision-making processes and outcomes (Deci and Ryan 1985; Martin and Marshall 1995). Also viewed synonymously with intrinsic motivation, individual choice and self-determination are both key elements in promoting independence (Davis and Strand 2001; Iyengar and Lepper 1999). McCombs (1997) and Ward (1988) suggest that people are self-determined if they are goal-directed and take the initiative to achieve these goals.

Perhaps the most valuable contribution to our contemporary understanding of self-determination as it relates to persons who are disabled has evolved from work by Michael Wehmeyer and associates. As a researcher of disability issues, Wehmeyer views self-determination as an educational outcome, characterized by actions or events, which involve "acting as the primary causal agent in one's life and making choices and decisions regarding one's quality of life free from undue external influence or interference" (Wehmeyer 1992, 1997).

Two phrases in this definition are particularly relevant to the notion of independence. A *causal agent*, as defined by Deci and Ryan (1985), is someone who makes or causes things to happen in their lives. At issue here is the importance afforded the *opportunity* to act as a causal agent in determining one's course of action. It is only after this opportunity arises that a sense of control over one's environment is likely to prevail. Importantly, the provision of opportunity, coupled with a perceived sense of control, does not guarantee success in one's actions. "It is one thing to be the causal agent in one's life, and it is yet another to be successful at that endeavour" (Wehmeyer 1996a, p. 122).

The term *undue* (as in "free from undue external influence or interference") is of particular significance because it reinforces the distinction between an individual who acts independently, as opposed to one who acts alone or separately from others. Wehmeyer (1996a) suggests that people are "interdependent," and autonomous actions reflect this interdependence through interactions with family, friends, and others. As a human condition, interdependence implies that individuals must have the rights and privileges to determine their own situation to be functionally autonomous (Condelucci 1995; Palmer and Wehmeyer 1998; Reindal 1999). This does not mean that people must make their decisions free of external input or directives. However, it does imply that the decision-making capabilities and the responsibilities, and consequences enacted by that choice,

ultimately belong to the learner despite the presence of others. "Self-determination does not reflect a complete lack of influence, or even interference from others, but instead reflects decisions made without undue interference or influence" (Wehmeyer 1996a, p. 117). It is a dynamic and adaptable construct that is highly susceptible to fluctuations, which is ultimately controlled by the individual. The truly self-determined individuals are ones who recognize the power they have in choosing to listen to, *and* deciding when and how to act upon, the voices of others who may be telling them what to do. While this comment holds true for any person, regardless of disability, it is important to recognize that people who are disabled are typically excluded from any personal control over their lives, and are often powerless as a result (Guess, Benson, and Seigel-Causey 1985; Oliver 1990; Mactavish, Mahon, and Lutfiyya 2000; Palmer and Wehmeyer 1998; Sands and Doll 1996).

Based upon the premise that self-determined individuals are causal agents in their lives, and causal agency requires certain skills and proficiencies, Wehmeyer, Kelchner, and Richards (1996) claim a person is self-determined if his or her actions reflect the following characteristics: autonomy, self-regulation, psychological empowerment, and self-realization. Definitions of each of these terms are provided at the end of this section. Briefly, a behaviour is *autonomous* if the person acts freely from undue external influence or pressure (in other words, independently), and according to his or her own preferences (Wehmeyer 1996b).

Self-regulating behaviour means that a person "decides how to act, acts according to that decision, evaluates the outcome of the actions, and modifies subsequent behaviour as necessary to improve the outcome" (Sands and Doll 1996, p.60). An individual's ability to self-regulate his or her own actions reflects the notion of causal agency and is supported by many leading self-regulation theorists. Zimmerman (1989) refers to the use of self-regulatory strategies as actions or skills that

Table 14.1 Component Elements of Self-determined Behaviour

- Choice-making
- Internal locus of control
- Decision-making
- Self-efficacy
- Problem-solving
- Self-awareness
- Goal-setting and attainment
- Self-knowledge
- Self-observation, evaluation, and reinforcement

involve "agency and purpose." Also referred to as self-control, self-regulation is a construct that has strong connections to self-determination because individuals must make decisions about what skills to use in what situation, and, in effect, carry out their plan of action. Self-regulation requires focussed attention and continuous decision-making among alternative responses (Kanfer and Gaelick 1986), and represents a complex system of self-monitoring, self-evaluation, and self-reinforcement (Whitman 1990).

Psychological empowerment refers to the multiple dimensions of perceived control, including cognitive (personal efficacy), personality (locus of control), and motivational domains of perceived control (Zimmerman 1990). Self-determined people behave in a psychologically empowered manner because they believe they have the capacity to perform behaviours needed to influence outcomes in their environment. They also believe desired outcomes will come about as a result of their actions (Wehmeyer, Kelchner, and Richards 1996).

Self-determined individuals are *self-realizing* people because of the self-knowledge they possess concerning their strength and limitations. Significantly, self-awareness develops as a result of one's experiences, combined with the evaluations and perceptions of others (Wehmeyer, Kelchner, and Richards 1996).

There are a number of skills or component elements crucial to the emergence of the characteristics of self-determination framed within Wehmeyer's model (1992, 1997).

Identified in table 14.1, these elements demonstrate that self-determination is a complex, lifelong process crucial to all individuals, regardless of age or ability.

Significantly, the facilitation of the four key characteristics and their related concepts is neither an automatic learning process nor one that is quickly, or easily, acquired. Section two will provide supporting evidence for the development of self-determination through instructional programmes that emphasize the importance of problem-solving skills, choice-making, goal-setting, and other component elements of self-determined behaviour identified by Wehmeyer (1992, 1997).

Not surprisingly, the instructor plays a key role in nudging the learner towards opportunities to develop and practice the skills of independence and self-determination. The opportunities to learn and apply the different skills of self-determination are critical early in instruction so that learners, even at a young age, can begin to appreciate the need to be active and present in their own learning (Butler 1995).

SUMMARY OF TERMS

Autonomy

Lewis and Taymans (1992): A complex concept involving an emotional separation from caregivers and a developing sense of personal control over one's life, the establishment of a personal value system, and the ability to enact behavioural tasks which are needed in the adult world.

Stainton (1994): The capacity of the individual to formulate and act on plans and purposes that are self-determined.

Wehmeyer and Palmer (2000): Within the framework of self-determined behaviour, a behaviour is autonomous if the person acts i) according to his or her own preferences, interests, and/or abilities, and, ii) independently, free from undue external influence or interference. The term is derived from the Greek words *autos* (meaning "self"), and *nomos* (meaning "rule").

Causal Agency

Deci and Ryan (1985): The act of making or causing things to happen in one's life. Causal agency implies an action and outcome that is purposefully performed to achieve that end.

Wehmeyer, Kelchner, and Richards (1996): One who makes or causes things to happen is known as a causal agent.

Empowerment

Lord (1991): The process whereby individuals feel increasingly in control of their own lives, and participate in the community with dignity.

World Health Organization (1987): The process of enabling people to increase control over, and to improve, aspects of their individual lives.

Zimmerman (1990): The multiple dimensions of perceived control, including cognitive (personal efficacy), personality-driven (locus of control), and motivational domains.

Independence

Reindal (1999). An ability to be in control of and make decisions about one's life. It involves obtaining assistance when and how one requires it, and does not involve (necessarily) doing things alone or without help.

Independent Living

Nosek (1992): Control over one's life based on the choice of acceptable options that minimize reliance on others in making decisions and in performing everyday activities.

Self-determination

Deci and Ryan (1985): The capacity to choose and have those choices (as opposed to reinforcement contingencies, drives, or any other forces or pressures) be the determinants of one's actions. Self-determination, when viewed as a motivational construct, is more than a capacity, it is a need.

Martin and Marshall (1995): A process that involves an individual knowing what they want and how to get it–in other words, knowing how to choose. Self-determined individuals are goal-directed and assert themselves by evaluating progress towards their goal(s), adjusting performance as needed, and creating the opportunities needed to solve problems.

Wehmeyer (1992; 1997): Acting as the primary causal agent in one's life and making choices and decisions regarding one's quality of life, free from undue external influence or interference.

Self-Regulated Learning

Butler and Winne (1995): Learning that infers a deliberate, judgemental, adaptive process.

Garcia (1995): A combined awareness of an individual's skill and will.

Wehmeyer and Berkobien (1991): The self-controlled mediation of one's behaviour.

Self-Regulated Behaviour

Sands and Doll (1996): Behaviour whereby individuals make a decision concerning how to act and act according to that decision, followed by an evaluation of the outcome of their actions, and modification of their behaviour to bring about the outcome.

Whitman (1990): Self-regulation includes the observation of one's social and physical environment, and one's actions in those environments (or *self-monitoring*); judgements about the acceptability of this behaviour through comparing what one is doing with what one ought to be doing (also known as *self-evaluation*); and the outcome of this evaluation (or *self-reinforcement*).

Self-Regulated Strategies

Zimmerman (1989): Actions or skills that involve agency and purpose.

Part Two: Supporting Evidence for Self-determination

Few would argue with the promotion of independence and its many related constructs as a desired goal of all learning. Indeed, instructional programmes that recognize the value of making choices, self-directed learning, and independent behaviour as precursors to autonomy and dignity for persons who have a disability are prevalent forces in the educational field (Agran, Blanchard, and Wehmeyer 2000; Guess, Benson and Siegel-Causey 1985; Gumple, Tappe, and Araki 2000; O'Reilly, Lancioni, and Kierans 2000; Mahon and Bullock 1992; Treece, Gregory, Ayres, and Mendis 1999; Wehmeyer, Agran, and Hughes 2000; Wehmeyer and Bolding 1999; Wehmeyer and Palmer 2000).

It is crucial that an instructor promote the skills of independence and self-determination in an active way and that learners be given the opportunity to 'try these skills out' in exploratory ways. In fact, Sowers and Powers (1995) identify three factors critical to the development of self-determination for individuals with a disability: 1) opportunity to participate, 2) available support systems (parents, caregivers, teachers), and 3) participation with same-age peers who are not disabled. Individual learners must develop the necessary inner resources and skills, *and* society must provide the necessary supports to nurture the development of these skills, and respond accordingly (Reindal 1999; Thoma, Rogan, and Baker 2001). As a shared partnership, the instructor and learner must actively create the opportunities for self-determined skills to grow and develop. It is through this collaboration that different opportunities to develop self-determination skills such as decision-making, problem-solving, and independence will emerge in the learner (Wehmeyer and Lawrence 1995).

While Wehmeyer's model of self-determination (1992, 1997) might seem an unrealistic achievement for people with disabilities, an increasing amount of research identifies just how viable the move towards independence truly is. Wehmeyer, Kelchner, and Richards (1996) tested the validity of the self-determination framework and examined the contribution of the characteristics of autonomy, psychological empowerment, self-awareness, and self-regulation to the achievement of behavioural outcomes associated with this construct. Using a series of structured interviews and self-report measures, self-regulation was identified by 407 adults with intellectual disabilities as one of the most potent predictors of self-determination.

A study by Gaudet and Dattilo (1994) examined the potential for increased leisure activity involvement amongst senior adults with dementia by using an intervention designed to promote independent behaviours. Although complete independence was not achieved, all of the participants who received the intervention attained a level of independence consistent with their individual ability level. Participants also showed a decreased tendency to rely on external prompts provided by an instructor. This same study also found that systematic instruction in problem-solving skills when applied to a recreation setting facilitated self-regulation, autonomy, and self-actualization and culminated in an enhanced sense of self-determination. As a component of self-regulation, arming individuals to become independent problem-solvers is important because they will develop an awareness and self-perception about their abilities and their role in choices.

A previous study by Dattilo and Kleiber (1993) concluded that self-determination, when achieved, leads to increased learning and perceptions of competence. Similar studies demonstrate that students who are disabled appear to perform better when they are involved in their own learning, such as choosing instructional tasks, methods, or materials (Brown and Gothelf 1996; Ferretti, Cavalier, Murphy and Murphy 1993; Wehmeyer, Palmer, Agran, Mithaug, and Martin 2000).

The emphasis upon fostering self-determination in individuals who are disabled, combined with the prevailing need to challenge long-held assumptions underlying commonly used instructional practices, reflects an emerging paradigm shift in the adapted physical activity field. According to Polloway, Patton, Smith, and Smith (1996), this shift will have profound implications for the future education, care, and treatment of people who are disabled. Indeed, the focus upon the individual with a disability as an active participant in his or her own learning marks a significant departure from traditional teacher-centred instructional environments.

Traditional instructional settings have reflected a top-down hierarchy in which individuals with a disability have typically been excluded from any personal control over their own learning. More often than not, persons with an intellectual disability (as an example) have been perceived as "mere objects of external manipulation," rather than viewed as "self-directing and purposeful human beings" (Guess and Siegel-Causey 1985, p. 234). Immersed in an externally directed learning environment, individuals who are intellectually disabled have rarely been taught to set their own performance goals, monitor their progress, or administer reinforcement contingent on their performance (Ferretti et al. 1993). Furthermore, research has demonstrated that the use of controlled instructional techniques, typical of externally driven teaching methods such as behaviourism, has actually encouraged learning helplessness rather than learning autonomy (Marsh 1993). Because they have been denied the opportunity to make decisions, choose options, or self-direct their own learning, individuals who are intellectually disabled often fall into a cycle of learned helplessness which, in turn, causes low motivation and a perceived lack of control (Deci and Ryan 1985; Mahon 1994; Seligman 1975; Shapiro 1981; Whitman 1990).

Another factor that has contributed to the stigmatization of individuals with a disability as being helpless is the prevailing attitude of individuals who perpetuate the medical model approach within special education. This approach, according to Lipsky and Gartner (1989) leads to the erroneous belief that individuals who are disabled are not capable of making choices or decisions. This preconception and single-mindedness has been the impetus behind a variety of research studies destined to prove otherwise (Bullock and Mahon 1992; Doll, Sands, Wehmeyer, and Palmer 1996; Henderson 1994; Mactavish, Mahon, and Lutfiyya 2000; Wehmeyer 1994), and has contributed greatly to the development of instructional programmes designed to facilitate self-determination and independent and active learners.

2 In what ways do medical models of disability contradict the focus upon self-determination and empowerment represented by the work of Wehmeyer and others writers in the disability field?

3 What mechanisms can organizations affiliated with disability put into place to collaborate with adapted physical activity researchers and practitioners to ensure that their voice is represented in an empowered manner?

Part Three: Instructional Implications

At this point, two crucial questions must be discussed: What are the skills of self-determination? How can they be taught to another individual? First and foremost, the learners must be involved in their learning process from the very beginning. The learner's individual needs and interests must be also be known by the instructor. As logical as this might sound, this key piece of information is often overlooked, or it is assumed that the needs of individuals who are disabled are collectively, and similarly, shared. In some situations, the learner's needs and interests are often secondary to the needs and interests of the instructors. At times, even the structure of the activity takes precedence over the learner him/herself. The best-intentioned instructors may assume that *they*, as the *expert*, know what the learner's abilities and limitations are and, as a result, know what is best for the learner. Basing activity choices upon assumptions, particularly ones that are uninformed and unfounded, can be detrimental to the success of an activity and undermine the skills and motivations of the learner. Even the smallest of opportunities to express one's own needs, interests, and abilities can encourage motivation levels, and contribute to increased feelings of self-worth.

As suggested by Mithaug, Martin, and Agran (1987), the failure of individuals with disabilities to exhibit active, independent behaviours may not be due to their inability to learn, but rather to the approach used by instructors to teach. More often than not, instructors choose the learning goal(s), decide how and where individuals with disabilities will be taught, and evaluate their performance accordingly (Guess and Siegel-Causey 1985). Because students are often peripheral to the problem-solving process (Butler 1995), it is possible that highly-controlled instructional programmes may contribute to the development of behaviours that are incompatible with independence (Mithaug et al. 1987). Wehmeyer (1996a) echoes these sentiments by suggesting that the greatest threats to self-determination for individuals who are disabled may, in fact, be external. It is crucial that we examine our instructional techniques and determine whether our inclinations towards highly structured programmes are contributing to the problem of dependency. Clearly, direct instruction, combined with the control orientation of the teacher, often undermines any opportunity for independence. Instructors of individuals who are disabled can foster independence in learners early on by first relinquishing the need for any unwarranted or excessive control in the teaching environment.

In an effort to avoid feelings of helplessness, individuals who are disabled need to experience some sense of control over their learning (Seligman 1975). This is particularly relevant in light of evidence which demonstrates that individuals in externally controlled situations report less enjoyment from the activity and are less likely to select this activity when given free choice activity (Ferretti 1989). Excessive repetition, over-learned tasks, and activities that are less than optimally challenging also result in decreased levels of motivation and self-determination (Deci and Chandler 1986). Conversely, instructional programmes that enhance self-determination by teaching self-management skills, problem-solving, and goal-setting, to name a few, have contributed to a sense of well-being and self-efficacy (Wall and Datillo 1995; Wehmeyer and Schwartz 1998; Wehmeyer and Lawrence 1998). Based upon the assumption that the capability to exercise some degree of control over one's learning is a function of self-determination, instructors must consciously and actively provide opportunities for students who are disabled to be causal agents in their own lives.

As mediators in the learning process acting as promoters of independent learning (Brown, Bransford, Ferrarra, and Campione 1983), instructors play a key role in nurturing the development of self-determination amongst people who are disabled. For example, consider the link between self-determination and problem-solving skills. Individuals who problem-solve effectively are ones who behave *and* act in a self-regulatory manner because they plan, select, correct, and monitor effective strategies for learning (Agran and Hughes 1997; Bouffard and Wall 1991; Corno and Mandinach 1983; Erez and Peled 2001). Research demonstrates that the problem-solving behaviours exhibited by those engaged in either motor or cognitive learning tasks are quite similar in that a goal is identified and an action plan is constructed, executed, and evaluated (Bouffard 1990; Bransford, Sherwood, Vye, and Reiser 1986). Solving a problem successfully requires that an individual consciously direct efforts in a self-regulatory manner, thereby acting as his or her own causal agent. Once again, instructors can facilitate the component elements of self-determined behaviour, such as choice-making, problem-solving, goal-setting, etc., by providing opportunities for individuals who are disabled to learn the skills they need to become as independent as possible. Instructors sensitive to the needs of individual learners also encourage the development of self-determined behaviours by providing hands-on experiences for the learner to apply the component skills to real-life situations.

Studies (Lee and Solomon 1992; Schunk 1996) demonstrate that teachers can assist learners in identifying what they can and cannot control by encouraging them to be consciously aware of their learning and by systematically directing their attention to environmental cues that provide this information helpful to learning. In this way, teaching self-determined behaviours is similar to good coaching. Students who are taught to be increasingly aware of their environment will be more effective performers and, as a result, will become more active in monitoring their own progress (Lee and Solomon 1992; Paris and Oka 1986). Another way instructors can directly promote this awareness is by teaching students about the use of problem-solving strategies and by explicitly discussing effective ways to improve students' own learning. Referred to as "consciousness raising" by Paris and Winograd (1990), taking the time to discuss learning with students has two benefits. Firstly, increasing one's personal level of awareness helps transfer the responsibility for monitoring progress to the student or, at the very least, conveys the message that they can affect their own learning. Secondly, including students in this process will help to promote positive feelings of self-worth and improved motivation. In turn, this motivation will help encourage students to make a personal commitment to their learning (Brown, 1988). Through the facilitation of independence, such as the use of self-regulated learning skills, students eventually become active managers of their own learning, which may also empower them to be inquisitive and persistent in their efforts (Paris and Oka 1986; Reid and Hresko 1981).

The work by Pressley and Levin (1986) and Brown, Campione, and Day (1981) demonstrates that studies designed to promote

self-determination must include explicit instruction in self-regulation and the use of problem-solving strategies to have long lasting effects. Similarly, Scardamalia and Bereiter (1983) state that self-regulated learning is possible only after students become directly aware of the connections and links between related concepts. According to Chi, Bassok, Lewis, Reimann and Glaser (1989), an inability to self-regulate may occur because students are not aware that they lack understanding or, conversely, because of a perception that falsely leads them to believe that they *do*.

Additional insight concerning the reasons for poor learning by students in an instructional setting are provided in a study conducted by Winne and Marx (1982). Among the possible reasons cited are: the students' lack of attention to instructions given by the teacher, the students' inappropriate knowledge base, the teachers' failure to convey instructions and expectations clearly to students, and finally, a lack of motivation exhibited by students.

The role instructors play as mediators in the learning process is crucial to the development of self-determined and independent learning (Campione, Brown, Ferrarra and Bryant 1984; Stone and Wertsch 1984; Vygotsky 1978). In an environment of inter-dependence, learning is simultaneously an individual and social construction, in that individuals contribute to their own learning as much as their teachers do (Vygotsky 1978). Instructors who act as mediators between the student and his or her external world, can help provide links, clarify meanings, and reinforce understanding with the learner's assistance. While this process may take some time and energy by the teacher, this kind of learning environment will ultimately contribute to the learner's development as a critical thinker.

It is important to recognize that learners construct meaning from their own experiences, *as well as* experiences shared under the guidance of an instructor. This perspective views teachers as agents who assist students in becoming aware of their own learning by actively involving them as collaborators in the problem solving enterprise and being supportive of these efforts (Brotherson et al. 1995; Moore, Rieth, and Ebeling 1993). The provision of instructional situations that facilitate the learner's ability to construct meaning is the ultimate goal of guidance and the foundation upon which students can construct additional knowledge. Arming students with problem-solving skills means empowering them with the ability to identify a problem, determine the most appropriate response, and evaluate the outcome. Accomplishing this will assist them in recognizing their potential as independent learners, and lead them to an increased sense of self-determination.

4 It what ways can an instructor facilitate a learner's understanding of the connection between choice and consequence?

5 How can choice be communicated and enacted by individuals for whom verbal articulation is not possible?

Summary of Instructional Strategies to Facilitate Independence

PROVIDE A CONTEXT OF CHOICE

- Offer alternatives (equipment, rules, number of rest periods, etc.).
- Build in opportunities for decision-making.
- Start with simple binary, 'this or that' decisions, and build up slowly.
- Gradually reduce teacher control in instructional settings.
- Structure the environment, not the activity.
- Establish boundaries, and let the activity unfold naturally.
- Learn to tolerate confusion and chaos.
- Safety and chaos are not always mutually exclusive terms.
- Celebrate exploration, personal creativity, and diversity.

ENCOURAGE MASTERY CLIMATES

- Emphasize personal improvement and progress.
- Increase self-awareness of personal goals.
- Praise efforts towards reaching/adjusting personal goals.
- Encourage realistic self-referenced evaluations.

ADOPT EMPOWERING INSTRUCTIONAL OBJECTIVES

- Explicitly teach self-regulation strategies and problem-solving skills.
- Increase levels of self-awareness.
- Identify the goal clearly and check for understanding.
- Increase awareness of critical features of the task through conscious attention.
- Encourage personal responsibility for actions and consequences.
- Provide explicit instructions in context-specific environments.
- Provide task challenges that emphasize the value of 'the try'.
- Actively respect the learner's decisions and choices.

USE EFFECTIVE INSTRUCTIONAL STRATEGIES

- Personalize strategies to increase their meaningfulness and memory value.
- Bring your bags of tricks to the gym! (Use mnemonics, visual cues, rhymes, etc.)
- Encourage self-talk, thinking out loud by being your own example.
- Promote conscious and active awareness of learning.
- Avoid heavy reliance on social reinforcement or external rewards.

Part Four: Case Studies, or Putting the 'I' Back into Independence

The scenarios presented here do not have one correct answer, nor do they have any automatic, guaranteed, or magic solution. In fact, only a few suggestions for instructional strategies are actually included in this section. It is up to **you** to fill in the blanks and provide possible instructional strategies, or ways to encourage independence, and improve the learning climate for the learner and the instructor.

As you read these case studies, remember that learning is a highly active, constructive process. The way we learn, including what and where we learn, depends upon many different factors. In light of this, careful consideration must be given to the individual learner, the task, and the environment, as well as any potential interactions between these components (Reid 1996). With each of the scenarios presented, ask yourself what is really happening and whether or not the instructor is fostering independence in any way. What golden opportunities, or valuable teachable moments is the instructor missing out on because of his or her own lack of awareness? Does the task/environment/or learner afford any opportunity for the occurrence of self-determined behaviour?

Reflect upon the ways in which independence may be facilitated in a practically applied manner. Do not forget to identify the key issues/problems from the learner's perspective, as well as the instructor's. Consider all of these variables in determining the best course of action to take in the following scenarios. Be creative, have fun, and activate your own learning!

CASE STUDY SCENARIOS

1. **You are a physical education teacher in an elementary school.** Following a lesson on throwing technique for a group of eight year olds, you have set up the following drill to practice this skill. A series of pylons have been set up about a metre apart. Small red rubber balls are balanced on top of each pylon as targets for children to aim at. Additional balls have been provided in a bin about five metres away for children to throw at the pylon targets. Craig is a student with a learning disability who is often teased by other children who taunt him by saying he "throws like a girl." Out of ten tries, Craig hits two targets. Frustrated, he loses his focus upon the activity at hand, and

starts to 'goof off' by throwing the ball in non-designated target zones.

COMMENTS?

- What is the goal of the task, and who decided the goal?
- What types of choices are available to the children (e.g., equipment, movement pattern, target zones)?
- What accommodations been made for different skill and ability levels?
- What are the motivations to succeed? What types of challenges are present?
- Teach self-regulatory strategies (or 'tricks') to encourage movement skill. Use imagery, cues, and symbols meaningful to the learner to reinforce the memory to move. Ask the learner to identify his or her own strategies (e.g., television heroes, computer game icons, or anything else children find interesting).

2. **You are an instructor of a large, inclusive play programme for children aged three to six with limited staff resources.** There are name tags for each child to wear as soon as they enter the gym area, but you are short on time and staff to accommodate so many children at once. As a result, too much time is taken individually pinning the name tag on each child's clothing, and the children are getting restless. Because you recognize the need to memorize each child's name as early as possible, you cannot do without the name tags.

COMMENTS?

- Consider making a name tag game. Place footprints on the floor for children to follow as soon as they enter the gym to help them find their name tag.
- To encourage independence, and honour decision-making, let children choose their own body part on which to place their name tag.

- Reinforce peer interactions.
- For time efficiency, incorporate motor skills and movement concepts into the search for name tags.
- Prompt children to explore a repertoire of movement skills by posing open questions: e.g., "Can you think of another way to get to the blue mat?" "What happens to your body when you stand on one foot?"

3. **As an instructor at a drop-in recreational programme for inner city teens, you face many obstacles but feel up to the challenge of your new job.** One of the most obvious obstacles is a severe lack of funding reflected in little available equipment. The equipment you can use (a set of basketballs, an old high jump standard, and floor hockey sticks) is old and in need of repair. Youth at the drop-in centre are tired of the same old games and want to try something new.

COMMENTS?
- Explicitly teach problem-solving skills: What is the problem? How can it be fixed?
- Build team cohesion and actively demonstrate respect for a variety of opinions. Collaborate!
- Encourage goal-directed behaviour, and identify realistic goals that can be prioritized.
- Identify measurable outcomes as indicated by the students.
- Encourage resourcefulness, promote initiative, have students develop themes for activities and plan accordingly.
- Relinquish instructor control of the activities, and provide opportunities for students to acquire leadership skills.
- Introduce activities that the students are motivated to learn.
- Introduce fund-raising as a collective effort to facilitate the inclusion of more relevant types of activities (e.g., wall climbing, roller blading, etc.).

4. **Susan is a young woman with a severe multiple disability who uses a motorized wheelchair and has little motor control.** She has expressed an interest in white water rafting and adamantly refuses to change her mind about her wish to go rafting.

COMMENTS?
- Respect the choice!
- Encourage conscious awareness about the activity; clearly identify what skills are required.
- Investigate existing rafting companies in the area to determine how well equipped they are to deal with varying ability levels.
- Visit an outdoor centre or the local white water rafting club together to educate each other.
- Explore alternative activities that may satisfy adventure seeking inclinations.
- Simulate risk-taking activities as a starting point to explicitly teach the importance of responsibility, safety, and consequences.

5. **John is a 20-year old man with Down's syndrome who lives at home with his mother.** Except for his job at the sheltered workshop and his friends there, John spends most of his time at home watching television. After watching a programme on bodybuilding, he tells his mother he wants to start working out at the local gym. His mother fears others at the gym will ridicule him. She also does not think he understands what 'working out' really means and is worried he is setting himself up for failure.

COMMENTS

_____

_____

_____

_____

6 It has been said that the only way to truly understand the present, or project into the future, is to reflect on the past. Project yourself and other individuals (practitioners, researchers, and persons with a disability) into the year 2010.

In your opinion, how will the present focus on self-determination and empowerment impact upon the adapted physical activity field?

7 What changes in the lives of persons with disabilities do you believe may occur in the future?

8 What factors may contribute to this change?

Summary

Many who work with the handicapped, impaired, disadvantaged, and aged tend to be overzealous in their attempts to "protect", "comfort", "keep safe", "take care", and "watch". Acting on these impulses, at the right time, can be benevolent, helpful, and developmental. But, if they are acted upon exclusively or excessively, without allowing for each [person's] individuality and growth potential, they will overprotect and emotionally smother the intended beneficiary. In fact, such overprotection endangers the client's human dignity, and tends to keep him [her] from experiencing the risk-taking of ordinary life which is necessary for normal human growth and development. (Perske 1972, p. 195)

The true challenge of self-determination is to involve individuals in exercising control over their own lives. What choices can be made, should be made, when, how, and by whom? These are just a few of the many questions facing adapted physical activity practitioners and researchers today. Providing individuals with the opportunity to make choices, enact decisions, and carry out a sense of responsible action over these decisions is crucial for all people. The presence of a disability does not make the attainment of independence and self-determination any less valuable or significant; nor does it excuse researchers and practitioners from the responsibility they have to promote self-determination in adapted physical activity.

Study Questions

1. Define self-determination.
2. Discuss why self-determination is considered a life long process.
3. Discuss the essential characteristics of self-determination as discussed in Wehmeyer's model.
4. Discuss the value of self-determination as an educational outcome from the learner's perspective.
5. Discuss the value of promoting self-determination as an educational outcome from the instructor's perspective.
6. Identify practical instructional strategies that may be incorporated by an instructor interested in facilitating independence for students in an adapted physical activity class.

References

Agran, M., Blanchard, C., and Wehmeyer, M.L. (2000). Promoting transition goals and self-determination through student self-directed learning: The self-determined learning model of instruction. *Education and Training in Mental Retardation and Developmental Disabilities, 35*(4), 351–64.

Agran, M., and Hughes, C. (1997). Problem solving. In M. Agran (Ed.), *Student directed learning: Teaching self-determination skills* (pp. 171–98). Pacific Grove, CA: Brooks/Cole.

Bosner, S.M., and Belfiore, P.J. (2001). Strategies and considerations for teaching an adolescent with Down's syndrome and type I diabetes to self-administer insulin. *Education and Training in Mental Retardation and Developmental Disabilities, 36*(1), 94–102.

Bouffard, M. (1990). Movement problem solutions by educable mentally handicapped individuals. *Adapted Physical Activity Quarterly, 7,* 183–97.

Bouffard, M., and Wall, A.E. (1991). Knowledge, decision-making, and performance in table tennis by educable mentally handicapped adolescents. *Adapted Physical Activity Quarterly, 8,* 57–90.

Bowman, B.D.V. (1999). Thinking outside the box: Use of invitational counseling to promote self-determination for people with disabilities. *Mental Retardation, 37*(6), 494–96.

Bransford, J., Sherwood, R., Vye, N., and Reiser, J. (1986). Teaching thinking and problem-solving. *American Psychologist, 41,* 1078–89.

Brotherson, M.J., Cook, C.C., Cunconan-Lahr, R., and Wehmeyer, M.L. (1995). Policy supporting choice and self-determination in the environments of persons with severe disabilities across the lifespan. *Education and Training in Mental Retardation and Developmental Disabilities, 30,* 3–14.

Brown, A. (1988). Motivation to learn and understand: On taking charge of one's own learning. *Cognition and Instruction, 5*(4), 311–21.

Brown, A.L., Bransford, J.D., Ferrara, R.A., and Campione, J.C. (1983). Learning, remembering, and understanding. In J.H. Flavell and E.M. Markman (Eds.), *Handbook of child psychology: Cognitive development Vol. 3* (pp. 77–166). New York: Wiley.

Brown, A.L., Campione, J.C., and Day, J.D. (1981). Learning to learn: On training students to learn from texts. *Educational Researcher, 10,* 14–21.

Brown, F., and Gothelf, C.R. (1996). Self-determination for all individuals. In D.H. Lehr and F. Brown (Eds.), *People with disabilities who challenge the system* (pp. 335–53). Baltimore: Brookes Cole.

Bullock, C.C., and Mahon, M. (1992). Decision-making in leisure: Empowerment for people with mental retardation. *Journal of Physical Education, Recreation, and Dance, 63*(8), 36–40.

Butler, D.L. (1995). Promoting strategic learning by postsecondary students with learning disabilities. *Journal of Learning Disabilities, 28*(3), 170–90.

Butler, D.L., and Winne, P.H. (1995). Feedback and self-regulated learning: A theoretical synthesis. *Review of Educational Research, 65*(3), 245–81.

Campione, J.C., Brown, A.L., Ferrara, R.A., and Bryant, N.R. (1984). The zone of proximal development: Implications for individual differences and learning. In B. Rogoff and J.V. Wertsch (Eds.), *Children's learning in the "zone of proximal development": New directions for child development* (pp. 77–92). San Francisco: Josey-Bass.

Chi, M.T.H., Bassok, M.W., Lewis, M., Reimann, P., and Glaser, R. (1989). Self-explanations: How students study and use examples in learning to solve problems. *Cognitive Science, 13,* 145–82.

Condelucci, A. (1995). *Interdependence: the route to community.* Winter Park, FL: GR Press.

Corno, L., and Mandinach, E. (1983). The role of cognitive engagement in classroom learning and motivation. *Educational Psychologist, 18,* 88–108.

Dattilo, J., and Kleiber, D. (1993). Psychological perspectives for therapeutic recreation research. In M. Malkin and C. Howe (Eds.), *Research in therapeutic recreation: Basic concepts and methods* (pp. 57–76). State College, PA: Venture.

Davis, W., and Strand, J. (2001). *Choices: The forgotten motivator in adapted physical activities.* Unpublished manuscript.

Deci, E.L., and Chandler, L.L. (1986). The importance of motivation for the future of the LD field. *Journal of Learning Disabilities, 19,* 587–94.

Deci, E.L., and Ryan, R.M. (1985). *Intrinsic motivation and self-determination in human behavior.* New York: Plenum.

DePauw, K., and Sherrill, C. (1994). Adapted physical activity: Present and future. *Physical Education Review, 17,* 135–43.

Doll, B., Sands, D.J., Wehmeyer, M.L., and Palmer, S. (1996). Promoting the development and acquisition of self-determined behavior. In D.J. Sands and M.L. Wehmeyer (Eds.), *Self-determination across the lifespan: Independence and choice for people with disabilities* (pp. 65–90). Baltimore: Brookes Cole.

Erez, G., and Peled, I. (2001). Cognition and metacognition: Evidence of higher thinking in problem-solving of adolescents with mental retardation. *Education and Training in Mental Retardation and Developmental Disabilities, 36*(1), 83–93.

Ferretti, R. (1989). Problem-solving and strategy production in mentally retarded persons. *Research in Developmental Disabilities, 10,* 19–31.

Ferretti, R.P., Cavalier, A.R., Murphy, M.J., and Murphy, R. (1993). The self-management of skills by persons with mental retardation. *Research in Development Disabilities, 14,* 189–205.

Garcia, T. (1995). The role of motivational strategies in self-regulated learning. *New Directions for Teaching and Learning, 63,* 29–42.

Gaudet, G., and Dattilo, J. (1994). Re-acquisition of a recreation skill by adults with cognitive impairments: Implications to self-determination. *Therapeutic Recreation Journal, 28*(3), 118–33.

Guess, D., Benson, H.A., and Siegel-Causey, E. (1985). Concepts and issues related to choice-making and autonomy among people with severe disabilities. *Journal of The Association for Persons with Severe Handicaps, 16,* 140–45.

Guess, D., and Siegel-Causey, E. (1985). Behavioral control and education of severely handicapped students: Who's doing what to whom and why? In D. Bricker and J. Filler (Eds.), *Severe mental retardation: From theory to practice* (pp. 230–43). Reston, VA: Division on Mental Retardation of the Council for Exceptional Children.

Gumple, T.P., Tappe, P., and Araki, C. (2000). Comparison of social problem-solving abilities among adults with and without developmental disabilities. *Education and Training in Mental Retardation and Developmental Disabilities, 35*(3), 259–68.

Henderson, K. (1994). An interpretive analysis of the teaching of decision-making in leisure to adolescents with mental retardation. *Therapeutic Recreation Journal, 28*(3), 133–46.

Iyengar, S.S., and Lepper, M.R. (1999). Rethinking the value of choice: A cultural perspective on intrinsic motivation. *Journal of Personality and Social Psychology, 76*(3), 349–66.

Kanfer, F.H., and Gaelick, L. (1986). Self-management methods. In F.H. Kanfer and A.P. Goldstein (Eds.), *Helping people change* (pp. 283-345). New York: Pergamon.

Lee, A.L., and Solomon, M.A. (1992). Cognitive conceptions of teaching and learning motor skills. *Quest, 44*, 57-71.

Lewis, K., and Taymans, J.M. (1992). An examination of autonomous functioning skills of adolescents with learning disabilities. *Career Development for Exceptional Individuals, 15*, 37-46.

Lipsky, D.K., and Gartner, A. (1989). Building the future. In D.K. Kipsky and A. Gartner (Eds.), *Beyond separate education: Quality education for all* (pp. 255-90). Baltimore: Paul H. Brookes.

Lord, J. (1991). *Lives in transition: The process of personal empowerment.* Kitchener, ON: Centre for Research and Education in Human Services.

Mactavish, J.B., Mahon, M.J., and Lutfiyya, Z.M. (2000). "I can speak for myself": Involving individuals with intellectual disabilities as research participants. *Mental Retardation, 38*(3), 216-27.

Mahon, M.J. (1994). The use of self-control techniques to facilitate self-direction skills during leisure in adolescents and young children with mild and moderate mental retardation. *Therapeutic Recreation Journal, 28*(2), 58-72.

Mahon, M.J., and Bullock, C.C. (1992). Teaching adolescents with mild mental retardation to make decisions in leisure through the use of self-control techniques. *Therapeutic Recreation Journal, 26*(1), 9-26.

Marsh, D.G. (1993). Friere, Vygotsky, special education, and me. BC *Journal of Special Education, 17*(2), 119-34.

Martin, J.E., and Marshall, L. (1995). Choicemaker: A comprehensive self-determination transition programme. *Intervention in School and Clinic, 30*, 147-56.

McCombs, B.L. (1997, June). Understanding the keys to motivation to learn [on-line]. Available: http:/www.mcrel.org/products/noteworthy/barbaram.html. (URL on October 21, 2002).

Mithaug, D.E., Martin, J.E., and Agran, M. (1987). Adaptability instruction: The goal of transitional programming. *Exceptional Children, 53*(6), 500-505.

Moore, P.R., Reith, H., and Ebeling, M. (1993). Considerations in teaching higher order thinking skills to students with mild disabilities. *Focus on Exceptional Children, 25*(7), 1-12.

Nirje, B. (1972). The right to self-determination. In W. Wolfensberger (Ed.), *Normalization* (pp. 176-93). Toronto: National Institute on Mental Retardation.

Nosek, M.A. (1992). Independent living. In R.M. Parker and E.M. Szymanski (Eds.), *Rehabilitation counseling: Basics and beyond* (2nd ed.) (pp. 103-33). Austin, TX: Pro-ed.

Oliver, M. (1990). *The politics of disablement.* London: Macmillan.

O'Reilly, M.F., Lancioni, G.E., and Kierans, I. (2000). Teaching leisure social skills to adults with moderate mental retardation: An analysis of acquisition, generalization, and maintenance. *Education and Training in Mental Retardation and Developmental Disabilities, 35*(3), 250-58.

Palmer, S.B., and Wehmeyer, M.L. (1998). Students' expectations of the future: Hopelessness as a barrier to self-determination. *Mental Retardation, 36*(2), 128-36.

Paris, S.G., and Oka, E.R. (1986). Self-regulated learning among exceptional children. *Exceptional Children, 53*(2), 103-8.

Paris, S.G., and Winograd, P. (1990). Promoting metacognition and motivation of exceptional children. *Remedial and Special Education, 11*(6), 7-15.

Perske, R. (1972). The dignity of risk. In W. Wolfensberger (Ed.), *Normalization* (pp. 195-200). Toronto: National Institute on Mental Retardation.

Polloway, E.A., Patton, J.R., Smith, J.D., and Smith, T.E.C. (1996). Historic changes in mental retardation and developmental disabilities. *Education and Training in Mental Retardation and Developmental Disabilities, 31*(1), 3-12.

Pressley, M., and Levin, J. (1986). Elaborative learning strategies for the inefficient learner. In C.J. Ceci (Ed.), *Handbook of cognitive, social, and neuropsychological aspects of learning disabilities* (pp. 175-211). Hillsdale, NJ: Erlbaum.

Rappaport, J. (1981). In praise of paradox: A social policy of empowerment over prevention. *American Journal of Community Psychology, 9*, 1-25.

Reid, D.K., and Hresko, W.P. (1981). *A cognitive approach to learning disabilities.* New York: McGraw-Hill.

Reid, G. (2000). Future directions of inquiry in adapted physical activity. *Quest, 52*, 369-81.

Reid, R. (1996). Research in self-monitoring with students with learning disabilities: The present, the prospects, and the pitfalls. *Journal of Learning Disabilities, 29*(3), 317-31.

Reindal, S.R. (1999). Independence, dependence, interdependence: Some reflections on the subject and personal autonomy. *Disability and Society, 14*(3), 353-67.

Ridley, D.S., McCombs, B., and Taylor, K. (1994). Walking the talk: Fostering self-regulated learning in the classroom. *Middle School Journal*, November, 52-57.

Sands, D.J., and Doll, B. (1996). Fostering self-determination is a developmental task. *The Journal of Special Education, 30*(1), 58-76.

Scardamalia, M., and Bereiter, C. (1983). Child as co-investigator: Helping children gain insights into their own mental processes. In S.G. Paris, G.M. Olson, and H.W. Stevenson (Eds.), *Learning and motivation in the classroom* (pp. 61-82). Hillsdale, NJ: Erlbaum.

Schunk, D.H. (1996, October). Students can motivate their way to success [on-line]. Available: http:/www.purdue.edu/UNS/html

Seligman, M.E.P. (1975). *Helplessness: On depression, development, and death.* New York: W.H. Freeman.

Shapiro, E.S. (1981). Self-control procedures with the mentally retarded. In M. Hersen, R.M. Eisler, and P.M. Miller (Eds.), *Progress in behavior modification* (Vol.12, pp. 265–97). New York: Academic Press.

Sowers, J., and Powers, L. (1995). Enhancing the participation and independence of students with severe physical and multiple disabilities in performing community activities. *Mental Retardation 33,* 209–20.

Stainton, T. (1994). Autonomy and social policy: Rights, mental handicap, and community care. Aldershot, UK: Avebury.

Stone, C.A., and Wertsch, J.V. (1984). A social interactional analysis of learning disabilities remediation. *Journal of Learning Disabilities, 17*(4), 194–99.

Thoma, C.A., Rogan, P., and Baker, S.R. (2001). Student involvement in transition planning. *Education and Training in Mental Retardation and Developmental Disabilities, 36*(1), 16–29.

Treece, A., Gregory, S., Ayres, B., and Mendis, K. (1999). I always do what they tell me to do: Choice-making opportunities in the lives of two older persons with severe learning difficulties living in a community setting. *Disability and Society, 14*(6), 791–804.

Vygotsky, L.S. (1978). *Mind in society.* Cambridge: MIT Press.

Wall, M.E., and Datillo, J. (1995). Creating option-rich learning environments: Facilitating self-determination. *Journal of Special Education, 29*(3), 276–94.

Ward, M. (1988). The many facets of self-determination. National Information Center for Children and Youth with Disabilities. *Transition Summary, 5,* 2–3.

Watkinson, J. (1994, October). *Empowering the individual for active living.* Keynote address presented at The North American Federation of Adapted Physical Activity Conference (NAFAPA), Michigan State University, Lansing.

Wehmeyer, M.L. (1992). Self-determination and the education of students with mental retardation. *Education and Training in Mental Retardation, 27*(4), 302–14.

Wehmeyer, M.L. (1994). Perceptions of self-determination and psychological empowerment of adolescents with mental retardation. *Education and Training in Mental Retardation and Developmental Disabilities, 29*(1), 9–21.

Wehmeyer, M.L. (1996a). Self-determination in youth with severe cognitive disabilities: From theory to practice. In L. Powers, G.H.S. Singer, and J. Sowers (Eds.), *On the road to autonomy: Promoting self-competence in children and youth with disabilities* (pp. 115–33). Baltimore: Paul H. Brookes.

Wehmeyer, M.L. (1996b). Self-determination as an educational outcome: Why is it important to children, youth, and adults with disabilities? In D.J. Sands and M.L. Wehmeyer (Eds.), *Self-determination across the lifespan: Independence and choice for people with disabilities* (pp. 17–36). Baltimore: Paul H. Brookes.

Wehmeyer, M.L. (1997). Student-directed learning and self-determination. In M. Agran (Ed.), *Student-directed learning: Teaching self-determination skills* (pp. 28–59). Pacific Grove, CA: Brookes Cole.

Wehmeyer, M.L., Agran, M., and Hughes, C. (2000). A national survey of teachers' promotion of self-determination and student-directed learning. *Journal of Special Education, 34*(2) 58–68.

Wehmeyer, M.L., and Berkobien, R. (1991). Self-determination and self-advocacy: A case of mistaken identity. *TASH Newsletter, 17*(7), 4.

Wehmeyer, M.L., and Bolding, N. (1999). Self-determination across living and working environments: A matched-samples study of adults with mental retardation: Interpersonal cognitive problem-solving skills of individuals with mental retardation. *Mental Retardation, 37*(5), 353–63.

Wehmeyer, M.L., and Kelchner, K. (1994). Interpersonal cognitive problem-solving skills of individuals with mental retardation. *Education and Training in Mental Retardation and Developmental Disabilities, 29,* 265–78.

Wehmeyer, M.L., Kelchner, K., and Richards, S. (1996). Essential characteristics of self-determined behavior of individuals with mental retardation. *American Journal on Mental Retardation, 100*(6), 632–42.

Wehmeyer, M.L., and Lawrence, M.M. (1995). Whose future is it anyway? Promoting student involvement in transition planning. *Career Development for Exceptional Individuals, 18,* 3–19.

Wehmeyer, M.L., and Palmer, S. (2000). Promoting the acquisition and development of self-determination in young children with disabilities. *Early Education and Development, 11*(4), 465–81.

Wehmeyer, M.L., Palmer, S.B., Agran, M., Mithaug, D.E., and Martin, J.E. (2000). Promoting causal agency: The self-determined learning model of instruction. *Exceptional Children, 66*(4), 439–53.

Wehmeyer, M.L., and Schwartz, M. (1998). The relationship between self-determination and quality of life for adults with mental retardation. *Education and Training in Mental Retardation and Developmental Disabilities, 33*(1), 3–12.

Whitman, T.L. (1990). Self-regulation and mental retardation. *American Journal on Mental Retardation, 94*(4), 347–62.

Winne, P.H., and Marx, R.W. (1982). Students' and teachers' views of thinking processes for classroom learning. *The Elementary School Journal, 82*(5), 493–518.

World Health Organization. (1987). Ottawa charter for health promotion. *Canadian Journal of Public Health 77*(6), 1.

Zimmerman, B.J. (1989). A social cognitive view of self-regulated academic learning. *Journal of Educational Psychology, 81*(3), 329–39.

Zimmerman, B.J. (1990). Toward a theory of learned hopefulness: A structural model analysis of participation and empowerment. *Journal of Research in Personality, 24,* 71–86.

CHAPTER 15

Applying Ecological Task Analysis to the Assessment of Playground Skills

E. Jane Watkinson
Janice Causgrove Dunn

Learning Objectives
- To understand the basic tenets of ETA as an approach to the assessment and prescription of instruction.
- To understand how ETA differs from stage theory, behaviourism, and individual difference or ability theory, and what the implications for these differences are in assessment.
- To be ready to construct an assessment device or protocol of your own based on ETA.
- To know how to manipulate constraints and affordances to allow the person assessed to demonstrate task solutions to a specific movement task goal.

Introduction

Assessment of movement skills can serve a number of purposes, as Bouffard has explained in Chapter 11. It can be used for screening, to determine placement and diagnosis, to provide information for student evaluation, and to provide information about programme effectiveness. This chapter will describe an approach to movement skill assessment for the purpose of prescribing instruction. The application is made to playground activities, but the approach can be used with any physical activity. Although playground activities are not typically considered for assessment and instruction, we contend that ensuring children have the skills to participate actively with peers in this setting should be our concern. The playground is the primary active living environment for most children until grades five or six, making it an ideal setting for an ecologically valid (in other words, valid in real settings) assessment approach.

The approach to assessment described in this chapter is a modification of ecological task analysis or ETA (Davis and van Emmerik

1995a; 1995b), which has been mentioned in a number of the chapters included in this book. Goodwin (Chapter 16) also provides an overview of this approach and its theoretical underpinnings. Finally, Bouffard (Chapter 11) introduces ETA as a form of functional skills assessment. This chapter will discuss the assumptions about movement that are at the heart of the ETA approach to assessment and instruction and will compare these briefly to the assumptions that other theorists hold. It will demonstrate how an ETA assessment differs from other current motor skill assessments and how to use ETA (with some modification) to develop an assessment instrument of your own. The process will be illustrated using material developed at the University of Alberta.

What Is Ecological Task Analysis?

Ecological psychologists think "movement patterns emerge from the mutual constraints of the task goal, environmental conditions and characteristics and intention of the performer" (Davis and van Emmerik 1995a, p. 25, citing Newell 1986). The person is conceptualized as a living system that is driven by information and constrained by physical and social structures and systems (Davis and van Emmerik 1995a). We are connected to, not separate from, nature in this way, and the systems in which we are embedded (social systems, physical systems) are central to how we move. Movement form is assumed to be an outcome of three factors: the task goal (what we are trying to do), the environmental conditions under which we are trying to do it, and our own characteristics (intentions, feelings, physical capacities). Figure 15.1, adapted from Davis and Burton (1991), illustrates the interaction of these three factors in the production of a movement skill on the playground.

If one element among these three factors is changed beyond a particular range or bandwidth, the movement outcome or movement choice is predicted to change. Think about the differences in your throwing pattern when you throw a ball for distance versus accuracy (a change in the task goal), and consider how

Figure 15.1 Ecological Task Analysis Model

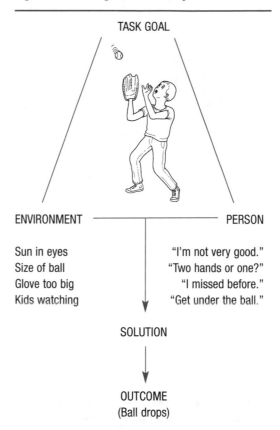

SOURCE: Adapted from "Ecological Task Analysis: Translating Movement Behaviour Theory into Practice: by W.E. Davis and A.W. Burton, 1991, *Adapted Physical Activity Quarterly, 8*(2), pp. 154–77. Adapted with permission.

a slippery surface might affect your running pattern and performance (a change in the physical environment). However, the environment is more than just physical (equipment, space, weather). There are also social and emotional (affective) environments influencing movement. You might be willing to try a new skill alone or with a supportive teacher but be unwilling to try it in front of your peers, who may make disparaging remarks (a change in the social environment). Similarly, movement performance on a physical test can change if motivation to take the test changes (a change in the individual). Have you ever felt differently about a task when you were told to do it, compared to when you chose to do it? Did your performance differ as a result?

Consider a situation where a child is out in the field playing softball and a fly ball comes within a few metres of her. She does not catch it. Why not? What reasons could there be for her to miss the ball? Was the ball dropping from such a height that it was too difficult for her to judge where it would land? Did no one ever teach her how to line up under the ball? Did she not move quickly enough to get to it? Is her glove too small to capture the softball? Could it be that she just did not want to? Was she so nervous from her last failure that she could not concentrate on the ball with so many people watching? Was the sun in her eyes? Was the ball spinning so that it was hard to predict where it would land? Did she deliberately drop it so that she would not have to play this position again? Was she busy talking to the other fielders when the ball came?

All of these are potential reasons, alone or in combination, for the failure to catch the ball. Some of the reasons have to do with the task itself, whether it is too difficult, new, or unpredictable. Other reasons have more to do with the environment: the weather, the glare of the sun, the size of the glove, the other players on the field, the crowd watching the performance. Finally, some of the reasons seem to reside in the child: her movement skill, her strength or stride length, her feelings, her motivation in this particular situation. See if you can think of any more reasons not included in those listed above. Now see if these reasons can be grouped into factors arising from the **task**, the **environment**, the **person**, or a combination of these factors. Are there any reasons that do not fit into one of these groups? Are these three factors **sufficient** to describe any influence on the performance that you can think of? Can you catch a fly ball without these elements having an influence? Davis and van Emmerik (1995a; 1995b) claim the three elements (i.e., task, environment, person) are both **necessary and sufficient** to describe the conditions that lead to a particular

movement performance. If this is true, then it follows that the three elements need to be considered in the assessment of performance.

Ecological task analysis is a method of assessment and instruction that encourages teachers and others to think about movement performance in terms of the independent and interactive influences of the task goal, the environment in which the goal is to be achieved, and the characteristics and predispositions of the learner or performer. ETA is based on the concept of "affordances" put forward by Gibson in 1977. Affordances are what an environment offers to a person in terms of action. This concept was once described by a seven year old, who said that "a soccer ball wants to be kicked" while "the cat doesn't want to be kicked at all." In other words, the soccer ball *affords* (or offers, or calls for) kicking, just as a chair *affords* sitting. Have you ever seen a group of young children arrive at the gym after a day in a classroom? They 'automatically' start to run because the large, empty space 'affords' it.

But the affordances of the environment are accompanied by 'constraints' as well. Constraints can be either temporary or enduring. In both cases, they limit the options perceived to be available, rather than actually causing a choice (Bouffard, Strean and Davis 1998). The result is that environments are not perceived exactly the same way by all people. The key notion here is that an individual perceives what an environment affords, but both social and affective constraints can impact what is afforded by the physical aspect of the environment for a particular person. A physical space may afford running, and most young children might run when they perceive an open gym space. Yet when a child lacks a positive perception of competence in running (an enduring affective constraint), or a child worries that his friend might trip him (a temporary affective or social constraint), the choice to run may not be perceived or acted upon. A different task goal (tying gym shoes again) may be acted upon instead. These perceptions and choices are not always conscious ones. Rather, they may be unconscious

Figure 15.2 *Sample Test Item from the Test of Gross Motor Development (TGMD)*

Skill	Equipment	Directions	Performance Criteria	1st	2nd
CATCH	A 4-inch plastic ball, 15 feet of clear space, and tape.	Mark off two lines 15 feet apart. The child stands on one line and the tosser on the other. Toss the ball underhand directly to the child with a slight arc aiming tell him/her to "catch it with your hands." Only count those tosses that are between the child's shoulders and belt. Repeat a second trial.	1. Preparation phase where hands are in front of the body and elbows are flexed 2. Arms extend while reaching for the ball as it arrives 3. Ball is caught by hands only		

Record of Scores

1st TESTING				2nd TESTING			
	Raw Score	Standard Score	Percentile	Age Equivalent	Raw Score	Standard Score	Percentile	Age Equivalent

1st TESTING				2nd TESTING			
Locomotor _____ _____ _____ _____				Locomotor _____ _____ _____ _____			
Object Control _____ _____ _____ _____				Object Control _____ _____ _____ _____			
Sum of Standard Scores _____				Sum of Standard Scores _____			
Gross Motor Quotient _____ _____				Gross Motor Quotient _____ _____			

SOURCE: From *Test of Gross Motor Development* (Second Edition) by D.A. Ulrich, 1985, Austin, TX: Pro-Ed. Reprinted with permission.

or tacit. Nevertheless, the performer perceives affordances of the environment along with constraints, selects a task goal (consciously or unconsciously), and attempts to meet that goal with a movement solution. The movement emerges from the complex relationships among these elements.

From an ETA perspective, motor development (that is, the changes that we see in growing children) arises from the experience of individuals' interactions with the environment and with the movement problems 'solved' as we achieve task goals that we perceive in our environment. As we solve more and more problems, and as the constraints and affordances change with age and size, we find better and better solutions. This is quite a different point of view from that of **stage theorists** who believe (or believed) that

movement patterns 'unfold' as children mature [see Roberton (1982) and Gallahue (1983) for examples of this view]. These scholars suggested that, except under very extreme environmental circumstances, mature motor patterns emerge from within the child if that child is genetically 'normal'. They assumed there are movement patterns that are universal, in that virtually everyone achieves them at some time, in the same order, and that these patterns will be used consistently once they are attained. It is progress towards these milestones, often reflected in our physical education curricula, that some developmentalists want to assess.

What should be apparent from the discussion above is that, while ecological psychologists and stage theorists acknowledge the significant similarities in movement patterns across people, the hypothesized source of these similarities differs according to the theory one holds. To a maturationist, or a stage theorist, the similarities are thought to be due to the genetic programming of our species, while to the ecological psychologist the similarities are presumed to be the outcome of similar solutions to movement problems that emerge under social, emotional, and environmental constraints. The influence of stage theory can be seen in the many assessment tools that describe stages of motor skill (see the test item from the TGMD in figure 15.2, for example). In this view children are assessed for their developmental stage in running, throwing, kicking, catching, and so forth, based on the movement patterns that have been documented in studies of many, many children followed over several years [for examples see Halverson and Williams (1985), Roberton (1985) and Wickstrom (1983)]. Certain skills such as running, jumping, hopping, skipping, throwing, catching, kicking, and striking, are seen to be 'fundamental' to overall motor development by stage theorists, because they are assumed to be the foundation on which other skills are built. This implies that they are basically prerequisites to further development, say, of sport skills. As such, our instructional efforts should be directed towards improving them. ETA would suggest that skills are only fundamental in the sense that they may be used frequently to solve movement problems in situations that arise with some regularity in a particular environment. In an environment where kicking is not required frequently, this approach would suggest that kicking not take up extensive instructional time.

The ETA approach differs also from the **individual difference** perspective in which people are assumed to have talents or abilities that are largely genetically determined and that influence the performance of many different tasks. Highly skilled performers are assumed to have more of the relevant abilities required for a skill than poorly skilled performers. ETA suggests instead that capacities and predispositions arise from previous interactions with tasks and environments, and constrain future interactions. In other words, our 'abilities' are not stable features of individuals. They are not talents that people were born with but arise from experience. Some may be predisposed to benefit more from these experiences than others (in other words, there is a genetic contribution to these interactions). But the ETA approach would suggest that individual differences are the outcomes of different interactions of a (different) person with the task and the environment, not simply the result of a difference in native (inherent) talent.

Few people are strict maturationists, strict behaviourists, or absolutely firm believers in genetically-determined abilities. Rather, most tend to believe in the interaction of genetics and experience (see Lerner 1976; Anastasi 1958). Despite this trend toward the combination of various theoretical approaches in explaining movement development, assessment instruments that are available today reflect a strong influence of one theoretical perspective or another. The approaches to assessment taken by maturationists (or stage theorists), behaviourists, and ability theorists differ considerably from that reflected in ETA. Let us consider the immediate differences that might be evident in assessment protocols as a way to more fully understand ETA.

ASSUMPTIONS ABOUT MOVEMENT INFLUENCE THE NATURE OF ASSESSMENT TOOLS

Assessment instruments that are most often used today typically include a relatively small number of performance items. The specific items are included for one of two reasons: (a) because they reflect developmental milestones (or stages of motor development) that have been described in studies of children's maturation, or (b) because they are assumed to be indicators of underlying 'abilities' that contribute to the performance of all childhood motor skills. The Test of Gross Motor Development or the TGMD (Ulrich 1985) is an example of the first (see figure 15.2). It contains skills that have been traditionally referred to as *phylogenetic* skills or developmental milestones that are eventually acquired by most individuals. They are grouped into locomotor skills and object control skills. The items on this test are assumed to be the developmental foundation for many complex sport and games skills (Ulrich, Ulrich and Branta 1988). The skills are task-analysed for movement form (arm action, leg action) according to developmental norms (how most children tend to perform as they grow), for the purposes of assessment and prescription. The assessor observes specific aspects of the child's performance and records whether they are present (i.e., observed) or not. For example, to assess the skill of catching, the assessor observes whether or not the child (1) prepares to catch the ball with elbows flexed and hands in front of the body, (2) extends arms in preparation for ball contact, (3) catches and controls the ball with hands only, and (4) bends the elbows to absorb the force of the ball. For each skill, the total number of skill characteristics present is compared to norms in order to determine if the child's performance is developmentally appropriate. A quotient, which is a combination of the scores on all the tests, is also determined (see figure 15.2).

The Movement Assessment Battery for Children or MABC (Henderson and Sugden 1992), and the Bruininks-Oseretsky Test of Motor Proficiency (Bruininks 1978) are examples of the second approach to assessment. These tests include items that measure performance outcomes (number of accurate trials, distance, time) that are assumed to be a reflection of abilities such as 'manual dexterity' or 'dynamic balance'. Test items are grouped into subtests to yield a score that is indicative of an underlying motor ability (Davis 1984; Riggen, Ulrich and Ozmun 1990). There is also a form to collect qualitative data. Examples of a test item for hopping (a subtest for dynamic balance) for nine and ten year olds in the MABC can be seen in figure 15.3. Figure 15.4 contains an example of a test item for bilateral coordination from the Bruininks-Oseretsky test. The actual test item is finger and foot tapping.

In virtually all of the currently available assessment tools (including those mentioned here), the authors have tried to reduce the number of tasks assessed in the belief that a performance on one task is predictive of performance on other similar tasks. In contrast to this, ETA suggests that tasks are highly specific, that performance on one does not predict performance on another. Therefore an ETA assessment might include only one or many tasks, depending on the interests or purposes of the assessor. It may not necessarily specify the exact skill to be assessed. An ETA assessment, based on the ETA approach, would identify a task goal only, thereby allowing the individuals being assessed to choose the skills with which they can meet it.

It is important to note that the assessments discussed thus far (excluding ETA) imply that the person who is being assessed has a set of 'characteristics' that are brought along wherever she or he goes. In other words, this means that individuals respond relatively the same way in every environment they encounter, because they have traits or talents or accomplishments that are stable features of themselves. Abilities, for example, are assumed to be fairly stable characteristics of the performer which influence performance across many contexts, and are not easily modifiable through practice (Burton and Miller 1998). In ability testing, "abilities are treated as if they are a possession of the performer which he/she takes from one context to another" (Davis 1984, p. 129). (Davis (1984), Davis and Burton (1991) and Bouffard (1997) have addressed the historical roots of these approaches to measurement and their underlying assumptions.) A corollary of this is the notion that in order to assess a person's movement skill we must eliminate all aspects of the environment that might affect the performance, so that we get down to the real issue: motor skill. Much energy has been devoted to the standardization of tests to reduce the influence on performance contributed by variance in the context. For example, the TGMD, the MABC, and the Bruininks are all conducted under standard

Figure 15.3 Sample Test Item from the Movement Assessment Battery for Children (MABC)

Dynamic Balance

Hopping in Squares (9 and 10 years)

Materials
Coloured tape

Set-up
Tape down six adjacent squares, each with an inside measurement of 18 x18 inches (0.45m), to give an overall length of 9 feet (2.7m).

Task
The child starts the task standing on one foot inside the first square. The child makes five continuous hops forward from square to square, stopping inside the last square. The last hop does not count if the child fails to finish in a balanced, controlled position, or makes an extra hop outside the square. Both legs are tested.

Demonstration
While demonstrating the task, emphasize:
- hopping inside the squares
- hopping once inside each square
- keeping the free foot from touching the ground
- finishing the series of hopes in a balanced, controlled position inside the last square — this is achieved by bending the knee to accommodate the hop, and controlling momentum

Practice phase
Give the child one practice attempt with each leg. If any fault of procedure is observed, the examiner should interrupt at the earliest opportunity and give a reminder or re-demonstrate.

Formal trials
THREE for each leg. Present the second and third trials only if needed to achieve the pass criterion. No assistance may be given during these trials.

Record
Number of correct consecutive hops (maximum 5) completed without committing a procedural fault, i.e.,
- hopping on or outside the lines
- hopping more than once in a square
- letting the free foot touch the floor

Quantitative data
Record number of correct hops; F for failure; R for refusal; I for inappropriate

Preferred leg		age 9	age 10		score		Nonpreferred leg		age 9	age 10
Trial 1 _____		5	5		0	0	Trial 1 _____		5	5
Trial 2 _____		–	–		1	1	Trial 2 _____		–	–
Trial 3 _____		–	–		2	2	Trial 3 _____		4	4
		4	4		3	3			3	3
		1–3	3		4	4			1–2	2
		0	0-2		5	5			0	0-1

*Item score

SOURCE: From *Movement Assessment Battery for Children* by S. Henderson and D. Sugden, 1992, Sidcup, Kent, England: The Psychological Corporation. Reprinted with permission.

Figure 15.4 Sample Test Item from the Bruininks-Oseretsky Test of Motor Proficiency

Subtest 3: Bilateral Coordination
Tapping – Foot and Finger on Same Side Synchronized
The subject simultaneously tapes the foot and index finger on one side of the body and then simultaneously taps the foot and index finger on the opposite side. The subject is given 90 seconds to complete 10 consecutive foot/finger taps correctly. The score is recorded as a pass or a fail.

TEST SCORE SUMMARY

Complete Battery:							
Subtest	Point Score		Standard Score		Percentile Rank	Stanine	Other
	Max	Subj	Test	Comp			Age Eq.
Gross Motor Subtests: 1. Running speed and agility 2. Balance 3. Bilateral coordination 4. Strength	15 32 20 42	____ ____ ____ ____	____ ____ ____ ____				
Gross Motor Composite			____ (Sum)	____	____	____	____

SOURCE: From *Bruininks-Oseretsky Test of Motor Proficiency, Examiners Manual*, by R.H. Bruininks, 1978, Circle Pines, MN: American Guidance Service. Reprinted with permission.

conditions as prescribed by the testing manuals to ensure that everyone does each test item in virtually the same way. The authors have tried to reduce or remove the role of the environment in performance by controlling it. The assumption here is that the testing environment is a sample of all environments and that performance is likely to be relatively stable across many environments. Do you agree with this assumption? This is consistent with the previous assumption that the responsibility for the performance lies with the child, that extraneous influences such as the tester, the environment, and the equipment must be reduced or minimized to get at the real characteristic of the child. Is this assumption consistent with ETA?

Skills are always performed within a context that is meaningful to the performance (Davis and van Emmerik 1995a). In other words, the performance is not done outside of a context, or in isolation, therefore contexts are a critical part of the assessment of performance. "Understanding the *context* in which human movement occurs is fundamental to ecological psychology.... The context provides not only constraints but is the catalyst for action" (Davis and van Emmerik 1995a, p. 12). For ETA theorists the context is critical, and it consists of more than just the physical environment, the size of the ball, or the space inside the gymnasium. It includes the other people as well (the social environment), and the performer's own emotions: his or her response to the people and the physical environment in which the performance is embedded. The aim of an ETA assessment is to understand what a child can do in a particular physical, social, and emotional context (Davis and van Emmerik 1995a).

A further element in these other approaches to assessment (and the last that will be discussed) is the assumption that people should be assessed on how they perform compared to others, that is, where they place with respect to other people, based on norms already established on the test items. (An exception to this might be criterion-referenced assessments that have been described by Bouffard in Chapter 11, though even in these cases the criteria are often based on normative expectations.) In effect, what most tests do is control the task and the controllable conditions under which a particular task is performed (by specifying the task itself, the way in which it is to be done, the number of trials, the size of the equipment). This is done so that one person's performance can be compared to another person's performance accurately. But is this what we really want to know from an assessment of skill if we are using it to prescribe instruction? Are we really interested in whether Mary can perform this better than Jack? Or that she can perform as well as 50 percent of North American kids? Or are we interested in what skills Mary and Jack **can and cannot do**, and the conditions under which they can or cannot perform these skills? This is the approach that is favoured in ETA.

Frequently, people choose assessment instruments without realizing that, in selecting a particular instrument, they are also selecting assumptions or beliefs about motor development. When you choose the Bruininks-Oseretsky assessment device you are buying into the belief that individuals have abilities that can be captured by testing sample skills. When you choose the TGMD you are adopting the belief that there are universal stages of motor development. When you choose the Movement ABC you are choosing to assess a child relative to his or her age-group peers (the child is compared to others of the same age). Some tests actually have conflicting assumptions embedded in them.

Similarly, when you choose the ETA approach to assessment you are buying into a number of philosophical assumptions, the most significant of which are as follows (See Bouffard, Strean and Davis 1998 and Davis and van Emmerik 1995a for a full explanation of these):

1. Humans make decisions and have goals and intentions that are revealed in their movement patterns (these patterns are not predetermined by their genetic endowment). Determinism (that is, the belief that human action is determined by external forces) is rejected, but since humans are constrained by their social, physical, and emotional environments, there cannot be absolute free will either (Davis and van Emmerik 1995a). For example, a boy may not be completely free to choose to engage in activities that are typically engaged in by girls.

2. There cannot be a single cause of any behaviour or behaviours (Davis and van Emmerik 1995a). Behaviours result from multiple causal factors.

3. Individuals with intellectual or other disabilities may experience social limitations that impact on their motor development. Thus their motor development cannot be attributed to the 'condition' they exhibit (for example Down's syndrome), but is, rather, influenced by the covariates of the condition (in other words, the enduring social and affective constraints they have experienced in relation to their condition). A child with Down's syndrome may experience years of low expectations from teachers that influence his or her perceptions of competence.

Using ETA in the Assessment of Motor Skills

Burton and Davis (1996) describe four basic steps for the use of ETA in the assessment and instruction of skills. The first step is to establish or identify the task goals that are of interest to the assessor or instructor. The second step is to allow choices of movement solutions by the performer to determine which solutions are currently in the child's repertoire, and to identify which solutions are preferred by the performer. The third step is to manipulate the environmental, person, or task variables to determine the conditions under which task solutions can be applied or chosen (they refer to these conditions as 'control variables'). Here the assessor wants to know which conditions are optimal for performance, and under which conditions the task goal or preferred solution cannot be met. The fourth step in the process is to introduce instruction, applying methods that maximize self-discovery to help children attain valued solutions to the task goal. Our assessment tool (Watkinson and Causgrove-Dunn 2001) is designed to help instructors through the first three steps by providing the task goals in the domain of playground activity and by providing suggested task solutions to each task goal.

Step One: Establish the task goals to be assessed

ETA requires the identification of a **functional task goal**, that is, what is to be accomplished. This differs from the notion of a **skill**, or what the performer does to meet the task goal. On the playground, going down the slide may be the desired task goal. It is the functional outcome that the child wants to perform or accomplish (other task goals might be shooting a basket, jumping rope, or riding a bicycle). Different children may exhibit different skills (often referred to as 'solutions') to accomplish this goal. One child may slide down safely on his or her bum while another goes head first. The affording and constraining features of the environment (external and internal), the task goal itself, and the child will determine the solution, if there is to be one. In other words, the child will perceive what the situation affords for him or her. The specific movement form (sliding on feet or sliding on knees) will be the

outcome. A straight slide with a gradual slope may afford a more 'risky' movement pattern than a swift spiral slide. A sore head from a previous attempt may constrain the child from going down head first, resulting in a choice to go feet first next time. These are simple examples of what is a very complex phenomenon.

How do you determine what the task goal is? How general or specific should it be? ETA theorists have not given a position on this. One important criterion worth consideration is whether or not the ability to perform a particular task goal will contribute to an individual's ability to engage in an active living lifestyle. Will the specific task goal ultimately contribute to an individual's ability to make choices about his or her active living? Culturally or socially relevant functional task goals that will prepare children for participation in inclusive settings, or in settings of their choice, are important. The social and physical setting includes opportunities for children to play on playgrounds and fields, to be active on the ice or the snow, to dance, to engage with balls, bats, hoops, clubs, baskets, or bicycles, and skateboards. These should be reflected in our functional task goals.

Consideration may also be given to the constraints and affordances that reside in the individual when choosing task goals to assess. In this case, the constraints imposed by an individual's specific disability may impact on performance in such a way that some task goals are more appropriate than others. For example, an individual who has a developmental disability may find that some inclusive environments require excessively demanding task goals (such as passing a puck to a teammate while skating backwards). Tasks of reduced complexity (but still of cultural relevance) that meet the demands of other inclusive or exclusive settings may be more appropriate for this person. The resulting level of social, psychological, and physiological demands should be such that full participation over the long term (that is, throughout childhood and into adulthood) is possible.

Certainly, ball skills have not been found to be the most common skills used on North American playgrounds by elementary school aged girls (Borman and Kurdek 1987). Canadian data on individuals over ten years of age indicate that golf was the only activity involving balls that was in the top ten list of popular activities for both males and females (Stephens and Craig 1990). Yet many of our movement skill assessments rely on ball tasks (see the MABC and the TGMD) and many of our programmes assume the cultural 'normativeness' (social relevance) of ball skills.

Block (1992) proposes a "functional life skills curricula" in the school system for individuals with profound disabilities which features adaptations to ball skills that can allow those with profound disabilities to experience partial participation (1992, p. 202). These adapted ball skills are self-paced and performed in a predictable environment whereas most ball games require rapid adaptations to changes in the environment, with little time for planning (Gentile 1987; Schmid 1999).

Within many instructional settings (e.g., school), a curriculum largely determines the task goals to be assessed. Nevertheless, prior to beginning an assessment, we encourage you to think independently about **why** certain skills are included in the assessment for a particular child. Our recommendation is to choose a relatively small number of task goals carefully. Ensure that children with disabilities have a repertoire that allows them to be active in an inclusive setting with peers and that allows them to be active in more protected environments such as home.

Burton and Davis (1996) acknowledge that goals are both conscious and unconscious, but say clearly that goals should be made explicit if they are to be the object of instruction and assessment. In instructional settings, task goals can be made explicit by setting up the environment to 'communicate' them. In other words, the physical environment can be prepared or arranged so that it affords certain functional goals and not others (the play space can afford volleyball and not badminton, or climbing activities and not running). If instructors are interested in knowing how well children can run and jump, then the physical environment can be set up to encourage these activities. On the playground, the physical environment is not usually modifiable. Unlike those in the gymnasium, physical structures on playgrounds are usually in place for years. These structures do 'afford' many different kinds of activities, but they are not easily manipulated by adults or children.

When the task goal can not be implicitly communicated, it can be made explicit to the child by the assessor. A statement can be made, or a question can be asked, or a demonstration can be given. The assessor may simply ask whether the child can throw the ball to a target, and then observe the degree to which the child can do this under the chosen circumstances. The child can choose the distance from the target, the kind of throw that will be used, and even the size of the ball to be thrown. The teacher may want to assess one or many task goals (all the task goals involved in the game of baseball for instance: base running, hitting, fielding, throwing). At first, the instructor may want to know if the task goals can be met under less

Figure 15.5 Task Goals for the Playground

What did you do at recess today?

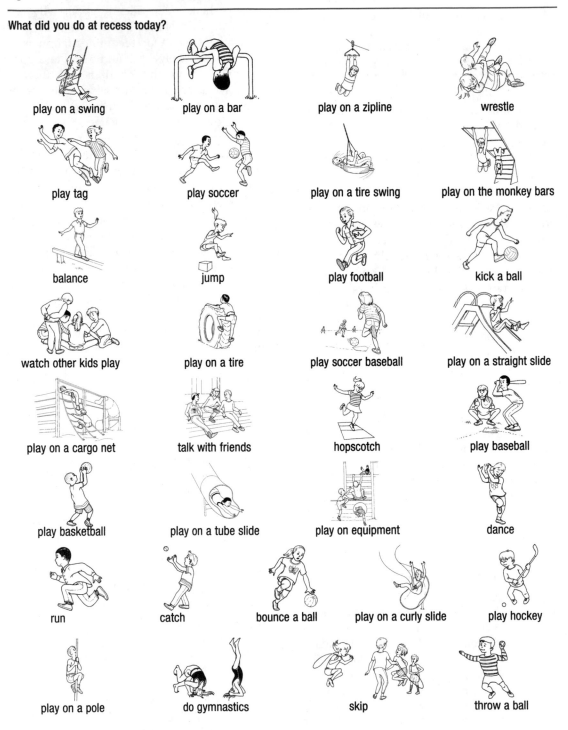

play on a swing   play on a bar   play on a zipline   wrestle

play tag   play soccer   play on a tire swing   play on the monkey bars

balance   jump   play football   kick a ball

watch other kids play   play on a tire   play soccer baseball   play on a straight slide

play on a cargo net   talk with friends   hopscotch   play baseball

play basketball   play on a tube slide   play on equipment   dance

run   catch   bounce a ball   play on a curly slide   play hockey

play on a pole   do gymnastics   skip   throw a ball

SOURCE: From "Assessing Criteria A and B for the Identification of DCD: A Context-specific Approach to Finding Children at Risk," by E.J. Watkinson and J. Causgrove Dunn, 2001, Paper presented at the 13th International Symposium for Adapted Physical Activity Vienna. Reprinted with permission.

demanding circumstances such as in a drill or a lead up game. Ultimately, the assessor may want to know if the child can respond within the game of baseball to the movement problems that are presented there.

In the assessment of playground activities, the task goals are determined by what children are actively doing on the playground. These goals have 'social relevance' because these are the activities that children want to be included in when there is free time on the playground. When we developed our reporting form (figure 15.5) we had children recall what they did at recess, and we identified task goals from their reports. We produced illustrations of the many possible activities on playgrounds, and children told us which ones they had chosen to do at recess. We observed a sample of children to be sure that most children in grades one to four could accurately report what they did (Watkinson et al. 2001). The results showed that the children had very accurate memories of the activities in which they had engaged.

The children's choices were different in almost every class. The grade one children did things that were different from the children in grade two. Children in one class of grade two spent their time in different activities than children in another grade two class in the same school! We chose the activities that were done by several children in the class as the task goals for that class. We did not want to assume that everyone should be doing exactly the same thing on the playground, but we did assume that the activities that were frequently chosen by at least a few members of the group were valuable activities in which to take part. These activities have social relevance for that age group.

For most classes, eight to twelve task goals were chosen as socially relevant because at least 20 percent of the children in the group did them. We only chose task goals that were active (talking with friends was not chosen, for example, even though a large percentage of the class reported doing it.) For one class of twenty-five students, the following task goals were chosen because they were done by at least five students in the class: swinging on a swing, climbing on a climber, going down a slide, using a zipline, running, and jumping. These tasks became the focus of assessment.

Step Two: Allow choices in movement solutions

Once task or functional goals have been determined, the child is given the freedom to choose the skill or form that will be used to meet the goal. These skills are referred to as 'solutions' to demonstrate that they arise from the child in response to a movement 'problem' (how to reach the task goal). This differs significantly from the other tests that we have discussed, where the particular skill or task to be completed is specifically communicated to the child. In fact, testers frequently demonstrate the test item and direct the child to attempt the very same skill. In ETA it is essential that the child is presented with a choice so that the assessor can determine whether or not the child has a solution to the task goal in hand. It is important to know whether the child can generate a skill in response to an environment, without a teacher there to demonstrate or prompt it. Children, with or without disabilities, who act only when they are shown exactly what to do will lack independence when they encounter inclusive settings with no demonstrator. Providing choice is also assumed to maximize motivation to perform, and to facilitate decision making as an educational goal in itself.

An attempt is made to observe both movement product and movement process when the environmental influences are systematically manipulated by the assessor. The movement product refers to the actual outcome, such as how far the ball went, while the movement process refers to how the outcome is produced. Did the child throw it overhand or underhand? Assessment becomes a process of identifying the conditions under which a performer can meet a movement goal (find a movement solution), and identifying the conditions under which the goal is seldom or never met.

Figure 15.6: Movement Solutions for the Task Goal of Sliding

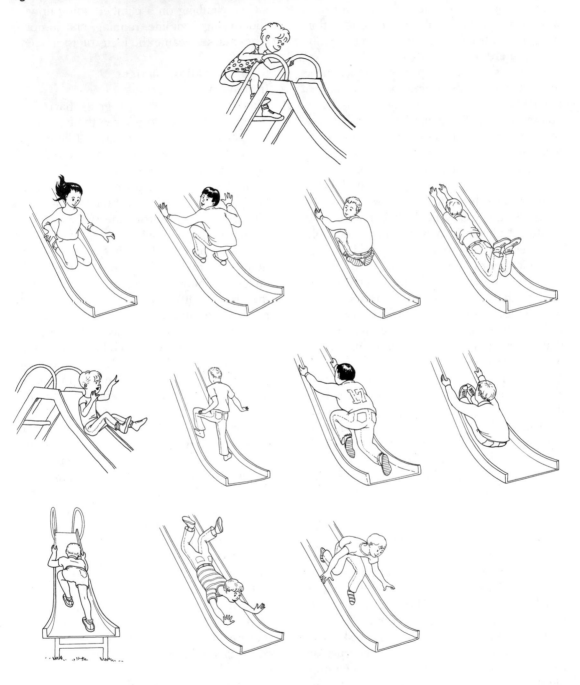

A key feature of this model is that the nature of the solution to the problem or goal is not as important as reaching the goal. For example, using this model a child could be assessed on his or her ability to climb a ladder and go down a slide. The movement process by which the goal is accomplished is not important (for example, does the child ascend on hands and knees, or on feet?), provided it results in goal accomplishment within the constraints of the physical, social, and affective environments. In other words, it is assumed that different, and equally valuable, solutions might lead to the goal rather than one particular solution or skill. If the goal is locomotion, then whether the locomotion is done through the skills of running or wheeling a wheelchair is unimportant. If the child is expected to throw a ball, then the throwing pattern that is used (overhand, underhand, 'mature' or not) is not important as long as the target is hit. This is different from the assessment and instructional approaches that recommend one (efficient and 'mature') way to throw a ball, run, or jump.

An ETA approach to assessment and, subsequently, to instruction may encourage children with disabilities to seek unique but highly effective ways to meet task goals. This would be a positive contribution to the inclusion of children with disabilities in physical activities. However, despite efforts to promote acceptance and appreciation of different skill sets, it may be that children **value** some task solutions more than others. It may be 'cool' to go down the slide in certain ways, but it may not be 'cool', for example, to go down the slide on your seat when you are in grade four. It may be socially desirable to use the same task solutions as those used by a sporting hero (i.e., Gretzky) when you do a particular skill (a shot on goal). In other words, we should acknowledge that children with disabilities may **want** to acquire the specific skills that are valued by the cohort, and that these skills may have an important impact on their perceptions of inclusion on the playground. In fact, there may be significant social and affective constraints that

cause one solution to be more desirable than another, and this should be kept in mind during assessment and instruction. Some task solutions may be considered optimal by an instructor because they are efficient, while others may be considered optimal by a child because they are socially accepted and/or desired.

In a study of children on the playground, we asked children to identify all the different ways in which they met the task goal (in other words we asked them what 'solutions' were possible for that activity). These possible solutions were put in a checklist so that future assessors would not need to record each specific solution. The children told us and showed us all the different ways they could slide on a slide, and we used these ideas to determine which solutions were viable ones for children with disabilities, or with lack of movement competence, to learn. Figure 15.6 has some samples of the solutions that were provided for a particular task goal. Once again, we put these into illustrations so they could be easily recognized by an instructor and checked off by a child in elementary school.

There are other solutions that are valuable, but these were most typical. To find out which of these task solutions is valued by a class or an age group, children can be asked which skill they use or want to use. If most of the children in the group like to go on the spiral slide, and go down face first on their stomachs, then this might be something worth helping all the children achieve. If children can do the task that is highly valued, they might be more likely to take part in that activity with their social group.

Step Three: Manipulate the variables that may influence performance in order to determine the conditions under which goals can be, and can not be, met

Identifying the conditions (affordances and constraints) under which a goal is achieved can be a huge task: an assessor must determine which 'conditions' are of interest. For example, an instructor may want to know which physical conditions allow goal attainment and may systematically manipulate the dimensions of equipment to determine where optimal performance can be achieved (height of bar, size of ball, angle of slide). She or he may also want to know the social conditions that are required for the goal to be met (does the child need the instructor there, or can she accomplish the task alone or with a friend, during free play?). Finally, while the emotional conditions under which the child performs may be much more difficult to describe or assess, the instructor or assessor may feel it is an important contributor to the performance and may want to identify affective factors that may afford or constrain the performance.

A key point is that while most assessment devices ask the assessor to determine how well a child can perform a specific skill under specific circumstances, the ETA approach **asks the assessor to determine the conditions under which a child can and can not accomplish a task.** This means that the ETA assessor must change the circumstances (or 'scale' the factors that are suspected of being relevant to the performance) during the assessment, or observe the child under naturally changing circumstances and describe what those circumstances are. For this reason, ETA assessments can be conducted in naturally occurring contexts, such as during free play, games, or instruction.

IDENTIFYING CONDITIONS IN THE PHYSICAL ENVIRONMENT

The physical environment can be analysed according to size or distance or other physical measures (time, weight). We can offer different sizes of balls if we want to assess the conditions under which catching is accomplished, and we can alter the height of baskets and the width of goals to determine the optimal conditions for target shooting. We can change the length of the rope for skipping, or the speed at which the rope is turning. An instructor may want to determine whether the child can hit a ball with a bat when the ball is thrown at the perfect height from an easy distance by a skilled thrower. The instructor may also want to know whether the task goal (hitting the ball) can be achieved when a peer throws the ball less than perfectly. In this case, the performer will have to make a decision about whether the pitch is good enough to strike at. The physical conditions under which a child can meet the functional task goal can be manipulated in these ways so that the assessor can determine which conditions lead to accomplishment of the goal and which do not.

Burton and Davis (1996) recommend that the performance be measured, or noted, along with the circumstances under which the performance was obtained. They particularly recommend that the physical attributes of the equipment and space be measured and recorded according to the performer's size (they refer to these as 'intrinsic' measures because they are made relative to the performer's body). Rather than, "Sonya can climb the six-rung ladder when the rungs are 20 cm. apart," the record might say (but perhaps in a briefer format!) "Sonya can climb a six-rung ladder when the rungs are shin-height apart, but not when the distance between the rungs is knee height." Scaling the physical environment in this way may be easier for some movement goals than others.

Clearly this level of measuring and recording could be time-consuming for instructors who are assessing large groups of children. Herkowitz's work on general and specific task analysis can be helpful in scaling the physical aspects of throwing, catching, running, dodging, and jumping, and you are encouraged to look at her assessment examples (Herkowitz 1978). In our playground application we have produced materials that make recording much easier, a matter of checking the appropriate box. In fact, we ask the children themselves to do some of the recording. In this way, full assessments by an instructor are reserved for children who give indications that they are unable to meet valued task goals.

IDENTIFYING THE SOCIAL CONTEXT

The social-emotional context can afford or constrain performance and should be assessed along with the performance to gain a meaningful understanding of the social-emotional conditions under which goals can be reached. "Social constraints have their effect mostly but not only upon the types of goals and activities selected out of the myriad of possibilities in the real world" (Davis and van Emmerik 1995a, p. 13). In other words, **social constraints and affordances may influence whether a child actually takes part and which task goal will be selected,** as well as the movement solution that is chosen to meet the goal. One social constraint may be group size. A child may be able to do an activity alone but not with others around. Another social constraint may be the make up of the group: friends or strangers. On the high horizontal ladder, a girl may choose a particular skill, perhaps hanging by one knee, if the kids around her are her friends and are interested in seeing her succeed at the task. If there are bigger kids there who are playing a tag game in which feet can not touch the ground, the girl may decide that she has to move along the bar more quickly and will choose a hand-over-hand skill. Describing or scaling social constraints is difficult, and may at first simply mean recording whether the child does (or can do) activities alone or with a partner or a small group.

Since the instructor or assessor will be part of the social environment, his or her presence during the assessment may constrain or afford different choices on the part of the child. For example, hanging upside down from a horizontal bar is a frequent activity (or task goal) on the playground. Kelly may be able to accomplish this goal if she is alone on the playground, or with her younger brother. However, she can not do so at recess with her classmates because the social context constrains her (she has to push through to get a space on the bar and then she feels uneasy about her proximity to others). If the social conditions change so that a teacher is there, Kelly may do it, especially if the teacher ensures that each child has enough room on the bar to be comfortable. The instructor assumes that Kelly can meet the task goal under these conditions, but she may not be able to do so under other social constraints. In our playground application, we suggest an assessment method that scales the assessor's involvement in the performance. In our case, the scale goes from relatively no involvement in the production of the movement solution, to significant physical support for the performance.

The discussion that follows suggests another way in which the social environment might be described to determine the conditions under which task goals can be met. It is based on whether the task goal has to be met in a cooperative or competitive activity. It could, for example, be relevant to the assessment of soccer tasks, or softball tasks, or to a game of tag. These are all common-sense ways in which the social environment 'affords' certain activities and not others, and constrains the performer to move in a particular way (or not to move at all). Assessors should explore those factors that are believed to have a particular influence on the task goals in which they are interested.

SCALING THE SOCIAL ENVIRONMENT

The social environment might prove constraining or facilitating to children in physical activity. One major aspect of the social environment is the nature of the activities we take part in. The goal structure of an activity is the essential organization that determines the relationship of children with each other and their relationship to the goal of the activity (Ames 1984; Ames and Ames 1984a; 1984b). (Note that 'goal' here is something bigger than a task goal).

Three goal structures are common in physical activities: **cooperative, competitive, and individualistic.**

---

4 What do you understand each of these words to mean when you say them? What kind of social-emotional environment do they establish?

In cooperative activities, children must rely on each other to reach the activity goal, but this demands the effortful and capable (though not necessarily equal) contribution of each member of the group. In competitive structures, comparison between individuals and groups is essential in determining which person or group reaches the goal. Once again, each person must make an effortful contribution, and the more capable one is the more likely one is to reach the goal (to win). For children who are less capable, competition can be demotivating and can lead to maladaptive decisions and behaviours, including complete withdrawal. Finally, individualistic settings provide for autonomous goals for each individual involved, so that if there is competition it is with oneself.

---

5 Which goal structure do you think is most conducive to movement skill assessment? Why do you think so?

An assumption is generally made that individualistic settings provide the best settings for individual assessment. Children are usually assessed alone, or in a setting where each child does the task without competition with others. Would you anticipate that an ETA approach would recommend this as a usual procedure?

From the point of view of ETA, one might want to know how a child responds in cooperative and competitive settings, and whether or not a behaviour is consistent across these settings. Some children may reach task goals in basketball (shooting, passing, dribbling, defending) when it is played with a parent or sibling in the driveway (a fairly cooperative setting depending on the parent and sibling), but be unable to do so in a more competitive setting with peers.

Since one principle of ETA is to determine the conditions under which a child can or can not perform a skill, assessors may want to test skills in individualistic, cooperative and competitive environments. In this way the assessor can determine where the child can respond optimally and what help is needed to facilitate performance in all three environments, especially those in which the task goals are most frequently used.

IDENTIFYING THE EMOTIONAL CONTEXT

Affect (how we feel) is also seen to be a source of information that affords and constrains the performances and choices of individuals (Davis and van Emmerik 1995a, p.7). In other approaches to assessment of movement skill, a child's feelings are not considered to be part of the assessment. Most assessment instruments look at the movement pattern (arm action, force production) or the movement outcome (number correct, distance covered), and do not pay attention to the emotional state of the performer except perhaps to provide extra trials to someone who is nervous.

Motivational theorists suggest that decisions to do something, and decisions to stick with it, and to exert effort, are largely determined by self-perceptions, perceptions of the difficulty of a task (expectations of success), and the degree to which the behaviour (or activity) is valued. In other words, these factors constrain movement choices even in situations where the physical and social environment affords them. However, how are the affective conditions that are involved in an assessment described or identified?

Including the affective conditions in the assessment is difficult in that we do not yet have easy ways to determine the emotional constraints and affordances to performance. However, since theories suggest that high perceptions of competence and high perceptions of the value of an activity will lead to optimal effort and choice (Eccles 1992; Eccles, Wigfield and Schiefele 1998; Wigfield 1994), these two factors can at least be taken into account in our assessments. (You might ask yourself if these are really affective/emotional factors, or cognitive factors. They may in fact be cognitions that lead to affective outcomes after successful or unsuccessful performance.) We should determine whether the task goals themselves are appealing and valuable to the children. Are the task goals ones that children want to be able to meet, or are the goals a chore? Is the task important to that child? We could also determine what the child's perceptions of self are with respect to that goal. Does the child feel competent? Are there conditions under which he or she would feel more competent? Seeking answers to these questions may be one way to recognise that there are emotional conditions (constraints and affordances) to movement solutions, though these may be difficult to measure or analyse. We can at least try to **optimize the emotional environment in which assessment is taking place,** or recognise that children's performances on tasks that are not valued may not be their best.

According to Davis and van Emmerik (1995a), the affective system is a higher-order system that perceives the emotional state of others, and it determines whether or not a particular action under these conditions will lead to a satisfactory internal emotional state (that is, will lead to the comfort, safety, or happiness of the mover). How we feel, and how we perceive others feel, will influence what we choose to do and how we do it. Clearly, the emotional and the social systems are closely linked, and hence we often hear the terms *social-emotional*, or *social-affective*. Our perceptions of our selves, and the value that we place on certain tasks, may be modified by the social conditions we are in. For example, we found that children would choose some task goals when they were with one friend, but not when they were in a larger group on the playground (Watkinson, Dwyer and Nielsen 2000). They lacked confidence in their performance when there were too many people around to see them, and they feared ridicule if they were to demonstrate incompetence. Their motivation to choose a task goal was constrained by the social environment and linked to the feelings they would have afterwards, indicating that these systems are related.

In summary, ETA calls for the identification of the conditions under which a task goal can and can not be reached. This implies that all of the conditions–physical, social, and emotional–can afford and constrain performance and should be measured along with the performance. This is difficult for the assessor, but the purpose of ETA is to alert instructors to these constraints and affordances, in the hope that they can be considered wherever possible in the assessment process. Assessors can not possibly describe all of the constraints that lead to the goal solution, but they may become aware of constraints or affordances that are most significant as they carry out their assessments. These can then be addressed through instruction so children are able to meet task goals under the conditions that arise in their natural environments, including play, school, and sport.

In our playground example, we decided that if the task goals involve balls and implements, the size and shape of these should be manipulated. Distances should also be changed. For task goals in which the physical structures are stable, these should be described. For instance, sliding on a straight slide should be differentiated from sliding on a spiral or tube slide. Swinging on a tire should be assessed as well as swinging on a regular swing.

The social environment should also be manipulated or described. It should be noted whether a child can perform in free play without a teacher, or only under supervision. It should be noted whether the child can meet the task goal in the presence of friends, or only when alone. Our procedure recommends that assessors also manipulate or describe how much assistance the child requires to provide a movement solution.

Step Four: Begin instruction on task goals that can not be met

This chapter does not specifically deal with instructional styles or programmes, but rather simply with assessment. Nonetheless, the ETA approach recommends the adoption of instructional methods that maximize independence and choice for children in climates that are free from social comparison. Other chapters in this textbook are rich sources of information on pedagogy.

Conducting an Assessment of a Particular Child Using the Playground Self-report

A self-report form is provided for the use of the assessor (see figure 15.5). In this instrument, the task goals are written and illustrated for easy reference by the assessor. The illustrations also make it possible for the children themselves to contribute to the assessment process, both to make sure the task goals that are selected for instruction are relevant to the group being assessed and to make the self-reporting process enjoyable.

The self-report form is first given to the child's whole group (a class or a play group) to determine which task goals are most socially relevant. Each child circles the activities he or she did that day on the playground. Using his or her own form, the instructor simply sums the number of children who chose each goal, putting a check mark beside a task goal for each child who reported doing that activity. Doing this over several playground periods provides a good idea of what the children in the group typically do. The task goals that have the most check marks are assumed to be the most socially relevant. The instructor can discover through this process if a particular child is not taking part in the common recess activities of his or her peers. Assessors then concentrate their assessments on the children who are not actively involved in the favoured activities of their peers. In a group of twenty-five children, this may mean only three to five children will need further assessment. For the others, the assessment is completed when it is clear that each child can reach the task goals that are socially relevant for the group, regardless of the task solution that is used to meet the task goal. If instructors have reason to suspect that a particular child may not be reliably reporting his or her activity, then an observation with the same checklist can be carried out, or the child can be further assessed. If instructors want to be sure that each child in the group can meet the task goal with a highly valued 'solution', then a complete assessment of that task goal can also be carried out with all children.

This method is planned so that each child can tell the instructor what he or she can do before a complete assessment is undertaken. This means the instructor **assesses only the children who are not taking active part in the socially relevant task goals, and then she assesses only the skills that children seem to be missing** or are afraid to try but are typically done by others. In fact, children need never know they are being assessed since the activities themselves, and the method of assessment, are enjoyable and simple and can be used with a whole class or group unobtrusively. In this approach, individual children are not 'tested' in a gym or a clinical setting, and many children can be assessed at once. The targeted child (targeted because he or she is not doing the activities that most of the others are doing) should then be assessed on each of the task goals in which he or she is not engaging.

---

6 Who should choose the task goals? It is often up to teachers or parents to decide which task goals should be tested and taught. But why do we assume that? Can you think of reasons why a child might be a good source of information about which task goals are important?

Sometimes children do not actively participate at recess because they lack the confidence to try new skills and activities that are part of the daily life of their classmates. Often children will tell you what the problem is if you are able to ask them directly. You can use the recording sheets to find out what children think about their own skills and whether they really want to be a part of the activities in which they currently do not engage. You can even start instruction on those task goals and solutions or skills that a child feels he or she does not perform well enough but really wants to learn. If the child is highly motivated, instruction and practice opportunities may have a more positive impact on the performance of these skills than on those in which the child shows little or no interest.

Figure 15.7 Assessor's Prompting Levels

Determining the conditions under which the goal can be reached: assessor's assistance

No Prompts	Complete free play
	Providing opportunity
Verbal Prompts	Specific cues
	General cues (directions or questions)
Visual Prompts	Gestures
	Partial demonstrations
	Full demonstrations
Physical Prompts	Minimal physical guidance
	Partial physical support
	Complete physical support

SOURCE: Adapted from *The PREP Programme: A Preschool Play Programme for Moderately Mentally Retarded Children*, by E.J. Watkinson and A.E. Wall, 1982, Ottawa: Canadian Association for Health, Physical Education and Recreation. Adapted with permission.

7 Is there an ethical question about putting a child into an instructional programme based on what other children are doing, that is, deciding for the child which playground skills are most important for him or her to learn or trying to get him or her to acquire the same skills as other children?

THE ASSESSOR'S ROLE DURING PERFORMANCE

Instructors themselves can be part of the 'physical' environment by giving physical aid to a child who is trying to accomplish a task. Instructors are also a social environmental constraint in this instance. It is not unusual for parents and instructors in instructional settings to give physical, visual, and verbal assistance to students as they are learning a new skill, by holding them, moving their limbs, or supporting them at the same time as they are using gestures, demonstrations, and instructions. In our model of assessment of playground skills, we are recommending the adoption of a prompting system (Watkinson and Wall 1982) to determine the conditions under which a child can or cannot do a playground skill. This model is comprised of systematic environmental prompts from the assessor as the child attempts the skill, beginning with the least intrusive (the least constraining) and moving to the most intrusive (that is, the most assistance) if the child is still unable to perform the skill.

The prompting model can be seen in figure 15.7. It is comprised of four 'levels' of environmental prompts. The first, least intrusive level is the **natural** one in which the assessor may be present but giving no specific help, simply making relevant aspects of the environment available to the child and observing which task goals are reached without any help at all. At this level we are trying to determine if a child can reach a task goal under the normal circumstances of free play. Even at this level we can 'scale,' or manipulate, the environment somewhat: the assessor at this level could control the use of the equipment by other children such that the child has the time required to attempt a task solution. This small modification to the natural environment should be noted so that

Figure 15.8 Assessment checklist for swinging on a swing

	Does it in free play	Does it when told or shown	Does it with physical help		Does it in free play	Does it when told or shown	Does it with physical help
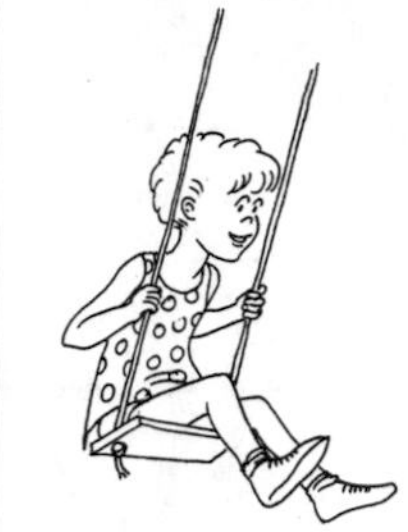				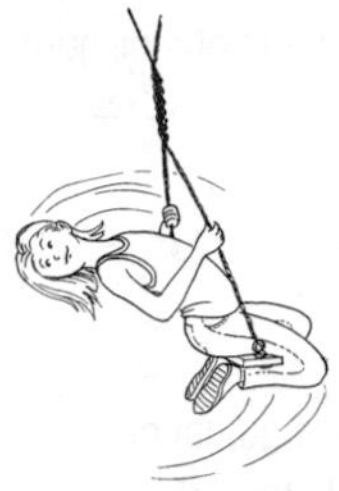			
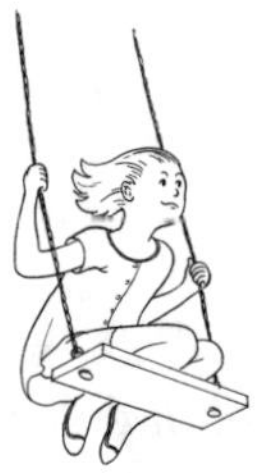				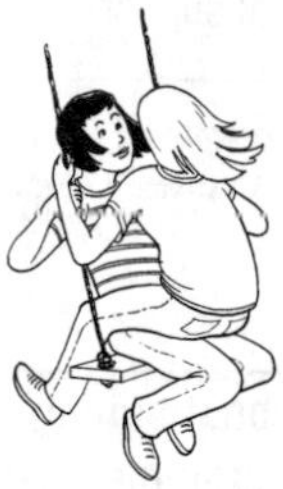			
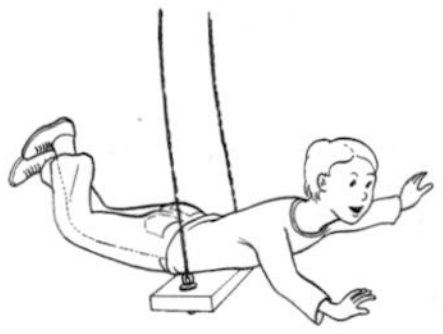				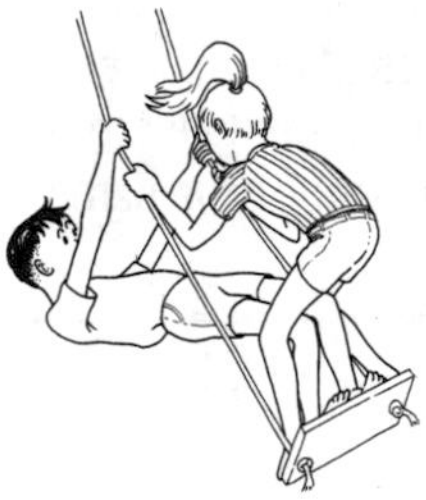			
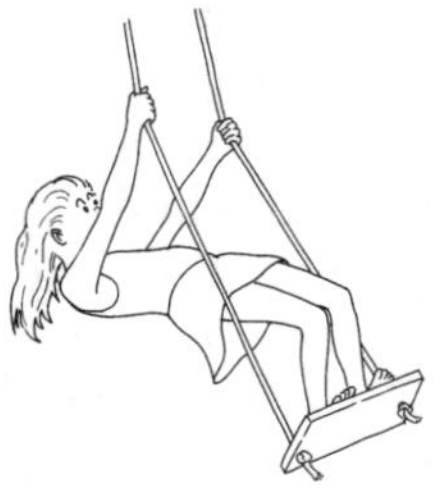				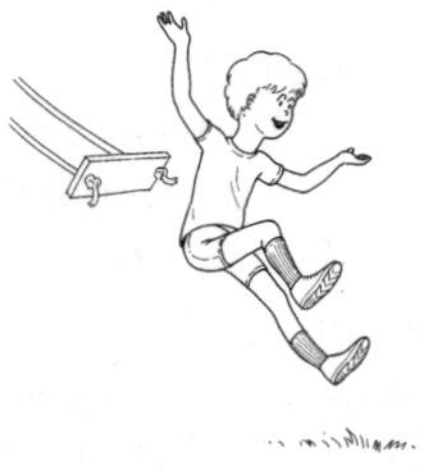			
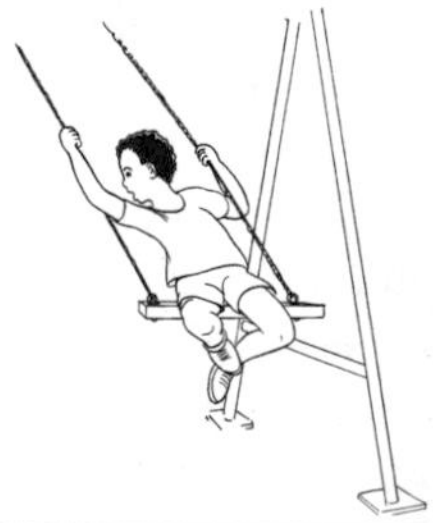				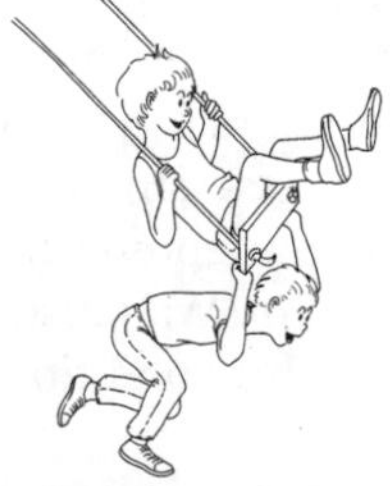			

the instructor is aware that the child can not do the task when there is no supervision but can do it when someone ensures she or he has time to try.

The second level is one in which the assessor **verbally prompts** the child towards a solution. This can be done through the provision of general suggestions as commands or questions ("Can you jump down from there?"), or specific suggestions about how to maximize the success of a solution ("Use both hands at once.").

The third level involves richer information provided to the child through **gestures or demonstrations** and can be coupled with verbal prompts to bring the child's attention to a specific aspect of the task ("Try it like this, Jamie, so that your knees are tucked up under you.").

The fourth, and most intrusive, level is one in which the assessor actually gives **physical assistance,** either partially or wholly, to help the child reach the task goal. The assistance may be minimal (catching the child at the bottom of the slide), or significant (holding the child's body weight as he or she hangs on a bar). The amount of physical help should be recorded so that it too can be reduced with instruction and practice.

It is recommended that during assessments assessors try to use the least intrusive prompts first to determine if the child can be relatively independent in performance. Once the instructor knows the conditions under which the task goal can be reached (the level of help required), then his or her job is to practice with the child until the goal can be reached independently. Specific teaching methods are described elsewhere in this textbook.

We would suggest using this framework to explore the conditions under which a child can and can not do a particularly valued solution to a task goal. For example, if a particular child does not report using the zipline though all the other members of his group do, the assessor may choose the zipline 'solutions' most valued (or used) by the cohort for

further assessment. She or he might give verbal directions and a demonstration first to see if the child can do the valued skills. If the child can not do the skill when asked or shown, then the assessor may want to give some slight physical support (perhaps holding the feet or knees). If this does not work, then more physical support or prompting can be used until the instructor finds a place at which to begin instruction. For a more complete discussion of these prompts please see Watkinson and Wall (1982).

A sample of an assessment checklist can be found in figure 15.8. The sample contains the task goal (swinging on a swing), and the skills or task solutions that have been seen most frequently on playgrounds. For each solution the assessor records whether the child can reach the task goal in free play alone, with a friend, or in a group. The assessor also records if the child can reach the task goal with the teacher present, with verbal prompts or instructions, with demonstrations or gestures, or with physical assistance. A further breakdown of these conditions can also be monitored using the definitions provided in Figure 15.7 (from Watkinson and Wall 1982). When instruction begins, the instructor can use these prompts to help the child attain the task solution he or she chooses.

Summary

The ecological task analysis model of assessment asks the assessor to be aware of the many factors that can influence performance and to record and monitor these during assessment. Unlike other assessment devices, an ETA assessment helps the instructor determine which task goals can be met and under what circumstances they can be met. It also provides for the acceptance of different task solutions to a movement problem. Used in conjunction with a prompting system such as the one described here, it can be used to determine which playground skills a child can do and can not do, and the circumstances in which they can and can not be done.

Study Questions

1. Choose a physical task in which you have recently engaged. Jot down all the factors that influence how well you can do this task at a particular time. Can you classify these as 'task', 'person', or 'environment' affordances and constraints? Are there any that can not be so classified? Justify these three categories as 'necessary and sufficient' to describe the influences on your performance.

2. What are the characteristics of an assessment device that is based on an assumption that we have abilities?

3. How do different tests and their protocols reflect the concern that performances vary according to the environment in which they are tested? How does an ETA approach address this 'problem'?

4. According to ETA, why is it problematic to attribute the performance of a child with disability to the disability itself? What does it mean to say there are 'covariates' of disability that can lead to poor motor performance?

References

Ames, C. (1984). Competitive and individualistic goal structures: A cognitive motivational analysis. In R. Ames and C. Ames (Eds.), *Research on motivation in education: student motivation* (pp. 177–207). New York: Academic Press.

Ames, C., and Ames, R. (1984a). Goal structures and motivation. *The Elementary School Journal, 85*(1), 39–52.

Ames, C., and Ames, R. (1984b). Systems of student and teacher motivation: Toward a qualitative definition. *Journal of Educational Psychology, 76*(4), 535–56.

Anastasi, A. (1958). Heredity, environment and the question 'How?'. *Psychological Review, 65*, 197–208.

Block, M.E. (1992). What is appropriate physical education for students with profound disabilities? *Adapted Physical Activity Quarterly, 9*, 197–213.

Borman, K.M., and Kurdek, L.A. (1987). Grade and gender differences in and the stability correlates of the structural complexity of children's playground games. *International Journal of Behavioural Development, 10*(2), 241–51.

Bouffard, M. (1997). Using old research ideas to study contemporary problems in adapted physical activity. *Measurement in Physical Education and Exercise Science, (1)*, 71–87.

Bouffard, M., Strean, W.B., and Davis, W.E. (1998). Questioning our philosophical and methodological research assumptions: Psychological perspectives. *Adapted Physical Activity Quarterly, 15*, 250–68.

Bruininks, R.H. (1978). *Bruininks-Oseretsky Test of Motor Proficiency, examiners manual.* Circle Pines, MN: American Guidance Service.

Burton, A.W., and Davis, W.E. (1996). Ecological task analysis: Utilizing intrinsic measures in research and practice. *Human Movement Science, 15*, 285–314.

Burton, A., and Miller, D. (1998). *Movement skill assessment.* Champaign, IL: Human Kinetics.

Davis, W.E. (1984). Motor ability assessment of populations with handicapping conditions: Challenging basic assumptions. *Adapted Physical Activity Quarterly, 1*(2), 125–40.

Davis, W.E., and Burton, A.W. (1991). Ecological task analysis: Translating movement behaviour theory into practice. *Adapted Physical Activity Quarterly, 8*(2), 154–77.

Davis, W., and van Emmerik, R. (1995a). An ecological task analysis approach for understanding motor development in mental retardation: Philosophical and theoretical underpinnings. In A. Vermeer and W. Davis (Eds.), *Physical and motor development in mental retardation* (pp. 1–32). Basel: Karger.

Davis, W., and van Emmerik, R. (1995b). An ecological task analysis approach for understanding motor development in mental retardation: Research questions and strategies. In A. Vermeer and W. Davis (Eds.), *Physical and motor development in mental retardation* (pp. 33–66). Basel: Karger.

Eccles, J. (1992). School and family effects on the ontogeny of children's interests, self-perceptions, and activity choices. In J. Jacobs (Ed.), *Nebraska Symposium on Motivation, 1992: Developmental perspectives on motivation* (pp. 97–132). Lincoln: University of Nebraska Press.

Eccles, J., Wigfield, A., and Schiefele, U. (1998). Motivation to succeed. In W. Damon and N. Eisenberg (Eds.), *Handbook of child psychology.* New York: Wiley.

Gallahue, D.L. (1983). Assessing motor development in young children. *Studies in Educational Evaluation, 8*, 247–52.

Gentile, A.M. (1987). Skill acquisition: Action, movement, and neuromotor processes. In J. H. Carr, R. B. Shepherd, J. Gordon, A. M. Gentile, and J. M. Held (Eds.), *Movement science: Foundations for physical therapy in rehabilitation* (pp. 93–154). Rockville, MD: Aspen.

Halverson, L.E., and Williams, K. (1985). Developmental sequences for hopping over distance: A prelongitudinal study. *Research Quarterly for Exercise and Sport, 56*, 37–44.

Henderson, S., and Sugden, D. (1992). *Movement assessment battery for children.* Sidcup, Kent, England: The Psychological Corporation.

Herkowitz, J. (1978). Developmental task analysis: The design of movement experiences and evaluation of motor development status. In M. Ridenour (Ed.), *Motor development: Issues and applications* (pp. 139–64). Princeton, NJ: Princeton Book Company.

Lerner, R.M. (1976). *Concepts and theories of human development*. Reading, MA: Addison-Wesley.

Magill, R. (1998). *Motor learning: Concepts and applications* (5th ed.). Boston: McGraw-Hill.

Riggen K.J., Ulrich, D., and Ozmun, J. (1990). Reliability and concurrent validity of the test of motor impairment: Henderson revision. *Adapted Physical Activity Quarterly, 7*, 249–58.

Roberton, M.A. (1985). Changing motor patterns during childhood. In J.K. Thomas (Ed.), *Motor development during childhood and adolescence*. Minneapolis, MN: Burgess.

Roberton, M.A. (1982). Describing stages within and across motor tasks. In J.A.S. Kelso and J.E. Clark (Eds.), *The development of movement control and co-ordination* (pp. 293–307). New York: Wiley.

Schmidt, R.A. (1999). *Motor control and learning: A behavioral emphasis*. Champaign, IL: Human Kinetics.

Stephens, T., and Craig, C. (1990). *The well-being of Canadians: Highlights of the 1988 Campbell's survey*. Ottawa: Canadian Fitness and Lifestyle Research Institute.

Sugden, D., and Sugden, L. (1991). The assessment of movement skill problems in 7- and 9-year-old children. *British Journal of Educational Psychology, 61*, 329–45.

Ulrich, D.A. (1985). *Test of gross motor development*. Austin, TX: Pro-Ed.

Ulrich, D.A., Ulrich, B.D., and Branta, C.F. (1988). Developmental gross motor skill ratings: A generalizability analysis. *Research Quarterly for Exercise and Sport, 59*(3), 203–9.

Watkinson, E.J., and Causgrove-Dunn, J. (2001, July). *Assessing Criteria A and B for the identification of DCD: A context-specific approach to finding children at risk*. Paper presented at the 13th International Symposium for Adapted Physical Activity, Vienna.

Watkinson, E.J., Causgrove-Dunn, J., Cavaliere, N., Calzonetti, K., Wilhelm, L., and Dwyer, S. (2001). Engagement in playground activities as a criterion for diagnosing developmental coordination disorder. *Adapted Physical Activity Quarterly, 18*, 18–34.

Watkinson, E.J., Dwyer S., and Nielsen, A.B. (February, 2000). *Children theorizing about recess: Testing Eccles' expectancy value theory*. Paper presented at the Qualitative Methods Conference, Edmonton, AB.

Watkinson, E.J., and Wall, A.E. (1982). *The PREP programme: A preschool play programme for moderately mentally retarded children*. Ottawa: Canadian Association for Health Physical Education and Recreation.

Wickstrom, R.L. (1983). *Fundamental motor patterns*. Philadelphia: Lea and Febiger.

Wigfield, A. (1994). Expectancy-value theory of achievement motivation: A developmental perspective. *Educational Psychology Review, 6*, 49–78.

CHAPTER 16

Instructional Approaches to the Teaching of Motor Skills

Donna L. Goodwin

Learning Objectives

- To identify the various instructional approaches that have been used in the teaching of motor skills.
- To discuss the relationship between the learner and the instructor within each of the instructional approaches.
- To distinguish between the various instructional approaches given the underlying assumptions upon which they are based.
- To illustrate how a particular instructional approach could be applied to the teaching of a specific motor skill.

Introduction

Various approaches to instruction have guided the teaching of motor skills in adapted physical activity (APA) over the past eighty years. Although seldom mutually exclusive in practice, each instructional approach reflects inherent assumptions about learning and about disability. The skill instruction approaches that have received the most attention are, (a) remedial therapy wherein medical knowledge is deemed necessary to the prescription of exercise, (b) a developmental perspective in which an assessment of the developmental level provides prerequisite information about skill instruction, (c) perceptual motor programming that purported movement to be the basis of academic success, (d) behavioural approaches which utilize response cueing, shaping, and reinforcement procedures, (e) a cognitive approach that conceptualizes human functioning as the processing of information, (f) an ecological approach that places learner processes within the context of the instructional environment and the task itself, and (g) a strategic orientation that emphasizes the instruction of self-regulatory cognitive behaviours.

The intent in reviewing each of the approaches is not to suggest that one is superior to another. The richness and depth of instruction required for successful motor skill acquisition by persons with disabilities may be the result of a sensitive blending of approaches depending upon the nature of the disability and the performer's stage of learning (i.e., early coordination or getting the idea of the movement stage versus the later control stage when the movement pattern is parameterized to the demands of the situation) (Magill 1998). The purpose of this chapter is to help us understand the various instructional approaches to the teaching of motor skills. The assumptions of each approach and the ensuing relationship between the instructor and the learner will be highlighted. Table 16.1 provides an overview of the role of the learner and the instructor for each instructional approach.

Each instructional approach has implicit ideas embedded within it. These embedded ideas take two forms, assumptions and implications. Assumptions refer to the historical roots of the idea (or theory) and how the world must be viewed for the idea to be true, whereas, implications refer to the consequences that logically follow if the idea is implemented (Slife and Williams 1995). By understanding what is embedded in each of the instructional approaches, teachers of APA can make informed choices about the techniques, strategies, and methods they select thereby making explicit their own assumptions about their teaching and the impact it may be having on the people with whom they are working. Table 16.2 provides a summary of how the various the instructional approaches can be applied to the teaching of kicking.

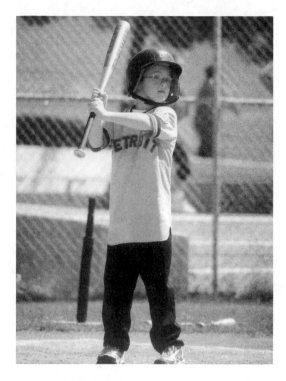

Remedial Therapy

The origins of APA can be traced back to corrective therapy and its roots in functional medicine or what was termed *medical gymnastics* (Sherrill 1988). The mid-1800s saw the prescription of passive, active, or resistive exercises prescribed by physicians or medical gymnasts. The purpose of the exercises was to develop and restore health to diseased body parts or to treat physical defects (Sherrill and DePauw 1997). Originating in Sweden, medical gymnastics was brought to North America in the late 1800s.

The medical model persisted into the 1950s in the form of corrective therapy. It was aimed at correcting orthopaedic and postural defects and other health conditions that prevented participation in vigorous physical activity (Sherrill and DePauw 1997). Corrective therapy also proved effective in meeting the needs of World War I and World War II veterans returning from combat. The human consequences of these wars provided the impetus to develop new orthopaedic surgical techniques, which precipitated the evolution of physical and rehabilitation medicine.

Table 16.1 A Comparison of Learner and Instructor Roles

Instructional approach	Role of the learner	Role of the instructor
Remedial therapy	Complete exercise routines prescribed by therapist	Ameliorate structural changes to the body
Developmental approach	Achieve tasks presented by instructor	Maximize performance by selecting and teaching task analysed learning objectives reflective of normal growth and development patterns to correct deficits in neural-maturation
Perceptual motor approach	Comply with prescribed perceptual motor activities	Enhance cognition by passively and engaging child in perceptual motor activities
Behavioural approach	Respond to external reinforcement and/or punishment schedules by approximating terminal motor behaviour	Shape desired motor behaviour by applying reinforcement and/or punishment procedures to sub-steps of desired terminal motor behaviour
Cognitive approach	Process and translate sensory information into temporally and sequentially organized movement patterns	Analyse the sensory, perceptual, and effector demands on the performer and provide practice at perceiving, storing, recalling, and outputting the desired response
Ecological systems approach	Solve the degrees of freedom problem through exploration and self-discovery	Within the context of the learner, adapt task and environmental constraints toward goal attainment
Strategic approach	Analyse, problem solve, and generalize task solving strategies	Teach metacognitive strategies such as readying, imaging, focussing, executing and evaluating

The physical medicine team at the time consisted of a physician, physical therapist, occupational therapist, and the new discipline of corrective therapy (Davis 1976).

The vision and pioneering work of Dr. Howard Rusk at the Veterans Administration Hospital in Perry Point, Maryland, led to the application of medically prescribed therapeutic exercises and activities to the treatment of combat injuries (Davis 1976; Stende 1975). Dr. Rusk explored the restorative effects of physical exercise and demonstrated its effectiveness by returning patients, who were previously confined to bed, to active service (Rusk 1966). In the event of permanent disabilities, the veterans could return to their home communities (Davis 1967).

The range and depth of the medically directed reconditioning procedures included exercises for mobilization, conditioning and reconditioning, and pre- and postoperative management. In addition, training was provided in postural alignment, gait management, cane and crutch walking, and ramp climbing techniques. Not only did the therapist demonstrate exercises and training procedures, but there was also an expectation that the patient would learn the exercises and be able to complete them unsupervised.

One of the first physicians to be actively involved in using retraining and reconditioning through sport was Sir Ludwig Guttmann of the National Spinal Injuries Centre, Stoke Mandeville Hospital, Aylesbury, England. He was commissioned by the British government during the Second World War to develop a programme "to maximize the physical and psychological equilibrium of the disabled person and thus enable him to come to terms with his physical defect and face up to daily life in spite of his disability" (Guttmann 1960, p. 29). Participation in sport as a natural rehabilitative process was found to be a more interesting form of rehabilitation than clinical exercises (Rosen 1973). In fact, sporting activities were included in the medical treatment of injured servicemen (Guttmann 1967). In addition to including sport as a component of the rehabilitation process while in hospital, it was believed that an opportunity to participate in sport after being discharged was also needed. In response, the first Stoke Mandeville Games were held on July 28, 1948, on the same day the Olympic Games opened in London (Guttmann 1975). From a small beginning of only sixteen ex-members of the British armed forces (fourteen men and two women), an international disability sport movement was born (see Chapter 26 (Steadward and Foster) for more information on the history and development of disability sport).

The increased public awareness that resulted from soldiers returning home forged new public attitudes toward persons with disabilities and their ability to be active members of their communities. The notion of reconditioning exercises expanded beyond veterans in rehabilitation hospitals to include those who experienced paralysis due to accidents or the polio epidemics of the thirties and forties (Clarke and Clarke 1978; Sherrill and DePauw 1997).

During this period, school personnel also recognized the health benefits of exercise and fitness activities and the educational value of games, dance, and gymnastics in the overall development of children (Brace 1949). Regular physical education emerged as school personnel became responsible, not for therapy or treatment, but for fitness, game, and sport skill development. Physical reconditioning exercises were taken beyond the therapy room and into the gymnasium within the context of games and sport (Sherrill and DePauw 1997).

During the 1950s physical education within special education programmes for children with disabilities developed, as the philosophies of corrective therapy and education began to merge (Sherrill 1998). Adapted physical education was first defined by the American Association of Health Physical Education, Recreation and Dance in 1952 as a "diversified program of developmental activities, games, sport, and rhythms suited to the interests, capacities, and limitations of students with disabilities who may not safely or successfully engage in unrestricted participation in the vigorous activities of the general physical education programs" (DePauw 1996, p. 103). The tradition of corrective therapy influenced early adapted physical education instruction (DePauw 1996). In fact, exercise for postural correction remains an integral component of our current APA professional preparation (Winnick 1990; Sherrill 1998). Readers are referred to Sherrill and DePauw (1997) for an exhaustive review of the evolution of medical and corrective therapy as it applies to the emergence of APA.

ASSUMPTIONS

A remedial approach to instruction assumes that a disability is largely biological in nature (Hedlund 2000). The resulting medical approach to exercise and physical activity for persons with disabilities separates the physiologic disease process or illness from the rest of the person. The illness or disability becomes disembodied or objectified as it is separated and distanced from the social self and the fullness of the human experience (Leder 1985). The resulting illness focus brings attention to the structural change in the body, rather than a disturbance in a person's ability to function

Table 16.2 Application of the Instructional Approaches to the Skill of Kicking

Instructional strategy	Application to kicking	
Remedial therapy	Resistance weight training exercises to restore quadriceps strength	
	Stretching activities to restore hamstring flexibility	
Developmental approach	Developmental task analysis Kick a 12-inch beach ball Kick a junior-sized soccer ball Kick a 4-inch rubber utility ball	Hierarchical task analysis Push stationary ball with straight knee Kick stationary ball with bent knee Kick stationary ball with bent knee and extended hip with follow through
Behavioural approach	Track the number of correct kicks completed, with positive reinforcement across instructional days	
Cognitive approach	Modify the state of the system to increase task complexity Stand and kick a stationary ball Stand and kick a rolling ball Run and kick a rolling ball	
Ecological systems approach	Allow performer to choose the skill and movement form to use to put ball in play in game of soccer Kick the ball the foot (while standing, while seated) Kick the ball with an implement (forearm crutch, floor hockey stick) Throw the ball (two-handed overhand throw, one-handed throw, roll the ball)	
Strategic approach	Teach a five-step process to improved kicking Get ready Imagine the kick Focus on ball contact Do it Evaluate the performance	

and relate to the world (Baron 1985). The primary focus becomes the biological and therapeutic processes, with less emphasis given to understanding the social and personal impact of the illness or disability (Wheeler 1998). In doing so, the body is handed over to the physician, clinician, or therapist and placed in his or her care. The person becomes somewhat passive in his or her own physical management as interventionists work to fix the problem (Conrad 1990; Leder 1985).

Although independence and the return to either active duty or the community were the rehabilitative goals, the person with a disability was still perceived to be a 'victim' of a severe misfortune. A state of dependency was assumed (Alger and Rusk 1955; Dembo, Ladieu Leviton, and Wright 1956). The disability was perceived to be biological in nature, and the protective setting of the hospital or other care facility was assumed to be most appropriate for 'patient' rehabilitation.

With prescribed bedrest, the sense of weakness increasingly reinforced the state of dependency; loss of function and ill health of the person became more firmly entrenched. Although the goal of hospital care was to return the patient to a functional existence, the hospital setting may have unwittingly undermined the socially valued behaviours of independence and self-reliance by assigning the role of patient to those with disabilities (Alger and Rusk 1955; Davis 1967).

To this point the discussion has not really addressed instruction. This is due in part to the lack of skill instruction that is inherent in the medical model. Intervention consisted of repeated exercises for the purposes of restoring function, with no view to the learning of new movement skills. It is a model that inherently removes personal responsibility for well-being by placing the individual in a setting of care and rehabilitation until such time as the person can resume care and responsibility for him- or herself (Condeluci 1991). There is a further assumption that the period of time will be relatively short, and that once the person has received a regiment of care, function will be returned and normal life activities will resume.

---

1 What was the purpose of rehabilitation exercises and why were they perceived to be important?

---

2 How does our current understanding of adapted physical education differ from the 1952 definition?

---

3 What is the consequence of objectifying illness or disability?

Developmental Approach

Early research by child psychologists on movement skills carefully documented the progressions of sitting, standing, walking, running, grasping, and throwing. Collectively, these studies provided the foundation for future research on human motor development (Ames 1937; Gesell 1930; Bayley 1935; McGraw 1941; Shirley 1931; Wild 1938). This research was descriptive in nature and done within the framework of developmental theory (Espenschade and Eckert 1967; Rarick 1973; Roberton 1982). In contrast to the medical approach of remedial therapy, a developmental approach to the teaching of motor skills explored the changing profiles of motor development that occur with age (Haywood 1993).

The developmental continuum, specific to the motor domain, encompasses the hierarchy of infant reflex activity (e.g., grasp, moro, walking reflex) through the development of fundamental motor skills (e.g., bouncing, kicking) in early childhood (Cowden, Sayers, and Torrey 1998). Fundamental motor skills are subsequently applied in lead up games or transitional motor activities (e.g., four square, kick ball) and finally utilized in culturally determined individual and group games and sports (e.g., basketball, soccer) (Haywood 1993).

Three further skill classifications are typically included in the fundamental level of the hierarchy: locomotion (e.g., running, leaping, jumping), nonlocomotion (e.g., twisting, curling, bending), and projection and reception of objects (e.g., throw, kick, catch, trap) (Wickstrom 1983; Davis and Burton 1991). These skills are considered to be fundamental because they are perceived necessary to the optimal development of more complex game and sport skills. What was termed a proficiency barrier (Rose and Heath 1990; Seefeldt 1980) prompted instructional interest in motor skills for children who appeared to demonstrate difficulty moving through the hierarchy of skill development (Seefeldt 1980).

In the 1960s, physical education scholars provided leadership in motor development, and the concept of stages emerged (Seefeldt and Haubenstricker 1982). Longitudinal and cross-sectional studies provided the foundation for the biomechanical labelling of fundamental motor skill stages (Halverson 1966; Hellebrandt, Rarick, Glassow, and Carns 1961; Roberton 1978; Seefeldt 1980), which are well summarized in the works of Espenschade and Eckert (1967) and Wickstrom (1983).

Although a great deal of information contributed to our understanding of the sequential progressions involved in motor development, little was offered by way of practical information for teachers of movement skills. It was not until teachers were asked to instruct children with developmental disabilities that the utility of motor skill stages for instructional purposes became evident (Seefeldt 1980; Ulrich 2000; Wessel 1975). The intent of motor skill instruction was to challenge the child to perform at maximum capacity within the naturally occurring framework of typical growth and development patterns. "It implies the process of generating a motor response with increasing complexity, appropriateness, accuracy, and specificity along the entire developmental continuum" (Seaman and DePauw 1982, p. 18).

Instruction in adapted physical education for children with developmental disabilities focussed on the achievement of movement patterns typical of children without disabilities and to the highest stage or level possible (Watkinson and Wall 1982). It became clear, however, that the criteria identified within the substages of fundamental motor skills were often too complex for children with disabilities to achieve. Numerous forms of task analysis evolved as a means of systematically breaking the subtasks down even further for the purpose of instruction, two of which will be discussed here.

DEVELOPMENTAL TASK ANALYSIS
Halverson (1966) described the influence of environmental conditions on the motor patterns of children. She noted that children's overarm throwing and striking regressed to earlier patterns when the demands of the environment placed too much stress on their present stage of motor development. At the same time, she purported that progress to a more mature pattern occurred when the stimulus was carefully considered so as to effectively stimulate performance just beyond the children's current level of achievement. Herkowitz (1978) and Morris (1980) later introduced *developmental task analysis* and

proposed that the environment can be analyzed according to its influence on motor development.

Herkowitz (1978) identified environmental variables that limit motor skill acquisition in the two categories of general task analysis (GTA) and specific task analysis (STA). GTA defines the task and environmental factors influencing movement behaviour, while STA more specifically defines the characteristics of these factors for instructional purposes. For example, the GTA indicates that ball size, weight, speed, and trajectory all influence the movement of striking (see figure 16.1). Each of these factors can, in turn, be further analyzed using the STA to reveal that the ball size can vary from two to twelve inches in diameter, the length of the implement can be changed, and finally the ball can be rolled, bounced, or tossed. Through the process of GTA and STA, instructors can assess motor skill development status and sequence movement experiences, presumably from less to more difficult tasks. Herkowitz (1978) acknowledged that intuition, and not empirical evidence, was used to formulate the ordering of variables. Davis and Burton (1991) provide a very good overview of the role of developmental task analysis strategies in adapted physical activity instruction.

HIERARCHICAL TASK ANALYSIS
Task analysis procedures, within the realm of APA, have been used primarily for two purposes: (a) to analyze complex skills so as to identify their component parts, and (b) to provide instructional content for their sequential acquisition (Block 2001; Kennedy, Esque, and Novak 1983; Reigeluth 1983). The process typically involves breaking the task down behaviourally into constituent elements, determining the instructional relationship among these subtasks, and outlining instructional strategies such as verbal, physical, and environmental prompting (Watkinson and Wall 1982; Winnick 1990). Referred to as *hierarchical task analysis* (Dick and Carey 1978), this approach typically places the terminal objective (the last skill the learner will perform)

Figure 16.1 General Task Analysis for Striking Behaviour

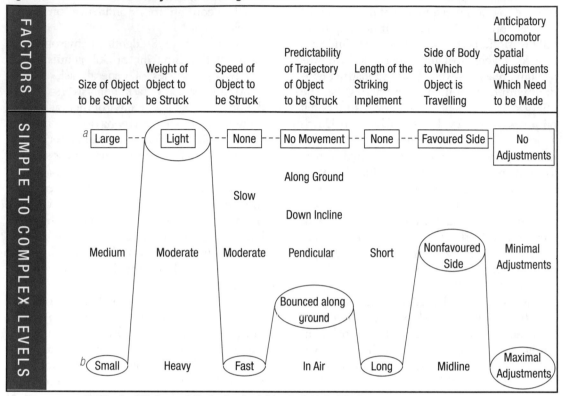

FACTORS	Size of Object to be Struck	Weight of Object to be Struck	Speed of Object to be Struck	Predictability of Trajectory of Object to be Struck	Length of the Striking Implement	Side of Body to Which Object is Travelling	Anticipatory Locomotor Spatial Adjustments Which Need to be Made

a Profile of a GTA for a relatively simple striking task (dotted line).
b Profile of a GTA for a relatively complex striking task (solid line).

SOURCE: From Developmental Task Analysis: The Design of Movement Experiences and Evaluation of Motor Development Status by J. Herkowitz, 1978, in M. Ridenour (Ed.), *Motor Development: Issues and Applications* (pp. 139–64). Princeton, NJ: Princeton Books Co. Reprinted with permission.

at the top of the hierarchy. Below the terminal behaviour are subordinate skills that must be achieved. Hierarchical task analysis provided a way in which to bring about behavioural change through the direct instruction of motor skills. However, breaking the task down into subtasks can, in essence, create new tasks that are different from the mature skill form.

A number of movement skill instructional programmes, based on developmental theory, and utilizing hierarchical task analysis, were designed and validated for use by instructors of children with disabilities. The work of Watkinson and Wall (1982) with the PREP programme and Wessel (1975) with the I CAN programme are two exemplary examples of

such programmes. The PREP Instructional Model was designed to facilitate the achievement of play skills by children (three to twelve years old) with developmental disabilities. Observational assessment of free play behaviour precedes a comprehensive criterion referenced assessment of the children's competencies. The resulting learner profile identifies the children's strengths and developmental weaknesses in the areas of locomotion (e.g., running, jumping, hopping, ascending and descending stairs), large play equipment (e.g., climbing, sliding down a slide), small play equipment (e.g., throwing, catching, kicking), and play vehicles (e.g., tricycles, scooters) (see figure 16.2). Based on the assessment information specific behaviourally

Figure 16.2 An Excerpt from the PREP Preschool Play Programme Individualized Student Profile

Individual Student Profile

Teacher's Name Student's NameDate

Skills for Locomotion	Performs with a Phyical Prompt	Performs witha Visual Prompt	Perofrms witha Verbal Prompt	Initiates in Free Play (No Prompt)
Running				
1. Walks quickly	□	□	□	□
2. Runs with instances of non-support	□	□	□	□
3. Runs with bent arms moving in opposition to legs	□	□	□	□
4. Runs quickly dodging obstacles	□	□	□	□
Ascending Stairs				
1. Crawls up stairs on hands and knees	□	□	□	□
2. Ascends stairs marking time with support	□	□	□	□
3. Ascends stairs alternating feet with support	□	□	□	□
4. Ascends stairs alternating feet without support	□	□	□	□
Descending Stairs				
1. Descends stairs on seat	□	□	□	□
2. Descends stairs marking time with support	□	□	□	□
3. Descends stairs alternating feet with support	□	□	□	□
4. Descends stairs alternating feet without support	□	□	□	□
Jumping Down				
1. Steps off box of shin height.	□	□	□	□
2. Jumps down off box of shin height, two foot take-off and landing	□	□	□	□
3. Jumps down off box of knee height, two foot take-off and landing	□	□	□	□
4. Jumps down off box of hip height, two foot take-off and landing	□	□	□	□

	Performs with a Phyical Prompt	Performs witha Visual Prompt	Perofrms witha Verbal Prompt	Initiates in Free Play (No Prompt)
Jumping Over				
1. Steps over a line on floor	□	□	□	□
2. Jumps over a line, one foot to other foot	□	□	□	□
3. Jumps over a line, two foot take-off and landing	□	□	□	□
Hopping on One Foot				
1. Stands momentarily on one foot	□	□	□	□
2. Bounces on one foot without leaving floor	□	□	□	□
3. Hops in place on one foot three times	□	□	□	□
4. Hops forward three times on one foot	□	□	□	□
Forward Roll				
1. Rolls into sitting position	□	□	□	□
2. Rolls into squatting position	□	□	□	□
Backward Roll				
1. Rocks backwars onto shoulders	□	□	□	□
2. Rolls over onto shins	□	□	□	□
3. Rolls over to crouch	□	□	□	□
Skills for Large Play Equipment				
Ascending an Inclined Bench on Stomach				
1. Slides along bench on stomach by pulling with hands	□	□	□	□
2. Slides up inclined bench on stomach by pulling with hands	□	□	□	□
Ascending an Inclined Bench on Hands and Knees				
1. Crawls along bench on hands and knees	□	□	□	□
2. Crawls up inclined bench on hands and knees	□	□	□	□

	Performs with a Phyical Prompt	Performs witha Visual Prompt	Perofrms witha Verbal Prompt	Initiates in Free Play (No Prompt)
Walking up an Inclined Bench				
1. Walks along a bench	□	□	□	□
2. Walks along a narrow bench or beam	□	□	□	□
3. Walks up an inclined bench	□	□	□	□
Jumps on a Trampoline				
1. Bounces on hands and knees	□	□	□	□
2. Bounces standing without leaving surface	□	□	□	□
3. Bounces with instances of feet leaving bed	□	□	□	□
4. Jumps consecutively	□	□	□	□
Seat Drop on a Trampoline				
1. Jumps, lands sitting on bed	□	□	□	□
2. Jumps, drops to seat, bounces back to feet	□	□	□	□
3. Drops to seat and continues jumping	□	□	□	□
Swivel Hips on a Trampoline				
1. Does seat drop, jumps and turns 90°	□	□	□	□
2. Does seat drop, jumps and turns 90° twice and does another seat drop	□	□	□	□
3. Does seat drop, jumps and turns 180°, jumps and does another seat drop	□	□	□	□
4. Does seat drop and turns 180° to go directly into another seat drop	□	□	□	□
Sliding Down a Slide				
1. Slide on seat	□	□	□	□
2. Slide on tummy, feet first	□	□	□	□
3. Slide on tummy, head first	□	□	□	□
Climbing on a Box				
1. Climbs onto hip high box	□	□	□	□
2. Climbs onto chest high box	□	□	□	□
Swinging on a Rope				
1. Holds on with hands while being swung	□	□	□	□
2. Holds on and locks legs while being swung	□	□	□	□
3. Swings on rope	□	□	□	□

	Performs with a Phyical Prompt	Performs witha Visual Prompt	Perofrms witha Verbal Prompt	Initiates in Free Play (No Prompt)
Swinging on a Bar				
1. Hangs from a bar with hands	□	□	□	□
2. Steps off (bench) to hang on bar	□	□	□	□
3. Swings on bar	□	□	□	□
4. Swings on bar, returns to (bench)	□	□	□	□
Swinging on a Swing				
1. Sits on seat and holds on while being pushed	□	□	□	□
2. Mounts swing and sits while being pushed	□	□	□	□
3. Pumps swing	□	□	□	□
Hanging from Knees on a Horizontal Ladder				
1. Hangs from hands and knees on adjacent rungs of horizontal ladder	□	□	□	□
2. Hangs from hands and knees on single rung of horizontal ladder	□	□	□	□
3. Hangs from knees on horizontal ladder	□	□	□	□
Rolling Around a Bar				
1. Supports himself grasping bar and flexing hips	□	□	□	□
2. Rolls over bar to sitting position on floor	□	□	□	□
3. Rolls over bar to land on feet	□	□	□	□
Ascending Ladder				
1. Ascends 5 rungs, marking time	□	□	□	□
2. Ascends 5 rungs, hands and feet alternately landing on same rung	□	□	□	□
3. Ascends 5 rungs, hands and feet alternately landing on next rung	□	□	□	□
4. Ascends 10 rungs, hands and feet alternately landing on next rung	□	□	□	□
5. Ascends 10 rungs, alternating hands and feet simultaneously	□	□	□	□

SOURCE: From PREP: *A Preschool Play Programme*, by E.J. Watkinson and A.E. Wall, 1982, Ottawa, ON: CAHPER. Reprinted with permission.

Figure 16.3 Individual Record of Progress for Basketball from the I CAN Program

I CAN						Individual Record of Progress			
SPORT, LEISURE, and RECREATION SKILLS						**BASKETBALL**			

STUDENT NAME_____

BIRTHDATE_____
month   year

Levels of Student Performance	Chest Pass	One-Hand Set Shot	Dribbling	Lay-Up	Rebounding	Guarding	Pivot	Participation
1	/	/	/	/	/	/	/	/
2	/	/	/	/	/	/	/	/
3	/	/	/	/	/	/	/	/
4	/	/	/	/	/	/	/	/
5	/	/	/	/	/	/	/	/
6	/	/	/	/	/	/	/	/
	mo. yr.*	mo. yr.	mo. yr.	mo. yr.	mo. yr.	mo. yr.	mo. yr.	mo. yr.

*Record month and year in which the level of performance was attained.

Permission is hereby granted to reproduce this form for use in connection with the I CAN Sport, Leisure, and Recreation Skills program.

SOURCE: From *I CAN Sport, Leisure, and Recreation Skills Program* by J.A. Wessel, 1978, East Lansing: Michigan State University. Reprinted with permission.

defined, task analysed skills are targeted for individualized instruction.

The I CAN Curriculum Project (Wessel 1975) also presents individualized physical education instructional materials by providing a system of diagnostic and prescriptive teaching based on task-analysed sequences of fundamental motor skills and fitness activities. Learner progress records are provided to facilitate the recording of entry-level performance, their progress, and rate of learning. Progress is measured and monitored by keeping daily performance data on instructional objectives (figure 16.3).

ASSUMPTIONS

An underlying assumption of a developmental approach is that neural-maturation is primarily responsible for the development of an individual (Thelan and Smith 1994). When applied to motor skill development, individual progress from simple movements to more complex movements occurs because of qualitative advancement in the biological make up of the person. This assumption resulted in limited effort to understand the processes involved in behavioural change for the forty-year period following the rich, descriptive work of the developmental psychologists of the 1930s and 1940s (Thelan and Smith 1994). From an instructional point of view, it meant that only when the naturally occurring maturation process fell behind to the degree that an individual experienced difficulty acquiring motor skills was an effort made to externally bring the system back "up to speed."

The developmental approach to motor skill acquisition was a systematic way for children with performance disorders to approximate developmental norms (Seaman and DePauw 1982). Accordingly, teaching physical activity from a developmental perspective means assigning instructional goals that have been defined by the developmental stages typical of normal motor development (Hellison 1991). An assumption of, and valuing of, normalcy is therefore implicit in the developmental approach to instruction (Shogan 1998). The emergence of typical progressions of motor skill acquisition serves to divide the population into standard and nonstandard populations (Shogan 1998). In-depth descriptive research provides a template of normal motor skill development with which we can compare the progress of most learners.

Deviations from the way things 'should be' create the need for intervention. Intervention, in turn, focusses on reducing the 'learner's' problem by modifying motor behaviour toward the norm. This implies a further assumption that learners with disabilities can replicate the stages of normal development. However, we know that learners whose development has been altered by neurological or structural influences may not be able to reproduce normative established movement forms behaviourally (Kalnins et al. 1999). Indeed, if motor skill acquisition is solely interpreted from a traditional motor development perspective, then the goal of motor skill acquisition may be unattainable by and inappropriate for some learners.

Learners' competence is therefore based upon their success or failure in meeting the template criteria (Jenkins and Jenkins 1985). Any "performance disorder" is perceived to lie clearly with the learner. "Whatever is found wrong with the student, or whatever the student hasn't learned, becomes the focus of special instruction" (Simpson, Poplin, and Stone 1992, p. 158). The role of the learner is to achieve predetermined tasks and subtasks as presented by the instructor. If successful, it is the responsibility of the learner to take the parts and reintegrate them into the whole and generalize that learning to other settings. Generalization of learning, or lack of it, is perceived to be a problem of the learner. This presumption has been so pervasive in our instructional practices within the developmental approach that the inability to generalize has become an accepted descriptor of children with disabilities (Simpson, Poplin, and Stone 1992). Consequently, a further inherent assumption of hierarchical task analysis is that learning of the subtasks will generalize to the acquisition of the terminal task and its subsequent application in other settings or times.

A final assumption of the developmental approach to the instruction of motor skills rests with the proficiency barrier. Lack of competence in fundamental skills was perceived to be a barrier to success in more advanced skills or those higher up the hierarchical chain of performance. The validity of the proficiency barrier has been recently questioned (Burton and Miller 1998). In an alternate taxonomy, Burton and Miller (1998) present six levels of motor skills, acknowledging that specialized skills may emerge before the movements of the early milestone or the fundamental skill levels are achieved. In their taxonomy, the first level, foundations of movement, includes such things as cognition, knowledge, motivation, and postural control. The second level consists of motor abilities. Assessments of abilities measures such constructs as balance, agility, and coordination. The next three levels of the taxonomy match the traditional developmental levels of early milestone movements, fundamental movements, and specialized movement skills. *Specialized skills*, in this instance, refers to skills that involve combinations or variations of one or more of the early movement milestones and/or fundamental movement skills.

The sixth and final level is termed *functional movement skills*. It refers to early, fundamental, or specialized skills that are performed in their natural setting and within a meaningful context. A functional movement skill, for example, may be a young child learning to sit up in a crib, or a youth engaged in throwing snowballs at a friend (Burton and Miller 1998).

The significant difference between the two taxonomies, from an instructional perspective, rests with the notion that children with disabilities do not need to achieve the underlying or prerequisite fundamental motor skills before receiving instruction in specialized skills. There is some support for the emergence of specialized skills before fundamental skills are achieved that has resulted from an investigation of the developmental validity of traditional learn-to-swim progressions (Gelinas and Reid 2000). In a study of forty children with physical disabilities, five to twelve years of age, it was determined that most children could achieve the specialized skill and functional task goal of front crawl. They were able to do so when they were free to make their own movement choices, while at the same time not achieving all of the prerequisite skills of rhythmic breathing, front float, and front glide.

In summary, in the developmental approach, the teaching and learning process is typically viewed as unidirectional. The instructor's role is to identify the learning objectives for those learners who are not progressing through the developmental stages or achieving the stage levels within a specified time period and to teach them directly using predetermined and standardized movement sequences (task analysed to reduce complexity). The teacher measures progress through daily performance records (criterion-referenced assessment and instruction).

4 What is the proficiency barrier and why has it been refuted?

5 What is the distinction between developmental and hierarchical task analysis?

6 Is it conceivable that all children with disabilities would benefit from a developmental approach to instruction? Why or why not?

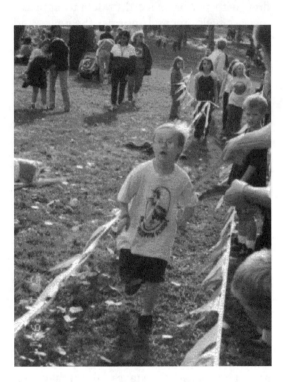

Perceptual Motor Programming

Motor skill instruction in the 1960s was strongly influenced by perceptual motor training programmes. Perceptual motor theory postulated that motor activities, when properly applied, could prepare children for spelling, reading, and other intellectual endeavours (Delacato 1963). Such theorists as Kephart (1960), Getman (1962), and Ayres (1965), representing the disciplines of psychology, optometry, and occupational therapy, respectively, influenced perceptual-motor practice. It was during this period that the proposed relationship between motor and academic proficiency resulted in perceptual motor programmes being the most popular intervention approach for children with learning disabilities. Clinicians noted that children's learning disabilities often had motor deficiencies concomitant with their academic difficulties (Reid 1981).

Delecato's theory of neurological organization provided the impetus for what was later determined to be unsubstantiated research claims regarding enhanced intelligence and corrective treatment for brain damage. The Institute for the Achievement of Human Potential proposed recapitulating or repeating the stages of motor development through which a child passes as remedial therapy for children with severe sensory or motor impairments (Freeman 1967). Referred to as *patterning*, passive and active activities often revolved around obstacle courses, balance beams, tunnels, visual tracking, body-image exercises, and jumping on trampolines (Reid 1981).

Bryant Cratty, a physical educator, contributed to the perceptual-motor training era and wrote numerous books in the area (e.g., 1969, 1970, 1973, and 1975). His underlying aim was to improve fitness and motor and physical development and not to enhance academic success (Sherrill and DePauw 1997). Cratty believed that perceptual motor programmes developed motor abilities and contributed to academic success only if the child was engaged in thinking of the academic task during that movement activity (Cratty 1973). One of the benefits of the perceptual-motor training era was an increased awareness of the motor skill development needs of children who were awkward (Reid 1981).

ASSUMPTIONS

Proponents of perceptual motor programming assumed that the hierarchical nature of stages meant that all tasks that develop before others were prerequisites for subsequent tasks. The further premise that motor and perceptual training could transfer to enhanced cognition was called into question as extravagant claims and demanding programmes for parents, educators, and clinicians resulted in limited outcomes (Cratty 1975). A meta-analysis of 180 studies assessing the efficacy of perceptual-motor training programmes concluded that the programmes were based on informal and subjective investigations and that, "perceptual-motor training is not effective and should be questioned as a feasible intervention technique for exceptional children" (Kavale and Mattson 1983, p. 165). For a comprehensive discussion of the controversy surrounding the validity of the claimed results of the Institute for the Achievement of Human Potential, you are referred to Freeman (1967), Kavale and Mattson (1983), Robbins (1966) and the Official Statement on The Doman-Delacato Treatment of Neurologically Handicapped Children (1968).

---

7 Why was perceptual motor programming abandoned as a treatment for children with brain damage?

---

8 What assumption lead to the practice of recapitulating early stages of motor development for children with severe sensory or motor impairment?

Behavioural Approach

Behaviourists assume that human behaviour does not just happen; it is conditioned by the consequences that result from our actions to certain stimuli (Rachlin 1991). This suggests that, although we are capable of responding to the environment in which we live, we do not need to carry out actions consciously or with purpose; "all human behaviours are essentially…automatic" (Slife and Williams 1995, p. 25). Our responses to the demands of the environment, or stimulus, are hence combinations of simpler responses that have been conditioned by their favourable consequence (reinforcement) or outcome. Because of reinforcement histories, or the strength of the connection between the stimulus and response, we are more likely to be conditioned to repeat some behaviour over others. When the response occurs in the presence of stimuli other than the one to which the behaviour was conditioned, it is considered to have generalized (Schunk 1996).

Three elements are essential to a behavioural approach: a stimulus, a response, and a reinforcing consequence to the behaviour (Schunk 1996). The stimulus, because of some quality, sets the occasion for the response. A response is emitted, thereby resulting in an observable behaviour that can be reinforced. The reinforcement, in turn, can become the stimulus for the behaviour to be repeated, thereby building the link between the stimulus and response and increasing the likelihood the response will occur in the future. There are four basic procedures used to change the likelihood or rate of occurrence of a response occurring:

a. positive reinforcement
b. negative reinforcement
c. positive punishment
d. negative punishment (Rachlin 1991)

In teaching and learning settings, differential reinforcement and punishment procedures and schedules can be used to shape our behaviour to the desired form or rate (Domjan 1993).

Positive reinforcement, also called *reward*, increases the likelihood that the response will occur in the future by providing a consequence that is perceived favourably by the person (e.g., performers' better use of arms results in praise from the coach). *Negative reinforcement*, also called *escape*, involves removing a consequence contingent upon a response that is negatively valued by the person (e.g., the coach's criticism of the poor arm use is withheld with improved performance). In this case, the young person avoids criticism by improving arm performance.

In contrast, *punishment* is a form of reinforcement that is used to weaken the connection between the stimulus and response and decrease the likelihood the response will occur in the future. Providing an aversive or

Figure 16.4 The Relationships Among the Four Basic Procedures That Can be Used to Influence Behaviour

	Stimulus presented	Stimulus removed
Positively valued stimulus	Reinforcement	Negative punishment
Negatively valued stimulus	Punishment	Negative reinforcement

SOURCE: Adapted from *Introduction to Modern Behaviorism* by H. Rachlin, 1991, New York: W.H. Freeman and Company. Reprinted with permission.

negatively valued consequence following behaviour is referred to as *positive punishment* (e.g., doing extra pushups for speaking out of turn). The punishment procedure can also be negative in that behaviour is followed by the removal of a stimulus that is positively valued by the individual (e.g., loss of facility privileges because of a curfew violation). *Negative reinforcement* has also been referred to as *omission* (Rachlin 1991; Schunk 1996). Figure 16.4 shows the relationships among the four basic procedures that can be used to influence behaviour.

When successive approximations of the required response are reinforced, the desired behaviour is referred to as *shaping* (Domjan 1993). Behavioural change brought about by shaping has often been paired with the successive approximations made possible by the task analysis approaches previously described. Because an action cannot be rewarded unless it occurs, complex patterns must emerge or be shaped from simpler structures. To shape a behaviour, the following sequence is commonly adhered to:

a. identify what the student can do (entry behaviour)
b. identify the desired (terminal) behaviour
c. identify potential reinforcers in the student's environment

d. break the terminal behaviour (task analyze) into small sub-steps to be mastered and

e. move the student from the entry behaviour to the terminal behaviour by successively reinforcing each approximation of the terminal behaviour (Schunk 1996, p. 77)

In summary, human motor action is complex and is often composed of actions that are chained together. A series of discrete skills may be chained together and thereby acquire a new functional utility when successfully implemented. Each component of the chain, once completed, becomes a stimulus for the next component (Keller 1969). For example, the terminal behaviour of tricycle riding can be broken down into the discrete tasks of skills of mounting, dismounting, pedaling, and steering. Learning how to get on the tricycle becomes the stimulus for pedaling the tricycle, which in turn becomes the stimulus for steering. Each of these discrete tasks can be shaped using reinforcement procedures and, when chained together, result in the skill of tricycle riding.

Behavioural shaping has been used successfully to teach leisure skills such as table games and bowling (Wall and Gast 1997; Chen, Zhang, Lange, Miko, and Joseph 2001), gross motor skills such as kicking, throwing, and striking (Dunn, Morehouse, and Fredericks 1986; Hanson and Harris 1986; Silliman and French 1993; Watkinson and Wall 1982; Zhang, Gast, Horvat, and Dattilo 1995), and increase uninterrupted time spent on motor tasks (Owlia, French, Ben-Ezra, and Silliman 1995; Silliman-French, French, Sherrill, and Gench 1998).

ASSUMPTIONS

Within a behavioural approach, human beings are essentially viewed as biological organisms that can be studied as any other biological organism, using the methods of natural science. That which is unobservable cannot be scientifically studied. As such, unobservable behaviours can not be controlled or used for the prediction of human behaviour and are overlooked (Schunk 1996). As learners, therefore, there is an assumption that we are not agents in our own learning, but rather that behaviour becomes associated with stimuli in precise and lawful ways because of external reinforcers (Slife and Williams 1995). In other words, behaviourist theory is strongly deterministic.

The behavioural approach, therefore, downgrades the importance of self-knowledge. Because attitudes, beliefs, opinions, values, personal will, and desires are "unobservable," the behavioural approach downgrades their importance. If we believe that learner responses are biologically determined and conditioned, as occurs with other biological organisms (animals), we further dismiss the notion of providing choice in how people learn and the meaning that learning brings to the learner.

Within adapted physical education instructional settings, a focus on conditioned responses to environmental stimuli may limit the educational experiences to which a person is exposed, while also disregarding responses that are not predicted by the instructor. In its strictest instructional form, a behaviourist teacher presents the stimulus to the learner based upon previously identified learning objectives, waits for the correct response given the presented stimulus and, once provided, controls the nature and frequency of the reinforcement that is provided. Responses that are creative, original, or alternate in form to that anticipated by the teacher may be disregarded or, in some cases, punished as being incorrect. Equating human learning to a more complex form of behaviour based upon operant conditioning experiments conducted on animals such as rats, pigeon, and apes has implications for the meaning we give to our teaching, how we think about our learners, and the meaning we give to the instructional relationship (Rachlin 1991).

9 What is the distinction between positive and negative reinforcement? Provide examples of each.

10 Identify the five steps commonly adhered to when shaping behaviour.

11 Why are the attitudes, beliefs, and values of the individual downgraded in a behavioural approach to instruction?

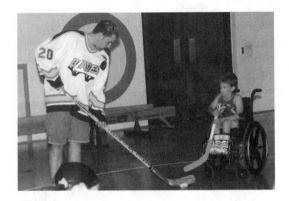

Cognitive Approach

Within a cognitive science approach to motor skill learning, we are conceptualized as processors of information (Fitts and Posner 1967; Magill 1998; Marteniuk 1976; Schmidt and Lee 1999). Information from the environment is taken into the human system through the perceptual system. Accepted information is held in a storage system (memory) and is processed or coded. Through a decision-making mechanism, the encoded information is combined with other information and an observable motor output or response is enacted. This model of information processing made reference to the "black box." The black box was considered to house the unobservable internal processes involved in transforming information into action (Schmidt and Lee 1999). By studying such things as reaction time and response patterns, inferences about events internal to the person inside the black box are made.

Whereas behavioural scientists are interested in the relationship between the stimulus (input into the black box) and the response (output from the black box), the cognitive scientist is interested in what occurs within the black box in terms of its capacity, its structure, and its function (Slife and Williams 1995). For example, within the motor domain, people have studied the effects of the manipulation of some of the input and output variables on performance and learning (e.g., use of selective attention or feedback specificity). Other people have studied what is in the black box indirectly by manipulating variables that isolate or demonstrate some aspect of the actual processing or the results of that processing (e.g., effects of contextual interference or variability within practice schedules) (Magill 1998). From the perspective of instruction in adapted physical education, cognitive science has provided a foundation upon which to analyze the demands of the motor task on the information process system (Robb 1972).

INFORMATION PROCESSING TASK ANALYSIS

Information processing task analysis goes beyond the objectives-based behavioural approach discussed earlier to specify the cognitive operations involved in solving a particular class of problems, in this instance, motor problems (Foshay 1983; Klahr 1992). In essence, the task structure is analysed rather than the task itself. Five different approaches to information processing task analysis have been undertaken:

a. environmental regulation
b. pacing of the movement
c. the state of the system prior to movement
d. the objective of the movement
e. information conservation, reduction, or creation (Robb 1972)

Figure 16.5 provides an illustration of how task structure can be analysed.

Keeping the environment stable or putting it into a state of flux can regulate the environment. Closed skills are performed in a predictable environment and require a habitual response (e.g., diving). Open skills are those that adjust to the demands of a changing environment (e.g., shooting a basketball during game play). In early skill learning, a predictable

Figure 16.5 Task Analysis Classification from an Information Processing Perspective

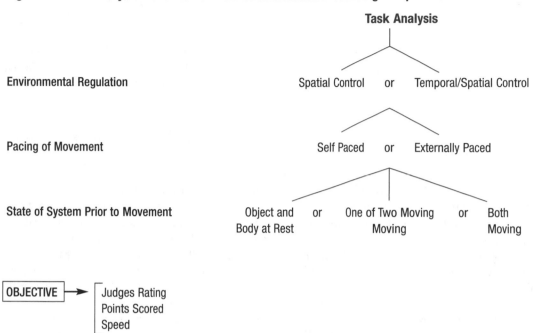

SOURCE: From "Task analysis: A consideration for teachers of skills" by M.D. Robb, 1972, *Research Quarterly, 43*(3), 362–73. Reprinted with permission.

environment decreases the cognitive demands on the learner, thereby allocating more attentional capacity to acquiring the appropriate movement form (Fitts and Posner 1967; Magill 1998; Schmidt and Lee 1999). Figure 16.6 illustrates how a single motor skill can be adapted from a closed environment to an open environment, thereby providing an instructional progression for skill development (Gentile, Higgins, Miller, and Rosen 1975).

The pacing of the movement makes reference to the rate of incoming information as well as its source. Self-paced activities allow the performer to initiate action (e.g., golf swing) while externally paced tasks require the performer to respond to the movements of an opponent or game object (e.g., catching). By creating a self-paced learning situation, the individual is not required to ignore or filter out information that is arriving too quickly to be processed. Many externally paced movements are initially practiced as if

self-paced, until they become habit (Singer and Cauraugh 1985).

The state of the system can be classified by answering the questions: is the performer at rest or in motion, is the object to be acted on at rest or in motion, or are both the performer and the object in motion? The degree of difficulty is inherent in the task, and not the skill level of the performer. A situation in which the performer and object are at rest is less complex than one in which the performer or object are moving, which, in turn, is less complex than one in which both the performer and object are moving (Magill 1998).

Feedback about performance outcomes must also be processed. The objective may be to score goals, earn judges' ratings, or outperform others with respect to speed or distance. Although the nature of the feedback cannot be manipulated, this information becomes the standard against which the final movement form is compared. An additional

Figure 16.6 Adapting Baseball Batting from a Closed Environment to an Open Environment

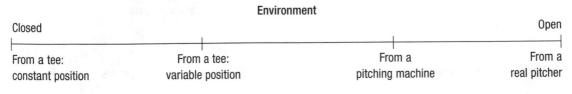

Environment

Closed			Open
From a tee: constant position	From a tee: variable position	From a pitching machine	From a real pitcher

Batting a Ball

SOURCE: From *Motor learning and control* by C.H. Shea, W.L. Shebilske, and S. Worchel, 1993, Boston, MA: Allyn and Bacon. Reprinted with permission.

demand is made when the learner is asked to conserve information for application at a later time, or to respond only when the situation calls for a response.

The role of the instructor within the information processing conceptualization of skill learning is to analyze the demands of the activity and provide information that is related to the capacities of the learner, given their stage of learning (Miller 1993). By manipulating the amount and rate of information received by the learner, it is purported that the instructor can facilitate the problem-solving process. The instructor can provide experiences that give learners practice at perceiving, storing and recalling, and outputting the response. Perceptual strategies such as "watch the ball all the way to the bat" for a striking task can be taught, as can memory-enhancing strategies such as "step, step, turn" for a dance step (Thomas 1996). Such strategies assist learners to gain conscious control over the learning process.

Information processing task analysis presents no clear guidelines for instruction (Foshay 1983). As with the developmental approach, the instructor is once again left to determine intuitively the variables, pacing of instruction, and sequencing of activities that will most significantly influence performance.

ASSUMPTIONS

The deterministic assumption of behaviourism is also purported to be inherent in cognitive theory (Slife and Williams 1995). Somehow information is taken in from the environment and the encoded information guides the ultimate response. The mechanistic view of human activity means that the natural context of behaviour is ignored or perceived to have little impact on the result (Bouffard, Strean, and Davis 1998). As with the behaviourist approach, the learner is perceived to be rational, without feelings, attitudes, or interests (Miller 1993; Slife and Williams 1995). The resulting impact has been a lack of interest in the motivation or affect people bring to motor skill acquisition (Bouffard, Strean, and Davis 1998).

Others suggest, however, that the mediating processes of cognition on the selection and modification of information entering into the system contravenes the deterministic nature of behaviourism. That is to say, whereas behaviourism was seen to be a representation of human behaviour void of conscious control and the result of reinforcement to stimuli, cognitive science purports that cognitive processes are in control of our behaviour (Slife and Williams 1995). In other words, the fundamental importance of information processing approaches is the capacity for self-modification (Klahr 1992). Further to the assumption of self-modification is the assumption that a learner's mental ability can be described in terms of processes that manipulate symbols and that these symbols in turn are representations of knowledge (Klahr 1992; Miller 1993).

Although the question as to whether cognitive theory is substantially different from behavioural theories' premise of determinism will continue to be debated, the contribution of cognitive science to our understanding of motor skill acquisition has been substantial and will continue to inform the instruction of motor skills.

12 Within information processing task analysis, to what is *state of the system prior to movement* referring? How can it be used to enhance motor skill learning?

13 To what does the "black box" refer and of what importance is it to instructors of motor skills?

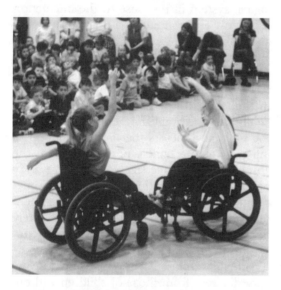

Ecological Systems Approach

The ecological approach to instruction focusses on the organism-environment synergy that occurs in coordinated action (Handford, Davids, Bennett, and Button 1997). Bronfenbrenner (1992) defined an ecological paradigm for the study of development in context by stating,

> The ecology of human development is the scientific study of the progressive, mutual accommodation, throughout the life course, between an active, growing human being, and the changing properties of the immediate settings in which the developing person lives, as this process is affected by the relations between these settings and by

the larger contexts in which the settings are embedded. (p. 188)

The notion of motor development being a fixed action pattern or motor programme that emerged with maturation independent of the performance context was challenged by such people as Bernstein (1967), Kugler, Kelso, and Turvey (1982), Newell (1986), and Thelan and Smith, (1994) as they explored the dynamic interaction of the biological organism with the constraints of the environment and the specific task context. Bernstein (1967) was fascinated with the ability of the neuromuscular and skeletal systems of the body to act as a single unit in light of the enormous number of mechanical variables operating within coordinated movement (Kelso 1998). He referred to the coordination of the "units of analysis" as the *degrees of freedom* problem. Bernstein identified the motor coordination and control problem this way:

> Given that the behaving organism is a dynamic creature, acting in an environment that is never exactly the same, how is stable and adaptive behaviour produced? How do the many organic (structural, physiological) elements cooperate to respond with functional activity in the physical and social world? (Thelan and Smith 1994, p. 76)

Dynamic system theory claims to provide an answer to Bernstein's problem. Movement is purported to be the consequence of the operation of the system's dynamics without regulation from an executive level of regulation. "Spontaneous change in behaviour is governed by natural laws and physical principles that constrain the nonlinear interactions of the components comprising the system" (Hodges, McGarry, and Franks 1998, p. 18). Dynamic system theory proposes that the neuromuscular, neural, and cognitive systems of the person interact with the person's motivation to perform the task within the constraints of the environment and the structure of the task to solve a movement problem (Missiuna, Mandich, Polatajko, and Malloy-Miller 2001).

The tenets of dynamic system theory are:

a. Coordination is perceived to be self-organizing and results from dynamic interaction of internal learner characteristics, environmental effects, and the task itself (Thelan 1987).

b. Essential collective or coordinative variables that characterize coordination are task specific (Thelan and Fogel 1989).

c. Control parameters lead the system through different coordinative states such that stable patterns of behaviour give way to unstable patterns and ultimately a new pattern (Thelan and Ulrich 1991).

d. Relative timing reflects temporal stability of coordinated states despite external perturbations to the system (Thelan 1992).

e. Coordination dynamics is a law-based mathematical structure describing and predicting the coordination activity of a system (Kelso 1998).

According to a dynamic systems perspective, the task of the learner is to solve the degrees of freedom problem (i.e., coordination of the limbs) to attain a certain goal (Hodges et al. 1998). The movement that best achieves the goal differs according to the uncertainty of the environment and the goal requirements. For example, in one instance, the goal may be to put the ball in play using a variety of techniques or solutions as would occur within an open skill setting. In another instance, the goal may be to perform to a predetermined standard of behaviour as occurs in the stable environment of gymnastics (Gentile 1972). In the first instance, the task goal is to use the best solution possible to reach the goal (e.g., project the ball over the net), while in the second instance, the goal is to reproduce another person's performance qualities. It has been suggested that instructors have confused these two goals and have over emphasized the 'how to' of movement, thereby detracting from goal attainment (e.g., how to kick the ball versus passing the ball to the intended location). It is further suggested that focussing only on what the final behaviour looks like may constrain the search for other solutions that may be better suited to the individual (Hodges et al. 1998).

Newell (1986), based on the work of Kugler, Kelso, and Turvey (1980, 1982), has also suggested that action was not the emergence of genetically encoded maturation or behavioural theory generated prescriptions for development, but rather the consequence of constraints imposed on action. Constraints, according to Newell, are boundaries or features that limit motion. Coordinated action then reflects the self-organization of the biological system in response to the interaction of its own constraints with environmental and task constraints.

Three categories of constraints interact to determine the optimal coordination pattern for any given activity: organismic, environmental, and task (Newell 1986; Newell and Scully 1987). Organismic constraints specify the biological factors that limit motion. The integrity of the child's nervous system, the absolute and relative size of respective body parts, and their resulting influence on biomechanical outputs constrain the development of coordinated movement. It immediately becomes evident that the organismic constraints imposed on the development of coordination in children with disabilities can be very different from those of children without disabilities. Even among children with disabilities, the constraints on coordinated movement can be very different depending upon the nature of the impairment (e.g., neurological or structural).

Environmental constraints are those that are external to the person. They may reflect temperature, lighting, gravity, or surface qualities. Although Newell indicated that the environment is generally not manipulated, the environment can be changed to lessen the constraining influence of an environment on movement. For example, the influence of gravity on movement can be modified by taking advantage of the buoyancy afforded by being submerged in water.

Task constraints, according to Newell include such things as the equipment that may be used in the completion of the task, as well as the complexity of the movement pattern itself. Task characteristics interact with the learner and the environment in the development of coordinated action.

The ecological psychology work of Gibson (1977, 1979) has provided insights into the affording qualities of the organism, the environment, and the task. Gibson suggested that an affordance links the functional utility or adaptive value of objects or events to the capabilities of the person. Some of his six environmental affordances, which include medium (e.g., air), surfaces (e.g., ramps), substances (e.g., water), objects (e.g., implements), places (e.g., gymnasium), and people (e.g., instructor) overlap with what Newell terms *task constraints*.

ECOLOGICAL TASK ANALYSIS

Davis and Burton (1991) brought together the task analysis accomplishments of Herkowitz (1978) and Morris (1980, 1981) with the dynamic system theory (Kugler et al. 1980, 1982; Newell 1986) and developed an assessment and instruction model they term *ecological task analysis*. Four steps are involved in ecological task analysis. The first is to identify the task in terms of function (e.g., moving from one place to another, propelling an object, receiving an object, or changing the position of the body or an object). The second step grants the learner choices in the determination of skills, which when carried out, will meet the task goal. For example, the goal of getting a ball over a volleyball net can be accomplished by serving, throwing, or volleying the ball. The third step involves the identification and manipulation of relevant task variables to determine the optimal skill choice and movement form in relation to performer variables. Finally, the instructor further manipulates the task variables (e.g., equipment use), thereby varying the complexity of the task to challenge the learner continually (Davis and Burton 1991).

The ecological task analysis view of motor skill instruction compels us to think of the goal in terms of function or the intended outcome of the movement. Consequently, achieving the outcome of the task (e.g., getting the ball into the opponent's court) takes precedence over achieving the 'correct' movement form.

Ecological task analysis provides important clues for instructional planning for learners with disabilities. The instructor can determine the conditions under which the learner is able to achieve the task, the most efficient and effective performance, the point at which the learner can no longer meet the task goal demands and must choose a different skill (boundary conditions), the range of movement solutions (skills) available to the learner, and finally, how they are applied (Balan and Davis 1993). The role of the instructor, then, is to adapt skillfully these task and environmental constraints within the context of the learner, so as to take advantage of the affordances presented, while minimizing the constraints. In doing so, the boundaries of the movement problem solution cannot be so tightly constrained as to limit self-discovery. Nor should the boundaries be so broad as to promote random unguided discovery that can be time consuming, possibly unsafe, or lead to losses in motivation and confidence (Handford et al. 1997).

Ecological task analysis presupposes that tasks should be categorized by function and intention (i.e., the task goal) and not by mechanism (i.e., specific component parts or processes). In this way, the same task goal remains the focus throughout the learning process. The instructional process consists of varying essential variables or those that are relevant to the goal, thereby linking properties of the performer, environmental, and task constraints (Balan and Davis 1993).

ASSUMPTIONS

According to ecological task analysis, three elements are always present in a performance:

  a. the task goal
  b. performer attributes and

c. the affordances of the physical and social context (Bouffard et al. 1998)

It is assumed that the three elements are distinct and yet connected, with connectedness implying causality. There is a further assumption that behaviour emanates from multiple causal factors that can be ranked according to the magnitude of their influence. And thirdly, that causality within the system is mutual and reciprocal, not linear. This implies that people can and do make choices that are guided, not determined, by physical or social laws (Bouffard et al. 1998).

Wherein traditional task analysis methods failed to account for performer capabilities relative to the requirements of the task (Davis and Burton 1991), instruction within an ecological framework transfers responsibility away from the instructor as the primary source of information regarding content, size of instructional units, pacing of material presentation, and evaluation of progress as it occurs with the developmental and behavioural approaches. In contrast to other approaches, it shares these responsibilities with the learner (McNaughton 1991). The movement solutions are collaboratively determined through exploration and self-discovery, led by the learner and guided by the instructor. Instruction, consequently, becomes a two-way interaction, taking on a learner-led rather than an instructor-led focus. The instructor becomes less concerned with controlling the learner's behaviour and more responsive to the movement experienced by the learner. Learners, in turn, are freed to discover the movement form that enables them to achieve the task goal.

A learner-led approach to assessment and instruction removes the onerous responsibility of having to know, or presuming to know, the best movement form for all learners. It is designed to provide strategies for individualizing instruction, providing learners with choices, and enhancing collaborative decision-making. Hence, this approach is well suited for inclusive physical education programmes, although it is equally applicable to learners without disabilities (Balan and Davis 1993).

By providing opportunities for learners to make choices and take an active role in the generation of solutions to movement problems, the capability and intent of the learner becomes fundamental to improvement of movement performance. Providing opportunities for choice-making presumes that the learners are able to link the properties of their own performance with that of environmental and task constraints. Further investigation into the degree to which learners with disabilities are active agents in their own learning, and the efficacy of ecological task analysis for assessment and instructional purposes, still is needed (Davis and Burton 1991). There are few, if any, published instructional programmes using this approach to date.

---

14 What three categories of constraints interact to determine the optimal coordination pattern for any given activity?

---

15 How is the premise that tasks should be categorized by function and intention reflected in the four steps of ecological task analysis?

---

16 What is meant when it is said that an ecological approach to instruction is learner-led rather than instructor-led?

Strategic Approach

Learning how to learn within an instructional setting has become the focus of recent research on motor skill acquisition (Yang and Porretta 1999). Self-knowledge has been referred to as *metacognition*. Metacognitive knowledge is defined as "the learners' self-awareness of their own cognitional knowledge through which they acquire information, gain understanding, and learn in the classroom" (Peterson 1988 p. 7). Only recently have we attempted to describe the knowledge that children possess about the mental

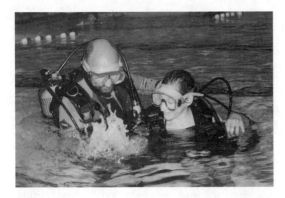

processes they use to acquire motor skills (Reid 1986).

The metacognitive approach to motor skill acquisition emphasizes the processes by which individuals learn how to analyse, problem solve, and generalize their task-solving strategies to future performance situations (Singer and Cauraugh 1985). This approach is a departure from the instructional approaches that emphasize mastery of specific performance skills or 'content', and largely ignore the role of self-knowledge, motivation, attitudes, beliefs, and affect in movement skill learning (Bouffard 1990; Bouffard and Dunn 1993). Rather than resulting in learning, instructor behaviour within the metacognitive approach is seen to impact on learning only to the extent that the individuals are engaged in their own learning process (Lee and Solomon 1992).

A self-regulation approach to learning purports that by becoming metacognitively aware of their own learning process, learners can control their own behaviour, motivation, and affect by exercising various cognitive strategies (Alexander 1995; Boekaerts 1995; Pintrich 1995). A *strategy* refers to a self-initiated or externally imposed way of directing information leading to decisions for purposeful behaviour. Within the domain of motor skill performance, strategy use has emphasized such techniques as mental mastery, self-monitoring, self-instruction, attentional focus, biofeedback, and positive self-talk (Kirschenbaum 1987).

The regulation of movement activities requires the solving of problems created by the interplay of the performer and the environment (Bouffard 1990; Bouffard and Wall 1991). The problem-solving process can be broken down into five interrelated steps. The first step is the identification of a problem. Once identified, the second step is to define the problem within the confines of the ultimate movement goal. The person must be able to identify the current situation and note the difference between what is and what is desired. The third step is to construct a plan to eliminate the perceived difference. Both inference and memory resources can be used in the plan construction. Once the plan is formulated, the fourth step is to execute the plan. Finally, each stage of the process as well as the overall outcome of the plan are evaluated.

The extent to which persons with developmental disabilities can utilize a problem-solving process has been the focus of recent research, with deficiencies being reported in all of the five steps (Bouffard 1990). Deficiencies have been related to the knowledge base available to the learner, failure to use appropriate strategies, lack of metacognitive knowledge and understanding, lack of ability to judge the appropriateness of strategy selection, and finally, lack of motivation and practice (Bouffard 1990). "In summary, numerous studies have shown that mentally retarded persons do not spontaneously use appropriate strategies to solve memory problems. When appropriate strategies are taught to these people, and they are required to use them, their performance is frequently better" (Bouffard and Wall 1990, p. 116).

Bouffard (1990) outlines a number of implications for instructors of learners with developmental disabilities. It is important to know what strategies to teach. This knowledge can be gained by studying the strategic use of others who are learning the task, or through a process of strategic task analysis such as outlined by Singer and Cauraugh (1985). They advocate a five-step procedure that is applicable to any self-paced activity. Based on athlete interviews, personal experience, and research, they recommend the procedure of readying, imaging, focussing, executing, and evaluating.

Secondly, it is important to know the knowledge, beliefs, and strategies each learner brings to the task (Ferrari, Pinard, Reid, and Bouffard-Bouchard 1991). It may also be necessary to teach the movement skill explicitly, using one of the previously mentioned instructional approaches, so as not to overwhelm the learner initially. Strategies should also be taught, as should the conditions under which they should be applied. Using multiple contexts for the instruction of the task can enhance strategy utilization as can an instruction setting that as closely as possible resembles the environment in which the strategy will be used. Feedback about the effectiveness of strategy use by the learner is also important.

A strategic approach to the teaching and learning of motor skills seems particularly well suited to the needs of children with developmental coordination disorder (DCD). Children with DCD, although not intellectually impaired, have difficulty achieving the same level of skill proficiency as their peers (Missiuna 1994). In a break from developmentally sequenced activities aimed at the amelioration of underlying sensory, sensorimotor, or sensory integrative deficits, a programme that actively engages the children in solving performance problems and testing out solutions was developed. The Cognitive Orientation to Daily Occupational Performance (CO-OP) programme emphasizes the importance of the interaction of the person, the task, and the environment and advocates that children learn the processes involved in discovering the solution to movement problems for themselves (Missiuna, Mandich, Polatajko, and Malloy-Miller 2001; Polatajko, Mandich, Missiuna, Macnab, Malloy-Miller, and Kinsella 2001; Polatajko, Mandich, Miller, and Macnab 2001). The CO-OP programme teaches a four-step global problem-solving strategy that encourages the children to identify a goal, state the plan they will use, do the activity, and check how successful they were in its completion (Polatajko,

Mandich, Miller, and Macnab 2001). The results of this programme have been encouraging, as children have successfully used strategies to effect change on their performances (Miller, Polatajko, Missiuna, Mandich, and Macnab 2001; Polatajko, Mandich, Miller, and Macnab 2001).

ASSUMPTIONS

Several assumptions underlie the application of self-regulation strategies to motor skill instruction and persons with disabilities. Firstly, persons with disabilities can learn metacognitive skills and, once learned, they can be controlled or regulated. In other words, self-regulation is something that is "teachable" (Pintrich 1995). It is also presumed that those who acquire and utilize self-regulatory processes will retain and transfer their learning once the initial instructional period is concluded (Singer and Cauraugh 1985). Reid (1986) correctly states that further investigation is needed into such variables as task selection (ecologically meaningful coordination tasks), identification of strategies to instruct (what are the learners to be strategic about), the need to demonstrate the subsequent efficacy of strategic instruction (empirical verification), and who will be the recipients of such instruction (heterogeneous nature of disability).

17 What is *metacognition* and how has it been applied to instruction in adapted physical activity?

18 What is unique to the strategic approach to instruction that has been largely absent from the previously discussed strategies?

19 The problem-solving process has been broken down into a number of steps. What are they?

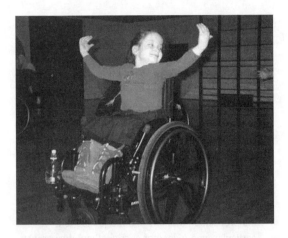

Summary

Seven instructional approaches have been utilized in adapted physical education instruction, namely remedial therapy, the developmental approach, perceptual motor programming, a behavioural approach, a cognitive orientation, an ecological approach, and a metacognitive or strategic orientation. Each approach reflects inherent assumptions about learning and about disability. The medical orientation speaks to the very roots of adapted physical education. The human consequence of the two world wars provided impetus for the development of new surgical techniques. Corrective therapy, a member of the ensuing physical medicine team, prepared the veterans to return to combat or their home communities by demonstrating and teaching medically prescribed reconditioning exercises. The therapist took responsibility for restoring useful activity to veterans who were perceived to be weak or unable to complete useful activities. The 'patient's' role was to comply with the prescribed exercise regime.

The benefits of medically prescribed exercises were eventually taken beyond the therapy room and into the school gymnasium. Disability was no longer viewed solely as an illness, but also as a social value judgement about individual potential.

The developmental approach to the teaching of physical education, in contrast to the medical approach, recognized the changing profiles of development that occur with age. According to developmental theorists, people progress through a series of qualitatively different stages. Adapted physical education instruction focussed on the achievement of movement patterns typical of children without disabilities to the highest stage or level possible. The instructor's role was to identify learners who were not progressing at the same rate as their age-matched peers and to teach specific movement sequences. Developmental, hierarchical, and information processing task analysis techniques were utilized as a way of decreasing the complexity of the task for the learner.

Learner progress was measured against the template of normal development as outlined by developmental stages. Leisure skill development, enhanced gross motor skill performance, and time spent on task have been the targets of behavioural programming.

Perceptual motor programming, although found to be unsubstantiated in its claim to enhance academic performance, brought instructional focus to children who were experiencing motor difficulties. The benefits of perceptual motor programming were found in programming that improved fitness, physical development, and motor skills.

The cognitive approach, although considered to be mechanistic in its view of human learning and performance, provided instructors of motor skills with a framework from which to assist learners to process environmental information and solve movement problems. By analyzing the motor task, the instructor could moderate the environment, pace movements, vary the degree of task difficulty, or provide feedback in accordance with the cognitive needs of the learner.

The ecological approach to instruction focusses on the organism-environment synergy that occurs in coordinated action, rather than on internalized knowledge structures or executive regulators. The notion of motor development being a fixed pattern, or motor programme, that emerges with maturation was challenged as scholars explored the dynamic interaction of the biological organism with the constraints of the environment and the specific task context. Ecological

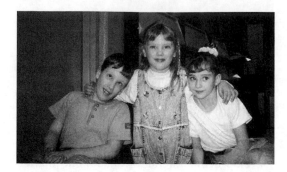

task analysis links ecological theory with practice by providing a systematic way of assessing and instructing motor skills. The task is identified in terms of function and the learner chooses skill and movement forms that will meet the goal requirements. Task constraints are then varied to ascertain the optimal movement form and to challenge the learner. The appealing aspect of this approach is the choice and decision-making responsibilities assumed by the learner.

The metacognitive approach to motor skill acquisition emphasizes the processes by which individuals learn how to analyse, problem solve, and generalize their task solving strategies to future performance situations. This is a departure from performance- or outcome-based models of instruction as it emphasizes the role of learner knowledge, self-regulation, motivation, and affect. Although our understanding of metacognition and self-regulation, as it applies to adapted physical education instruction, has yet to be fully explored, the study of cognitive structures offers promise in the promotion of independent learning.

The relationships between the learner and the instructor in the instructional approaches we use in the teaching of motor skills to people with disabilities reflects our beliefs and knowledge about the capability of our learners, their learning processes, and our perceptions of disability. The evidence needed to bring credibility to our instructional intuition is mounting and will continue with the combined efforts of theorists, researchers, instructors, and the learners.

Study Questions

1. Why is it important to consider the assumptions underlying our instructional approaches when instructing motor skills?
2. Given your understanding of motor skill acquisition, is it reasonable to accept the notion of the blending of instructional approaches for a particular learner when the underlying assumptions of the approaches may be in conflict? Support your answer.
3. How do the roles of the learner compare in the behavioural approach to motor skill instruction to that of the strategic approach? Would you support the proposition that one is better suited to a particular type of learner over another? Why or why not?
4. To what does *determinism* refer and to what instructional approach(es) does it apply?
5. What is the role of the instructor in an ecological task analysis approach to instruction?

Acknowledgment

The author acknowledges the input of Dr. David Fitzpatrick, Physical Activity and Sport Studies, University of Winnipeg, and the parents who generously allowed the use of personal photos of their children.

References

Alexander, P.A. (1995). Superimposing a situation-specific and domain-specific perspective on an account of self-regulated learning. *Educational Psychologist, 30*(4), 189–93.

Alger, I., and Rusk, H.A. (1955). The rejection of help by some disabled people. *Archives of Physical Medicine and Rehabilitation, 36,* 281–97.

Ames, L. (1937). The sequential patterning of prone progression in the human infant. *Genetic Psychology Monographs, 19,* 409–60.

Ayers, J.A. (1965). Patterns of perceptual-motor dysfunction in children: A factor analytic study. *Perceptual Motor Skills, Monograph Supplement, I–V20.*

Balan, C.M., and Davis, W.E. (1993). Ecological task analysis: An approach to teaching physical education. *Journal of Physical Education, Recreation, and Dance, 64*(9), 54–61.

Baron, R.J. (1985). An introduction to medical phenomenology: I can't hear you while I'm listening. *Annuals of Internal Medicine, 103,* 606–11.

Bayley, N. (1935). Development of motor abilities during the first three years. *Monographs of the Society for Research in Child Development, 1,* 1–26.

Bernstein, N.A. (1967). *The coordination and regulation of movements.* Oxford: Pergamon.

Block, M.E. (2001). *A teacher's guide to including students with disabilities in regular physical education.* Baltimore: Paul H. Brookes.

Boekaerts, M. (1995). Self-regulated learning: Bridging the gap between metacognitive and metamotivation theories. *Educational Psychologist, 30*(4), 195–220.

Bouffard, M. (1990). Movement problem solutions by educable mentally handicapped individuals. *Adapted Physical Activity Quarterly, 7,* 183–97.

Bouffard, M., and Dunn, J. (1993). Children's self-regulated learning of movement sequences. *Research Quarterly for Exercise and Sport, 64*(4), 393–403.

Bouffard, M., Strean, W.B., and Davis, W.E. (1998). Questioning our philosophical and methodological research assumptions: Psychological perspectives. *Adapted Physical Activity Quarterly, 15*(3), 250–68.

Bouffard, M., and Wall, A.E. (1990). A problem-solving approach to movement skill acquisition: Implications for special populations. In G. Reid (Ed.), *Problems in movement control* (pp. 107–31). New York: Elsevier Science Publishers.

Bouffard, M., and Wall, A.E. (1991). Knowledge, decision-making, and performance in table tennis by educable mentally handicapped adolescents. *Adapted Physical Activity Quarterly, 8,* 57–90.

Brace, D.K. (1949). The contributions of physical education to total education. *Journal of the Association for Health, Physical Education, and Recreation, 20*(10), 635–37.

Bronfenbrenner, U. (1992). Ecological systems theory. In R. Vasta (Ed.), *Six theories of child development* (pp. 187–249). London: Jessica Kingsley.

Burton, A.W., and Miller, D.E. (1998). *Movement skill assessment.* Champaign, IL: Human Kinetics.

Chen, S., Zhang, J., Lange, E., Miko, P., and Joseph, D. (2001). Progressive time delay procedure for teaching motor skills to adults with severe mental retardation. *Adapted Physical Activity Quarterly, 18*(1), 35–48.

Clarke, H.H., and Clarke, D.H. (1978). *Developmental and adapted physical education.* Englewood Cliffs, NJ: Prentice-Hall.

Condeluci, A. (1991). *Interdependence: The route to community* (2nd ed.). Winter Park, FL: GR Press.

Conrad, P. (1990). Qualitative research on chronic illness: A commentary on method and conceptual development. *Social Science and Medicine, 30*(11), 1257–63.

Cowden, J.E., Sayers, L.K., and Torrey, C.C. (1998). *Pediatric adapted motor development and exercise: An innovative, multisystem approach for professionals and families.* Springfield, IL: Charles C. Thomas.

Cratty, B.J. (1969). *Developmental games for physically handicapped children.* Palo Alto, CA: Peek.

Cratty, B.J. (1970). *Perceptual and motor development in infants and children.* Los Angeles: Macmillan.

Cratty, B.J. (1973). *Teaching motor skills.* Englewood Cliffs, NJ: Prentice-Hall.

Cratty, B.J. (1975). *Remedial motor activity for children.* London: Lea and Febiger.

Davis, J.E. (1967). The historic promise of corrective therapy in American culture. *Journal of the Association for Physical and Mental Rehabilitation, 21*(2), 4–53.

Davis, J.E. (1976). The golden heritage of corrective therapy. *American Corrective Therapy Journal, 30*(4), 122–27.

Davis, W.E., and Burton, A.W. (1991). Ecological task analysis: Translating movement behaviour theory into practice. *Adapted Physical Activity Quarterly, 8,* 154–77.

Delacato, C.H. (1963). *The diagnosis and treatment of speech and reading problems.* Springfield, IL: Charles C. Thomas.

Dembo, T., Ladieu Leviton, G., and Wright, B. (1956). Adjustment to misfortune: A problem of social-psychological rehabilitation. *Artificial Limbs, 3,* 4–62.

DePauw, K.P. (1996). Students with disabilities in physical education. In S.J. Silverman and C.D. Ennis (Eds.), *Student learning in physical education: Applying research to enhance instruction* (pp. 101–24). Windsor, ON: Human Kinetics.

Dick, W., and Carey, L. (1978). *The systematic design of instruction.* Glenview, IL: Scott Foresman.

The Doman-Delacato Treatment of neurologically handicapped children: Official statement. (1968). *Archives of Physical Medicine and Rehabilitation, April,* 183–85.

Domjan, M. (1993). *The principles of learning and behavior.* Pacific Grove, CA: Brooks Cole.

Dunn, J.M., Morehouse, J.W., and Fredericks, H.D.B. (1986). *Physical education for the severely handicapped: A systematic approach to a data based gymnasium.* Austin, TX: Pro-Ed.

Espenschade, A.S., and Eckert, H.M. (1967). *Motor development.* Columbus, OH: Charles E. Merrill.

Ferrari, M., Pinard, A., Reid, L., and Bouffard-Bouchard, T. (1991). The relationship between expertise and self-regulation in movement performance: Some theoretical issues. *Perceptual and Motor Skills, 72,* 139–50.

Fitts, P.M., and Posner, M.I. (1967). *Human performance.* Belmont, CA: Brooks/Cole.

Foshay, W.R. (1983). Alternative methods of task analysis. *Journal of Instructional Development, 6*(4), 2–9.

Freeman, R.D. (1967). Controversy over "patterning" as a treatment for brain damage in children. *Journal of the American Medical Association, 202,* 385–88.

Gelinas, J., and Reid, G. (2000). The developmental validity of traditional learn-to-swim progressions for children with physical disabilities. *Adapted Physical Activity Quarterly, 17*(3), 269–85.

Gentile, A.M. (1972). A working model of skill acquisition with application to teaching. *Quest, 17,* 3–23.

Gentile, A.M., Higgins, J.R., Miller, E.A., and Rosen, B.M. (1975). The structure of motor tasks. *Movement, 7*, 11–28.

Gesell, A. (1930). Reciprocal interweaving in neuromotor development. *Journal of Comparative Neurology, 70*, 161–80.

Getman, G.M. (1962). *How to develop your child's intelligence.* Wayne, PA: Research Publications.

Gibson, J.J. (1977). The theory of affordances. In R. Shaw and J. Bransford (Eds.), *Perceiving, acting, and knowing* (pp. 67–82). Hillsdale, NJ: Lawrence Erlbaum.

Gibson, J.J. (1979). *The ecological approach to visual perception.* Hopewell, NJ: Houghton Mifflin.

Guttmann, Sir L. (1960). Sport for the disabled as a world problem. *Rehabilitation, 68*, 29–43.

Guttmann, Sir L. (1967). History of the National Spinal Injuries Centre, Stoke Mandeville Hospital, Aylesbury. *Paraplegia, 4-5*, 115–26.

Guttmann, Sir L. (1975). Development of sport for the spinal paralyzed. *Hexagon, 7*, 6–13.

Halverson, L. (1966). Development of motor patterns in young children. *Quest, 6*, 44–53.

Handford, C., Davids, K., Bennett, S., and Button, C. (1997). Skill acquisition in sport: Some applications of an evolving practice ecology. *Journal of Sports Sciences, 15*, 621–40.

Hanson, M.J., and Harris, S.R. (1986). *Teaching the young child with motor delays.* Austin, TX: Pro-Ed.

Haywood, K. (1993). *Life span motor development.* Champaign, IL: Human Kinetics.

Hedlund, M. (2000). Disability as phenomenon: A discourse of social and biological understanding. *Disability and Society, 15*(5), 765–80.

Hellebrandt, F.A., Rarick, G.L., Glassow, R., and Carns, M.L. (1961). Physiological analysis of basic motor skills: Growth and development of jumping. *American Journal of Physical Medicine, 40*, 14–25.

Hellison, D. (1991). The whole person in physical education scholarship: Toward integration. *Quest, 43*, 307–18.

Herkowitz, J. (1978). Developmental task analysis: The design of movement experiences and evaluation of motor development status. In M. Ridenour (Ed.), *Motor development: Issues and applications* (pp. 139–64). Princeton: Princeton Books.

Hodges, N.J., McGarry, T., and Franks, I.M. (1998). A dynamical system's approach to the examination of sport behaviour. *Avante, 4*(3), 16–38.

Jenkins, J., and Jenkins, L. (1985). Peer tutoring in elementary and secondary programmes. *Focus on Exceptional Children, 17*(6), 1–12.

Kalnins, I.V., Steele, C., Stevens, E., Rossen, B., Biggar, D., Jutai, J., and Bortolussi, J. (1999). Health survey research on children with physical disabilities in Canada. *Health Promotion International, 14*(3), 251–59.

Kavale, K., and Mattson, P.D. (1983). "One jumped off the balance beam": Meta-analysis of perceptual-motor training. *Journal of Learning Disabilities, 16*(3), 165–71.

Keller, F.S. (1969). *Learning: Reinforcement theory.* New York: Random House.

Kelso, J.A.S. (1998). From Bernstein's physiology of activity to coordination dynamics. In M.L. Latash (Ed.), *Progress in motor control: Bernstein's traditions in movement studies* (pp. 203–19). Champaign, IL: Human Kinetics.

Kennedy, P., Esque, T., and Novak, J. (1983). A functional analysis of task analysis procedures for instructional design. *Journal of Instructional Development, 6*(4), 10–16.

Kephart, N.C. (1960). *The slow learner in the classroom.* Columbus, OH: Merrill.

Kirschenbaum, D.S. (1987). Self-regulation of sport performance. *Medicine and Science in Sports and Exercise, 19*(5), S106–S113.

Klahr, D. (1992). Information-processing approaches. In R. Vasta (Ed.), *Six theories of child development* (pp. 133–85). London: Jessica Kingsley.

Kugler, P.N., Kelso, J.A., and Turvey, M.T. (1980). On the concept of coordinative structures as dissipative structures: Theoretical lines of convergence. In G.E. Stelmack and J. Requin (Eds.), *Tutorials in motor behavior.* Amsterdam: North-Holland.

Kugler, P.N., Kelso, J.A., and Turvey, M.T. (1982). On the control and co-ordination of naturally developing systems. In J.A. Kelso and J.E. Clark (Eds.), *The development of movement control and coordination* (pp. 5–78). New York: John Wiley.

Leder, D. (1985). Medicine and paradigms of embodiment. *The Journal of Medicine and Philosophy, 9*, 29–43.

Lee, A.M., and Solomon, M.A. (1992). Cognitive conceptions of teaching and learning motor skills. *Quest, 44*, 57–71.

Magill, R.A. (1998). *Motor learning: Concepts and applications.* Dubuque, IA: WCB McGraw-Hill.

Marteniuk, R.G. (1976). *Information processing in motor skills.* New York: Holt, Rinehart and Winston.

McGraw, M.B. (1941). Development of neuro-muscular mechanism as reflected in the crawling-creeping behavior of the human infant. *Journal of Genetic Psychology, 58*, 83–111.

McNaughton, S. (1991). The faces of instruction: Models of how children learn from tutors. In J. Morse and T. Linzey (Eds.), *Growing up: The politics of human learning* (pp. 135–50). Auckland: Longman Paul.

Miller, L.T., Polatajko, H.J., Missiuna, C., Mandich, A.D., and Macnab, J.J. (2001). A pilot trial of a cognitive treatment for children with developmental coordination disorder. *Human Movement Science, 20*, 183–210.

Miller, P.H. (1993). *Theories of developmental psychology.* New York: W.H. Freeman.

Missiuna, C. (1994). Motor skill acquisition in children with developmental coordination disorder. *Adapted Physical Activity Quarterly, 11*(2), 214–35.

Missiuna, C., Mandich, A.D., Polatajko, H.J., and Malloy-Miller, T. (2001). Cognitive orientation to daily occupational performance (CO-OP): Part I: Theoretical foundations. *Physical and Occupational Therapy in Pediatrics, 20*(2/3), 69–81.

Morris, G.S. (1980). *How to change the games children play*. Minneapolis: Burgess.

Morris, G.S. (1981). Toward inclusion. In A.M. Morris (Ed.), *Motor development: Theory into practice (Monograph 3)*, 7–10. Newtown, CT: Motor Skills: Theory into Practice.

Newell, K.M. (1986). Constraints on the development of coordination. In M.G. Wade and H.T.A. Whiting (Eds.), *Motor development in children: Aspects of coordination and control* (pp. 341–60). Boston: Martinus Nijhoff.

Newell, K.M., and Scully, D.M. (1987). Steps in the development of coordination: Perception of relative motion. In J.E. Clark and J.H. Humphrey (Eds.), *Advances in motor development research* (pp. 153–70). New York: AMS Press.

Owlia, G., French, R., Ben-Ezra, V., and Silliman, L.M. (1995). Influence of reinforcers on the time-on-task performance of adolescents who are profoundly mentally retarded. *Adapted Physical Activity Quarterly, 12*(3), 275–88.

Peterson, P.L. (1988). Teachers' and students' cognitical knowledge for classroom teaching and learning. *Educational Researcher,* June/July, 5–14.

Pintrich, P.R. (1995). Understanding self-regulated learning. *New Directions for Teaching and Learning, 63*, 3–12.

Polatajko, H.J., Mandich, A.D., Miller, L.T., and Macnab, J.J. (2001). Cognitive orientation to daily occupational performance (CO-OP): Part II: The evidence. *Physical and Occupational Therapy in Pediatrics, 20*(2/3), 83–106.

Polatajko, H.J., Mandich, A.D., Missiuna, C., Macnab, J.J., Malloy-Miller, T., and Kinsella, E.A. (2001). Cognitive orientation to daily occupational performance (CO-OP): Part III: The protocol in brief. *Physical and Occupational Therapy in Pediatrics, 20*(2/3), 107–23.

Rachlin, H. (1991). *Introduction to modern behaviorism*. New York: W. H. Freeman.

Rarick, G.L. (1973). Motor performance of mentally retarded children. In G.L. Rarick (Ed.), *Physical activity: Human growth and development* (pp. 225–56). New York: Academic Press.

Reid, G. (1981). Perceptual-motor training: Has the term lost its utility? *Journal of Health, Physical Education, Recreation, and Dance, 52*(6), 38–39.

Reid, G. (1986). The trainability of motor processing strategies with developmentally delayed performers. In H.T.A. Whiting and M.G. Wade (Eds.), *Themes in motor development* (pp. 93–107). Boston: Martinus Nijhoff.

Reigeluth, C.M. (1983). Current trends in task analysis: The integration of task analysis and instructional design. *Journal of Instructional Development, 6*(4), 24–30.

Robb, M.D. (1972). Task analysis: A consideration for teachers of skills. *Research Quarterly, 43*(3), 362–73.

Robbins, M.P. (1966). A study of the validity of Delacato's theory of neurological organization. *Exceptional Children, 32*, 517–23.

Roberton, M.A. (1978). Longitudinal evidence for developmental stages in the forceful overarm throw. *Journal of Human Movement Studies, 4*, 167–75.

Roberton, M.A. (1982). Describing 'stages' within and across motor tasks. In S. Kelso and J.E. Clark (Eds.), *The development of movement control and co-ordination* (pp. 293–309). New York: John Wiley.

Rose, D.J., and Heath, E.M. (1990). The contribution of a fundamental motor skill to the performance and learning of a complex sport skill. *Journal of Human Movement Studies, 19*, 75–84.

Rosen, N.B. (1973). The role of sports in rehabilitation of the handicapped, Part 1A: Historical. *Maryland State Medical Journal, 22*(2), 30–32.

Rusk, H.A. (1966). Tomorrow is not yesterday. *Archives of Physical Medicine and Rehabilitation, 47*(1), 3–8.

Schmidt, R.A., and Lee, T.D. (1999). *Motor control and learning: A behavioral emphasis*. Champaign, IL: Human Kinetics.

Schunk, D.H. (1996). *Learning theories: An educational perspective*. Englewood Cliffs, NJ: Prentice Hall.

Seaman, J., and DePauw, K. (1982). *The new adapted physical education: A developmental approach*. Palo Alto, CA: Mayfield.

Seefeldt, V. (1980). Developmental motor patterns: Implications for elementary school physical education. In C. Nadeau, G. Roberts, and W. Halliwell (Eds.), *Psychology of motor behavior and sport* (pp. 314–23). Champaign, IL: Human Kinetics.

Seefeldt, V., and Haubenstricker, J. (1982). Patterns, phases, or stages: An analytical model for the study of developmental movement. In S. Kelso and J.E. Clark (Eds.), *The development of movement control and co-ordination* (pp. 309–18). New York: John Wiley.

Shea, C.H., Shebilske, W.L., and Worchel, S. (1993). *Motor learning and control*. Boston: Allyn and Bacon.

Sherrill, C. (1988). Personal preparation in adapted physical education: Early history. In C. Sherrill, (Ed.), *Leadership training in adapted physical education* (pp. 23–42). Champaign, IL: Human Kinetics.

Sherrill, C. (1998). *Adapted physical activity, recreation, and sport: Crossdisciplinary and lifespan* (5th ed.). Dubuque, IA: Brown and Benchmark.

Sherrill, C., and DePauw, K. (1997). Adapted physical activity and education. In J.D. Massengale and R.A. Swanson (Eds.), *The history of exercise and sport science* (pp. 39–108). Champaign, IL: Human Kinetics.

Shirley, M. (1931). *The first two years: A study of twenty-five babies*. Minneapolis: University of Minnesota Press.

Shogan, D. (1998). The social construction of disability: The impact of statistics and technology. *Adapted Physical Activity Quarterly, 15*(3), 269–77.

Silliman, L.M., and French, R. (1993). Use of selected reinforcers to improve the ball kicking of youths with profound mental retardation. *Adapted Physical Activity Quarterly, 10*(1), 52–69.

Silliman-French, L., French, R., Sherrill, C., and Gench, B. (1998). Auditory feedback and time-on-task of posture alignment of individuals with profound mental retardation. *Adapted Physical Activity Quarterly, 15*(1), 51–63.

Simpson Poplin, M., and Stone, S. (1992). Paradigm shifts in instructional strategies: From reductionism to holistic/constructivism. In W. Stainback and S. Stainback (Eds.), *Controversial issues confronting special education* (pp. 153–79). Boston: Allyn and Bacon.

Singer, R.N., and Cauraugh, J.H. (1985). The generalizability effect of learning strategies for categories of psychomotor skills. *Quest, 37*, 103–19.

Slife, B.D., and Williams, R.N. (1995). *What's behind the research? Discovering hidden assumption in the behavioral sciences.* Thousand Oaks, CA: Sage.

Stende, D.A. (1975). The scope of corrective therapy. *American Corrective Therapy Journal, 29*(3), 76–79.

Thelan, E. (1987). The role of motor development in developmental psychology: A view of the past and an agenda for the future. In N. Eisenberg (Ed.), *Contemporary topics in developmental psychology* (pp. 3–33). New York: John Wiley.

Thelan, E. (1992). Development as a dynamic system. *Current Directions in Psychological Science, 1*(6), 189–93.

Thelan, E. and Fogel, A. (1989). Toward an action-based theory of infant development. In J. Lockman and N. Hazen (Eds.), *Action in social context* (pp. 23–62). New York: Plenum.

Thelan, E., and Smith, L.B. (1994). *A dynamic systems approach to the development of cognition and action.* Cambridge: MIT Press.

Thelan, E. and Ulrich, D.A. (1991). Hidden skills: a dynamic systems analysis of treadmill stepping during the first year. *Monographs of the Society for Research in Child Development, 56*(1, Serial no. 223).

Thomas, R.M. (1996). *Comparing theories of motor development.* New York: Brooks/Cole.

Ulrich, D.A. (2000). *Test of gross motor development.* Austin, TX: Pro-ed.

Watkinson, E.J., and Wall, A.E. (1982). *PREP: A preschool play programme.* Ottawa: CAHPER.

Wall, M.E., and Gast, D.L. (1997). Caregivers' use of constant time delay to teach leisure skills to adolescents or young adults with moderate or severe intellectual disabilities. *Education and Training in Mental Retardation and Developmental Disabilities, 32*(4), 340–56.

Wessel, J.A. (1975). I CAN Curriculum Project. *Journal of Physical Education and Recreation, 46*(6), 50.

Wessel, J.A. (1978). *I CAN Sport, Leisure, and Recreation Skills Program.* East Lansing: Michigan State University.

Wheeler, G.D. (1998). Challenging our assumptions in the biological area of adapted physical activity: A reaction to Shephard. *Adapted Physical Activity Quarterly, 15*(3), 236–49.

Wickstrom, R.L. (1983). *Fundamental motor patterns* (3rd ed.). Philadelphia: Lea and Febiger.

Wild, M.R. (1938). The behavior pattern of throwing and some observations concerning its course of development in children. *Research Quarterly for Exercise and Sport, 9*, 20–24.

Winnick, J.P. (1990). *Adapted physical education and sport.* Champaign, IL: Human Kinetics.

Yang, J.J., and Porretta, D.L. (1999). Sport/leisure skill learning by adolescents with mild mentally retardation: A four-step strategy. *Adapted Physical Activity Quarterly, 16*(3), 300–315.

Zhang, J., Gast, D., Horvat, M., and Dattilo J. (1995). The effectiveness of a constant time delay procedure on teaching lifetime sport skills to adolescent with severe to profound intellectual disabilities. *Education and Training in Mental Retardation and Developmental Disabilities 30*, 51–64.

CHAPTER 17

Culturally Relevant Physical Education for Students Who Experience Emotional and Behavioural Difficulties

Joannie M. Halas

Learning Objectives

- To explore the socio-cultural and economic factors that contribute to a young person's emotional and behavioural difficulties.
- To explore the socially constructed nature of categories and labels used to define and describe students who experience emotional and behavioural difficulties and how these descriptive labels are used within the school system.
- To explore culturally relevant means for addressing the needs of youth who have emotional and behavioural difficulties in a physical education context.

Introduction

Students who present as angry, difficult to control, hyperactive, withdrawn, with low self-esteem, poor concentration, and so forth are often identified (for funding or treatment purposes) as having emotional or behavioural 'dis-orders'. The use of the word *disorder* to describe behaviour has negative connotations. By hyphenating the word *dis-order*, attention is focussed on the social construction of words and how the language that is used to define individuals can be problematic. While acknowledging that identifying labels and categories have specific purposes within an educational discourse, this chapter will focus on the *teacher practices* that are culturally relevant to the landscape of everyday life challenges that face many young people in Canadian society. Throughout this chapter, I will explore various means by which physical educators might develop culturally relevant, 'reclaiming', gymnasium climates for students who experience emotional and behavioural difficulties. In particular, I will draw attention to the need for teachers to understand the cultural landscape of their students' day-to-day life challenges as a means to develop a meaningful and relevant physical education curriculum that positively connects students to the gym environment.

By focussing on the teacher-student relationship, and exploring ways to provide students more control over their physical education experience, I hope to show how the construction of safe and inviting physical education environments for all students is a key factor in determining how effective physical education programmes can be. The chapter concludes with the example of a successful active-living programme that has been designed specifically for students who have been diagnosed as having severe emotional and behavioural disorders. Although not all readers of this textbook will work in a segregated school environment for severely troubled youth, the example provided by the Macdonald School active-living programme illustrates how physical education can provide many personally and socially relevant health outcomes for young people.

Understanding the Cultural Landscape

> Our culture is producing a growing population of hostile, unattached children with weak conscience development. Reared in severely abusive environments, they have learned to reject all attempts to form positive human bonds. Leaving a trail of broken relationships, they are bounced from placement to placement, becoming evermore angry and unlovable.
> (Brendtro and Long 1994, p. 3)

THE EFFECTS OF INTERNALIZED OPPRESSION ON A YOUNG PERSON'S PERFORMANCE IN SCHOOL

As the Roman calendar stretches into its third millenium, physical education teachers in schools across North America will certainly encounter a number of students who experience emotional and behavioural difficulties in their classes. These students will present themselves in a myriad of ways. Their personal behaviours, individual characteristics, and unique life stories are highly diverse yet so completely entwined within a complex matrix of socio-cultural and economical factors that any discussion of effective educational programmes designed to help these young people will always be incomplete. This group is often referred to as *youth at risk, emotionally and behaviourally disordered students, juvenile delinquents*, or *deviants* (see table 17.1 for other terms).

One characteristic that commonly defines many students who experience difficulty either emotionally or behaviourally in our classrooms and gymnasiums is that they can be experts at isolating themselves from adults. For many of these young people, whom I will call *troubled youth*, their anger, resistance, failure to conform to expectations, disinterest in school, *apparent* lack of motivation, *apparent* lack of remorse over the hurt they may have caused others, and generally poor social skills are but a few of the characteristics that contribute to making them become, as Brendtro and Long suggest "evermore angry and unlovable."

Nonetheless, to be effective, physical educators must find ways to connect with and *accept* these young people, even when it becomes a challenge to do so. Teachers must find ways to build nurturing relationships of trust and respect that will encourage troubled youth to connect positively with their teachers, their classmates, and their school. But how do we build these relationships without a comprehensive understanding of the underlying factors that contribute to a student's difficulties in school? That is, how do teachers learn to understand the day-to-day challenges that make up what I will call the *cultural landscape of oppression* that a growing number of North American children face today? By *cultural landscape*, I refer to Usher and Edwards (1994) who explain how students' lifeworlds are "forged" in history and by "culture"; their experiences and perspectives are influenced daily by issues such

Table 17.1 Some Terms Used to Describe Students Who Have Experienced Emotional and Behavioural Difficulties

Juvenile delinquents, alienated youth, gang members, young offenders, young criminals, deviants, dropouts, marginalized, on the edge, social pathology, children with mental health problems, children with learning disabilities, drug and alcohol dependent youth, sexually promiscuous youth, postmodern youth culture, violent youth, adolescents, disenfranchised youth, aggressive youth, maltreated children, children with emotional and behavioural disorders, emotionally disturbed children, chronic deviants, children on the edge, 'bad boys', 'underserved' youth, throw away kids, severely 'unwanted kids', sexually and physically abused youth, neglected youth, abandoned youth, poor kids, kids in poverty, homeless youth, youth in care, troubled youth, youth at risk…

as socio-economic class, race, gender, sexuality, and so forth.

Let me present an example: if a student lives in a home where the adults are consumed by the debilitating effects of poverty and have little leftover time and energy to pay attention to their children, how will you, as a teacher, provide the necessary emotional attention that communicates the message "I care about you" in your classes? What type of physical education programme will you create for the angry child, feeling unloved, who might really benefit from the stress release opportunities that being playful in your gym might offer? (Peter McLaren's (1998) personal journal, *Life in Schools*, describes what it is like to teach in a low-income suburban Toronto school and highlights, in graphic detail, how children respond to the struggles their parents are enduring.)

The *ITP Nelson* (1997) Canadian dictionary defines *oppression* as "a feeling of being weighted down in mind or body." As a form of internalized oppression, the experience of poverty weighs heavily on the senses and spirit, and in Canada and the United States the number of families living under the weight of poverty is growing (Hubka 1992; Lawson 1997). The relationship between poverty and education is two-way; poverty rates are highest for those with low levels of education, and those who live in poverty experience severe educational problems (Wotherspoon 1998). Similarly, low economic status is considered a significant contributor to high school drop-out rates (Brady 1996), and low-income parents do not have

adequate time (e.g., paid work leave or flexible work schedules) to address their children's school and developmental needs (Heymann and Earle 2000).

We, as physical educators, need to acknowledge that our students are connected to very real social, cultural, economic, and historical issues that affect their home lives and school experiences. We need to recognize that in Canada the cultural landscape of daily life is affected by social inequality. It has been shown that the divisions of gender, class, race, ethnicity, region, age, and other factors will affect how students perform in schools (Wotherspoon 1998). To be effective, we can no longer ignore the complex social and economic factors that impact daily on our students' and their families' lives, and lead to difficulty in school.

Yet the reality remains that, for the most part, our educational systems continue to deal with students with emotional and behavioural difficulties by focussing attention entirely on the individual's behaviour and *pathology* and not on the complex web of interconnected factors that are beyond a young person's control (e.g., growing up in poverty or experiencing emotional, physical, or sexual abuse). The most common method used to determine educational resources for troubled youth in the school system is based solely on the student's ability to conform to set behaviour expectations in the classroom. I am speaking about the social construction of emotional and behavioural disorders, and how these descriptive labels are used to help schools identify students who may be in need of extra funding and resources to meet their educational needs. *Social construction* means how theories and ideas about reality and truth depend on social attitudes as opposed to biological or physical facts.

---

1 Historically, who have been the marginalized groups within Canadian society?

---

2 How might your own position within Canadian society influence how you interpret such issues as poverty, racism, sexism, classism, homophobia, and so on?

Emotional and Behavioural Dis-orders

The cross section of students who present themselves as angry, difficult to control, hyperactive, withdrawn, with low self-esteem, poor concentration, and so forth are often identified for funding or treatment purposes as having emotional or behavioural disorders. The terms *emotional disorders* and *behavioural disorders* are psychiatric labels that arise from biophysical, pyschodynamic, behavioural, and ecological models. The American Psychiatric Association's (1994) *Diagnostic and Statistical Manual of Mental Disorders–IV* locates emotional and behavioural dis-orders within two major categories, externalizing (e.g., attention deficit hyperactivity disorder, conduct disorder, oppositional defiance disorder) and internalizing (e.g., depression, anxiety disorder) (American Psychological Association; Coleman 1996). For a description of the categories used to describe children and youth with emotional and behavioural difficulties, see Squair and Groeneveld (Chapter 4).

The use of identifying labels and categories is helpful in that extra educational funding can be targeted for a student who is experiencing difficulty. These labels may allow particular students to receive additional educational resources, as in the assignment of a teacher's assistant. However practical this might sound, as teachers we must realize that these categories also serve a *normalizing*

discourse that reinforces socially-constructed ideas that assume what 'normal' means in our society. For example, definitions of 'normal' and 'deviant' behaviour in the classroom are based on criteria that apply to a middle-class, whitestream reference point. Denis (1997) states that Canadian society, although fundamentally structured on the European, white experience, is more than a 'white' society in socio-demographic, cultural, and economic terms. The descriptive term *whitestream* is meant to capture this evolving diversity of Canadian society, while acknowledging a continuity of privilege and hierarchy. Stated otherwise, normal behaviour is defined based on expectations for a child growing up in a 'normal' family. How appropriate (or ethical) is it to create categories of deviance based on socially-constructed definitions of normal when we know that normal does not apply to all families?

---

3 What is the normal way to respond to oppression? Is there an appropriately normal (or natural) response for how to behave in harsh environmental conditions that deviate from societal norms, such as being born into economic poverty, having to deal with systemic racism, or needing to deal with the breakdown of your family?

Most categories of emotional and behavioural dis-orders describe behaviour that deviates from socially-constructed conceptions of order in the classroom. Those who disrupt the order of the class can be targeted for extra resources as a means to help normalize their behaviour such that they can succeed in school. A major concern about these categories is 'who' decides what is a dis-order (i.e., the teacher is often the first person to identify the symptoms, which begs the question: how might this identification process differ amongst different teachers with differing classroom management styles?), and how the label might be utilized *inappropriately* to control *inappropriate* behaviour in the classroom. Currently, the intervention of choice for many students identified as having ADHD often involves the psychostimulant Ritalin or other pharmaceutical medications. Is it wise to medicate children based on personal characteristics in absence of an analysis of the social factors that might affect their behaviour (see Christian 1997; Halas and Hanson 2001)?

Similarly, students diagnosed as having other behaviour problems such as depression, anxiety-related dis-orders, sleep dis-orders, lack of motivation, and obsessive-compulsive dis-orders are receiving pharmaceutical interventions as part of the treatment process, despite the limited research evidence of their efficacy with children and adolescents (e.g., antidepressent medications such as Norpramin, Tofranil, Pamelor; serotonin re-uptake inhibitors such as Prozac, Paxil, and Zoloft; antiseizure medications such as Tegretal, Depakote; and drugs that lower blood pressure such as Inderal (see Hyman and Snook 1999). In many cases, behaviour problems are being controlled by feeding children a chemical soup that, when mixed with all the other known and unknown toxins in our foods, water, and environment, raises a simple question: is it harmful or helpful for a student to be categorized as having an emotional or behavioural dis-order? As Debra Shogan suggests in Chapter 5, identifying labels must be used with caution (see also Shogan 1998), and teachers must be aware of the effects that a diagnosis can have on a student, particularly given North America's attraction to the quick and cost-effective remedies that technology can provide (i.e., pharmaceutical intervention).

THE PROBLEMATIC NATURE OF LABELS AND LABELLING

After a class discussion about the issues facing troubled youth, a group of my second year physical education students at the University of Manitoba provided their own understanding of the meaning of the hyphenated term *'emotional and behavioural dis-order'*.

The following represents some of their responses:

- Detached, so it doesn't label them as hopeless.

- Because 'Dis' stands for disrespecting someone, and if we label people with a *disorder* we are putting them down.
- *Dis-order* shouldn't be a word to describe all children. All kids are socialized differently.
- This word is used as a label or stereotype. The way they perform day-to-day tasks is 'their order' of doing things.
- By displaying the word this way, it makes it look more positive than negative. For some it might be disorder, but it might be normal for others.
- Everybody shows signs or symptoms of a disorder.
- Dis/engage themselves from the norm.
- Dis/ruptive, go against authority, interrupt class. Dis/rupt others from learning.
- *Dis* is a negative connotation that has no part in teaching kids. It is a negative word that has no place for the confidence level of children.
- No slash = can't be cured (sounds that way).
- Labels them with an abnormality. Classifies as 'bad' or 'problem'.
- Because then it's being compared to normal and then you have to define normal.
- What meaning do you give to the word *dis-order*?

---

4 What are the dangers of using socially-constructed categories to target students for educational interventions?

Recognizing Troubled Youth and the Signals They Send in the Class

Given the widespread use of the emotional and behavioural dis-order classification systems, physical education teachers may at some point be called upon to assist in the identification of a student whose behaviour matches one of the dis-order categories. Once identified, a team may be formed to determine how the student's needs might best be met, and in some cases, an Individual Education Plan (IEP) might be drawn up. Presently, the options for students who experience more severe emotional and behavioural difficulties include the following continuum of placements: 1) full integration within the regular programme, no supports; 2) full integration within the regular programme, with support (e.g., a teacher's assistant); 3) partial integration: segregation within a special programme housed within the regular school (e.g., resource room, behaviour modification programme), participation in some regular classes (e.g., physical education, art, music); and, 4) segregation in a special school. In Canada, this is sometimes referred to as a *more habilitative environment* (e.g., treatment centre, community learning centre; see Hallenbeck and Kauffman 1996). Poor schooling also results in students dropping out of the system altogether.

As a physical education teacher, you can expect to have students who experience some difficulty in any one of your classes. Whatever the institution, and however the programme is offered, you will be challenged to build a meaningful physical activity programme that will help these students deal with the real, stressful life challenges that they face on a daily basis. The greater your understanding of these oppressive conditions, the more you may be able to develop a meaningful and relevant curriculum that respects their cultural landscape in terms of gender, class, ethnicity, family experience, and so forth. And the better your relationship with students, the more effective you will be in recognizing the existence of a problem that might be affecting student performance.

Personal Safety Issues: Signs of Emotional, Physical, and Sexual Abuse

In comparison to other school teachers, physical education teachers must be particularly vigilant regarding the signs and signals of abuse that may be conveyed by students participating in the gym. The enhanced social nature of the physical education class often allows physical education teachers to get to know their students on a more informal level,

which may open up increased opportunities for a student to disclose the existence of a current abusive situation. Signs of self-destructive behaviour, such as eating dis-orders, self-abuse, and suicide ideation, can be detected by alert teachers who know what to look for with regard to their students' behaviour. Warning signs might include a loss of appetite or weight, covering up arms or legs excessively to hide the presence of self-inflicted cuts, or verbal comments about death (for more information on self-injury, visit the SAFE in Canada Web site at http://www.safeincanada.ca).

Changing for class is one aspect of the physical education experience that might expose a student's vulnerabilities regarding the existence or expression of a prior abuse (e.g., wearing shorts might expose physical bruises; changing in front of others may threaten the self esteem and body image of an individual who is dealing with the leftover trauma of a past abuse or reveal self-inflicted wounds or scars on a student's arms). In some school programmes, changing for class is optional, and teachers encourage but do not force students to change for class (see Halas 2002). Recognizing a sudden change in the student's behaviour (e.g., when a typically happy child is suddenly quiet and withdrawn, or uncharacteristically refuses to change for class) might be a talking point to approach a student to ask if "everything is okay."

All teachers and caregivers are required by law to follow designated procedures within the school with regard to the reporting of any suspicion or disclosure of abuse involving a student. As a first step, new teachers to a school should be informed of this reporting protocol so that they are prepared should the disclosure of abuse occur. In the event that a student does take a teacher in her or his confidence, it is imperative that the teacher let the student know that the law compels all suspicions or disclosures of abuse to be reported. In these situations, the teacher and student must negotiate the tensions involved, which may include the student feeling that the teacher has betrayed her or him. The better the relationship between the teacher and the student, the greater the opportunity that these tensions can somehow be resolved.

Other Adolescent Issues Affecting the Students in Your Class

Other issues affecting young people in your physical education classes will include: dropping out, sexual activity (including teen pregnancy), prostitution, substance abuse (alcohol, drugs, and solvents), gangs, delinquency, and criminal involvement. Information is available in all school districts that provide guidelines or protocols relevant to each one of these areas. It is important, as an example, to recognize the identifiable signs and symbols used by criminal gangs in order to maintain a 'gang-free' climate within the school. Teachers are encouraged to contact their community police for information on the signs and symbols of local gang activity, which might include recognizable graffiti, specific hand gestures, and colours of clothing.

It is also important to recognize signs of alcohol, drugs, or solvent use by your students (e.g., the smell of alcohol, bloodshot eyes, unusual behaviour), and to be vigilant regarding the presence of any of these substances within your gymnasium or change rooms. Being aware of what is happening with your students is not a call for more police; rather, it is a reminder that teaching is about looking after the well-being of your students. It is a call to demonstrate your respect for children and youth by acknowledging that the issues and challenges they may be facing are real, and that their personal choices in relation to these challenges (e.g., choosing to come to school drunk or high on drugs) reflect the cultural landscape of their life beyond the classroom.

To summarize, students entering into the gym tell stories about their lives through the way that they present themselves in class. Teachers must be vigilant to read the signs and symbols of a student's life. How they are dressed, whom they interact with, what they are saying, how they respond to your lesson plan, are all bits of information that can help teachers better determine meaningful educational objectives that are contextualized within the present-day cultural landscape of each student. For these young people, finding a caring, trustworthy adult to support them sensitively and respectfully requires courage on the part of the student, and understanding on the part of the adult. Again, developing a caring, supportive relationship with your students will allow you to determine the most effective way for addressing some of these more difficult adolescent issues.

---

5 Explain why it is important for the physical education teacher to develop a good relationship with students who are experiencing difficulty.

Building the Teacher-Student Relationship

THE CONTACT ZONE

Schools are hierarchical organizations that have rules and procedures which ensure that students and teachers interact in asymmetrical relations of power in what can be referred to as 'the contact zone', the space where cultures interact with each other in highly unequal relations of power, often to the detriment of the less dominant culture (Pratt, as cited in Brown 1998). In the following case, the term *exercise power* is a key phrase: physical education teachers exercise power with regard to the students in their class. Darrell enters the gym during free time and his eyes immediately zoom in on two students who are playing twenty-one at the basketball net. He walks right up to one of them and says, "Get lost, this is my basket." Darrell is bigger than both of these two students, and his intimidation works. They drop the ball and saunter over to the far side of the gym, looking for something else to do. You have expelled Darrell from the last two gym classes for this type of aggressive behaviour, and you decide that it's time to try something new.

Why might Darrell be acting this way? What alternative strategies could you use? What would be the effects of continually expelling Darrell from the class, as opposed to attempting a different strategy? Should the teacher evict Darrell for his aggressive behaviour, or should attempts be made to work with about him, to create ways in which he can express the energy he brings with him to class in a more postive way? How might the rules of the gym, teacher practices, and procedures be used to enable Darrell to succeed in the class? How might the choice of how to respond to Darrell's aggressive behaviour be influenced by knowing more about him? Suppose that after the second time you send Darrell from class, his homeroom teacher tells you that Darrell recently learned that his mother, who is his sole caregiver, is dying of cancer? Would this information change the way you choose to deal with the situation?

The choice of which rules, strategies, or procedures to use when exercising power is referred to as *teacher practices*. In culturally relevant educational programmes (Ladson-Billings 1994, 1997), teachers try to disrupt the hierarchical nature of the school by using teacher practices that build *humanely equitable* and *fluid* relationships with students. A fluid teacher relationship is one that involves an approach to the use of rules, procedures, and teaching strategies based on the specific needs of individual students. For example, rules can be enforced differentially but fairly for different students as a means to promote rehabilitative, as opposed to punitive, consequences. Research indicates that zero tolerance programmes that control and punish students are not only ineffective but contribute to increased violence within schools.

In a well-managed gymnasium, rules of conduct are established in the very first class. These rules, when clearly communicated and reinforced (e.g., respect each other, respect the teacher, respect the equipment and facility) are meant to shape/constrain student behaviour in order that all students can participate in class activities knowing that they will be physically and emotionally (or psychologically) safe from harm. Procedures are used to reinforce these expectations: for example, at the start of the instructional part of a class activity, all students are asked to gather in one area of the gym in order to

listen to the teacher's lesson. When a student doesn't respond to the teacher's request to meet in the middle or listen while she or he is speaking, the teacher can pick from a repertoire of procedural strategies to help bring the student in line with the class activity (see Problem Solving: Kelly Refuses to Join the Group Activity). Teacher practices with regard to the use of rules, procedures, and strategies will have varying effects, which will not be static but, in turn, will vary depending on each situation and student. Incorporating past results into present and future lessons is a means to transform teacher practice.

Problem Solving: Kelly Refuses to Join The Group Activity

Let us use the example of a student, Kelly, who refuses to join the class activity and continues doing her own thing at the far end of the gym. What would you, as a teacher, do in this scenario? Perhaps you could use a second request, or wait for the student to respond, or cajole the student into responding, or focus positive attention on the student, or focus negative attention on the student. What effects might the following two responses produce?

1. "C'mon Kelly, we really need you for this part of the class."
2. "Kelly! Everybody is waiting for you. What right do you have to hold everyone up?"

When students resist the rules, teachers can respond in a variety of ways. They can use a warning ("If you're not here in three seconds…"), prescribe a time-out ("Kelly, take a time-out on the side of the gym"), or modify the time-out ("Take a time-out and when you're ready to join the class activity, come sit down quietly"). Teachers can ignore the student and carry on with the class while the student carries on with whatever activity she or he was doing, or the teacher could eliminate the student altogether from class ("Go to the office"). If possible, the teacher can ask a teacher's assistant to talk with Kelly while the larger group is organized into the next activity. Or, the teacher can switch positions, whereby the teacher's assistant supervises the larger class while the teacher speaks to Kelly quietly on the side. How might your relationship with a student influence the way in which you respond to her or his classroom behaviour?

The suggestions offered in the problem-solving scenario are not exhaustive, and there is not a 'one size fits all' solution. You may have come up with an entirely different response. What is more certain is that *how* a teacher decides to interact with this student will affect the outcomes: the student might react positively and choose to join the class, or she or he might continue to disrupt the rules and teacher authority, thus resulting in a more punitive consequence (e.g., a time-out, or being sent from class). If the student is made to feel humiliated in any way (e.g., suppose the teacher yells or uses sarcasm that is not well-received by the student), the humiliation may have carry-over affects. To be sure, the student's relationship with the teacher will be influenced by the decisions made, and the other students will be watching to see how the teacher deals with this situation.

6 How do you deal with a conflict without humiliating the student?

In traditional gymnasium settings that reinforce the dominance of the teacher, teacher practice favours the use of threats, punishment, or exclusion (e.g., a time-out, expulsion from class, expulsion from school, expulsion from extracurricular school activities, poor evaluations) as a means to control student behaviour. An alternative to punishment and control is to recognize the unequal relations of power that exist between the teacher (who is in the more privileged position) and the student (who, because of behaviour difficulties, might find herself or himself already caught within the web of rules and procedures, meaning, therefore, that the student is also more often affected by teacher practice), and to devise ways to disrupt the hierarchy by allowing students to exercise more control over their environment in this 'contact zone'.

One strategy that minimizes the unequal relations of power between a teacher and student is to allow the student the opportunity to express feelings, likes, and dislikes about the class in the areas of content, structure, environment, and even teacher involvement. Students can help determine the rules of the physical education class. They can provide input regarding what procedures are most effective in maintaining these rules. They can be asked what activities they like and for how long the activity unit should last. Although choice of activity in the gymnasium is often limited by such factors as availability of equipment, amount of supervised space available for multiple activities, and the number of differing student likes and dislikes, effort can be made to accommodate a student's primary interests at some point. At the end of a lesson, students can provide feedback regarding how they feel about a class or activity, and this feedback can be used to determine future lessons. By reflecting on their own experiences, students can provide the necessary information that teachers need to construct more relevant and inviting physical activity programmes.

A second teacher practice involves what is commonly referred to as *reflective practice*. Reflective practice is a process of self-reflection that questions the assumptions underlying our observations of a situation, event, student, or student conflict. It is a process that is on-going, one that continually seeks to construct improved and varied ways of interacting with students. It is one that continually questions the rules and procedures used to produce certain student behaviours. It is a process that seeks to understand the reasons for our successes in order to improve our practice. It is also a process that questions our own complicity in our students' failures. Reflective practice means that the teacher is also and always the learner, approaching each new situation with a desire to learn from the multiple messages that students are sending our way in every class, be they positive or negative. It is the conscious effort to question our own assumptions regarding our teacher practices and their effects on the successes and failures of our students.

7 The kids do not come with instructions…how do we know what to do with them? How would you give the troubled student attention without ignoring the rest of the class? I want my students to know they can talk to me when they have a problem…how can I communicate to them that I am willing to listen?

READING RESISTANCE

If a student tells a teacher to "fuck off," she or he is expressing any number of messages that we, as teachers, may not understand unless we take the time to sit down and talk to the student about the meaning behind the words. As a form of reflective practice, one question that I often use in this situation is to first ask myself: "What might I be doing to cause this act of disrespect?" If I can provide answers to that question, I would then talk to the student about what I think I may have done wrong and, if necessary, apologize. If I can not come up with any idea of how my actions might have encouraged a negative response from a student, I then approach the student and ask the following question: "What have I done to cause you to disrespect me?" For me, this simple practice has worked over and again with students. The student's answer to that question usually provides essential information that relates directly to the conflict. If I was perceived as the cause of the problem, I would attempt to adapt or modify my ways to acknowledge and show respect for the student's interpretation, even if I didn't always agree with her or him.

If other issues were the cause of the problem (e.g., pressures from sources outside the gym, such as problems at home or a conflict from the previous class), I would then explore methods that the student could use to express herself or himself more effectively in our interactions. For instance, she or he could forewarn me at the start of class that it was a "bad day." We could negotiate a means to deal with any potential conflict situations (e.g., having the student self-determine a time out or, in some cases, choose to opt out from the activity entirely). The idea is to allow the student to make this choice, and to respect the decision once made. As with other key concepts from the inclusion literature (e.g., empowerment, self-determination, self-regulation), students need to exercise as much control as possible over the rules and procedures affecting their lives in the gymnasium. The more control students have, the less they may seek to disrupt the rules. Effective teachers will learn to devise ways to disrupt the power differential by allowing students to exercise more control over their environment in this 'contact zone'.

In summary, teachers and students can collaborate to construct a physical activity environment where the entanglement of rules, procedures, and teacher practices communicate to young people that they are valued, no matter what their resistance. The real-life scenario in physical education and physical activity settings across North America suggests that the number of children who experience emotional and behavioural difficulties is rising. No matter where we teach or instruct a physical activity programme (e.g., the public school, the treatment centre, the community club) we should be prepared to work with these young people in a nurturing and meaningful way. Those adults who genuinely like children and youth and exercise power self-reflexively will be more likely to negotiate outcomes that best serve the needs of the individual student.

8 Do *all* your students like phys. ed.? Are they on time at the start of class, eager to get going? Do they say "Hi" to you in the hallways? Do they ask "What are we doing today?" Does everyone participate, including those who are less talented? If you can answer "yes" to these questions, chances are you have succeeded in creating an emotionally safe, inclusive, and culturally relevant physical education class.

1. Ask a student who is struggling: "What can I do to help you succeed in this class?"
2. Pass on the compliment: When a student has done something really good, tell her or him, tell the class, tell the other teachers, tell their parents…
3. Take time to be 'playful' with students: having fun with your students lets them know you by the way you play and interact in competitive and non-competitive physical activities.

Building a Culturally Relevant Physical Education Programme

DIS-RUPTING TRADITIONAL PRACTICES TO RECLAIM TROUBLED YOUTH

Culturally relevant and gender relevant educational programmes include teaching practices that encourage students to develop multiple identities that are consistent with personal and social constructions of self (Ennis 1999; Ladson-Billings 1994). All students are socialized differently, and we, as teachers, need to be aware of how our own practices in the gym can and will produce different outcomes with respect to our students' cultural landscapes. For example, assimilationist teaching practices reproduce traditional gender, ethnic, and academic stereotypes that favour the dominant (whitestream) society by excluding females, minorities, the dis-abled, homosexuals, the poor, et cetera. In these classes, it remains that boys are better skilled at sports than girls, that sports based on the whitestream European experience are emphasized in curriculum content (e.g., golf, tennis), and only the skilled succeed in physical education. These types of programmes do not provide much room for students who fall outside the dominant group, unless, of course, the non-dominant students learn to perform appropriately, that is, sit quietly on the sidelines.

In their extensive work with American youth at risk, Brendtro and Brokenleg (1993) promote the need for "reclaiming school environments" that incorporate Native American empowerment values such as belonging, mastery, independence, and generosity. To design this type of reclaiming programme, teachers would need to disrupt Western civilization's patriarchal values of hierarchy, individualism, winning, dominance, affluence, and other such values that are reproduced and rewarded through traditional physical activity and sports programmes. Traditional physical education programmes that offer a few days of skill practice followed by weeks of competitive game play often reproduce a scenario by which the skilled succeed and are reinforced through winning while the less-skilled (often girls and smaller or weaker boys who have not been provided enough instruction and opportunity to develop skills) are marginalized off the playing court (Ennis et al. 1997; Humbert 1995).

An alternative to this type of programme is exemplified in the Sport for Peace programme, where boys and girls of varying skill levels are encouraged to collaborate by assuming different roles (e.g., player, coach, referree, score keeper) during each class (Ennis 1999). Using the students' preferred activity choice in an *extended* unit (in this case, basketball), students take responsibility for each other by actively engaging in the process of skill development (through peer teaching) and game organization. In this type of learning climate, students become real participants in the "community of learners," their effort in class improves, and the values of belonging (to the team), mastery (of the skills), independence (in learning, as students become the teacher), and generosity (where the better-skilled participants pay attention to the less-skilled players) replace the importance of winning and losing.

Reclaiming environments also respects the multiple identities that students construct for themselves inside and beyond the walls of the gymnasium. If a student presents herself as angry, that anger is accepted as an essential aspect of her current life. It is not dismissed as inappropriate or controlled through punishment. Rather, efforts are made to allow the student to express that anger safely through social interaction and the expenditure of physical energy. If a student is sad and withdrawn and chooses to avoid physical activity, that choice is honoured. Students are encouraged, but *never forced* to join the gymnasium activity. Students are not expected to fit into one mold, and they are not punished if they deviate from accepted social standards of behaviour. Rather, teachers work with the student to construct gymnasium experiences that will be meaningful and relevant to their present-day life, however daunting a task that may seem to be.

9 Compare and contrast assimilationist teaching practices to culturally relevant teaching practices.

10 What is the value of having students participate in an extended activity unit of their own choosing? Discuss possible outcomes in terms of physical, social, emotional, and cognitive outcomes.

11 What are the benefits of being a 'peer teacher' in the gymnasium?

12 Think back to your own high school physical education programme. Who were the marginalized kids? How culturally relevant was it for students who did not fit into the mainstream or had trouble in class? Did all kids feel safe in the gym? Were sexist, racist, and homophobic comments tolerated, or was there a respectful climate that all students adhered to? Did girls participate as much as boys? How about the kids who hung out back of the school smoking between classes? Were they a part of the phys.ed. class? What kind of programme do you want to be known for?

PHYSICALLY AND PSYCHOLOGICALLY SAFE PHYSICAL EDUCATION

The gymnasium, when constructed as a physically and emotionally safe and inclusive environment that provides meaningful and relevant activity choices, can provide opportunities for students to experience many positive interconnected physical, social, and emotional outcomes. Conversely, gymnasium environments that favour some (e.g., those with excellent physical ability) while excluding others (e.g., girls, the unskilled, the 'difficult' students) can negatively impact on a young person's desire to participate actively in the physical education class. In the latter type of learning climates, the opportunity to use the gymnasium as a means to engage students positively who have emotional and behavioural difficulties is wasted.

In physical education, the movement focus requires the suspension of many classroom formalities. The contingencies of game play in team sports requires that students cooperate with each other in order to achieve team goals; students can choose to meet this challenge in a variety of ways, by encouraging and including one another in the game or by putting each other down and marginalizing the less skilled or unpopular players. When negative social interactions are allowed to happen and go unchecked by the teacher, the number of physical education students who are being picked on, ignored, excluded, or harassed in our school gymnasiums increases.

Conversely, when social skill development is planned for and reinforced through pedagogically sensitive teacher involvement, troubled youth can be encouraged to interact positively and successfully in the physical education class. At all times, the teacher needs to be present to the activity (i.e., watching the students' body language and verbal expressions) in order to evaluate continually how students are interacting. The moment that a conflict arises, the teacher must be ready to step in immediately to intervene. In some cases, this might involve breaking up a physical fight, negotiating a truce in an argument, stopping an activity altogether, or interacting one on one with a student who is making sexist, racist, classist, homophobic, or other disrespectful comments. Strategies such as the Fair Play programme, Don Hellison's (1990, 1995) social responsibility levels system, using directed time-outs to deal with moral dilemmas (e.g., having students problem solve how to share equipment), and/or stopping an entire class to deal with disrespectful behaviour will reinforce the social skill development goals that you set as a class (see also Herbal and Parker 1997). Non-violent Crisis Intervention Training provides safe and effective methods for interacting with students during conflict situations. Check with school division officials to see if there is a training programme offered to teachers in your area.

In summary, the inclusion of students with emotional and behavioural difficulties in the highly interactive gymnasium environment presents both challenges and opportunities. In a space where body contact often occurs and bodily emotions can be freely expressed (e.g., jumping for joy after scoring a goal, throwing a stick/racquet/bat after making a bad play), the challenge is to create a safe and respectful climate for students to express themselves positively through active participation. The opportunity for this type of self-expression opens the door to many potential physical, social, and emotional outcomes that result from active participation (e.g., see Nobes 1996). If you develop a programme that students will want to be a part of, such that they will arrive on time for each class, eager to participate without the influence of alcohol and other substances, then you have most likely succeeded in creating a programme that is meaningful and nurturing for students, one that is culturally relevant for troubled youth.

13 Now that we have an idea of the cultural landscape of troubled youth, what next? Can we ever fully understand why these young people struggle in our schools? Are we as willing to adapt and modify our programmes for students who struggle to perform socially and/or behaviourally in school in the same way as we modify and adapt our programmes for students who are physically or intellectually challenged? Or, by ignoring these factors, will our teacher practices and programmes reproduce the conditions that will further marginalize these students within our gymnasiums?

In the following section, I will describe an outstanding active living programme at Macdonald School (a pseudonym), which is associated with an adolescent treatment centre designed for students who experience severe emotional and behavioural difficulties (including alcohol and substance abuse; emotional, physical and sexual abuse; and conflict with the juvenile justice system) (Halas 2002). Many of the students at the school have been diagnosed as having such dis-orders as ADHD, conduct dis-order, and in some cases, fetal alcohol syndrome and fetal alcohol effects. This school is of interest because a high percentage of the very diverse student population (in terms of ethnic background, socio-economic class, problems that were being addressed at the centre) was engaged in the school's active living programme on a daily basis. In this physical education programme, there were more students running to the gym, as opposed to away from it, for a variety of reasons. The following is a short description of life in the gymnasium at that treatment centre.

Learning by Example:
Tales from the Real World

WHEN TROY MEETS RONDA

It's fifteen minutes into free time, the start of phys. ed. class where students choose the activities they want to do and work on their own. Sensing a small change in the flow of 'free time' energy, Ronda, the teacher, calls everyone in and they randomly drop to the floor in the space around her. As she waits for the students to settle in, Troy, who's been on edge since the start of class, walks right up to Ronda's face and yells "FU…!!" Ronda is half expecting the unexpected from Troy, and she immediately voices her own quick reply: "Fun! Emphasis on the *n*. Is that what you wanted to say?" As hard as he tries to bug her, Ronda won't be rattled today. Sensing this, Troy wanders off to the side of the gym and slouches against the wall.

Ronda focusses her attention on the students directly in front of her and asks "What do you want to do?" One voice immediately calls for Octopus, a low-organized tag game that they've been playing since the beginning of the term, and five hands shoot up in agreement. Consensus is formed without much complaint, and the chosen activity is greeted with yelps as the boys jump up and run toward the end wall. Troy slams his body into the protective mats that line the end walls under the basket, and he bounces in a forward spinning motion, each contact dispersing energy as one by one, the mats fall from the velcro attachment. Ronda instructs Troy to put the mats back up "cause we don't want people flying into the wall." She quickly calls over to Alex to ask if he knows the rules of Octopus. Some students are talking which forces Ronda to speak louder. She then asks, "Are you ready?" The game begins, and ends six rounds later when the students decide to finish the five minutes left in class with a game of basketball. They organize themselves quickly and play until 'last basket' is called. When Ronda signals the end of class, the students stop playing and turn toward the exit door. They leave the gym knowing they'll be back sooner than later, and that makes leaving not such a bad thing.

Providing Opportunities to Play:
An Active Living Success Story

Macdonald School offers a "more restrictive environment" that has as its primary goal to reconnect students with a school environment. A large number of the students at this crosscultural school are Aboriginal, and the oppression their families and communities endured through colonization has left many students the victims of abject poverty. Most of the students (forty-five female and male students, aged ten to seventeen), have experienced some form of school failure, and it is not uncommon for many students to have attended multiple schools prior to arriving at the treatment centre/school. In fact, the school population might turn over as many as two to three times in one school year. Many students present as having very low self-esteem, thus challenging teachers to find creative ways of motivating their students to attend and perform in school.

One method that teachers have found to be effective is to offer their students the opportunity to participate in a daily active living programme, which the students have enthusiastically embraced (Halas 2001; Halas and Watkinson 1999). *Active living* is defined as a way of life in which physical activity is valued and integrated into daily life. With an average school attendance of 75 percent for a population of students at high risk for truancy or dropping out, the school appears to be highly effective in its goal of attracting kids to school and away from the other attractions out on the street (e.g., drugs, prostitution, hanging out). Unlike other more restrictive/habilitative schools, this school incorporates active living as an integral aspect of what a nurturing and relevant curriculum is for all its students.

HOW THE ACTIVE LIVING PROGRAMME WORKS

At Macdonald School, lack of competence, either physically or socially, was never positioned as a bad thing; rather it was presented by the teachers as an opportunity to learn. An example is basketball. Although basketball (considered a traditional sport) dominated the games that were played, the games were organized such that the winning was de-emphasized and task mastery (e.g., getting the ball in the basket, making a good pass) was celebrated. Some of the loudest lunchtime cheers were reserved for the newer players as they scored their first-ever basket. As they turned to run back down the court, they would receive high-fives from the better players who had learned from the onset that the game was 'just for fun', and part of the fun was celebrating the accomplishments of others. Taking part was what was important, and yet, no one was ever forced to play. Students who opted out of the day's activity were gently encouraged by the teachers to join in, and a student's decision to engage in the gym activity was often celebrated in and of itself. Again, just taking part was framed as an accomplishment, particularly as students who were struggling with difficult issues in their life (see table 17.2 for the highlights of this programme).

HOW THE PROGRAMME HELPS

The quality and quantity of the active living programme was considered to help student performance in terms of school attendance, behaviour in class, improved student-teacher relationships, ability to focus on academic tasks, ability to integrate socially with peers, and a decrease in conflict issues. Both students and teachers commented at how important it was for students to have opportunities just to be playful, as many of the young people had not had the opportunity to experience the benefits of play in their childhoods.

Students who were interviewed in the study identified a number of personally relevant health benefits arising from their participation, which included release or relief from stress, anger, aggression, tension, and boredom. Perceived social benefits included the development of appropriate social skills (e.g., cooperation, teamwork) and a sense of belonging through the experience and development of social bonds on the playing field (which combated feelings of loneliness and isolation). The contingencies of games (e.g., they are highly interactive with lots of hands-on practice) allowed students the opportunity to experience improvement and success across a variety of skills and activities.

The experiential nature of the play experience (i.e., involving all the senses) was perceived to allow students greater control and responsibility over their learning. The immediacy of performance feedback allowed for self-correction (as opposed to relying on the teacher to know if you had performed the task correctly or now). The structure of games and the public celebration of accomplishment in the gymnasium was considered to affect the student's self-esteem positively. It is interesting to note that a similar public celebration of accomplishment was not perceived to be socially-acceptable in the classroom. For students who present as 'angry', both students and teachers described examples of how the gym allows a transformation of negative energy into more positive energy (e.g., engaging actively with a peer through play) that often carried over into other parts of the school (thus contributing to school performance). According to many teachers and students, physical education contributed a positive energy to the overall school climate.

Summary: 'Nurturing' Resistance, Exercising Power and Transforming Practice

As mentioned at the onset of this chapter, building a relationship is not always easy, particularly when working with students who are resistant to teachers' efforts to engage them in a class activity. Students who present as angry, difficult to control, hyperactive, withdrawn, with low self-esteem, poor concentration, and so forth are often identified (for funding or treatment purposes) as having emotional or behavioural dis-orders. Although identifying labels may serve a purpose, labels can also have negative effects, especially when used to focus on individual *pathology* and not the complex web of interconnected factors (often beyond the student's control) which will impact on how she or he performs in school. While acknowledging that identifying labels and categories have specific purposes within an educational discourse, this chapter has focussed on the *teacher practices* that promote non-traditional

Table 17.2 Active Living at the Treatment Centre: How the Programme Works and How It Helps

How the programme works	How the programme helps
Lots of time: up to 700 min/week or 140 min/day of physical activity time is used.	**Playtime for big kids:** for some students, playtime in the gym is an opportunity to make up for the childhood play experiences (and benefits) they missed out on.
Motto: lack of competence is not a bad thing; it's an opportunity to learn and improve.	**Play is experiential:** physical play involves all the senses: you see the ball go through the hoop, hear your name called for a pass, feel the expansion of your lungs in a run; smell the humidity and sweat…
Inclusive: students of all ability levels are included and encouraged in all gym activities.	
Teachers: they are easy-going and caring; use gentle interventions ("c'mon, let's get going…") to encourage participation.	**Feedback is immediate:** students can interpret their own performance feedback (e.g., the ball hits the target or doesn't, you make a good or bad pass).
A safe climate: low student:teacher ratio (including two female teacher's aides); always well-supervised; time-outs used to settle conflicts; fights immediately broken up; students not forced to participate if they don't want to or if they don't feel safe.	**Self-correction:** students do not need to rely on a teacher to tell them if a mistake has been made, they can correct their own skills.
Flexible: students allowed lots of activity choice.	**Sense of belonging:** the structure of games necessitates student interaction; teamwork (e.g., good communication) is essential to succeed in the activity.
Class content: experiential games focus; learn by watching others, limited skill instruction accommodated by generous amount of time students spend in activities they like.	**Public celebration of accomplishment:** successful performance is culturally acceptable in the gym; students are reinforced through high-fives, slaps on the back, hugs; "gets the self-esteem up."
Social skill development: gym used as a means to teach social skills and help newer students to meet classmates and teachers.	**Positive circulation of energy:** students can blow off steam, feel good, laugh, have fun, work up a sweat, etc.
Changing for class: encouraged, but not enforced (many students are dealing with personal safety and body image issues).	**Eases tension:** cathartic effects of physical expenditure of energy and social interaction; students who see themselves as angry can use the gym as a means of managing their anger so that their energy is expended positively, not negatively.

How the programme works

Picking teams: emphasis on choosing even-sided, fair teams; students involved in the choices; rotation of captains to include all students of all abilities.

Evaluation: based on participation, effort, attitude.

Daily physical education: promotes social skill development, fun, fair play.

Daily lunch hour basketball (and other activities): the gym is always open at lunch, supervised by teachers and treatment centre staff; all students (male/female; ages 10-17; all ability levels) invited to take part.

Physical activity option class: students who have performed well (i.e., been good) in the day's physical education class and other classes can opt into an extra gym activity at the end of the day.

Weekly swimming: optional class at a community pool, emphasis on recreational swimming/diving.

Active living breaks: regular or spontaneous physical activity breaks (e.g., a walk in the neighbourhood) organized by the classroom teachers; often used to motivate students to "work for awhile, then we'll play…"

Large group activities/special events: e.g., Friday afternoon school-wide baseball, winter carnival, tobogganing; wall-climbing; some inter-school activities; students often involved in the organization of these events (e.g., they make up the teams, schedule, rules, etc.).

How the programme helps

Effects of fun: students can forget about their problems for awhile.

Performance aid in class: for some students, knowing that the gym will offer a break from the classroom routine helps keep them on task; catalyst for social development: students meet new friends, interact differently than in the regular classroom.

Transforms student-teacher relationships: students get to know their teachers differently when they play together in games and activities (i.e., students see teachers making mistakes, missing a shot, not knowing how to perform a skill); equalizes the student-teacher relationship; carry-over effect in the classroom: "they've seen you see them" on a different level (e.g., being scared going downhill on the toboggan), which changes the way teachers and students communicate and connect when back in the class.

Motivates school attendance: according to some students, the only reason they came to school was "for the gym."

SOURCE: From *Physical Education/Physical Activity for Troubled Youth at an Adolescent Treatment Centre: An Interpretive Case Study.* Unpublished doctoral dissertation, by J. Halas, Edmonton: University of Alberta. Adapted with permission.

curricular outcomes (e.g., such as fun and enjoyment) as a means to connect all students positively to a school environment.

Children and youth who have experienced negative attachments to society, family, friends, care-givers, and teachers need opportunities to develop trusting relationships with caring adults who are prepared to stick with them through both the good and bad times. These students have lived through a thousand different 'contact zones', many of which have left them feeling broken and betrayed. It is up to you, as the teacher, through your own teacher practices with regard to the circulation of power (e.g., rules and procedures), to convince students that you are there for them. This takes time and energy and the repetition of consistent teacher practices that say to the student, over and over and over again, "you are important to me."

The challenges presented by young people who experience emotional and behavioural difficulties oblige the promotion of physical activity programmes that are designed to be emotionally safe and culturally relevant. Teachers exercise power daily as they interact with students in the 'contact zone'. As I have tried to show, how teachers relate to their students will have a major impact on how successful their physical education programme will be. In some cases, it may be necessary to modify the existing rules and procedures, class content, and curriculum to promote values and experiences that are more meaningful and relevant to your students. At all times, teachers must respect young people and create opportunities for them to exercise control regarding their involvement in the physical education programme.

For some teachers, this might require what has been called the "conversion" process (Pratt, as cited in Brown 1998): simply said, it is the teacher who changes her or his ways to meet the needs of the students, and not the reverse (Halas 1998). In so doing, we may see a greater movement from one that is a curriculum of control and patriarchal, to one of social inclusion, belonging, mastery, generosity, and responsibility, that reclaims troubled youth who have experienced emotional and behavioural difficulties.

Listen to your students, and when they look at what you are offering and reply with a very matter-of-fact "this sucks," try and find out what you can do better. Keep searching for new ways by which we can build relationships and programmes that will bring young people running to our gymnasiums, excited by the opportunities to be playful in a safe environment where each individual knows she or he can be respected for who she or he is and be cared for by the adults who run the programme. And, to borrow from a little bit of practice wisdom, if you don't like your students or your job, look for something else to do. Students who have experienced emotional and behavioural difficulties deserve the very best that a culturally relevant, emotionally safe, and inclusive physical activity environment can offer.

Study Questions

1. Explain the problematic nature of using emotional and behavioural categories to identify students who experience emotional and behavioural difficulties in the school.

2. How might teachers who ignore the socio-cultural and economic factors affecting their students contribute to the continued oppression of children and youth?

3. Why is the relationship between the physical education teacher and the student with emotional and behavioural difficulties so important?

4. What are the characteristics of a culturally relevant physical education programme?

5. You have applied to teach at a new inner-city school with a high population of students who have emotional and behavioural difficulties. In the interview, the principal asks you why you think physical education is important for troubled youth; she also asks you to explain the type of programme you would organize in the school. How would you respond?

References

American Psychiatric Association. (1994). *Diagnostic and statistical manual of mental disorders-* N *(DSM-IV)* (4th ed.). Washington, DC: Author.

Brady, P. (1996). Native dropouts and non-Native dropouts in Canada: Two solitudes or a solitude shared? *Journal of American Indian Culture, Winter,* 10–20.

Brendtro. L., and Brokenleg, M. (1993). Beyond the curriculum of control: Reclaiming children and youth. *Journal of Emotional and Behavioral Problem, Winter,* 5–11.

Brendtro, L., and Long, N. (1994). Violence begets violence: Breaking conflict cycles. *Journal of Emotional and Behavioral Problems, Spring,* 3–7.

Brown, S. (1998). The Bush teacher as cultural thief: The politics of pedagogy in the land of the indigene. *The Review of Education/Pedagogy/Cultural Studies, 20*(2), 121–39.

Christian, J. (1997). The body as a site of reproduction and resistance: Attention deficit hyperactivity disorder and the classroom. *Interchange, 28*(1), 31–43.

Coleman, M.C. (1996). *Emotional and behavioral disorders: Theory and practice* (3rd. ed). Boston: Allyn and Bacon.

Denis, C. (1997). *We are not you: First Nations and Canadian modernity.* Peterborough, ON: Broadview Press.

Ennis, C. (1999). Creating a culturally relevant curriculum for disengaged girls. *Sport, Education, and Society, 4*(1), 31–49.

Ennis, C., Cothran, D., Davidson, K., Loftus, S., Owens, L., Swanson, L., and Hopsicker, P. (1997). Implementing curriculum within a context of fear and disengagement. *Journal of Teaching in Physical Education, 17,* 52–71.

Halas, J. (2002). Engaging troubled youth in physical education: An alternative program with lessons for the traditional class. *Journal of Teaching in Physical Education, 21,* 267–86.

Halas, J. (2001). Playtime at the treatment centre: Hour physical activity helps troubled youth. *Avante, 7*(2), 1–13.

Halas, J. (1998). Runners in the gym: Tales of resistance and conversion at an adolescent treatment center. *Journal of Native Education, 22*(2), 21–221.

Halas, J., and Hanson, L. (2001). Pathologizing Billy: Enabling and constraining the body of the condemned. *Sociology of Sport Journal* (1), 115–26.

Halas, J., and Watkinson, J. (1999). "Everyone gets a chance": A group of "at risk" students describe what's it like at their "active living" school. *Runner, 37*(1), 14–22.

Hallenbeck, B., and Kauffman, J. (1996). Constructing habilitative environments for students with emotional or behavioural disorders: Conclusion to the special issue. *Canadian Journal of Special Education, 11*(1), 101–8.

Hellison, D. (1995). *Teaching responsibility through physical activity.* Champaign, IL: Human Kinetics.

Hellison, D. (1990). Making a difference: Reflections on teaching urban at-risk youth. *Journal of Physical Education, Recreation and Dance, August,* 44–45.

Herbal, K., and Parker, M. (1997). Youth, basketball and responsibility: A fairy tale ending? *Research Quarterly for Exercise and Sport, 68*(1), March 1997 Supplement, A-81.

Heymann, S., and Earle, A. (2000). Low-income parents: How do working conditions affect their opportunity to help school-age children at risk? *American Educational Research Journal, 37*(4), 833–48.

Hubka, D. (1992). Reporting on child poverty: The efforts of campaign 2000. *Perception, 16*(4), 17–20.

Humbert, L. (1995a). On the sidelines: The experiences of young women in physical education class. *Avante, 1*(2), 58–77.

Hyman, I., and Snook, P. (1999). *Dangerous schools: What we can do about the physical and emotional abuse of our children.* San Francisco: Jossey-Bass.

ITP Nelson Canadian dictionary of the English language: An encyclopedic reference. (1997). Toronto: ITP Nelson.

Ladson-Billings, G. (1994). *The Dreamkeepers: Successful teachers of African-American Children.* San Francisco: Jossey-Bass.

Ladson-Billings, G. (1997). Culturally relevant pedagogy. In C.A. Grant and G. Ladson-Billings (Eds.), *Dictionary of multicultural education,* pp. 62–63. Phoenix: Oryx Press.

Lawson, H. (1997). Children in crisis, the helping professions, and the social responsibilities of universities. *Quest, 49,* 8–33.

Maunder, M. (1998, October 9). Every student is special: No shortage of appalling statistics for Native youth. *Winnipeg Free Press,* pp. A12–A13.

McLaren, P. (1998). *Life in schools: An introduction to critical pedagogy in the foundations of education* (3rd ed.). New York: Longman.

Nobes, S. (1996). In praise of new teachers and athletics for all. *ATA Magazine, 79*(1), 4–5.

Shogan, D. (1998). The social construction of disability: The impact of statistics and technology. *Adapted Physical Activity Quarterly, 15*(3), 269–78.

Usher, R., and Edwards, R. (1994). *Postmodernism and education.* London: Routledge.

Wotherspoon, T. (1998). *The sociology of education in Canada: Critical perspectives.* Don Mills, ON: Oxford University Press.

CHAPTER 18

The Role of Adapted Physical Education Consultants

Patricia C. Nearingburg
Laurie Clifford

Learning Objectives

- To define the roles and responsibilities of an adapted physical education consultant.
- To outline the overall school-based adapted physical education consultative process.
- To discuss how a referral for an adapted physical education consultant may be initiated.
- To describe some concerns raised by teachers, which may prompt the initiation of a referral to an adapted physical education consultant.
- To discuss why one would conduct a needs assessment prior to a school visit
- To reflect on the information that may be gleaned from each aspect of the on-site visit, which typically involves a number of activities.
- To complete an outline for a consultative and/or assessment report.

Introduction

Although most universities in Canada include adapted physical education (APE) classes in their undergraduate and graduate physical education programmes, few consultative employment positions have been established outside of the university setting. Graduates often seek teaching positions and apply their personal expertise within their individual classes. Unfortunately, very few school boards have identified the need to employ APE consultants as a specialized resource for their districts. This may be due to a variety of factors, including the limited number of students identified with special needs, the priority given to physical education by a school board, funding availability, or reliance upon allied professionals addressing physical education needs. Unlike the US, Canada has not embraced the idea of identifying professional competencies and regulating APE specialists in a manner similar to the one we have created for the recreational therapy field.

Consequently, many teachers and administrators are unaware of the expertise adapted physical education graduates possess. Consultants in private practice can also provide an alternative service delivery model for schools. This is a tremendously viable opportunity for professionals trained in this area to market their skills and expertise. It may also provide the best case scenario for school boards to purchase and provide service without having to establish formal full time equivalency (FTE) positions in this time of fiscal restraint.

Research is continuing to show the relationship between physical activity levels of children and adults. Unfortunately, our children and youth of late have been inundated with sedentary activities such as home-based computer activities and both hand-held and television-based video games. Outside free play is on the decline. According to a number of North American studies, (Tremblay and Willms 2000) and the Surgeon General's report (1996), the fitness levels of children and adults are declining and obesity is on the rise. Fitness levels of the majority of persons with disabilities are even more dismal. "People with disabilities are less likely to engage in regular moderate physical activity than people without disabilities, yet they have similar needs to promote their health and prevent unnecessary disease." The Surgeon General's report also provides some encouraging key messages. For example, "significant health benefits can be obtained with a moderate amount of physical activity. These benefits can include a reduction in death from coronary heart disease or from developing high blood pressure, colon cancer or diabetes."

In response to the latest research, newly revised physical education curricula (e.g., Alberta and British Columbia) have adopted more of an active living approach toward physical activity. Skill development is still a central focus; however, there is greater emphasis on personal growth and individual activity preference. This evolution of curricular focus has allowed for more tailoring of programming to meet individual abilities and challenges. Adapted physical education consultants can assist in this regard.

Within Canada, each province establishes the curriculum, and schools have a legal responsibility to meet the mandate of the curriculum, for every student. It is our society's expectation that all children will be exposed to the same breadth of information and opportunities. With respect to physical education, this would require all students to develop some understanding of the various dimensions of the curriculum. Physical education experiences emphasize development in the cognitive, motoric, and affective domains. Even though practicing the skills associated with basketball may be inappropriate for those students who are totally blind, an understanding of the equipment, skills, and strategies associated with this sport are appropriate. In addition to the standard activity dimensions, physical education curricula can encourage knowledge of disability specific activities and sport (e.g., goal ball or wheelchair basketball).

1 Do children with special needs have the 'right' to acquire skill and experience in the games that are played by others with similar functional ability, rather than fitting in to the games typically associated with physical education for the able-bodied? Put more specifically, do children who have a visual impairment have a right to learn goal ball instead of basketball, in their phys. ed. class?

A number of changes in regard to societal attitudes have also prompted a need for consultations by specialists in the area of special education and, specifically, adapted physical education. For example, with the occurrence of deinstitutionalization, students with disabilities are attending, and are being included in, their neighbourhood school or other regular school settings. Inclusive programming is becoming increasingly common. However, students within each class with significantly varied cognitive, psychological, and motor abilities are making even greater demands on teachers.

Another attitudinal change is the societal emphasis on student academic achievement and excellence in core areas of study. This focus has resulted in a move away from physical education being a priority. Elementary physical education specialists have, in many places, been replaced by regular classroom or generalist teachers who may or may not have a background or interest in physical education. As a result of all of these societal trends, many teachers have minimal training or experience in dealing with students with special needs in a physical education setting and, therefore, can benefit from consultative support.

The Consultative Process

WHAT IS A CONSULTANT?

According to the *Dictionary New Webster Encyclopedia of the English Language* (1985) a consultant is described as "one who consults". "Consulting is the process of giving advice." "Consultation is defined as deliberation of two or more persons with a view to some decision; a meeting of experts…to consult about a specific case." *Webster's New World Dictionary* (1995) defines a consultant as "an expert who gives professional or technical advice." An adapted physical education consultant provides advice and assistance to teachers who are legally responsible for meeting the educational needs and goals of his or her students.

More specific roles of an APE consultant include:

- Assisting teachers in meeting the physical education curricular requirements of their students appropriately and safely.
- Discussing with teachers their specific concerns regarding instruction, assessment, individual education plan (IEP) development, or equipment.
- Providing teachers with methods of class/setting organization that will maximize participation and performance.
- Observing student/s participating in their regular physical education and/or recess environments and, subsequently, providing relevant programming suggestions that will facilitate activity.

- Modelling appropriate teaching and/or assessment practices.
- Providing school-based consultative assistance on a one-time, intermittent, or regular basis.
- Conducting gross motor assessments.
- Consulting as member of multi-disciplinary team (e.g., occupational or physical therapists).
- Liaising with community-based recreational and/or professional agencies.

Topics to be outlined and discussed within this chapter are related to school-based APE consultative assistance. The first section (Phase I) examines the consultative process.

- Need for assistance identified by school staff
- Referral initiated by school
- Initial contact between consultant and school staff
- Needs assessment conducted.
- Visit scheduled (must meet school's timetabling needs re: physical education class times and days of the week)
- On site visit:
  · file review
  · classroom/hallway/playground/ gymnasium observations
  · individualized assessment
  · debriefing with school staff and parents, as deemed necessary
- Report preparation:
  · organizing resources/handouts
  · liaising with community agencies or other professionals
  · follow-up service provision

The second section (Phase II) provides readers with three case studies. Examples of two consultative and one assessment report are presented. The entire consultative process, as well as examples of follow-up written reports, are clearly outlined. Readers are also provided with an additional case study, which they may then independently follow through the entire process.

Need for Assistance Identified by School Staff

When APE consultative services have been established in a community, teachers seek service for the following reasons:

1. The teacher of physical education (generalist or specialist) recognizes that a student or group of students is experiencing difficulties meeting the appropriate curricular grade level expectations. The student may be having difficulty with skill development, or in the application of skills in the game setting (see figure 18.1).

2. A student has a medical diagnosis with which staff is unfamiliar (e.g., osteogenesis imperfecta, spina bifida, or autism). In these cases the school is very concerned about providing a safe physical education experience for the student. Consequently, the APE consultant must be able to provide specific contraindications to physical activity relevant to each syndrome or medical diagnosis.

3. Allied professionals such as psychologists, physical or occupational therapists, physicians, recreation therapists, or parents may suggest to school staff that APE consultative services would be beneficial.

Referrals

Referrals may be received in the form of a written request or a telephone conversation. In our experience, as employees of the district, it is the school's responsibility to inform parents regarding professional interventions which may affect their child(ren). Each school jurisdiction has its own process for meeting the needs of students with special needs. For example, the recent trend toward school-based budgeting has forwarded the responsibility of accessing services directly to the principal. Other jurisdictions may still use a centralized model for purchasing consultative or inservice assistance. As noted on the referral form, identification of other professionals associated with the student results in the potential for a collaborative approach to service.

2 Given today's financial constraints in education, how do we ensure that the physical education needs of students with disabilities are being addressed?

A referral form should include the following information:

Referral Form

Student's name:
Grade:
Teacher's name:
School:
School address and jurisdiction:
School telephone number:
Referral submitted by:
Medical concerns:
Assistance requested:
Funding qualification:
Parents' names and contact information:
Other agencies involved:

Needs Assessment

A needs assessment discussion should occur upon receipt of the written referral or may be conducted simultaneously with the initial telephone contact. Through this discussion, the specific needs of the school are clearly identified, for example, ascertaining the impact of the student's disability on her inclusion in physical education and/or recess activities, specific contraindications to physical activity based upon the student's disability, or community activities to supplement the physical education programme. Teachers also seek assistance to modify games, equipment, and specific curricular dimensions to promote skill development. Professional opinions regarding the selection of appropriate assistive devices for specific units (i.e., walker or wheelchair), determining accessibility access into the gymnasium, and developing appropriate

Figure 18.1 Physical Education Guide to Implementation (K–12) Sample Evaluation Strategies

Sample Evaluation Strategies

CHECKLIST SAMPLES

Basic Skills Checklist

Locomotor Skills	Criteria	1st Observation — Working to Achieve (yes / no)	1st Observation — Has Achieved (yes / no)	2nd Observation — Working to Achieve (yes / no)	2nd Observation — Has Achieved (yes / no)
Walking	• reflexive arm swing • little vertical lift • definite heel–toe action				
Running	• brief period where both feet are off the ground • arms in opposition to legs, elbows bent • slight body lean, even rhythm • support leg extends completely • nonsupport leg bent 90° • recovery thigh is parallel to the ground • little rotary action of recovery leg				
Hopping	• able to hop on either foot, land on same foot • nonsupport leg flexed with the foot further back than the knee • rhythmical, pendulum-like action of nonsupport leg to produce force • arms bent and swing to produce force • arms are not needed for balance				
Leaping	• take off on one foot and land on the opposite foot • a period where both feet are off the ground • forward reach with arm opposite the lead foot				
Forward Jump	• preparatory movement includes flexion of both knees with arms extended behind the body • arms extend forcefully forward and upward, reaching full extension above head • take off and land on both feet simultaneously • arms are brought downward during landing • body weight at landing moves forward				
Sliding	• body faces sideways to direction of travel • step sideways, followed by a slide of the trailing foot to a point next to the lead foot • a short period where both feet are off the floor • able to slide left or right				

Physical Education Guide to Implementation (K–12)
©Alberta Learning, Alberta, Canada
Appendix B /241
(2000)

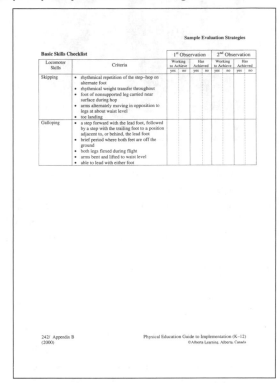

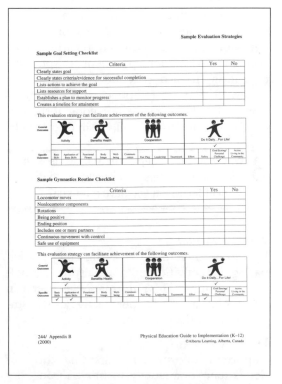

Sample Evaluation Strategies

Basic Skills Checklist

Manipulatives	Criteria	1st Observation — Working to Achieve (yes / no)	1st Observation — Has Achieved (yes / no)	2nd Observation — Working to Achieve (yes / no)	2nd Observation — Has Achieved (yes / no)
Overhead Throw	• arm is swung backward with elbow at shoulder height or higher • rotation of hip and shoulder to a point where the nondominant side faces the target • step with opposite foot to the throwing hand • follow through with the throwing hand moving diagonally across the body • lead with the elbow during the throwing action • thumb ends up pointing down on the follow-through				
Catching	• hands are held with fingers pointing up and the thumbs close for a ball caught above the waist, and the little fingers close and fingers pointing down for a ball caught below the waist • arms are held relaxed at sides and forearms are held in front of the body • arms reach for the ball just prior to contact • ball is caught by the hands • elbows bend to absorb the force				
Kicking	• movement of kicking is initiated at the hip • support leg bends slightly at contact • slight backward lean of the trunk during contact • forward swing of the arm opposite kicking leg • full extension of leg on follow-through				
Batting	• dominant hand grips the bat above the nondominant hand • stand sideways with nondominant side facing the object to be struck • weight shifts to back foot • arms swing backward • hips and spine rotate • weight shifts to forward foot at contact				

This evaluation strategy can facilitate achievement of the following outcomes.

Physical Education Guide to Implementation (K–12)
©Alberta Learning, Alberta, Canada
Appendix B /243
(2000)

SOURCE: From *Physical Education: Guide to Implementation, Kindergarten to Grade 12*, 2000, Edmonton: Alberta Learning, Learning and Teaching Resources Branch. Reprinted with permission.

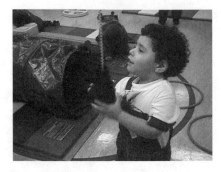

individualized programme plan (IPP) goals are also frequently requested. Teachers may also ask consultants to provide inservice sessions to staff on any of the topics mentioned above or disability awareness sessions to students.

On Site Visit

1. FILE REVIEW

It is important to conduct a file review upon arrival at the school to ensure that you do not replicate any recent testing which may have previously been completed. The student's cumulative (CUM) file also includes copies of report cards which may give you information about previous physical education experiences or recent medical reports which may contain information pertinent to physical education. It also may be clear from this review that cross referrals to allied professionals may be warranted. A copy of the student's IPP will also be available in the CUM file.

3 Why would it be important to dialogue with allied professionals also involved with the student for whom you have a referral?

2. OBSERVATIONS

It is important to observe the child participating in activities in a variety of school-based settings. This information is useful in developing a broader perspective of the student's strengths and challenges.

HALLWAYS

Important information regarding the student's functional ability to move throughout the school can be determined by observing him or her travelling in the school hallways. Questions such as, "Can the student safely negotiate hallway travel during class transitions with other students?" or "Can she propel a walker and/or wheelchair with appropriate speed and control?" are best answered by these kinds of observations. Other good questions include, "Does the student have the ability to ascend and descend stairs or ramps safely and independently?", "Does she have sufficient endurance for covering relatively long distances with or without support?", or, "Is the student distractible in the hallway setting?"

CLASSROOM

Movement about the classroom can reveal the student's ability to change levels, (e.g., rising from the floor if seated at 'circle time') and to successfully negotiate obstacles (e.g., desks or items on the floor). Postural anomalies and trunk stability can also be noted while the student is seated at a desk. Also noteworthy is the student's ability to follow the teacher's and/or programme assistant's directions and classroom routines such as retrieval of materials, interaction with peers, social skills, and appropriateness of behaviour.

RECESS

Recess provides the opportunity to observe the student's organizational skills related to dressing, such as finding one's own shoes, mittens, hat, locker, buttoning or zippering coats, tying/untying shoes, and adjusting sleeves of jackets. It also provides a wonderful opportunity to observe the child in unstructured play. Selection of activities, equipment preferences, choice of friends, willingness to cooperate with others, and level of independence are important factors that help determine the student's physical activity profile and skill repertoire. By viewing a child on the playground, it becomes very clear if the play space is barrier-free, accessible, and appropriate for their skill repertoire.

GYMNASIUM

It is important to see how the child follows the established gymnasium routine. Consequently, the consultant must arrive at the gym

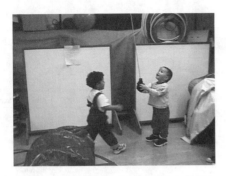

either prior to, or simultaneously with, the student. A typical physical education class is comprised of three components, including warm-up, skill instruction and development, and application or final activity. Students may be particularly challenged or skilled in one or all aspects of the class. Typically, all students with special needs can be easily accommodated in the warm-up portion of every class. For example, most upper-body stretching exercises can be performed while sitting. This would allow students with balance challenges to participate actively. Students and/or their programme assistants should be encouraged to select and substitute stretches that will address their personal functional needs and abilities.

4 Are there times during a physical education class that participation in a physical therapy stretching or range of motion programme would be more beneficial than participation in the regular physical education activity?

A skilled teacher of physical education will be more easily able to accommodate the varying skill levels presented in the skill development portion of the class.

More comprehensive modifications or activity choices may need to occur during the final activity. During culminating games, the activity becomes more complex in nature as a result of the need to assimilate a variety of factors. In order to be actively included, a student must be able to control his or her own actions, anticipate actions of others, predict trajectories of equipment, select and utilize appropriate strategies, and so forth.

There will undoubtedly be situations that arise where it is inappropriate for a student to be involved. Reasons for exclusion may be medical, behavioural, or educational in nature. For example, it is inappropriate for a power wheelchair user to participate in a three-week ice-skating unit. An initial visit to the rink, however, is recommended, as this allows the child to gain an understanding of the activity. It is during these alternate times that a student may perhaps participate in lead-up physical activities for upcoming units. This allows for some initial skill development to occur prior to the actual unit, thereby increasing the likelihood of that student's subsequent success. Students may also direct their attention toward expanding their knowledge of culturally typical leisure activities or local sporting teams. This activity provides an opportunity to demonstrate their knowledge to peers, in a social setting.

5 One of the recommendations that is commonly put forth by APE consultants is inclusion in the regular physical education setting. Does this inclusive attitude practically detract from the integrity of the physical education programme for the other students?

3. INDIVIDUALIZED ASSESSMENT

Individualized assessment is conducted when additional information is requested or required by school staff. Initial assessments are also very important in determining baseline motor skill status. This information can be referred to during report card or IPP preparation and review.

Standardized Gross Motor Assessments: A wide variety of standardized tests and screening instruments are available for assessing children's gross motor development. These tests are typically norm-referenced to the general population. As a result, most children with a disability will always score well below anticipated age levels. In these situations, information gleaned from the assessment should best be used for establishing an individualized test/retest protocol.

Figure 18.2 One page of Locomotor TGMD-2

Preferred Hand: Right ☐ Left ☐ Not Established ☐
Preferred Foot: Right ☐ Left ☐ Not Established ☐

Locomotor Subtest

Skill	Materials	Directions	Performance Criteria	Trial 1	Trial 2	Score
1. Run	60 feet of clear space, and two cones	Place two cones 50 feet apart. Make sure there is at least 8 to 10 feet of space beyond the second cone for a safe stopping distance. Tell the child to run as fast as he or she can from one cone to the other when you say "Go." Repeat a second trial.	1. Arms move in opposition to legs, elbows bent			
			2. Brief period where both feet are off the ground			
			3. Narrow foot placement landing on heel or toe (i.e., not flat footed)			
			4. Nonsupport leg bent approximately 90 degrees (i.e., close to buttocks)			
			Skill Score			
2. Gallop	25 feet of clear space, and tape or two cones	Mark off a distance of 25 feet with two cones or tape. Tell the child to gallop from one cone to the other. Repeat a second trial by galloping back to the original cone.	1. Arms bent and lifted to waist level at takeoff			
			2. A step forward with the lead foot followed by a step with the trailing foot to a position adjacent to or behind the lead foot			
			3. Brief period when both feet are off the floor			
			4. Maintains a rhythmic pattern for four consecutive gallops			
			Skill Score			
3. Hop	A minimum of 15 feet of clear space	Tell the child to hop three times on his or her preferred foot (established before testing) and then three times on the other foot. Repeat a second trial.	1. Nonsupport leg swings forward in pendular fashion to produce force			
			2. Foot of nonsupport leg remains behind body			
			3. Arms flexed and swing forward to produce force			
			4. Takes off and lands three consecutive times on preferred foot			
			5. Takes off and lands three consecutive times on nonpreferred foot			
			Skill Score			
4. Leap	A minimum of 20 feet of clear space, a beanbag, and tape	Place a beanbag on the floor. Attach a piece of tape on the floor so it is parallel to and 10 feet away from the beanbag. Have the child stand on the tape and run up and leap over the beanbag. Repeat a second trial.	1. Take off on one foot and land on the opposite foot			
			2. A period where both feet are off the ground longer than running			
			3. Forward reach with the arm opposite the lead foot			
			Skill Score			

SOURCE: From *Test of Gross Motor Development,* by D.A. Ulrich, 2000, Austin, TX: Pro-Ed. Reprinted with permission.

Consequently, reporting of the percentile rank may be irrelevant. Many standard gross motor assessments, however, do contain items that can tap the specific skill of a wide variety of students with special needs. Items that are not appropriate may be modified to reflect the student's abilities. Other new items may be substituted for those which will never be mastered. For example, most students with hemiplegia cerebral palsy will be unable to complete all of the items presented in the locomotor skills subtest of the Test of Gross Motor Development (TGMD-2, 2000), because of their neurological impairment. Running, hopping, and skipping skills require adequate hamstring strength in each leg for mastery. As a result of the hemiplegia, these students usually are unable to meet the standardized criterion. Alternately, these same students will be able to master galloping and sliding with their dominant leg leading and, in this case, their performance results can be compared to the norms. The APE consultant will assist teachers as they review their available test materials to determine the appropriateness of items and to suggest alternate skill items which are more relevant to the individual student and can be measured (e.g., wheeling in lieu of running).

4. DEBRIEFING

Each consultation visit must include the opportunity to meet directly with the physical education teacher and other relevant staff. During this meeting, observations and preliminary assessment results will be shared. This is yet another opportunity to further discuss the needs or concerns of the staff regarding the student's participation in physical education. These meetings are also an excellent opportunity to brainstorm ideas for upcoming physical education units and gross motor school-wide events (e.g., winter carnival). Suggestions regarding appropriate equipment modifications and purchases can also be discussed during this meeting.

Depending upon the school's wishes, parents may be invited to attend the debriefing session or a separate session may be scheduled. Parents can provide wonderful insights into the interests and leisure time experiences of their children. Check with families to determine whether they have any specialized equipment that could be used during specific physical education units (e.g., a sledge for use during the ice-skating unit).

6 Should parents be invited or expected to be present during their child's assessment and consultation?

Report Preparation

When schools purchase APE services, there is an expectation that a report outlining the various aspects of the visit and all relevant recommendations be completed in a timely fashion. This report should be positive in tenor, emphasizing the students' abilities and achievements rather than simply focussing on the weaknesses of their performances. It should be easily interpreted by school staff and parents. The report typically includes the following information:

BACKGROUND INFORMATION

This section should provide the reader with a general impression of the student's abilities and challenges. All relevant medical information, including diagnosis and previous interventions, is included as well as information pertaining to the number and type of assistive devices used (i.e., manual wheelchair, walker, communication systems). It may also be appropriate to include the number of scheduled physical education experiences in which the student participates each week.

PURPOSE OF VISIT

It is important to clarify the expectations of the school staff regarding your service. This should be clearly outlined in the report (i.e., assessment, consultation, file review, IPP goals).

OBSERVATIONS

Within this section include curriculum-based, observational impressions determined from the variety of settings in which the child participated (i.e., hallways, playground, classroom, and gymnasium). Observations should reflect the student's performance rather than the teacher's ability.

ASSESSMENT INFORMATION

In this section outline both the standardized and supplementary assessment tools utilized and provide a brief summary of the student's results. Complete assessment information is best provided in appendix format.

PROGRAMMING SUGGESTIONS

Teachers appreciate programming suggestions that are tied to specific activity units. Although teachers often ask for new 'games' that are inclusive in nature, we have found that providing minor modifications to the classes' already established games will be most useful to the teacher. Practical suggestions pertaining to equipment, skill, task complexity, and instructional delivery should be included. Specialized equipment catalogues available to schools are best used to identify equipment possibilities. Physical education distributors often carry the same items at a lower cost. Toy and department stores are another alternative for these purchases. In addition, remember that creative school staff may modify regular physical education equipment. For example, a tail ball for throwing and catching activities can be made by attaching a length of surveyor's tape to a whiffle ball.

COMMUNITY LIAISON

It is important to determine the agencies and individuals within your community that provide services to individuals with specific special needs. Contact your rehabilitation hospitals, service groups, and foundations tied to specific disability groups to gain a better understanding of local services available to families. Supplementary extracurricular physical activity experiences are important for all students.

SUMMARY

This brief section should highlight the important aspects of the student and the visit. Directions regarding report distribution should be outlined and follow-up services presented. This also may be an opportunity to suggest that teachers videotape future student performance concerns and forward these on to the APE consultant for review.

APPENDIX

Within this section, teachers may find comprehensive testing results information and/or supplementary resources and handout material. The *Moving to Inclusion Resource* (1994), which was distributed to schools nationwide, is an excellent resource to utilize. Additional resource materials may be accessed through disability specific agencies, libraries, hospitals, other professionals, and the Internet.

PHASE I

Case Studies

The following section will provide the reader with three hypothetical case studies. The purpose of including these examples is to demonstrate how an APE consultation is typically documented and subsequently reported to the school. Case studies should also provide the teacher with ideas pertaining to appropriate interventions.

CASE STUDY 1

The school requested a visit from an adapted physical education consultant to provide the teacher with programming suggestions that would facilitate physical education inclusion of a student with special needs. The male student is five years of age and has a medical diagnosis of spastic diplegia cerebral palsy. This student had not been seen previously by an adapted physical education consultant.

The following is our consultative report developed after the visit.

Consultation Report

Student's name:	Ben Smith
Address:	16 Active Lane
Date of birth:	April 10, 1996
Postal code:	T6G 2E1
Parents:	Mr. and Mrs. Smith
Telephone:	555-1111
Date seen:	May 10, 2001
Teacher:	Ms. Connor
School:	Creekside
Classroom	
Teaching Assistant:	Mary Jo Green
Grade:	Four–Intermediate Opportunity
Referral source:	Principal–Rod Woods
Referral date:	March 4, 2001

Ben is a five-year-old boy who presents with spastic diplegia cerebral palsy. Ben participates in a French immersion kindergarten class at his neighbourhood school. He wears ankle and foot orthoses but otherwise does not use mobility aids. Ben is scheduled for further physical review at the Community Rehabilitation Hospital in early June 1999.

Summary of Visit

During the visit today, I had the opportunity to observe Ben both in his classroom and during his regular physical education class. The following observations were made:

- prefers to use left hand
- attempts mirroring or 'copycat' activities; however, has difficulty with rapid transitions and activities involving weight transfer and static balance
- sat on a high-backed chair during 'calendar' time; quite fidgety in his chair
- often distracted and would initiate conversation with nearby peers
- not an active participant in 'show and share'
- keen to go to physical education class
- uses two hands on rail to assist with ascending and descending stairs; overuses arms to pull up
- exhibits a flight phase when running

- balance can be precarious at times, especially during rapid change of direction or sudden stops
- purposefully bumps into other children and pulls their hair at times
- rises quickly from the floor, although when this action is repeated, it is obviously quite fatiguing for him
- watches other children for cues rather than listening to verbal instructions
- repeatedly off-task while in the gym and especially during the 'clear out' game situation where the object is to kick the balls into the opposition's area
- independently selects an appropriate strategy of using his hands to slow the ball down when it is difficult to stop the ball with his feet
- kicks with his left foot but demonstrates an immature kick; however, this is expected due to balance complications which make a proper weight shift difficult

Further Observations After Class

CATCHING/BALL SKILLS
- becomes off-balance when attempting to catch a medium-sized playground ball; has marked difficulty if oncoming ball has a high-arched trajectory
- places arms appropriately in anticipation of oncoming ball
- tracks oncoming ball until close by and then turns head
- has difficulty bouncing and catching a ball; difficulty gauging appropriate force

THROWING
- Ben presently 'hurls' a bean bag; however, this is developmentally appropriate for him. When an oppositional throw was demonstrated for him, Ben was able to place his right foot forward and throw with his left hand. He commented that he would like to learn to throw and catch better.

STRIKING
- He was able to strike a medium-sized ball off the top of stacked traffic cones by using his hand and then a plastic bat.
- Ben exhibited great difficulty in successfully tracking and contacting a small, pitched ball. He experienced greater success when using a larger, softer ball.

MIRRORING
- Ben was able to copy simple arm and leg actions; some delay was apparent when more challenging combinations were presented such as those involving contra-lateral limbs.

ATTITUDE
- Ben was compliant and eager to try the various activities; however, when unsuccessful at an activity it seemed to bother him a great deal. At these times, physical assistance (hand-over-hand) was provided to ensure success and to assist in the development of the proper motor programme. This worked particularly well in the bouncing and catching activity. In addition to receiving physical assistance, Ben was encouraged to verbalize his actions (i.e., 'bounce-catch, bounce-catch').

Programming Suggestions

1. Ben will continue to benefit from participation in his regular physical education setting, with modifications provided only as necessary to ensure success. The four general curricular Physical Education Outcomes (Alberta Learning 2000) include:

   - Students will acquire skills through a variety of developmentally appropriate movement activities.
   - Students will understand, experience, and appreciate the health benefits that result from physical activity.
   - Students will interact positively with others.

- Students will assume personal responsibility to lead an active way of life.

These outcomes pertain to all students in Ben's class.

2. Due to Ben's medical diagnosis of cerebral palsy (diplegia), he presents with increased tone in his lower limbs (*diplegia* means that the legs are more involved than the arms) and therefore he counteracts that posturally in his upper body. Ben does ambulate quite well across even terrain, despite his inward rotation and subsequent scissor gait. However, activities such as floor hockey or tag that require rapid stops and changes of direction will be especially challenging for Ben. Reinforcing this notion of personal space will be very important for Ben and his classmates, in the gym, on the playground, and in the classroom. Ben will also be particularly challenged by crossing uneven terrain such as at the playground or on snowy fields.

3. It will be important to experiment with various sizes and weights of manipulative equipment. For example, Ben may find it easier to kick a lighter ball–one that does not require much force to travel, thereby reducing the balancing challenges. When dribbling a soccer ball, he may find it easier to use a heavier, slightly deflated ball as it will travel more slowly across the gym floor, thereby increasing his ability to stay with the ball.

4. Many children with cerebral palsy exhibit perceptual difficulties, thereby making such activities as striking a pitched ball difficult. Tee-ball stands or using stacked pylons may be used to eliminate the flight phase of the ball should Ben exhibit marked difficulties with these types of activities. Of course, he should always be initially given the opportunity to try all of the various activities in the physical education programme, but modifications may be necessary to encourage success and enjoyment. Another strategy is to suspend a ball from a basketball hoop.

This allows children with tracking difficulties an easier method of practicing their striking and/or catching skills. Tethering also eliminates the wasted time spent chasing a dropped or miss-hit ball.

5. With respect to assessment in physical education, it will be important that Ben also be challenged to improve his motor skills and abilities. Baseline information of the various motor skills and activities and periodic review of his skill development in these areas will readily reveal which areas require additional remediation both in class and at home.

6. Ben may become fatigued sooner than his peers may due to his increased expenditure of energy associated with cerebral palsy. This should be respected when establishing distances for relays or other locomotor activities. Travelling about the school can also be physically taxing for Ben. It will be important to monitor this factor on an ongoing basis, as fatigue can also impact his posture, attention, and fine motor work.

Ms. Connor indicated that Ben is experiencing great difficulty with fine motor skills. A referral for occupational therapy has been made to Consulting Services (Belvedere Office) and a follow-up telephone call has been made regarding scheduling. In addition, a review by the school board physical therapy consultant may be warranted depending on the upcoming general medical review.

7. An ability awareness session, presented by the adapted physical education consultant took place May 25, 2001. The purpose of this session was to increase the knowledge and understanding of Ben's peers concerning cerebral palsy and allow them the opportunity to experience some of the associated challenges. A video pertaining to cerebral palsy sports was loaned to the school for a period of one week. This video clearly depicts the athletic prowess of many local athletes with cerebral palsy.

8. A variety of handout materials are provided with this report. Game adaptations, equipment suggestions, and medical information pertaining to cerebral palsy are also included. A video outlining the different types of cerebral palsy will also be loaned to Ms. Green and Ms. Connor to increase their medical understanding of this disability.

9. Ben will benefit from participation in regular community leisure pursuits such as Cubs, swimming, and horseback riding. The Cerebral Palsy Sports Association offers a variety of activities, including floor hockey, skiing, and skating. Contact information is included with the brochure.

It has been a pleasure meeting Ben and Ms. Connor. Please share the contents of this report with Ben's family. It is recommended that a copy of this report accompany Ben to his upcoming medical appointment at the Rehabilitation Hospital. A follow-up consultation is recommended in the fall of 2001. Should additional concerns arise prior to the time, please do not hesitate to contact me at 555-1234.

> Patt Nearingburg, Ph.D.
> Adapted Physical Education Consultant
> cc: Rod Wood, principal, Creekside School
> Attn: Ms. Connor, teacher

CASE STUDY 2

Mr. Jones, principal at Spruce Hollow Elementary School, requested that an adapted physical education consultant review Mark Blue's participation in physical education. Mark is an eight-year-old boy who has a medical diagnosis of Down's syndrome and hearing impairment. He is included in a regular grade two class and his progress is monitored by an IPP. Mark's physical education teacher wants to ensure that she is meeting his gross motor needs and has requested assistance to ensure that he participates in the programme as actively as possible.

Consultation Report

Student's name:	Mark Blue
Date of birth:	June 1, 1993
Address:	1, Elm Lane, Spruce Hollow
Postal code:	T6G 2E1
Telephone:	555-4444
Consultant:	Laurie Clifford MA
Discipline:	Adapted Physical Education
Date seen:	February 1, 2002
Reason for visit:	To review Mark's participation in physical education
Teacher:	Mrs. Smith
TA:	Mrs. Black
School:	Spruce Hollow
Grade:	Two
Referral source:	Mr. Jones, principal
Referral date:	September 23, 2001

Background Information

Mark is an eight-year-old student who attends Mrs. Smith's grade two class at Spruce Hollow School in Spruce Hollow. Mark has a medical diagnosis of Down's syndrome with a moderate hearing loss in his left ear and moderate-to-severe hearing loss in the right ear. He wears two hearing aids, amplified with an FM system for classroom use. Mark receives full-time teaching assistant support from Mrs. Black. Upon the request of Mr. Jones, principal, and in conjunction with Mrs. Smith, physical education teacher and vice principal, and Mrs. Baxter, a visit was made to Spruce Hollow School on February 1, 2002. The purpose of the visit was to review Mark's file, to observe him participating with his classmates in a physical education lesson, and to provide programming and/or equipment recommendations if required.

File Review

Mark's IPP outlined the following gross motor goals:

- to walk using the heel-toe pattern
- to develop his throwing and catching skills using balls, beanbags
- to demonstrate increased confidence using outside playground equipment

Mark has mastered the locomotor skills of walking, running, galloping, jumping down, and jumping on the spot.

Strategies that staff have identified to assist Mark develop his gross motor skills include using peer partners for gross motor activities, limiting the distance Mark is expected to travel during locomotor activities, and providing adequate adult supervision while Mark is on the playground.

Physical Education Observations

Mark was observed participating in a physical education lesson designed to develop and refine a number of locomotor skills. The following observations were noted:

Upon arrival into the gymnasium, Mark positioned himself close to the equipment storage room rather than seating himself in the circular formation, which Mrs. Smith had established as the classes' gymnasium routine.

After introducing myself to Mark, I asked him if he could perform the warm-up activities being presented to the class by Mrs. Smith. Mark willingly performed three consecutive and mature stride jumps, three leg raises, three abdominal crunches, five push-ups, shoulder shrugs, shoulder circles in the backwards action, and half-neck circles upon my request. Mark did not require any assistance from Mrs. Black in order for him to comply with my requests. Mark appeared to be eager to demonstrate his skills to me. Mrs. Black reported that she had prepared Mark for my visit by explaining to him that I was coming to see him participating in his physical education class.

While the class was performing individual skills, Mrs. Smith purposefully communicated with Mrs. Black that a transition was about to

occur and the students would be expected to find a partner for the next activity. Mrs. Black then forewarned Mark that he would need to find a partner, and Mark began searching for one before Mrs. Smith asked the class to do so. This was a very effective strategy for Mark. Mark chose to position his skipping rope in the form of a circle. Other options available to the class-included rectangles, triangles, and diamonds.

Mark eagerly jumped over his skipping rope circle placed on the floor. He signed to Mrs. Black that water was inside his circle. On one attempt he slipped and fell with his buttocks landing inside the circle. Mark laughed and pretended that he was wet from falling in the water.

Mrs. Smith requested that the students perform a number of different locomotor activities into and out of the skipping rope shapes placed on the floor. Mark refused to jump into his circle. We then made a second target for Mark to use; however, Mark continued to refuse to step inside the target because it had water in it. Consequently, Mark experienced limited practice of the skills presented to his class. Mark did attempt to jump backwards two-foot to two-foot across one of the lines painted on the gym floor.

Programme Restrictions

The following programme recommendations were shared with Mrs. Smith during a meeting that followed Mark's physical education class.

1. Mark's continued participation in his grade-appropriate physical education class is highly recommended since it provides the best opportunity for him to develop and refine age appropriate gross motor, fitness, and social skills.
2. In order for Mark to continue to develop gross motor skills it is important that he be encouraged to maximize his practice opportunities during each physical education lesson. During ball activities, one method of maximizing practice opportunities is to limit ball retrieval time. This can be accomplished by:

- Providing Mark with a number of balls during throwing activities so that a number of practice opportunities can occur without the requirement of repositioning due to ball retrieval movements.
- Positioning Mark with his back to the corner of the gym during partner activities so that the walls can limit the distance travelled by stray balls.
- Using benches and walls to form lanes to trap stray balls.
- Tethering balls from wall-mounted basketball hoop for throwing, catching, and striking activities.
- Tethering a ball to Mark's waist or wrist during kicking act.

3. Try pairing two students with Mark, including one who is very skilled, as this will optimize practice opportunities.

4. The *Moving to Inclusion Resource: Including Students with Intellectual Disabilities* (1994), addresses compliance issues typical to this population. This resource is available on loan from our office, or for purchase from CAHPERD at a cost of $25.00. Order forms for the entire Moving to Inclusion resource package is included with his report. To borrow this resource, please call Milly Apple at 555–4444.

5. Participation in a gross motor centre such as an obstacle course during an indoor recess might also facilitate Mark's locomotor and manipulative skill development. Activity ideas included with this report may also be followed up at home.

6. Ensuring that Mark is always provided with physical education equipment that is in good working order and fits his body type is still another means of maximizing skill development. Unfortunately, slower moving students are often the last to pick equipment and may receive the 'left-over' objects.

7. During a telephone conversation with Mrs. Blue we discussed the medical condition of atlanto-axial instability which is a concern for children having Down's syndrome. Mrs. Blue reported that Mark has had two x-rays, both of which have not indicated the presence of this condition. After some discussion, we agreed that it is better to err on the side of caution with respect to the possibility of this condition. Consequently, the following contraindications to physical activity should be followed for Mark.

- Avoid all neck exercises (including half-neck circles).
- Do not permit Mark to perform forwards, backwards, or shoulder rolls.
- Do not permit Mark to assume any inverted position where the possibility exists of him falling on his head (e.g., cartwheels, head or hand stands, hanging upside down from gymnasium apparatus, or playground equipment).
- Avoid all contact sports including wrestling.
- Do not permit Mark to 'head' a soccer ball.
- Do not permit Mark to dive or perform the butterfly swimming stroke.
- Do not allow Mark to stand under basketball hoops where he could inadvertently be struck on the head by a basketball.
- Avoid all other exercises that place pressure on the neck and head.

Should Mark develop a keen interest in mastering any one of the skills mentioned above, school staff and Mark's family should seek medical advice before agreeing to the activity.

Included with this report is a recent article on this condition and its prevalence in children with Down's syndrome. Please forward this article to Mark's family.

Included with this report are some ideas for teaching bike riding. Please forward them to Mark's family. Michelle North, a physical education teacher at Muller School, has had remarkable success teaching students with a variety of disabling conditions how to ride a bike. She can be reached by phone at 555-1111 or e-mail at zzz@zzzz.

Please share the contents of this report with Mark's family.

It was a pleasure providing service to Spruce Hollow School. Follow-up adapted physical education consultation is available upon request. Should any questions or concern arise from the contents of this report, please contact me at 555-3333.

Laurie Clifford, MA, Adapted Physical Education Consultant
cc: Bill Bob, Coordinator of Special Education
Tim Thomson, principal, Spruce Hollow School
Attn: Mrs. Black

CASE STUDY 3

The adapted physical education consultant was contacted by the principal of Happydale School and requested to conduct a gross motor assessment of an early education student. This five-year-old girl was reported to be experiencing difficulties with meeting the expectations of the physical education curriculum. Activities involving balance and coordination were noted to be especially challenging for her. She also was reported to exhibit fine motor and speech delays.

Gross Motor Assessment Report

Student: Kate Smith
Date of birth: November 20, 1996
School: Happydale
Teacher: Mrs. Jones
Date of assessment: May 2, 2001
Referral source: Principal, Mr. White
Purpose of visit: To conduct gross motor assessment and to provide programming suggestions

Kate was assessed today using the Test of Gross Motor Development (TGMD-2, 2000). This criterion-based test evaluates the gross motor functioning of children between the ages of three and ten. Emphasis is placed upon the individual's mastery of the mature skill criteria.

Quantitative elements, such as distance or speed, are not factored in to the scoring. There are two sub-tests within this test:

Locomotor skills include: run, gallop, hop, leap, horizontal jump, and slide
Object control skills include: throw, catch, kick, stationary dribble, underhand roll, and strike.

	Raw Scores	Percentiles	Standard Scores
Locomotor skills	25	25	8
Object control skills	9	2	4
Sum of standard scores:			12
Gross motor quotient:	76 (5th percentile)		

According to the TGMD, Kate's motor skills are described as poor. Her locomotor skills are at approximately a four-year level, and her object motor skills are below the three-year level.

Kate was compliant and happy throughout the evaluation.

Locomotor—Stability Information

Kate is able to balance on her left foot for a period of two seconds and on her right for three seconds. She is able to walk backward across level flooring, without falling. When focussed, Kate is able to walk along close to a narrow line (not heel to toe) taking six steps. She is able to walk along a low beam (four steps) raised approximately four inches. Kate is able to tip-toe. At the time of testing, Kate was able to hop three times on her left foot but unable to hop on her right.

As this activity requires both balance, coordination, and leg strength, it is a challenging activity for Kate. When attempting to jump horizontally, Kate appropriately uses a two-to-two foot pattern. She does not yet use her arms for lift and/or propulsion. When jumping down from a mat six inches high, Kate was initially tentative, yet with encouragement she was able to successfully jump (one-to-two foot), maintaining her balance upon landing. Kate is competent on stairs. Kate is tentative when crossing a squishy mat. Kate is presently able to gallop with her left foot leading, however is unable with her right foot leading. She is not yet using her arms for lift and/or propulsion. When sliding sideways, Kate is generally able to travel in both directions, maintaining a sideways position. Kate is able to run around obstacles and run to an object, retrieve it, and return to start. She runs flat-footed and slowly in comparison to her peers. Kate is unable to skip. Kate is able to ride a tricycle. Kate is able to copy simple body movement actions, however continues to have some difficulty with more complex actions involving contra-lateral limbs. She scans the upper body of the demonstrator and then the lower portion. Kate exhibits great difficulty performing two jumping jacks.

Object Control Information

When asked to run up and kick a stationary ball, Kate instead walks up to or around the ball, stops and then kicks the ball, exhibiting a brief transfer of weight. When gently tossed a light, medium-sized ball, Kate is inconsistent in catching it (distance of one metre). She does not consistently or appropriately place her hands out in front of her body and does not move appropriately in relation to an oncoming object which is travelling off midline. After viewing a demonstration of an overhand throw, Kate attempted this skill. She keeps her feet stationary, uses her left hand, and generally looks in the direction of the target. Kate was unsure as to how far to stand back from the wall in order to successfully strike a target. Kate uses a 'shot put' technique. Kate exhibits difficulty rolling a ball toward a target. She tends to bend at the waist rather than bend her knees. Kate has great difficulty successfully bouncing and catching a ball. When presented with a bat, Kate is able to position herself appropriately in relation to a pitched ball. When striking a suspended ball, she had difficulty anticipating the trajectory of the ball.

Summary

When observing Kate's gross motor skills and relating this performance to the evaluative criterion of the TGMD-2, it is apparent that she exhibits motor delay. Kate frequently exhibits associated facial reactions when attempting complex tasks.

She has difficulty generalizing skills from one setting to another. Kate's ability to sustain motor skill competence is inconsistent. For example, she may perform a proper overhand throw one minute and then in the next minute appear confused as to what is expected of her.

Programming Recommendations

Kate benefits from participation in her regular daily physical education class. This setting provides her with gross motor instruction and practice opportunities. It is anticipated that Kate will continue to develop her motoric competency through programming at school, play at home, and in the community. Given her delays, it is recommended that a neurodevelopmental follow-up occur either through the Grey Nun's Hospital or the Glenrose. In addition, re-evaluation of her gross motor skills, as they relate to the physical education curriculum, is recommended to occur annually by an adapted physical education consultant.

Specific Skill Suggestions

It is important that Kate is provided with numerous practice opportunities with typical playground activities and games. Knowledge of these activities and competency in them will facilitate her socialization and inclusion at school and in the community.

It will be important that when demonstrations are provided Kate is positioned to be facing away from the busy section of the gym. It is also recommended that a multisensory approach be taken when providing instruction and feedback, combining visual, verbal, and physical assistance. The combined approach will help Kate develop a more appropriate motor programme. Practice in front of a mirror is also helpful for children who experience coordination and/or body awareness difficulties.

THROWING

Kate should be encouraged to practice throwing objects of various sizes, shapes, and textures. Work on throwing high, low, hard, underhand, or overhand. Accuracy is not a focus at this stage but may be incorporated for motivation.

CATCHING

Larger, lighter balls, such as a beach ball, are easier to catch than a small tennis ball or bean bag. Children enjoy catching scarves as they float slowly through the air and they have a large surface area. Kate may be challenged by initially sitting on the floor with legs in a V-position, tossing a ball up to herself. Once successful with this, she may kneel or stand. Suspending a ball from a basketball hoop using a piece of sewing elastic can provide an easier means of tracking an oncoming ball and may be used as a catching or striking station.

DRIBBLING BALL USING FEET

Slightly deflating a ball allows it to roll more slowly across the floor, thereby increasing control.

DRIBBLING A BASKETBALL

It is important that the ball is well-inflated so that it rebounds appropriately. Kate will be more successful if she initially bounces and catches a ball while standing still, then progresses to walking and bouncing and catching the ball. Then attempt dribbling with one hand while standing still, adding movement once successful.

BALANCE AND BODY MANAGEMENT

Some enjoyable ideas that assist children who are experiencing difficulty in these areas include such activities as stepping *over* little objects (obstacle course format), or *into* objects such as shoe boxes, moving to music at various heights or speeds and then

'freezing' on cue, walking on a ladder that is placed on the floor, and so forth. Physical assistance may be gradually reduced.

MOTOR PLANNING

Obstacle courses that require children to crawl, or to move under, over, through, or around, or to cross low beams, and so forth are appropriate. Periodically reverse the direction of travel so that, for example, children must roll up an inclined mat. Another idea is to scatter small obstacles such as mats on the floor. Challenge the children to move between and around the objects by twirling, walking backward, sideways on backs or stomachs.

Classroom Assistance

Staff within the early education programme have been assisted by the adapted physical education consultant during the past year in creating a developmentally appropriate preschool physical activity programme. Handout material such as the *Step by Step Motor Skills Programme* from the University of Winnipeg has been provided to the school and to the family during home visits. This material contains activity ideas pertaining to locomotor, balance, and stability skills. Additional ideas will be shared with family regarding summer activities.

With respect to community based programmes, the University of Alberta offers a motor development programme on Saturday mornings (492-5644). Information regarding this programme has been shared with the school and family. This programme will resume in September 2001 and fee reduction programmes are available. Kate would also benefit, in terms of strength and motor competence, from regular involvement in enjoyable leisure activities such as this U of A programme or perhaps swimming, dance class, tricycle riding, and playground play.

It is a pleasure working with Kate and the dedicated staff at Happydale Elementary School. Please share the contents of this report with Kate's family. If I may be of further assistance please do not hesitate to contact me at 555-4478.

Patt Nearingburg, Ph.D.
Adapted Physical Education Consultant

Original: Special Needs Coordinator
(to be put on student's file)
Susan Cameron

CASE STUDY 4

7 Using the following case study, outline the consultation process you would use in addressing the school's needs.

Susan Martin, special education co-ordinator at Lyndale School, has forwarded a written request for adapted physical education consultation. Sean Philips is a nine-year-old grade four student who has a medical diagnosis of Duchenne muscular dystrophy. Over the summer, between grades three and four, he has acquired a manual wheelchair and uses it for most of his school day. Sean is able to walk using Lofstrand crutches for short distances. Maintaining his ability to walk with assistance is very important for his medical progress. Physical education staff is seeking assistance to determine the most appropriate times for Sean to use his crutches and his wheelchair during physical education. The physical education teacher would also appreciate strategies for safely including Sean in the fast-paced activities typically presented in the grade four programme of studies.

Summary

This chapter has outlined the roles and responsibilities of an adapted physical education consultant. It has provided a process for conducting an on-site consultation and the reporting thereof. Case studies have been presented so that students may gain a better understanding of the range of students whom they may encounter when serving in the role of an adapted physical education consultant. These case studies have also offered a sampling

of relevant programming suggestions. Upon review of this chapter, it is clear that an adapted physical education consultant is an important member of an educational consultative/assessment team for students with special needs.

Study Question

How will you use the information from this chapter to address the needs of students with disabilities in physical education?

References

Active Living Alliance for Canadians with a Disability. (1994). *Moving to inclusion: Active living through physical education: Maximizing opportunities for students with a disability.* Ottawa: CIRA/CAHPER.

Alberta Learning and Teaching Resources Branch. (2000). *Physical Education: Guide to implementation, kindergarten to grade 12.* Edmonton: Alberta Learning, Learning and Teaching Resources Branch.

Neufeldt, V. (Ed.). (1995). *Webster's new world dictionary.* New York: Macmillan.

Thatcher, V.S. (Ed.). (1985). *The new Webster encyclopedic dictionary.* New York: Macmillan.

Tremblay, M.S., and Willms, J.D. (2000). Secular trends in the body mass index of Canadian children. *Canadian Medical Association Journal, 163*(11): 1429–33.

Ulrich, D.A. (2000). *Test of gross motor development.* Austin, TX: Pro-Ed.

United States. Public Health Service. Office of the Surgeon General. National Center for Chronic Disease Prevention and Health Promotion (U.S.). (1996). *Physical activity and health: A report of the surgeon general: Executive summary.* Washington: U.S. Department of Health and Human Services.

CHAPTER 19

Considering Motivation

Janice Causgrove Dunn

Learning Objectives

- To examine motivated behaviour in the context of adapted physical activity.
- To understand several motivation theories that are currently popular in physical activity and sport.
- To predict the implications of poor motor skills or qualitatively different motor skills on motivation and achievement in physical activity, based on these theories.
- To suggest potential strategies to enhance or maintain motivation of persons with disabilities in physical activity, with particular emphasis on children with movement difficulties.

Introduction

Motivation is an important consideration in adapted physical activity because it underlies participation, performance, and achievement in physical activity and sport. Motivation is what activates behaviour, gives it direction and energy, and maintains it. Motivation theories attempt to explain why people think and act the way they do. In doing so, these theories help to answer questions regarding individuals' behaviours in physical activity situations. For example, why do people choose to engage in some activities but not in others? Why do some individuals participate in a particular activity with intensity and vigour, while others look as if they are simply 'going through the motions'? Why do some people persist in activities they are obviously not very good at, while other highly skilled individuals give up at the first signs of difficulty?

WHAT IS MOTIVATION?

What does it mean to be motivated? What does motivation 'look' like? Can you observe someone participating in an activity and, based on what you see, determine the direction and level of motivation the individual has? The term *motivation* is used to refer to personality factors, social variables, thoughts, and beliefs that are presumed to underlie the behaviours we observe (Roberts 1992, 2001). Motivation has been described as an individual's personal investment in a particular activity (Maehr and Meyer 1997). Because we cannot see or measure an individual's motivation directly, we make inferences about it based on observations of the direction, intensity, persistence, and quality of an individual's actions and behaviours.

In the context of physical activity and sport, we typically assess the *direction* of behaviour from observations of individuals' choices to participate actively in (i.e., approach) or withdraw from (i.e., avoid) participation in an activity, and individuals' choices to participate in one activity over another. *Intensity* may be seen in the amount of effort expended and through observations of focus or concentration. *Persistence* typically refers to time spent engaged in an activity. *Quality* of investment may be observed in an individual's 'venturesomeness' or willingness to engage in challenging tasks (i.e., tasks in which the individual is unsure of his or her competence) and in the quality of his or her strategic engagement (Maehr and Meyer 1997). In addition, motivation has also been inferred from assessments of *performance outcomes*, although outcomes are influenced by multiple factors (not just motivation).

What is the impact of impaired motor performance on motivation in physical activity contexts? Are there any particular motivational concerns associated with impaired motor performance, or with qualitatively different motor performances, in physical activity and sport settings? Theories of motivation are potentially important sources of information to answer these questions because they seek to provide greater understanding about why individuals are, or are not, motivated to act and achieve. There are many theoretical approaches to understanding motivation. Research in physical activity and sport has been dominated in the past thirty years or so by theories that adopt a social cognitive approach (Roberts 2001). The social cognitive approach to motivation assumes that: (a) individuals have psychological needs that they seek to fulfill (e.g., a need for competence, a need for relatedness); (b) the degree to which these needs are satisfied affects individuals' perceptions, affect, and behaviours, and; (c) the social context significantly influences how well these needs are satisfied (Osterman 2000). Three theoretical frameworks that adopt the social cognitive approach will be considered in this chapter in the context of persons with disabilities. These include competence motivation theory (Harter 1978, 1981), achievement goal theory (Nicholls 1984, 1989), and self-determination theory (Deci and Ryan 1985, 2000).

Harter's Competence Motivation Theory

Harter's theory of competence motivation (1978, 1981, 1999) has been one of the most widely used motivation theories in adapted physical activity research. The focus of this theory is the concept of *perceived competence*, which is an individual's self-assessment of his or her ability to accomplish the skills necessary to meet environmental demands (Roberts 2001). Research has shown that perceived competence is a powerful mediator of individuals' decisions to participate, exert effort, and persist in physical activities (Duda 1992; Nicholls 1989; Roberts 1992; Roberts, Kleiber, and Duda 1981; Vallerand and Reid 1990; Yun and Ulrich 1997). It affects whether the individual adopts behaviours that are adaptive or maladaptive in relation to future skill development, social development, fitness, and overall health. Examples of adaptive behaviours include maximal effort and persistence, while examples of maladaptive behaviours include avoidance and withdrawal.

Harter's (1978, 1981) theory is based upon the earlier work of White (1959), who

Figure 19.1 Factors Affecting Perceived Competence

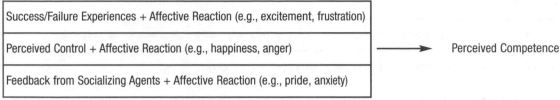

Success/Failure Experiences + Affective Reaction (e.g., excitement, frustration)	
Perceived Control + Affective Reaction (e.g., happiness, anger)	→ Perceived Competence
Feedback from Socializing Agents + Affective Reaction (e.g., pride, anxiety)	

SOURCE: From *The Relationship Between Perceived Competence, Affect, and Motivational Orientation within the Classroom, Processes and Patterns of Change*, by S. Harter, 1992, p. 79, Cambridge University Press. Adapted with permission.

introduced the concept of *effectance* (or competence) motivation as an intrinsic propensity, or predisposition, to have an effect on the environment and achieve valued outcomes within it (i.e., to demonstrate competence in valued skills). Unlike White, who saw effectance motivation as a *global* construct, Harter introduced a *multidimensional* view of competence motivation that includes distinct domains (e.g., athletic or physical, scholastic, social) (Harter 1985). A multidimensional perspective implies that people make distinctions in their perceptions of competence across different domains. Therefore, individuals can be motivated to engage in mastery attempts in some domains but not in others.

Harter's theory predicts that competence motivation leads individuals to engage in mastery attempts. These attempts result in: (a) some degree of success or failure, and accompanying affective reactions such as excitement about success or frustration about failure; (b) perceptions of control over outcomes and accompanying affective reactions, such as happiness about the perception of internal control over the outcome or anger about the lack of control; and (c) feedback from socializing agents (parents, teachers, coaches, or peers) plus accompanying affective reactions, such as pride and excitement or anxiety and shame. As shown in figure 19.1, each of these consequences directly impacts on an individual's perceptions of competence in the domain associated with the activity or behaviour (e.g., physical, cognitive, social). Perceived competence, in turn, is an important determinant of an individual's

motivation to engage in the behaviour in the future. Generally, people choose to participate in activities for which they have high perceptions of competence and avoid activities that are associated with low perceptions of competence.

---

1 Use Harter's competence motivation theory to develop a hypothesis about the likely impact of poor motor skills on a child's perceptions of competence and participation in the physical domain. What do you predict?

THE RELATIONSHIP BETWEEN PERCEIVED AND ACTUAL COMPETENCE

Based on the findings of research into the relationship between perceived and actual motor competence in children without disabilities, we know that perceived competence is positively associated with actual competence, and that older children tend to be more accurate than younger children in evaluating their own competence (Horn and Weiss 1991; Rudisill, Mahar, and Meaney 1993; Ulrich 1987; Weiss and Horn 1990). The more accurate perceptions of competence in older children are attributed to their increased cognitive ability to evaluate performance and to the sources of competence information that they use.

Developmental Changes in the Evaluation of Performance
The work of Nicholls and his colleagues in the classroom setting (see Nicholls 1989 for a review) and the more recent application of this work in the physical domain (Fry 2001;

Table 19.1 Possible Reactions to Failed Mastery Attempts by Children at Different Levels of Understanding of the Concept of Ability

Level 1	I was unable to do it because it is too hard for me. I will try something easier next time.
Level 2	I was unable to do it because I did not work hard enough. If I try harder next time I will be able to do it.
Level 3	I am not very good at this because I am the only one who was unable to do it. Maybe if I work harder I will be able to do it next time.
Level 4	I am not very good at this because I am the only one who was unable to do it. I do not want to do this anymore. I am going to try something that I am good at instead.

Fry and Duda 1997) suggests that the accuracy of children's evaluations of their own competence is partly dependent upon developmental changes in their understanding of the concept of ability. Up to about seven years of age, children do not differentiate between effort, ability, and task outcomes as cause-and-effect. Instead, they tend to believe that effort or outcome *is* ability. In other words, they believe that people with higher ability are those who try harder or score better. The idea that a person can try hard and *not* achieve success is beyond their understanding. In addition, young children do not fully comprehend the concept of normative difficulty (i.e., that the difficulty of a task is best judged with reference to the performance of others). Rather, they evaluate task difficulty in an egocentric (or subjective, self-referenced) manner. Difficult tasks are those that are *hard for me to do* and simple tasks are *easy for me to do*.

As children develop cognitively, they begin to recognize the cause-and-effect relationship between effort and outcome. In fact, effort is believed to be the main cause of outcomes (i.e., equal effort is expected to lead to equal outcomes). Beginning around age seven, and continuing until age eleven in some children, situations where two people have achieved equal outcomes with unequal effort are viewed as inexplicable, or attributed to insufficient or misdirected effort (Nicholls

1989). In any case, this level of understanding implies that failure outcomes (if they are perceived as such) are not likely to have the same negative affect on motivation as they will later in the child's development, due to the expectation that increased effort will result in success in the future (see table 19.1).

The third level in this developmental process represents a transition between the second and fourth levels of understanding, because children begin to show signs of a mature understanding of ability as *current capacity* (the fourth level), but not consistently. They now understand that effort is not the only cause of outcomes, and they evaluate their ability normatively (in relation to the performance of others). When asked to explain why two people achieve equal outcomes following unequal effort, a child at this level of understanding will likely focus on the idea that the person who worked harder is not as smart or skilled as the person who expended less effort. However, these explanations are still not applied consistently across situations, and they may not be followed through in predicting future outcomes. For example, after identifying the best athlete on the team as the person who did not have to try as hard to achieve a similar outcome as his or her teammates on a test of physical skill, a child at this level may still assert that all team members would achieve equally if they applied equal effort (Nicholls 1989).

Children at the fourth and final developmental level are those who have acquired the mature understanding of ability as current capacity. Almost all children have reached this point by twelve years of age, although many reach this mature understanding at an earlier age (Nicholls 1978). Children now understand that effort affects performance, but performance is ultimately constrained by ability. In other words, increased effort can improve performance up to the limit of current capacity. From this perspective, positive perceptions of competence arise in a child who performs better than others. Feelings of incompetence are fostered in a child who can not do something that others can do, or in a child who can achieve the same outcome as others who expended less effort.

---

2 Can you think of any reason why the presence of a movement difficulty might have an impact on the development of children's understanding of ability? Or would you expect the developmental changes described to be true for children who have poor movement skills? What do you think the impact of an intellectual impairment might be on an individual's understanding of the concept of ability?

We might predict that children with developmentally delayed intellectual abilities follow a similar developmental sequence as children who develop typically, but their rate of progress is slower. Alternatively, the sequence itself may be altered. Although there have not yet been any investigations specifically examining this question, there is some limited evidence of a similar, but slower, developmental sequence. A study of the relationship between perceived physical competence and actual competence in preschool children who were identified as being at risk of school failure or developmental delay found no significant relationship between actual and perceived physical competence (Goodway and Rudisill 1997). However, Yun and Ulrich (1997) reported a significantly positive relationship between perceived and actual physical competence

(r=.55) in eleven- to twelve-year-old children with mild mental retardation (MMR). A similar positive relationship was reported by Shapiro and Dummer (1998) in adolescents (twelve to fifteen years old) with MMR (r=.46).

Yun and Ulrich's (1997) study also revealed significant positive relationships between age and perceived competence (r=.31) and between age and actual competence (r=.61) in seven to twelve year olds with MMR. This indicates that although older children with MMR were generally more competent than their younger counterparts, the younger children with MMR tended to think they were more competent than the older children did. As a result, the authors suggested that "children with MMR must reach a certain cognitive level that comes with increasing age before they can construct their self-perception based on actual skill levels in the physical domain" (Yun and Ulrich 1997, p. 293).

Sources of Competence Information

The accuracy of children's perceptions of competence has also been linked to the information children use to evaluate their success and failure (Horn and Hasbrook 1986; Weiss and Horn 1990). Sources of competence information can be internal (i.e., sources that reside within the individual), such as the amount of effort exerted (e.g., *I tried hard*), whether or not self-set goals were achieved (e.g., *I'm getting better; I learned it*), and the type of affect experienced (e.g., *I had fun*). However, competence information is also available from external sources, primarily in the form of feedback and reinforcement from significant others (e.g., *my coach said I was good; no one made fun of my performance*), social comparison (e.g., *I had more hits than almost everyone else; I had fewer intercepted passes than anyone*), and sport or game outcomes (e.g., *we won*).

Researchers have consistently found developmental changes in the sources of competence information used by children between the ages of eight and seventeen years (Horn, Glenn, and Wentzel 1993; Horn and Hasbrook 1986; Horn and Weiss 1991; Weiss, Ebbeck, and Horn 1997). Younger children (eight to nine years old) tend to depend on evaluative feedback from significant adults (e.g., parents, coaches, teachers) for competence information, whereas children in middle to late childhood tend to rely on evaluative feedback from peers and peer comparison. This reliance on evaluative feedback from others in younger children highlights the important influence of the socializing environment on the development of competence motivation. Harter contends that if children receive positive reinforcement for their mastery attempts during early to late childhood, their attention to this evaluative information facilitates the internalization of performance standards based on effort, participation, persistence, and cooperation, and the development of a self-reward system. During adolescence there is a shift toward a preference for self-comparison information that, Harter (1978) contends, is necessary for older children to maintain positive perceptions of competence. She states that the continued need for external approval and dependence on externally defined goals has negative consequences for self-perceptions and behaviours because "this dependence may… lead to the perception that one has little control over the outcomes in one's life" (Harter 1978, p. 53). In contrast, the use of internal competence information sources enables older children and adolescents to praise themselves when they achieve their internal performance standards. When these performance standards are founded upon criteria such as effort, participation, and persistence, then positive perceptions of competence are likely to result even in individuals who are unskilled relative to their peers (Harter 1978; Nicholls 1989; Weiss and Horn 1990).

IMPLICATIONS FOR MOTIVATION IN ADAPTED PHYSICAL ACTIVITY

Based on Harter's theory, it is typically assumed that individuals with motor impairments will develop perceptions that they lack competence in physical activities, games, and sports. The mastery attempts of individuals with poor motor skills in physical activity and sport are expected to result predominantly in failure outcomes. In addition, because trying hard does not seem to make a difference to the outcome, individuals with poor motor skills are expected to develop low perceptions of control over performance (e.g., *I try as hard as I can, but no matter what I do, I can't seem to do it*), leading to unhappiness, frustration, and perhaps anger. Harter (1978) suggests that poor performance and lack of success are typically accompanied by (a) negative evaluative feedback from others, such as the lack of positive reinforcement or disapproval, and (b) anxiety caused by worry about disappointing parents and friends or being the target of ridicule. As a result of the negative perceptions and experiences associated with failed mastery attempts, persons with motor impairments are predicted to develop low perceptions of competence in the physical or athletic domain, and to be less inclined to seek out or take up future challenges and opportunities in physical activity or sports.

Research findings generally support these predictions, indicating that motor impairments do indeed introduce particular motivational concerns in physical activity situations. On average, children and adolescents with movement difficulties (such as developmental coordination disorder or clumsiness) have lower perceptions of physical or athletic competence than peers without movement difficulties (e.g., Cantell, Smyth, and Ahonen 1994; Piek, Dworkan, Barrett, and Coleman 2000; Schoemaker and Kalverboer 1994; Skinner and Piek 2001). The impact of these perceptions on behaviour are seen in research findings showing that children with movement difficulties do not often play or participate in games with peers, or in team sports (Cantell et al. 1994; Evans and Roberts 1987; Sandahl Christiansen 2000; Smyth and Anderson 2000). When they do participate, these children spend proportionally more time engaged in maladaptive (i.e., off task, inactive) behaviours than their movement competent peers (Bouffard, Watkinson, Thompson, Causgrove Dunn, and Romanow 1996; Causgrove Dunn 1997; Skinner and Piek 2001; Thompson, Bouffard, Watkinson, and Causgrove Dunn 1994). Children and adolescents with movement difficulties also tend to report lower levels of perceived social support and more anxiety than their movement competent peers (Rose, Larkin, and Berger 1994; Schoemaker and Kalverboer 1994; Skinner and Piek 2001).

Can the negative self-perceptions and maladaptive behaviours associated with low perceived competence in children with motor impairments be prevented or remediated? Harter's (1978) theory proposes that while actual competence does not directly affect motivated behaviour, it is a precursor to perceived competence. This is because actual competence influences the amount of success and failure experienced, perceptions of control, and feedback received from others. Therefore, interventions intended to improve children's actual motor skills should, if successful, also improve their perceptions of physical competence. This prediction has been supported by research findings from studies involving preschool children at risk of developmental delay (Goodway and Rudisill 1996) and children with developmental coordination disorder (Miller, Polatajko, Missiuna, Mandich, and Macnab 2001). Individualized activities that provide optimal challenge for children with motor impairments (i.e., where effortful participation leads to successful outcomes, skill improvement, and learning) should effectively maximize perceptions of success and internal control, leading to positive perceptions of physical competence.

Harter (1978) also suggests that perceived competence is directly influenced by feedback from socializing agents (e.g., parents, teachers, coaches, and peers). She states that the provision of positive reinforcement to young children for independent mastery *attempts* in physical activity (i.e., effort exerted, persistence, improvement) results in the internalization of a self-reward system and performance standards based on personal effort and improvement. The use of these self-referenced standards will presumably enable even individuals who recognize that they are less skilled than their peers to (a) perceive their interactions with the environment as successful, provided that effortful participation produces at least minimal improvements in performance, (b) feel that they have internal control over these interactions, and (c) develop positive physical self-perceptions.

3 Are positive perceptions of competence in children who have motor impairments necessarily adaptive for motivation and behaviour in physical activity?

Several researchers in adapted physical activity have suggested that children who overestimate their competence (such as children with movement difficulties who have positive perceptions of physical competence) will have a tendency to set unrealistic performance expectations for themselves, resulting in negative self-perceptions and maladaptive motivational consequences in the long run (Shapiro and Dummer 1998; Ulrich 1987; Yun and Ulrich 1997). As described by Yun and Ulrich (1997, p. 286),

> overestimation of the child's ability may lead to unsuccessful outcomes due to unrealistic expectations.... For example, if James cannot hit a baseball well, but he perceives his ability as good, James will likely set higher expectations. Because of the unrealistic higher expectation, James may experience an unsuccessful outcome in terms of task achievement. Overestimation of actual competence negatively influences the level of perceived competence over time.

The implication seems to be that, for individuals with motor impairments, perceptions of competence that accurately reflect actual competence will be more adaptive in the long run (than high perceptions of competence), because low and accurate perceptions will lead to more realistic expectations and more frequent success outcomes. While this appears to be a reasonable argument, consider the case of a child with a motor impairment who has high perceptions of physical competence resulting from the use of internal, self-referenced criteria (effort, improvement, and skill mastery) to evaluate his or her performance.

4 If a child's high perceptions of physical competence are based on improvements in his or her skills that have occurred as a result of effort and practice, should we describe these perceptions as inaccurate and overestimated? Furthermore, would you expect this child to set unrealistic performance expectations and select tasks that are beyond his or her capability?

Achievement Goal Theory

Another concept that is very useful to understanding motivation and behaviour in physical activity and sport is an individual's *goal perspective*. This concept comes from achievement goal theory (Nicholls 1984, 1989) and generally refers to *how* people evaluate their competence. Similar to Harter's (1978) competence motivation theory, achievement goal theory assumes that individuals are driven to demonstrate competence, and that perceptions of competence are a critical determinant of motivated behaviour. However, in contrast to Harter's theory, achievement goal theory assumes that individual differences in goal perspectives, or the "ways in which individuals judge their competence and define successful accomplishment" (Duda 2001, p. 129), lead to differences in motivation and behaviour.

According to achievement goal theory, there are two main goal perspectives that individuals adopt in their achievement strivings (Nicholls 1989). First, a *task goal perspective* refers to an individual's focus on exhibiting effort, completing a task, improving performance, or learning new skills. Therefore, perceptions of success or failure and perceptions of competence are based on self-evaluations of how well these aims were achieved: *Did I work hard? Did I finish? Am I getting better? Did I learn it? Can I do it now?* In other words, perceptions of success and competence are based on subjective, self-referenced assessments of personal achievement and mastery.

Nicholls (1989) relates task goals to the use of the undifferentiated concept of ability described earlier in this chapter. He states,

"when our aim is to solve a problem, to learn, or to increase our understanding, we become like little children for whom competence is signalled by gains in level of performance or by increases in the sense of certainty that they can understand or do something" (p. 85). Because the achievement of tasks that require great effort imply more learning or accomplishment than those achieved with little effort, individuals who are task-involved will seek to develop their competence through the selection of optimally challenging tasks (i.e., moderately difficult tasks that are perceived as achievable through significant effort). Furthermore, because an undifferentiated concept of ability leads to the expectation that greater effort will lead to more learning or greater skill development, "the more effort expended in completing a task, the higher the perceived ability" (Nicholls 1989, p. 85).

The second goal perspective is an *ego goal perspective*, which refers to a focus on demonstrating superior ability relative to others or, failing that, to avoid demonstrating low ability relative to others. This goal perspective is related to the use of a differentiated (or mature) conception of ability described earlier (Nicholls 1989). People who emphasize an ego goal perspective evaluate success and failure through social comparison by comparing their own ability to that of others. Effort is viewed as a 'double-edged sword'. The combination of effort and success on a moderately difficult task leads to high perceptions of competence. However, the combination of effort and failure, or effort and success when others succeed with less effort (i.e., effortful success on a normatively easy task), results in low perceptions of competence.

The goal perspective that an individual holds in a particular situation is referred to as the individual's *goal involvement* (Nicholls 1989). *Task involvement* is the psychological state of holding a task goal perspective, while *ego involvement* is the psychological state of holding an ego goal perspective. The degree to which an individual is task-involved or ego-involved depends upon developmental, dispositional, and situational factors.

DEVELOPMENTAL INFLUENCE

According to Nicholls (1989), young children's undeveloped (i.e., undifferentiated) conceptions of ability cause them to maintain a task-involved approach to their interactions with the environment. At the same time, however, a child's understanding of the concept of ability does not wholly determine which goal perspective is adopted in a particular situation. Research indicates that, although young children do not typically use norm-referenced information to evaluate their performance, they can be induced to do so if another person's performance is emphasized as the performance standard (Nicholls 1989). In addition, although virtually all children have developed a mature conception of ability as current capacity by about twelve years of age, there continues to be considerable variation in the extent to which individuals view superior ability as necessary for success. In other words, people who are capable of judging their performance outcomes and competence from a more mature or differentiated perspective do not always choose to do so (Nicholls 1989).

GOAL ORIENTATION

The second factor that influences an individual's goal involvement is his or her dispositional preference for task and ego goals (Nicholls 1989). Nicholls refers to this dispositional preference for certain types of goals as *goal orientation* (Nicholls 1989). Goal orientation is viewed as a stable, but not fixed, tendency to approach situations or tasks with certain achievement goals in mind. A person high in task orientation is one who tends to approach activities with task goals in mind. A person high in ego orientation, on the other hand, tends to approach activities with the goal of demonstrating superior performance relative to others. However, task orientation and ego orientation are not two ends of a continuum, but rather are independent constructs. This means that people have varying levels of dispositional tendencies toward both goal perspectives. Individuals may have high levels of both task and ego orientation (high task/high ego), high task and low ego

orientation (high task/low ego), low task and high ego orientation (low task/high ego), low levels of task and ego orientation (low task/low ego), or any combination of the two.

Research examining different combinations of task and ego orientation (i.e., different goal orientation profiles) has often found that the most adaptive combination is high task/high ego, and the least adaptive combination is low task/low ego (e.g., Fox, Goudas, Biddle, Duda, and Armstrong 1994; Walling and Duda 1995). Duda (2001) suggests that the high task/high ego goal orientation profile enables individuals to respond flexibly or adjust to different performance outcomes in different situations by focussing on either task-involved or ego-involved goals. "Researchers have suggested that a high task orientation might, to some degree, insulate highly ego-oriented individuals from the negative consequences of low perceived ability when they are performing poorly and, thus, be motivationally advantageous 'over the long haul' (Duda 1992; Nicholls 1989; Roberts et al. 1996)" (Duda and Treasure 2001, p. 53). Individuals with a low task/low ego orientation profile have been described as amotivated (Deci and Ryan 1985) because they do not appear to be concerned or interested in demonstrating competence in physical activity at all (Duda 2001).

Goal orientations are thought to develop through socialization experiences at home, school, and in physical activities (Ames 1992; Nicholls 1989; Nicholls, Patashnick, and Nolen 1985). Socializing agents (parents, teachers, and coaches) communicate their own definitions of success and achievement to children by making approval dependent upon winning and outperforming others or, alternatively, upon trying hard and demonstrating personal improvement (Treasure and Roberts 1994, 1995).

PERCEIVED MOTIVATIONAL CLIMATE

The third factor that influences the goal perspective adopted in a particular situation is an individual's perceptions of the goals emphasized within the environment. This is referred to as the *perceived motivational climate*. Motivational climates are structured through the provision of instructions, feedback, rewards, and explicit expectations that emphasize either task-involving goals (called a *mastery motivational climate*) or ego-involving goals (called a *performance motivational climate*) (Ames 1992; Nicholls 1989). For example, situations devoid of evaluative cues in which the emphasis is on performing a specific task, skill development, problem solving, or learning, will likely promote task involvement. In contrast, situations that emphasize evaluation (e.g., tests of highly-valued skills, interpersonal competition, social comparison, and the use of normative feedback) and factors that increase one's public self-awareness (e.g., the presence of an audience or video camera) tend to promote ego involvement (Nicholls 1989).

It is unlikely, however, that one general motivational climate is created for all individuals within a particular situation. Cues and demands are not usually the same for everyone, with particular differences in at least the perceptions of how high and low achievers are treated (Martinek and Karper 1984, 1986; Papaioannou 1995). And even when instructions and feedback are identical for everyone in a specific setting, different individuals select and attend to different cues, and there are differences across people in how those cues are interpreted (Ames and Archer 1988). Nicholls (1989) maintains that an individual's goal orientation affects the situational cues that the person selects and how they are interpreted. Individuals who are highly task oriented generally notice or select cues that reinforce task goals (Causgrove Dunn 2000; Ebbeck and Becker 1994; Kavussanu and Roberts 1996; Seifriz, Duda, and Chi 1992). Individuals high in ego orientation, on the other hand, tend to select and process cues related to their dispositional preference for interpersonal competition and normative comparison (Causgrove Dunn 2000; Kavussanu and Roberts 1996; Seifriz et al. 1992). There is also evidence that individuals request evaluative information that is congruent with their goal orientation (Butler 1993).

In situations where participants' goal orientations match the motivational climate, goal involvement is fairly easy to predict.

However, when goal orientations are in conflict with the motivational climate (e.g., when a person with high task/low ego orientation enters a highly performance oriented climate), researchers have suggested that goal involvement will depend upon the relative strength of the individual's dispositional goals in relation to the strength of the motivational climate (Roberts and Treasure 1992; Treasure and Roberts 1995). The stronger an individual's predisposition toward task or ego goals, the less likely that situational cues will override it. This suggests that the motivational climate may be most influential in determining the goal involvement of children and young adolescents because they have not yet developed personal theories of achievement and strong goal orientations (Treasure and Roberts 1995).

MOTIVATIONAL PREDICTIONS OF ACHIEVEMENT GOAL THEORY

Task involvement is generally considered to be a more adaptive goal perspective than ego involvement, because it is expected to foster positive self-perceptions and behaviours (e.g., enjoyment, interest, positive perceptions of competence and self-efficacy, intrinsic motivation, effort, the use of problem-solving strategies, a preference for challenging tasks, persistence in the face of failure) in individuals of all skill levels. Under task involvement, competence is evaluated according to subjective, self-referenced assessments of effort, improvement, and personal mastery. Therefore, normative perceptions of competence are irrelevant and individuals are expected to engage in adaptive behaviours regardless of their perceptions of how skilled they are compared to others.

In contrast, ego involvement is predicted to have differential effects on behaviour, depending upon participants' normative perceptions of ability (see figure 19.2). Because individuals who are ego-involved strive to demonstrate superior normative ability, adaptive behaviours are predicted for those who perceive their ability as high in relation to others. In fact, various achievement goal

Figure 19.2   The Predicted Impact of Ego Involvement and High Versus Low (Normative) Perceived Competence on Behaviour

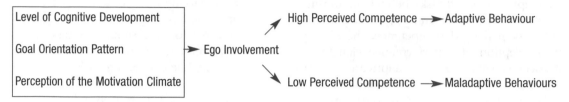

theorists have suggested that the behaviour of an ego-involved individual with high perceptions of competence will be similar to that of a task-involved individual (Nicholls 1989; Roberts 1992).

However, for ego-involved individuals who believe that they have low skills compared to others, maladaptive behaviours (i.e., behaviours that do not contribute to long-term achievement) are expected. In this case, low perceptions of competence lead individuals to expect that they will not be able to achieve the goal of demonstrating superior ability relative to others. Consequently, their focus shifts to avoiding the demonstration of incompetence. In situations that afford activity choices, an individual may avoid looking incompetent by selecting tasks that are (normatively) too easy or too difficult. Tasks that are too easy will result in success, thereby hiding the performer's lack of competence (or at least leaving it in doubt). Tasks that are too difficult will almost certainly lead to failure but will still enable the individual to avoid the implication of low ability because everyone would be expected to fail such a difficult task.

IMPLICATIONS FOR MOTIVATION

Achievement goal theory predicts that when an individual is task-involved (whether due to developmental factors, dispositional factors, situational factors, or some combination of all three), the presence of a movement difficulty is unlikely to be associated with motivational concerns. However, in situations where an individual with poor motor skills is ego-involved, he or she is at risk for low perceptions

of competence and maladaptive behaviours including withdrawal from participation.

In order to assess the validity of these predictions, we can examine the findings of several studies that have used achievement goal theory as a theoretical framework to investigate motivational factors in sport and physical activity of wheelchair basketball players (Duda and White 1992; Skordilis et al. 2001; White and Duda 1993), wheelchair marathoners (Skordilis et al. 2001), Paralympic athletes (Pensgaard, Roberts, and Ursin 1999), and children with movement difficulties (Causgrove Dunn 2000). For example, Causgrove Dunn (2000) examined the goal orientations, perceptions of the motivational climate, and perceptions of competence in physical education of children with movement difficulties from grades four to six. Positive relationships were found between children's levels of task orientation and their perceptions of mastery motivational climate, and between perceptions of a mastery climate and their perceptions of competence in physical education. Ego orientation was positively related to perceptions of a performance motivational climate, but the perception of a performance climate was negatively related to perceived competence. In other words, the higher the perception of a performance climate, the lower the perception of competence in physical education (Causgrove Dunn 2000). Further, findings of a related study involving the same participants found that children's perceptions of competence in physical education were (a) positively related to the amount of time they spent appropriately engaged in assigned tasks during the class, and (b) negatively related to the amount of time they spent engaged in maladaptive (i.e., off-task) behaviours during the class (Causgrove Dunn 1997). For children with low perceived competence, the higher the perception of a performance climate in physical education, the less adaptive and more maladaptive their behaviours tended to be.

Based on the theoretical predications and research findings of studies involving individuals with and without disabilities, it is recommended that physical activity settings be structured to emphasize a mastery motivational climate (Causgrove Dunn 2000; Nicholls, Cheung, Lauer, and Patashnick 1989; Treasure and Roberts 1995). Children participating in mastery motivational climates should be more likely to perceive the climate as mastery oriented, enabling higher perceptions of competence and engagement in more adaptive participation behaviours. At the same time, a mastery motivational climate may decrease perceptions of a performance climate and the frequency of maladaptive behaviours.

This recommendation may be particularly important for some persons with disabilities who participate in integrated settings and activities. As illustrated by an athlete in the study by Pensgaard et al. (1999):

> I started to train in an ordinary sports club, and I became used to being last also at the training sessions. And I had to work hard with my own psyche and to learn to set up goals based on my own standards.
> (p. 245–46)

According to Ames (1992) and Treasure (2001), careful attention to the structural features or 'building blocks' of the setting is required to emphasize a mastery motivational climate (i.e., to increase the salience of task involving goals relative to ego involving goals). Ames and Treasure refer to the work of Epstein (1988, 1989), which identifies structural features that define the motivational climate in the classroom. Based on this work, six recommendations are made to create a mastery motivational climate in physical activity settings:

a. Provide a diversity of meaningful tasks, drills, exercises, and learning activities with varying levels of difficulty for individual participants to choose from in order to increase interest, task involvement, and perceived competence while decreasing social comparison.

b. Shift the locus of responsibility for learning to involve participants by providing them with activity choices that are perceived as being of equal value.

c. Provide private (rather than public) recognition for achievements and improvement.

d. Use varied and heterogeneous groups (i.e., group individuals with different ability levels together) to increase cooperative learning and peer interaction while de-emphasizing the salience of social comparison within and between groups.

e. Emphasize self-evaluations of effort, improvement, participation, and mastery.

f. Individualize the pace of instruction and time allotted for practice or task completion.

Although there is some support for the use of these guidelines to facilitate a mastery motivational climate and to foster adaptive achievement-related perceptions and behaviours in physical activity (Solmon 1996; Theeboom, DeKnop, and Weiss 1995), none of this research has involved individuals with disabilities as yet.

Finally, let us reconsider the case of James from the earlier discussion of Harter's (1978) competence motivation theory, in light of the theory and research related to goal perspectives. James' situation was introduced to illustrate the hypothesis that positive self-perceptions of physical competence in individuals who lack actual competence (i.e., overestimate their actual physical competence) leads to unrealistic performance expectations (Shapiro and Dummer 1998; Yun and Ulrich, 1997).

5 However, if positive self-perceptions are based on the use of self-referenced performance standards (i.e., effort, improvement, mastery) rather than normative or social comparison, are they necessarily inaccurate or distorted?

Based on the criteria used to evaluate successful performance, self-referenced performance standards are likely to result in positive perceptions of competence, even in individuals who lack skill compared to others (Nicholls 1989). Therefore, the use of mastery performance standards can lead to positive self-perceptions in individuals with motor impairments who are well aware of their lack of ability relative to peers without disabilities. If this is the case in James's situation, then why would we expect him to determine his performance expectations more or less accurately than other children who use a different set of criteria for judging success and competence?

Self-determination Theory

The last theory to be considered in this chapter is self-determination theory (SDT) (Deci and Ryan 1985, 2000). Unlike other theories that view motivation as a unidimensional construct that varies in amount (i.e., high to low), SDT conceptualizes motivation as multidimensional. That is, Deci and Ryan (1985, 2000) propose that motivation can be intrinsic or extrinsic. Intrinsically motivated behaviours are those that are engaged in for their own sake–for the inherent satisfaction of the activity itself (Deci and Ryan 1985; Ryan and Deci 2000a, 2000b). Extrinsically motivated behaviours, on the other hand, are behaviours that are done for the purpose of attaining a separable, externally regulated outcome (e.g., recognition, money, a trophy).

According to SDT, intrinsic motivation is associated with more positive affect, such as interest, excitement, enjoyment, and satisfaction, and more adaptive behaviours, including effort, persistence, creativity, and strategic engagement (see Ryan and Deci 2000a, 2000b; Vallerand and Lossier 1999; Vallerand and Reid 1990). The degree to which a

person is intrinsically motivated is a function of the degree to which three psychological needs are satisfied. These are the needs for competence, autonomy, and relatedness (Deci and Ryan, 1985, 2000). Within SDT, the need for competence is conceptualized as an individual's innate psychological need to interact effectively with the environment and to achieve valued outcomes within it. The need for autonomy refers to the need for self-initiated regulation of one's own actions and behaviours. Finally, the need for relatedness is conceptualized as the need for secure and satisfying connections with others in the social context, or as a sense of belongingness. Activities that lead an individual to experience feelings of competence, autonomy, and relatedness are perceived as intrinsically rewarding and likely to be performed with effort and enjoyment, and to be selected for participation in the future. From this perspective, choice is important. A freely chosen behaviour or activity is more likely to be intrinsically motivated than a behaviour or activity that is externally imposed.

INTRINSIC AND EXTRINSIC MOTIVATION

Both intrinsically and extrinsically motivated behaviours can be described as highly motivated, but they differ in the extent to which they are self-determined. Behaviours that lack either intrinsic or extrinsic motivation are called *amotivated behaviours.* Amotivated behaviours are nonmotivated (Vallerand and Reid 1990). "Amotivation results from not valuing an activity (Ryan 1995), not feeling competent to do it (Deci 1975), or not believing it will yield a desired outcome (Seligman 1975)" (Ryan and Deci 2000b, p. 61). Individuals who are amotivated are predicted to engage in maladaptive behaviour patterns and eventually to cease participation altogether.

As shown in figure 19.3, the different types of motivation identified by Deci and Ryan can be placed along a continuum of self-determination, with intrinsic motivation and amotivation located on opposite ends of the continuum. Extrinsic motivation is situated in

Figure 19.3 The Psychological Needs, Types of Motivation, and Types of Regulation Underlying Behaviour

Psychological Needs	Motivation	Type of Regulation
	Intrinsic	Intrinsic: behaviour is self-determined, inspired by inherent interest and enjoyment of the activity.
Competence		Integrated: behaviour is self-determined and is part of the person's self-identity, but is still instrumental in nature.
Autonomy	Extrinsic	Identified: behaviour is internally regulated, its personal value is recognized and accepted.
Relatedness		Introjected: regulation of behaviour is partially internalized because internal contingencies are self-administered (e.g., pride, guilt, shame).
		External: behaviour is controlled by external contingencies (e.g., tangible rewards or threatened punishment).
	Amotivation	Non-regulated: No perceived reason for engaging in the behaviour.

(Vertical label between columns: Continuum of Self-Determination)

SOURCE: From *Intrinsic Motivation and Self-Determination in Behaviour,* by E.L. Deci and R.M. Ryan, 1985, New York: Plenum, and "Self-determination Theory and the Faciliation of Intrinsic Motiviation, Social Development, and Well-being" by R.M. Ryan and E.L. Deci, 2000, *American Psychologist, 55*, pp. 68–78.

the middle of this continuum, but even extrinsic motivation can vary in the degree to which it is self-determined (Deci and Ryan, 1985, 2000).

External regulation is the least self-determined form of extrinsic motivation. Externally regulated behaviours are those that are controlled by external contingencies. In other words, the reason for the behaviour is outside of the behaviour itself. For example, a child who is physically inactive may agree to engage in daily exercise after being promised a new computer game. The motivation is extrinsic because the behaviour is entirely contingent upon a tangible reward. Another example is a child who attends soccer practice to avoid being criticized or punished (e.g., benched) by the coach. In this case, the behaviour occurs solely to avoid negative consequences. Whether the reason for the

behaviour is to obtain a reward or to avoid a threatened punishment, the individual experiences feelings of obligation and of being controlled (Deci and Ryan 1985; Vallerand and Reid 1990). Not surprisingly, externally regulated behaviours are unlikely to be maintained once the reward or punishment contingencies are removed.

Introjected regulation is slightly more self-determined than external regulation because it refers to behaviours that are regulated by self-administered contingencies (rewards or punishments), rather than those administered externally. An example of this type of regulation is exercising in order to avoid feelings of guilt. In addition, "a classic form of introjection…[occurs when]…a person performs an act in order to enhance or maintain self-esteem and the feeling of worth" (Ryan and Deci 2000b, p. 62). Because introjected behaviours are regulated by internal contingencies, they are more likely to be maintained than externally regulated behaviours. However, these behaviours are still relatively unstable.

Behaviours that are *regulated through identification* are those that are personally valued and important to the individual, and thus are perceived as being self-selected (Deci and Ryan 2000; Vallerand and Reid 1990). For example, a person who recognizes and accepts the value of exercise for personal health and well-being would be said to identify with this behaviour, and is likely to participate as a result. Similarly, a child who recognizes that attending soccer practices will lead to improved performance can be said to identify with practicing and is likely to engage in it. However, these behaviours (exercising and practicing) are still considered to be extrinsically motivated because they are performed to achieve a separable outcome (i.e., to be healthier or more skilled), rather than for enjoyment and satisfaction in and of themselves.

Finally, *integrated regulation* is the most self-determined form of extrinsic motivation. Behaviours in this category are congruent with other values that the individual holds, are part of his or her self-concept, and are engaged out of personal choice. An example is a person who sees him or herself as an athlete (i.e., it is part of the self-concept) and chooses to attend a competition with athletes of much greater skill (i.e., that he or she has no chance of winning, or even placing well) due to the perceived value that the experience will have for the individual's continued development as an athlete. The behaviour is still considered extrinsic because it is "done for its presumed instrumental value with respect to some outcome that is separate from the behaviour, even though it is volitional and valued by the self" (Ryan and Deci 2000b, p. 62).

It should be noted that the continuum of self-determination in figure 19.3 is not a developmental continuum such that people must progress through each stage in order to achieve or experience intrinsic motivation (Ryan and Deci 2000a). While there is a general tendency for behaviours to become progressively more self-determined with increasing time, they can become internalized from any point along the continuum.

IMPLICATIONS

A great deal of research with typical populations has supported the predictions of SDT, that the more an individual's needs for competence, autonomy, and relatedness are satisfied in a particular setting, the more internalized his or her motivation becomes (see Ryan and Deci 2000a, 2000b). There is evidence that intrinsic motivation and the more internalized forms of extrinsic motivation are positively associated with interest, enjoyment, effort, positive coping styles, persistence, performance, and quality of learning (Ryan and Deci 2000a). Unfortunately, there have been relatively few studies examining SDT in the context of physical activity and sport, and fewer still that involve persons with disabilities.

The importance of perceptions of competence, autonomy, and belongingness to children with physical disabilities in inclusive physical education is revealed in a study by Goodwin and Watkinson (2000). These researchers conducted focus group interviews with nine children with physical disabilities (either spina bifida, cerebral palsy, or amputation) about their experiences in inclusive physical education. A number of themes were identified in the children's responses, revealing a dichotomy in their experiences. This dichotomy was named 'bad days' and 'good days'. Bad days were days in which the children felt (a) socially isolated (i.e., were ridiculed by classmates, ignored, or perceived as objects of curiosity), (b) that their competence was questioned, or (c) that they were limited in their ability to participate (either through a lack of support by the teacher, lack of engagement by classmates, or constraints imposed by the equipment or facilities). In contrast, good days were described by the themes of skillful participation and a sense of belonging. Although Goodwin and Watkinson (2000) did not set out to examine the relationship between the three psychological needs (competence, autonomy, and relatedness) and children's enjoyment of inclusive physical education, their findings suggest these basic needs play a very important role. It seems that bad days and good days in physical education are associated with conditions that either thwart or satisfy the basic needs identified in SDT.

In the interest of increasing individuals' intrinsic motivation, Ryan and Deci (2000a, 2000b) offer general guidelines aimed at increasing individuals' perceptions of competence, autonomy, and relatedness. Suggestions for increasing perceived competence are similar to those included in the earlier discussions of competence motivation theory and achievement goal theory. For instance, interventions intended to increase skill levels, the amount of success experienced in optimally challenging tasks, the provision of positive feedback for mastery attempts, and freedom from negative or demeaning feedback are all predicted to facilitate intrinsic motivation through increased perceptions of competence.

Conditions that promote perceptions of autonomy include the provision of choices and opportunities for self-direction, acknowledgement of participants' feelings, and freedom from threats and rewards. The use of extrinsic rewards are often not recommended, due to research findings showing that the use of extrinsic rewards and reinforcements can reduce intrinsic motivation due to the perception of increased external control (and decreased internal control) over behaviour (Vallerand, Deci, and Ryan 1987). However, it should be noted that extrinsic rewards can be used to facilitate intrinsic motivation. As suggested by Duda and Treasure (2001), a reward that is provided contingent upon personal performance communicates information about competence. As such, receiving the reward should increase perceptions of competence without undermining perceptions of autonomy and self-determination.

An interesting issue in relation to perceived autonomy and the provision of choice is the influence of perceived competence on perceptions of choice and autonomy. For example, a teacher in an inclusive physical education programme may attempt to increase students' perceptions of autonomy by setting up different activity options (or activity stations) around the gymnasium and then allowing each child to select an activity from the available options. Can we be certain, however, that all of the children in the environment perceive the same number of options?

6 If a child believes that he or she cannot do an activity successfully, or cannot do it the same way that his or her peers do it, then is that activity perceived as a real activity option? Or is the simple fact that the child does not *have* to do an activity (i.e., can choose to not do it) enough to facilitate perceptions of choice and autonomy, and increase intrinsic motivation?

Perceptions of relatedness are influenced by individuals' perceptions of connectedness and caring (Deci and Ryan 2000). For example, Ryan and Grolnick (1986) found that students who perceived their teachers as warm and caring reported greater intrinsic motivation. Unfortunately, recent research in inclusive physical education settings suggests that the relatedness perceptions of participants with disabilities are not always positive. Studies by Goodwin and Watkinson (2000) and Place and Hodge (2001) reveal that students with physical disabilities are sometimes excluded, neglected, teased or called names, and viewed as objects of curiosity by their classmates without disabilities. Moreover, observations of interactions between three eighth-grade girls with physical disabilities and their classmates without disabilities over three physical education classes revealed there were no interactions an average of 96 percent of the time (Place and Hodge 2001).

7 What might teachers do to encourage positive interactions and friendships among students with and without disabilities?

Sherrill (1998) has suggested that teachers design activities to afford structured contacts. Moreover, these "contacts must be frequent, interactive, pleasant, and focussed on common, meaningful goals that promote respect" (p. 227). Interactions of this nature, based on common interests and goals, are expected to promote equal status relationships between peers with and without disabilities. An equal status relationship is a mutually satisfying association in which both individuals contribute equally, building on each other's strengths (Sherrill 1998).

Generally speaking, it seems that steps taken to provide a mastery motivational climate (outlined in the previous section on goal perspectives) should also facilitate intrinsic motivation. These include a focus on task goals, the provision of choice from an array of activities of equal value but varying in difficulty, and groupings to facilitate interaction and cooperation among members. In addition, curricular adaptations, instructional modifications, and human resources (e.g., appropriately trained peer tutors, specialists) are also necessary (Place and Hodge 2001).

Summary and Considerations

As stated at the beginning of this chapter, there has been relatively little research examining the motivation of individuals with disabilities in physical activity and sport. It is important to acknowledge, however, that motivation research in adapted physical activity has certainly increased in recent years due largely to the increasing profile of disability sport and the corresponding interest in factors influencing the performance of athletes with disabilities (Reid and Prupas 1998).

Based on the theoretical predictions and research evidence presented in this chapter, it appears that the presence of a movement disability or a cognitive disability (or both) in a physical activity or sport environment may introduce particular motivational concerns. All three of the theories examined in this chapter suggest that individuals who *perceive* themselves to be competent in physical activity are more likely to be motivated to participate than those who have perceptions of low ability, regardless of their actual ability levels. Whether individuals with poor (or at least different) movement skills feel compe-

tent is influenced not only by their actual skill levels, but also by their cognitive development, their goals for participation, and by factors related to the task or the environment. Also important to motivation are perceptions of autonomy and internal control, and the feelings of connectedness with others within physical activity and sport environments (Deci and Ryan 1985, 2000; Harter 1978, 1981).

Study Questions

1. What behaviours are typically associated with high motivation to participate in physical activities? What behaviours are associated with low motivation?

2. Use Harter's competence motivation theory (or either of the other two theories) to develop predictions about the motivation to participate in an organized physical activity (e.g., physical education class) for a child with a disability that negatively affects motor skills.

3. What can you do to increase the motivation of an individual who has a disability that negatively affects the performance of motor skills during physical activities or sport? Develop separate recommendations based on competence motivation theory, achievement goal theory, and self-determination theory.

4. Based on each of the three motivation theories included in this chapter, what could you do to decrease the motivation of an individual who has a disability that negatively affects the performance of motor skills in physical activities or sport?

5. Select an activity of your choice and describe how you would structure it to encourage perceptions of a mastery climate. How would you change it to encourage perceptions of a performance climate?

6. Does the impact of failure on motivation to participate vary with the age of the individual? Explain why or why not.

7. Would you expect repeated failure outcomes to have the same impact on a child with an intellectual disability and a child without an intellectual disability, both of whom are the same chronological age? Explain why or why not.

8. Describe how the concept of motivation in self-determination theory differs from the other two theories in this chapter.

References

Ames, C. (1992). Achievement goals, motivational climate, and motivational processes. In G.C. Roberts (Ed.), *Motivation in sport and exercise* (pp. 161–76). Champaign, IL: Human Kinetics.

Ames, C., and Archer, J. (1988). Achievement goals in the classroom: Students' learning strategies and motivational processes. *Journal of Educational Psychology, 80,* 260–67.

Bouffard, M., Watkinson, E.J., Thompson, L.P., Causgrove Dunn, J., and Romanow, S.K.E. (1996). A test of the activity deficit hypothesis with children with movement difficulties. *Adapted Physical Activity Quarterly, 13,* 61–73.

Butler, R. (1993). Effects of task- and ego-achievement goals on information seeking during task engagement. *Journal of Personality and Social Psychology, 65,* 18–31.

Cantell, M.H., Smyth, M.M., and Ahonen, T.P. (1994). Clumsiness in adolescence: Educational, motor, and social outcomes of motor delay detected at 5 years. *Adapted Physical Activity Quarterly, 13,* 115–29.

Causgrove Dunn, J. (1997). *Individual differences in personal and situational factors related to motivation and achievement behaviour in physically awkward children.* Unpublished doctoral dissertation, University of Alberta.

Causgrove Dunn, J. (2000). Goal orientations, perceptions of the motivational climate, and perceived competence of children with movement difficulties. *Adapted Physical Activity Quarterly, 17,* 1–19.

Deci, E.L., and Ryan, R.M. (1985). *Intrinsic motivation and self-determination in behavior.* New York: Plenum.

Deci, E.L., and Ryan, R.M. (2000). The "what" and "why" of goal pursuits: Human needs and the self-determination of behaviour. *Psychological Inquiry, 11,* 227–68.

Duda, J.L. (1992). Motivation in sport settings: A goal perspective approach. In G. C. Roberts (Ed.), *Motivation in sport and exercise* (pp. 57–91). Champaign, IL: Human Kinetics.

Duda, J.L. (2001). Achievement goal research in sport: Pushing the boundaries and clarifying some misunderstandings. In G.C. Roberts (Ed.), *Advances in motivation in sport and exercise* (pp. 129–82). Champaign, IL: Human Kinetics.

Duda, J.L., Olson, L.K., and Templin, T.J. (1991). The relationship of task and ego orientation to sportsmanship attitudes and the perceived legitimacy of injurious acts. *Research Quarterly for Exercise and Sport, 62,* 79–87.

Duda, J.L., and Treasure, D. (2001). Toward optimal motivation in sport: Fostering athletes' competence and sense of control. In J.M. Williams (Ed.), *Applied sport psychology: Personal growth to peak performance* (4th ed.) (pp. 43–62). Mountain View, CA: Mayfield.

Duda, J.L., and White, S.A. (1992). Goal orientations and beliefs about the causes of sport success among elite skiers. *The Sport Psychologist, 6,* 334–43.

Ebbeck, V., and Becker, S.L. (1994). Psychosocial predictors of goal orientations in youth soccer. *Research Quarterly for Exercise and Sport, 65,* 355–62.

Elliot, A.J., and Dweck, C.S. (1988). Goals: An approach to motivation and achievement. *Journal of Personality and Social Psychology, 54,* 5–12.

Epstein, J. (1988). Effective schools or effective students? Dealing with diversity. In R. Haskins and B. MacRae (Eds.), *Policies for America's public schools* (pp. 89–126). Norwood, NJ: Ablex.

Epstein, J. (1989). Family structures and student motivation: A developmental perspective. In C. Ames and R. Ames (Eds.), *Research on motivation in education* (Vol. 3, pp. 259–95). New York: Academic Press.

Evans, J., and Roberts, G.C. (1987). Physical competence and the development of children's peer relations. *Quest, 39,* 23–35.

Fox, D., Goudas, M., Biddle, S., Duda, J., and Armstrong, N. (1994). Children's task and ego goal profiles in sport. *British Journal of Educational Psychology, 64,* 253–61.

Fry, M.D. (2001). The development of motivation in children. In G.C. Roberts (Ed.), *Advances in motivation in sport and exercise* (pp. 51–78). Champaign, IL: Human Kinetics.

Fry, M.D., and Duda, J.L. (1997). A developmental examination of children's understanding of effort and ability in the physical and academic domains. *Research Quarterly for Exercise and Sport, 68,* 331–44.

Goodway, J.D., and Rudisill, M.E. (1996). Influence of a motor skill intervention program on perceived competence of at-risk African American preschoolers. *Adapted Physical Activity Quarterly, 13,* 288–301.

Goodway, J.D., and Rudisill, M.E. (1997). Perceived physical competence and actual motor skill competence of African American preschool children. *Adapted Physical Activity Quarterly, 14,* 314–26.

Goodwin, D.L., and Watkinson, E.J. (2000). Inclusive physical education from the perspective of students with physical disabilities. *Adapted Physical Activity Quarterly, 17,* 144–60.

Harter, S. (1978). Effectance motivation reconsidered: Toward a developmental model. *Human Development, 21,* 34–64.

Harter, S. (1981). The development of competence motivation in the mastery of cognitive and physical skills: Is there a place for joy? In G.C. Roberts and D.M. Landers (Eds.), *Psychology of motor behavior and sport: 1980* (pp. 3–29). Champaign, IL: Human Kinetics.

Harter, S. (1985). *Manual for the self-perception profile for children: Revision of the Perceived Competence Scale for Children.* Denver, CO: University of Denver.

Harter, S. (1992). The relationship between perceived competence, affect, and motivational orientation within the classroom: Processes and patterns of change. In A.K. Boggiano and T.S. Pittman (Eds.), *Achievement and motivation* (pp. 77–114). Cambridge, UK: Cambridge University Press.

Harter, S. (1999). *The construction of the self: A developmental perspective.* New York: Guilford Press.

Horn, T.S., Glenn, S.D., and Wentzel, A.B. (1993). Sources of information underlying personal ability judgements in high school athletes. *Pediatric Exercise Science, 5,* 263–74.

Horn, T.S., and Hasbrook, C. (1986). Informational components influencing children's perceptions of their physical competence. In M.R. Weiss and D. Gould (Eds.), *Sport for children and youths* (pp. 81–88). Champaign, IL: Human Kinetics.

Horn T.S., and Weiss, M.R. (1991). A developmental analysis of children's self-ability judgements in the physical domain. *Pediatric Exercise Science, 3,* 310–26.

Kavussanu, M., and Roberts, G.C. (1996). Motivation in physical activity contexts: The relationship of perceived motivational climate to intrinsic motivation and self-efficacy. *Journal of Sport and Exercise Psychology, 18,* 264–80.

Klein, S., and Magill-Evans, J. (1998). Perceptions of competence and peer acceptance in young children with motor and learning difficulties. *Physical and Occupational Therapy in Pediatrics, 18*(3/4), 39–52.

Losse, A., Henderson, S.E., Elliman, D., Hall, D., Knight, E., and Jongmans, M. (1991). Clumsiness in children: Do they grow out of it?: A 10-year follow-up study. *Developmental Medicine and Child Neurology, 33,* 55–68.

Maehr, M.L., and Meyer, H.A. (1997). Understanding motivation and schooling: Where we've been, where we are, and where we need to go. *Educational Psychology Review, 9,* 371–409.

Maeland, A.F. (1992). Self esteem in children with and without motor coordination problems. *Scandinavian Journal of Educational Research, 36,* 313–21.

Martinek, T., and Karper, W. (1984). The effects of non-competitive and competitive instructional climates on teacher expectancy effects in elementary physical education classes. *Journal of Sport Psychology, 6,* 408–21.

Martinek, T., and Karper, W. (1986). Motor ability and instructional contexts: Effects on teacher expectation and dyadic interactions in elementary physical education classes. *Journal of Classroom Interaction, 21,* 16–25.

Miller, L.T., Polatajko, H.J., Missiuna, C., Mandich, A.D., and Macnab, J.J. (2001). A pilot trial of a cognitive treatment for children with developmental coordination disorder. *Human Movement Science, 20,* 183–210.

Nicholls, J.G. (1978). The development of the concepts of effort and ability, perception of academic attainment, and the understanding that difficult tasks require more ability. *Child Development, 49,* 800–14.

Nicholls, J.G. (1984). Conceptions of ability and achievement motivation. In R.E. Ames and C. Ames (Eds.), *Research on motivation in education: Vol. 1. Student motivation* (pp. 39–73). Orlando, FL: Academic Press.

Nicholls, J.G. (1989). *The competitive ethos and democratic education.* Cambridge, MA: Harvard University Press.

Nicholls, J.G., Cheung, P.C., Lauer, J., and Patashnick, M. (1989). Individual differences in academic motivation: Perceived ability, goals, beliefs, and values. *Learning and Individual Differences, 1,* 63–84.

Nicholls, J.G., Patashnick, M., and Nolen, S.B. (1985). Adolescents' theories of education. *Journal of Educational Psychology, 77,* 683–92.

Osterman, K.F. (2000). Students' need for belonging in the school community. *Review of Educational Research, 70,* 323–67.

Papaioannou, A. (1995). Differential perceptual and motivational patterns when different goals are adopted. *Journal of Sport and Exercise Psychology, 17,* 18–34.

Pensgaard, A.M., Roberts, G.C., and Ursin, H. (1999). Motivational factors and coping strategies of Norwegian Paralympic and Olympic winter sport athletes. *Adapted Physical Activity Quarterly, 16,* 238–50.

Piek, J.P., Dworkan, M., Barrett, N.C., and Coleman, R. (2000). Determinants of self-worth in children with and without developmental coordination disorder. *The International Journal of Disability Development and Education, 47,* 259–71.

Place, K., and Hodge, S.R. (2001). Social inclusion of students with physical disabilities in general physical education: A behavioral analysis. *Adapted Physical Activity Quarterly, 18,* 389–404.

Portman, P.A. (1995). Who is having fun in physical education classes? Experiences of sixth-grade students in elementary and middle schools. *Journal of Teaching in Physical Education, 14,* 445–53.

Reid, G., and Prupas, A. (1998). A documentary analysis of research priorities in disability sport. *Adapted Physical Activity Quarterly, 15,* 168–78.

Roberts, G.C. (1992). Motivation in sport and exercise: Conceptual constraints and convergence. In G.C. Roberts (Ed.), *Motivation in sport and exercise* (pp. 3–29). Champaign, IL: Human Kinetics.

Roberts, G.C. (2001). Understanding the dynamics of motivation in physical activity: The influence of achievement goals on motivational processes. In G.C. Roberts (Ed.), *Advances in motivation in sport and exercise* (pp. 1–50). Champaign, IL: Human Kinetics.

Roberts, G.C., Kleiber, D.A., and Duda, J.L. (1981). An analysis of motivation in children's sport: The role of perceived competence in participation. *Journal of Sport Psychology, 3,* 206–16.

Roberts, G.C., and Treasure, D.C. (1992). Children in sport. *Sport Science Review, 1,* 46–64.

Rose, B., Larkin, D., and Berger, B.G. (1994). Perceptions of social support in children of low, moderate, and high levels of coordination. *ACHPER Healthy Lifestyles Journal, 41*(4), 18–21.

Rose, B., Larkin, D., and Berger, B.G. (1997). Coordination and gender influences on the perceived competence of children. *Adapted Physical Activity Quarterly, 14,* 210–21.

Rudisill, M.E, Mahar, M.T, and Meaney, K.S. (1993). The relationship between children's perceived and actual motor competence. *Perceptual and Motor Skills, 76*, 895–906.

Ryan, R.M., and Deci, E.L. (2000a). Self-determination theory and the facilitation of intrinsic motivation, social development, and well-being. *American Psychologist, 55*, 68–78.

Ryan, R.M., and Deci, E.L. (2000b). Intrinsic and extrinsic motivations: Classic definitions and new directions. *Contemporary Educational Psychology, 25*, 54–67.

Ryan, R.M., and Grolnick, W.S. (1986). Origins and pawns in the classroom: Self-report and projective assessments of individual differences in children's perceptions. *Journal of Personality and Social Psychology, 50*, 550–58.

Sandahl Christiansen, A. (2000). Persisting motor control problems in 11- to 12-year-old boys previously diagnosed with deficits in attention, motor control and perception (DAMP). *Developmental Medicine and Child Neurology, 42*, 4–7.

Schoemaker, M., and Kalverboer, A. (1994). Social and affective problems of children who are clumsy: How early do they begin? *Adapted Physical Activity Quarterly, 11*, 130–40.

Seifriz, J.J., Duda, J.L., and Chi, L. (1992). The relationship of perceived motivational climate to intrinsic motivation and beliefs about success in basketball. *Journal of Sport and Exercise Psychology, 14*, 375–91.

Shapiro, D.R., and Dummer, G.M. (1998). Perceived and actual basketball competence of adolescent males with mild mental retardation. *Adapted Physical Activity Quarterly, 15*, 179–90.

Sherrill, C. (1998). *Adapted physical activity, recreation and sport: Crossdisciplinary and lifespan* (5th ed.). Boston: WCB/McGraw Hill.

Skinner, R.A., and Piek, J.P. (2001). Psychosocial implications of poor motor coordination in children and adolescents. *Human Movement Science, 20*, 73–94.

Skordilis, E.K., Koutsouki, D., Asonitou, K, Evans, E., Jensen, B., and Wall, K. (2001). Sport orientations and goal perspectives of wheelchair athletes. *Adapted Physical Activity Quarterly, 18*, 304–15.

Smyth, M.M, and Anderson, H.I. (2000). Coping with clumsiness in the school playground: Social and physical play in children with coordination impairments. *British Journal of Developmental Psychology, 18*, 389–413.

Solmon, M.A. (1996). Impact of motivational climate on students: Behaviors and perceptions of a physical education setting. *Journal of Educational Psychology, 88*, 731–38.

Theeboom, M., De Knop, P., and Weiss, M.R. (1995). Motivational climate, psychological responses, and motor skill development in children's sport: A field-based intervention study. *Journal of Sport and Exercise Psychology, 17*, 294–311.

Thompson, L.P., Bouffard, M., Watkinson, E.J., and Causgrove Dunn, J. (1994). Teaching children with movement difficulties: Highlighting the need for individualised instruction in regular physical education. *Physical Education Review, 17*, 152–59.

Treasure, D.C. (2001). Enhancing young people's motivation in youth sport: An achievement goal approach. In G.C. Roberts (Ed.), *Advances in motivation in sport and exercise* (pp. 79–100). Champaign, IL: Human Kinetics.

Treasure, D.C., and Roberts, G.C. (1994). Cognitive and affective concomitants of task and ego goal orientations during the middle school years. *Journal of Sport and Exercise Psychology, 16*, 15–28.

Treasure, D.C., and Roberts, G.C. (1995). Applications of achievement goal theory to physical education: Implications for enhancing motivation. *Quest, 47*, 475–89.

Ulrich, B.D. (1987). Perceptions of physical competence, motor competence, and participation in organized sport: Their interrelationships in young children. *Research Quarterly for Exercise and Sport, 58*, 57–67.

Vallerand, R., Deci, E.L., and Ryan, R.M. (1987). Intrinsic motivation in sport. In K. Pandolf (Ed.), *Exercise and sport science reviews* (Vol. 15, pp. 389–425). New York: Macmillan.

Vallerand, R.J., and Lossier, G.F. (1999). An integrative analysis of intrinsic and extrinsic motivation in sport. *Journal of Applied Sport Psychology, 11*, 142–69.

Vallerand, R.J, and Reid, G. (1990). Motivation and special populations: Theory, research, and implications regarding motor behaviour. In G. Reid (Ed.), *Problems in movement control* (pp. 159–97). New York: Elsevier Science Publishers.

van Rossum, J.H.A., and Vermeer, A. (1990). Perceived competence: A validation study in the field of motoric remedial teaching. *International Journal of Disability, Development and Education, 37*, 71–81.

Walling, M.D., and Duda, J.L. (1995). Goals and their associations with beliefs about success in and perceptions of the purposes of physical education. *Journal of Teaching in Physical Education, 14*, 140–56.

Weiss, M.R., Ebbeck, V., and Horn, T.S. (1997). Children's self-perceptions and sources of physical competence information: A cluster analysis. *Journal of Sport and Exercise Psychology, 19*, 52–70.

Weiss, M.R., and Horn, T.S. (1990). The relation between children's accuracy estimates of their physical competence and achievement-related characteristics. *Research Quarterly for Exercise and Sport, 61*, 250–58.

White, R.W. (1959). Motivation reconsidered: The concept of competence. *Psychological Review, 66*, 297–333.

White, S.A., and Duda, J.L. (1993). Dimensions of goals and beliefs among adolescent athletes with physical disabilities. *Adapted Physical Activity Quarterly, 10*, 125–36.

Yun, J., and Ulrich, D. (1997). Perceived and actual physical competence in children with mild mental retardation. *Adapted Physical Activity Quarterly, 14*, 285–97.

VI ■ THE ACTIVE LIVING DOMAIN

CHAPTER 20

Leisure Education

Promoting Quality of Life

Michael J. Mahon

Learning Objectives

- To understand the definition of person-centred leisure education and its relationship with other contemporary definitions of leisure education.
- To explore the relationship between leisure education, quality of life, and other concepts such as social role valorization, self-determination, and interdependence
- To determine the key components of a conceptual model for person-centred leisure education.
- To understand the relationship between leisure education and adapted physical education.

Introduction

The past half-century has seen the emergence of leisure as an important facet in North American society. In the 1960s, the United Nations Educational, Scientific, and Cultural Organization (UNESCO) adopted a Charter for Leisure. It emphasized each person's right to leisure, recognizing that leisure provides the freedom for individuals to experience quality of life beyond the stresses of work and other such activities. While the predictions made during the 1960s and 1970s of decreased work weeks and more time for leisure have never materialized, there has been ever-increasing attention paid to leisure and tourism by various sectors of society (Godbey 1999).

Why so much focus on leisure? A lot has to do with the contribution of leisure to our quality of life. Leisure has been conceptualized in a variety of ways, each of which has a strong connection to quality of life. Sometimes thought of as specific recreation activities, leisure is often considered synonymous with the activities people engage in for enjoyment and satisfaction. Alternatively, people associate leisure with discretionary time, during which we have the opportunity to choose non-subsistence activities. While both of these conceptualizations are quite common, many leisure scholars such as Kelly (1996) argue that both are too limiting. Kelly and others such as Mannell and Kleiber (1997) suggest that the term *leisure* describes an individual's perception that he or she is free to choose to participate in meaningful, enjoyable, and satisfying experiences. For the most part, there appears to be consensus that perceived freedom and intrinsic motivation are the critical regulators that serve to define an experience as being leisure, or not (Bullock and Mahon 2000).

What of people with a disability? While the UNESCO Charter for Leisure did assert that leisure is a right for all, there is strong agreement that people with disabilities have not had the same opportunities for leisure (Mahon and Bullock 1992a). While it is certainly the case that adults with disabilities have more non-work time because of higher levels of unemployment than the norm, this time is not often used for leisure. Bender, Brannon, and Verhoven (1984) described this time as "forced leisure," meaning that it is free time forced upon individuals because of the constraints related to employment and other forms of community participation. People with disabilities are often systematically excluded from community participation or social integration at all points of the lifespan. Often this exclusion is directly related to leisure pursuits and very directly affects the quality of life of people with disabilities (Mahon, Mactavish, and Bockstael 2000).

Recent findings in a 1998 National Organization on Disability/Harris Survey provide critical evidence of the need to consider quality of life within the field of disability (Harris and Associates 1998). The results of this survey indicated that only about one in three Americans with disabilities say that they are satisfied with their life, compared to six out of ten non-disabled Americans. This gap has widened in the last four years. In addition, fewer than half of people with disabilities living in the United States believe that their

quality of life will improve over the next four years. For these reasons, quality of life is a concept that has received increasing attention by people with disabilities, families, and service providers. According to Schalock (1996, p. vii), however, it is a concept that has been around for many years, but has gained prominence as we have come to recognize the disparities regarding the quality of life of people with and without a disability:

> What makes the concept of quality of life so important to our field is our attempt to use this concept as a process and an overriding principle to improve the lives of persons with mental retardation and closely related disabilities.

Leisure education is a process that has the capacity to empower individuals with disabilities to experience quality of life through leisure.

What Is Leisure Education?

The concept of leisure education has been around for many years. Mundy and Odum (1979) trace leisure education back to ancient Greek times during which men participated in education that included physical training, intellectual pursuits, and the arts. However, John Dewey (1917) should be credited with introducing the concept of leisure education. Dewey argued strongly that educational pursuits needed to be enhanced through the integration of such things as music, singing, storytelling, games, and exercise into the academic environment:

> Education has no more serious responsibility than making adequate provision for enjoyment of recreative leisure, not only for the sake of the immediate health, but still more if possible for the sake of its lasting effect upon habits of mind. (Dewey 1917, p. 1)

Krause (1964) was one of the first people to emphasize the need for community agencies to share in the responsibilities for leisure education. His work was the earliest comprehensive description of leisure education. At about the same time, Brightbill (1961) completed a landmark book on the philosophical underpinnings of leisure education.

Discussions about the value and place of leisure education became quite widespread by the mid-1970s. Chinn and Joswiak (1981) provided a cogent analysis of the concept of leisure education in a special issue of *Therapeutic Recreation Journal* dedicated to leisure education. They define leisure education in the following way:

> It is proposed that the term leisure education be applied to the use of comprehensive models focussing on the educational process which helps to develop the leisure lifestyles of an individual, as well as any single aspect of that approach. (p. 6)

Chinn and Joswiak interpret *leisure education* to mean both comprehensive models as well as any single aspect of a model. Most leisure education models include a number of components such as leisure awareness, decision-making, and skill development. The majority of these models imply or explicitly state an order and process for the implementation of these components. For example, Dattilo and Murphy's (1991) text on leisure education depicts a set of stairs, with different components of their model on each step. The stairs ultimately reach the top step, which represents a meaningful leisure experience. Implied in this figure is a particular order and process for the components of the model. In contrast, Chinn and Joswiak's definition suggests that, while one person may need all of the stairs in a certain order, another person may need only one or two steps. A painting class or a programme that teaches decision-making may each represent leisure education, separately or taken together. Leisure education can thus be comprehensive, focussing on a multitude of goals, or more narrowly focussed on one or two goals.

The definition of leisure education proposed by Chinn and Joswiak (1981) is very much in keeping with most of the definitions proposed during the sixties and seventies. Peterson and Gunn (1984) and Mundy and Odum (1979) both agreed that leisure education consists of broad-based comprehensive programmes that include a number of process components including leisure counselling. Mundy and Odum (1979, p. 377) state that leisure education is

> process rather than content. It is viewed as a total development process through which individuals develop an understanding of self, leisure, and the relationship of leisure to their own lifestyles and the fabric of society.

This and other definitions that have appeared in the literature from the mid-seventies up to the present time provide unique perspectives on leisure education. Most of the definitions, such as those cited above, situate leisure education within the context of the broad community. There have also been a number of conceptualizations of leisure education for people with disabilities proposed during the past decade (Dattilo and Murphy 1991; Peterson and Gunn 1984; Mundy 1998; Stumbo and Thompson 1986). Only recently has the concept of person-centred leisure education been proposed within the literature.

---

1 Discuss why leisure education may not have been embraced by adapted physical educators.

Person-centred Leisure Education

Quality of life is foundational to the person-centred approach. In many ways, our recognition of the importance of quality of life helps us to understand the essence of the person-centered approach. This is because quality of life is rooted in the person. According to Taylor and Bogdan (1996, p. 11), "quality of life is an elusive concept." There is really no agreed upon standard for measuring quality of life. Yet, there is strong agreement that the achievement of quality of life is a central goal for most human beings. There is also no accepted definition of quality of life. Schalock (1996) suggests that there are eight core dimensions of quality of life: emotional

Table 20.1 Principles of Quality of Life Central to the Person-centred Approach

Quality of life for persons with disabilities is...

- composed of those same factors and relationships that are important to all persons

- experienced when person's basic needs are met and when he or she has the same opportunities as anyone else to pursue and achieve goals in the major life settings of home, community, school, and work

- a multidimensional concept that can be consensually validated by a wide range of persons representing a variety of viewpoints of consumers and their families, advocates, professionals, and providers

- enhanced by empowering persons to participate in decisions that affect their lives

- enhanced by the acceptance and full integration of persons in their local communities

- an organizing concept that can be used for a number of purposes including evaluating those core dimensions associated with a life of quality, providing direction and reference in approaching customer services, and assessing persons' feelings of satisfaction and well-being

SOURCE: Adapted from "Reconsidering the Conceptualization and Measurement of Quality of Life," by R.L. Schalock, 1996, in *Quality of Life: Vol. I: Conceptualization and measurement*, pp.123–39, Washington: American Association on Mental Retardation. Adapted with permission.

well-being, interpersonal relations, material well-being, personal development, physical well-being, self-determination, social inclusion, and rights. Schalock (1996) also outlines some of the core principles of quality of life for people with disabilities. Those that are most germane to our discussion appear in table 20.1.

The core principles outlined in table 20.1 provide a useful frame of reference for the remainder of this chapter. We will discuss several other concepts that are imbedded within the dimensions of quality of life discussed by Schalock (1996). In addition to the over-arching framework of quality of life, the concepts of normalization, social role valorization, self-determination, and interdependence provide the conceptual cornerstones for person-centred leisure education.

With the above in mind, we proposed that person-centred leisure education is

an individualized and contextualized process through which a person develops an understanding of self and leisure and identifies and learns the cluster of skills necessary to participate in freely chosen activities which lead to an optimally satisfying life. (Bullock and Mahon 2000, p. 332)

Bullock and Mahon (2000) provide a full explanation for this definition. What follows is a summary of this explanation.

The Bullock and Mahon (2000) definition of person-centred leisure education describes the process as both individualized and con-textualized. Leisure education is designed to meet the needs of the individual. This point is crucial because it underscores the relationship between leisure education and leisure. Leisure is a personal construct which is inextricably linked to freedom of choice and personal or intrinsic motivation. In order for leisure education to facilitate the true leisure needs of a given individual, the process must encourage self-determination in leisure. Any leisure education process must, therefore, be closely connected and tailored to the needs of the individual, as opposed to their classification of disability and/or particular age within the lifecycle. Most of us would argue that we provide individualized services. Some of the situations that we find ourselves in, however, do not allow us to be as individualized as we would like to be. The leisure education process must be based on the person's needs and aspirations, as understood by that person.

Contextualization is often overlooked within services for people with disabilties, though this is a very important part of individualized service. The best way to explain contexualization is by way of an example. Consider a person who is in a psychiatric hospital. His or her sole reason for being there is so that he or she can get out and go home. A person-centred leisure education programme must be conceptualized with this in mind. The contextualized process is one that takes into consideration who those people are, where they have come from, where they're going to be returning, and their support systems.

Another key component of our definition of leisure education is that it is an educational process. The word *education* is defined in various ways. The *Concise Oxford Dictionary* (Allen 1990) defines it in the following manner:

1 the act or process of educating or being educated; systematic instruction.
2a particular kind or stage in education.
3a the development of character or mental powers. b a stage in or aspect of this.

This suggests that leisure education is ongoing or continuous. The use of the term *education* juxtaposed with leisure suggests that leisure education facilitates knowledge gain and personal development within the domain of leisure. It is a process that is systematic in nature and has a variety of different outcomes. In addition, according to our definition of education, leisure education can consist of one stage or any aspect of the educational process. This is in keeping with the definition of leisure education by Chinn and Joswiak (1981).

It is also important to understand that through leisure education a person develops an understanding of self and leisure. Leisure education helps a person to understand what leisure means to him or her in the context of his or her present life circumstances. Our understanding of the concept of leisure changes over the course of our lifespan. As such, leisure education must be a dynamic process, able to meet individuals where they are, but also able to change over time as individuals' perspectives grow and change.

Beyond awareness of leisure, the leisure education process can help a person to identify and learn a cluster of skills necessary to participate in activity. This may relate to the learning of a new skill related to a game or activity. In addition, there are other types of skills fundamental to leisure experiences. In the case of a person with a severe intellectual disability, this might include a skill such as money management or transportation skills such as riding a bus to and from the activity. Most often these types of skills are best learned in the context within which they will eventually need to be executed. This very often requires individualized instruction. In other words, the cluster of skills must be taught using an individualized and contextualized approach.

The final element should be self-evident. The leisure education process should contribute to life satisfaction. What is important when all is said and done is that the person experiences enhanced quality of life through leisure.

---

2 How might the concepts contained within the definition of person-centered leisure education be incorporated in adapted physical activity?

A Conceptual Model for Leisure Education

In the text, *Introduction to Recreation Services for People with Disabilities: A Person Centred Approach* (Bullock and Mahon 2000), we provide an overview of our conceptual model for leisure education (see figure 20.1). This model has been developed over a number of years while conducting research in the area of leisure education (e.g., Bullock and Howe 1991;

Bullock and Luken 1994; Mahon and Bullock 1992a; Mahon and Bullock 1992b; Mahon, Bullock, and Luken 1993; Mahon and Searle 1994; Searle, Mahon, Iso-Ahola, Sdrolias, and Dyck 1995, 1998; Searle and Mahon 1991). The model we have created incorporates what we believe to be the domains and corresponding components most germane to a conceptual model for leisure education.

Before presenting this model, it is important to discuss briefly the importance of providing both conceptual and practice models as a means of furthering leisure education as a process for people with a disability. A conceptual model is a simplified description of a system that assists us in understanding what are often abstract ideas. In the case of leisure education, a conceptual model helps us to understand the various concepts that come together to form our understanding of the process of leisure education. In contrast, a practice model typically presents a process for operationalizing a concept. In our case, a practice model for leisure education would present a process for operationalizing the concept of leisure education. We have published a number of practice models that we will not review in this chapter which you may wish to review on your own (Bullock and Howe 1991; Bullock, Morris, Mahon, and Jones 1992).

In keeping with our concern with hierarchical models of leisure education, this conceptual model is not intended to be directional in nature. The beginning, middle, and end of each process is determined by the individual in concert with the leisure education specialist. The two individuals function in an interdependent manner to achieve the goals identified by the individual. So, if an individual expresses a very specific goal that relates to only one domain of the model, the leisure education process would only include that one domain. Thus, at the top of figure 20.1 we indicate that the individual and his or her aspirations and needs provide unique input into the development of the individualized leisure education process. There are three domains within the leisure education conceptual model: awareness, skill learning and

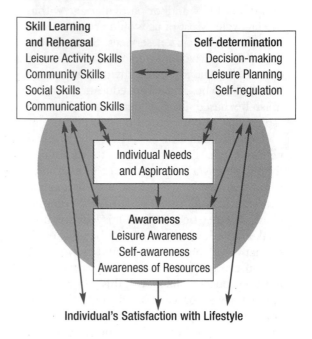

Figure 20.1 A Conceptual Model for Person-centred Leisure Education

Skill Learning and Rehearsal
Leisure Activity Skills
Community Skills
Social Skills
Communication Skills

Self-determination
Decision-making
Leisure Planning
Self-regulation

Individual Needs and Aspirations

Awareness
Leisure Awareness
Self-awareness
Awareness of Resources

Individual's Satisfaction with Lifestyle

rehearsal, and self-determination. Though each are presented as separate, there will always be overlap and connection between each. It is the individual and the leisure education specialist who determine which domains and corresponding components he or she will access during the individualized process. As with our definition of leisure education, the ultimate goal of the leisure education process is personal satisfaction with one's lifestyle. In the following section, each of the domains and corresponding components will be briefly discussed. Underlying the entire process are the interrelated concepts of normalization/social role valorization, self-determination, and interdependence. These surround the individual in our model, because they represent concepts that enable the process of leisure education to empower individuals with a disability to experience quality of life through leisure.

Conceptual Cornerstones of Leisure Education

NORMALIZATION

The principle of normalization was first defined by Nirje in a series of papers which he presented during the late 1960s and early 1970s while lecturing across Sweden, the United States, and Canada. This principle has become an internationally influential paradigm that has served as a cornerstone for service delivery (including recreation) for persons with a disability (Howe-Murphy and Charboneau 1987). Nirje (1992, p. 16) wrote the following contemporary version of his original definition:

> The normalization principle means that you act right when making available to persons with intellectual and other impairments or disabilities patterns of life and conditions of everyday living which are as close as possible to or indeed the same as the regular circumstances and ways of life of their communities.

The attractiveness of Nirje's definition is that it is written in very basic language. His definition clearly underscores that normalization is a value that should be adopted by all. In one of his very early works, Nirje (1969) described in great detail what he meant by patterns of life and conditions of everyday living.

SOCIAL ROLE VALORIZATION

While the principle of normalization was instrumental in changing the lives of people with disabilities in what was for the most part a positive direction, quite often the principle was misinterpreted. Normalization was miscontrued to be synonymous with the word *normal*. This lead many people to assume that *normalization* meant to strive to make people with disabilities 'normal'. As a result of the misrepresentation/interpretation of the normalization principle, Wolfensberger (1983) reconceptualized the principle into that of the theory of *social role valorization*. Briggs (1977) proposed a dynamic and multifaceted model of the self-concept in which one's perceptions

of self come from interactions with significant others, the conclusions drawn from those interactions, self-attributions, and previous life experiences. Wolfensberger applied this idea of self-concept to individuals with disabilities emphasizing

> that the most explicit and highest goal of normalization must be the creation, support, and defense of *valued social roles* [emphasis added] for people who are at risk of social devaluation. (Wolfensberger 1983, p. 234)

Social role valorization theory advocates for each individual's right and responsibility to assume a valued social role in society and for society's obligation to allow individuals to pursue that role without constraint.

Rancourt (1990) posed the dilemma and the challenge that social role valorization theory presents for recreation and physical activity. Neither the identification with disability nor leisure are generally socially valued roles. Yet, often persons with a disability have large amounts of time free from normative constraints such as work. Rancourt (1990) urged professionals to "demonstrate the worth of that which is presently culturally deemed as worth less" (p. 52). By this, Rancourt suggests that we must work to facilitate positive images of people with a disability experiencing leisure. Such images will serve to create positive social roles for people with a disability.

SELF-DETERMINATION

Self-determination and decision-making have been described as important considerations related to the facilitation of community-based recreation and leisure opportunities for persons with disabilities (Brown 1988; Dattilo and St. Peter 1991). This is based to some extent on the contemporary definition of leisure, which suggests that choice is a critical regulator for what we do or do not define as leisure (Iso-Ahola 1980; Neulinger 1981). In addition, Coleman and Iso-Ahola (1993) have recently suggested that leisure-generated self-determination dispositions may act as a buffer against stress and serve to decrease the likelihood of illness. According to these authors, people who perceive their actions as self-determined are less likely to experience illness and disease, and leisure very often provides important avenues for developing one's sense of self-determination.

In recent years, a number of definitions have been proposed for self-determination and for persons with a disability. Ward (1988) has suggested that self-determination consists of two critical components: (a) the attitude that leads people to define goals for themselves, and (b) the ability to take the initiative to achieve these goals. Fields and Hoffman (1991) have indicated that a critical underlying skill necessary for self-determination is decision-making. Wehmeyer (1992) suggested that self-determination not only consists of the capacity to choose and to carry out such choices, but also is linked to the individual's ability to self-regulate his or her behaviour.

The long-held assumption that individuals with disabilities are not capable of making their own decisions about what to do for recreation must be dispelled. This is an important implication for those responsible for designing and implementing recreation programmes and services. Numerous studies have demonstrated the capacity of a leisure education process for facilitating decision-making (Mahon and Bullock 1992b; Mahon 1994; Mahon and Martens 1996).

INTERDEPENDENCE

As we have suggested, self-determination is an important concept relative to facilitating the leisure needs of persons with disabilities. Condeluci (1991) notes, however, that a state of interdependence between persons with and without a disability is most conducive to facilitating social inclusion and quality of life. Interdependence focusses on relationships that lead to a mutual acceptance and respect between persons with and without disabilities. Interdependence is only achieved by those who are independent. Covey (1989, p. 186) describes interdependence in this way:

Interdependence is a choice only independent people can make. Dependent people cannot choose to become interdependent. They don't have the character to do it; they don't own enough of themselves…. As you become truly independent, you have the foundation for effective interdependence.

Thus, according to Covey, self-determination is a precursor to interdependence. If an individual is self-determined and independent, he or she is capable of being interdependent.

Why do we want people with a disability to be interdependent? Schoeller (1993/94) suggests that our brain, our spirit, our emotions, our psyche, and our sexuality all function better in social interaction than in isolation. Positive interaction, facilitated through an interdependent relationship, can in fact allow people to experience more choices and opportunities, leading to a determined spirit.

---

3 Defend or refute the following statement: interdependence is more important than self-determination in the lives of people with disabilities.

DOMAINS OF LEISURE EDUCATION

Within our leisure education conceptual model there are three domains: awareness, skill learning and rehearsal, and self-determination. As we previously indicated, the model does not imply a specific order, as the order of any process is determined by the needs of the individual. At the same time, our review of the literature found that most leisure education models begin with a focus on awareness, followed by some level of skill learning and rehearsal, and ending with an independent or supported initiation, with decision-making being filtered in throughout the process. Our own research suggests that it is a mistake to assume that one domain should necessarily proceed the other within leisure education. Some individuals may have many skills but little awareness of how to achieve a satisfying leisure lifestyle, while others may need a great deal of skill rehearsal. This is why it is essential that leisure education is a person-centred process. We discuss each of the three domains in detail in Bullock and Mahon (2000). We will highlight each briefly in the following sections.

Awareness

The opportunity for individuals to develop a deeper understanding of themselves and their personal lifestyles within the context of leisure is a key to any leisure education process. This process of enhancing one's personal awareness is extremely important for achieving a satisfying leisure lifestyle. The awareness domain within our conceptual model consists of the following three components: (1) leisure awareness, (2) self-awareness, and (3) awareness of resources.

Leisure awareness centres on helping an individual to understand the concept of leisure. Depending upon the individual, this may include helping the individual to understand the difference between work and leisure and when and where leisure can happen. For example, individuals with a cognitive impairment often have a difficult time distinguishing between work and leisure. A key aspect of the leisure awareness component is also exposing the individual to the various types of leisure pursuits. These types of pursuits are often grouped under the following five headings: social, relaxation, sports, crafts, and outdoors. One other important element of leisure awareness focusses on the benefits of leisure participation.

While it is possible to use picture cues and videos to support the process of leisure awareness we have found personal exposure to actual activities to be the most fruitful method. Borrowing from the field of supported employment, we have often described this process as 'leisure sampling'. By exposing individuals to activities in their natural setting, they are able to get a much better idea of whether or not the activity and its related setting are suited to their interests and their personal circumstances. The issue of personal circumstances relates to the next aspect of the awareness domain, which is self-awareness.

Table 20.2 Things I Can Ask Myself About Leisure

1. What are my past and present leisure pursuits?
2. Am I satisfied with what I am currently doing for leisure?
3. What benefits do I desire from leisure?
4. What new activities would I like to try?

Self-awareness helps the individual to personalize his/her understanding of leisure. A central goal of the self-awareness component is to help the individual become cognizant of preferred leisure experiences. To articulate leisure preferences requires that the individual consider a number of factors. These factors are presented in the form of questions in table 20.2.

In addition to the identification of leisure preferences, the self-awareness component is also designed to facilitate exploration of leisure attitudes, values, and motivations for participating in leisure. This requires a good deal of introspection on the part of the participant. Such introspection is easier for some than for others. The job of the leisure education specialist is to help the participant through this process by creating an environment that is best able to facilitate the reflection necessary for the identification of attitudes, values, and motivations. This may take the form of paper and pencil exercises, open-ended discussion with the specialist, or individual reflection.

The final component of this domain is awareness of resources. This component is intended to help focus the participant on the more pragmatic aspects of leisure participation. The resources that are addressed are both personal and community-based. Some of the issues that are dealt with in this component are:

1. home and community leisure activities
2. budgeting and money management
3. people and relationships
4. communication
5. transportation
6. leisure skills
7. personal routines

The purpose of this component is to help individuals identify the resources that will enable them to participate in their chosen leisure pursuit(s) and the barriers they face because of either a lack of personal resources within certain areas or a lack of community-based resources. Each individual is blessed with strengths within the area of resources, and most individuals who access a leisure education programme are also faced with resource-based barriers. This component enables the individual and leisure education specialist to clearly articulate both strengths and barriers as a precursor to developing strategies for the utilization of identified strengths and methods of either reducing the impact of or negating barriers. The remainder of the leisure education process is designed to enable the individual to work with these strengths and barriers in order to facilitate a satisfying lifestyle.

Skill Learning and Rehearsal

Skill learning and rehearsal is an equally important domain within our leisure education conceptual model. This domain consists of four components: leisure activity skills, community skills, social skills, and communication skills. Each of the areas within skill learning and rehearsal are important for facilitating the leisure goals of an individual. Whether some or all become a part of a programme depends upon the capacities and needs of the individual. In most cases, the areas of focus within this domain are closely associated with the barriers/areas of needs identified within the awareness section. For example, if an individual decides that he or she is interested in trying out rock climbing, it is likely that he or she will require some leisure activity skill instruction. Each of the four components of skill learning and rehearsal will be briefly discussed.

Leisure activity skills form the basis for leisure participation. Any leisure activity requires some level of skill. The complexity of the skills required depends upon the activity. Once an individual has chosen an activity or a few activities in which he or she wishes to participate, it then becomes important to determine whether she/he possesses the necessary skills for the activity. For example, if Bill, who has a visual impairment, decides that he wants to kayak, he must first identify whether he has the necessary skills. In order to help answer this question, activity analysis and/or task analysis procedures are often used. These two procedures are discussed in depth in Bullock and Mahon (2000). Those individuals who do not possess the skills to participate in a chosen activity must be taught. This is a very important part of the leisure education process. Just as important as the instruction, however, is the opportunity to practice. According to Bullock and Luken (1994, p. 224):

> The goal [of a leisure education programme] is skill development and mastery. Far too often, clients are offered minimal opportunities to develop and master a selected activity skill, and thus lack the self-confidence to continue their involvement without professional assistance. Activity skill mastery requires that sufficient time be devoted to skill development, rehearsal, and application in the "real environment".

It is crucial that a lack of skill not be seen as an insurmountable barrier to a person participating in a chosen leisure pursuit. Leisure education must be seen as a mechanism for teaching new leisure activity skills or upgrading previously learned skills.

Community skills are those skills that enable a person to participate in community-based programmes. Within the field of mental disabilities, these skills are often described as adaptive skills. One example of a community skill is transportation. In order to access many community-based leisure opportunities, individuals must have access to different types of transportation and knowledge of how to use them. The type of transportation individuals may use will depend on such things as their disability, whether they live in a rural or urban setting, their financial situation, where the programme is located, and what forms of transportation are readily available. For some individuals, learning how to get to a new programme may be quite straightforward—as easy as knowing where the programme is located so that they can choose the correct bus line or the correct route to drive themselves. Other individuals may need much more assistance in this area. Though transportation is not necessarily a leisure-based skill, it may mean the difference between a person attending or not attending a programme. Other related community skills include such things as money management and time management.

Social and communication skills are crucial for inclusion in community-based leisure programmes. Social skills are those skills that enable an individual to interact with another individual or to integrate into a social group or the larger community. A wealth of literature has identified that people with a disability and, in particular, persons with a developmental disability, often lack social skills necessary for social inclusion (Siperstain, Bak, and O'Keefe 1988; Taylor, Asher, and Williams 1987). According to Datillo and Murphy (1991, p. 31), "Absence of social skills is particularly noticeable during leisure participation and frequently leads to isolation and inability to function successfully." In addition, other research has determined that, in general, social isolation and, as a result, more limited social networks and limited friendships are also very common in persons with a disability (Abery, Thurlow, Johnson, and Bruininks 1990; Horner, Dunlop, and Koegel 1988; Bogdan and Taylor 1987). Given this, it is important for leisure education programmes to include a component focussed on enhancing social skills.

A social skills component can deal with a number of issues, including learning valued behaviours within different leisure settings. A particular challenge for some individuals with a disability is learning that some behaviours are valued within one leisure setting, while in others they are completely inappropriate. Another social skill area that is strongly associated with play and leisure is cooperation.

Some cooperative behaviours that are important for successful leisure participation are sharing toys and games appropriately, taking turns in structured activities, initiating an activity with a partner, and getting along with others during an activity. Bullock et. al. (1992) have a module in their leisure education programme called "Getting Along With Others." This module uses cooperative games as a means of teaching cooperation skills.

One other skill area that is crucial is communication. Communication is vital within games and activities that include more than one person. Communication, both verbal and non-verbal, is also strongly associated with the extent to which persons with a disability connect with other people within a programme and are able to develop relationships. A number of strategies for facilitating communication have been incorporated within leisure education programmes (Bullock et al. 1992; Dattilo and Murphy 1991).

Self-determination

The importance of self-determination has already been discussed on a conceptual level. Unfortunately, many individuals with a disability have little opportunity to be self-determining within the context of leisure. Because of this, a focus on self-determination in any leisure education model is crucial. Our self-determination domain is divided into decision-making, leisure planning, and self-regulation. This is consistent with the definitions of self-determination proposed by both Ward (1988) and Wehmeyer (1992).

The majority of recent literature concurs that one of the most significant ways in which society can empower individuals with a disability to become more self-determining is through enabling them to make decisions for themselves (Brown 1988, Mitchell 1988; Kennedy and Killius 1987; and Ward 1988). Most of the research on decision-making has been related to work and daily living skills, but few studies have focussed their inquiry in the leisure domain. Recently, Mahon and colleagues have developed a process for facilitating decision-making in leisure for persons with a mental disability (Bullock et al. 1992; Mahon 1994; Mahon and Bullock 1992a; Mahon and Bullock 1992b). The central focus of this process is on enhancing decision-making in leisure through the use of self-talk, a common cognitive-behavioural strategy.

The Decision-Making in Leisure model (DML) (Mahon 1990) is based on the theoretical single choice open model proposed by Wilson and Alexis (1962). The structure of the DML model is adapted from Mithaug and Martin's (1987) Adaptability Instructional Model. The leisure activity areas identified in the DML model are derived from Nash's (1953) original list. The DML model is composed of the following four steps:

A. Identify a desired leisure experience such as a spectator activity, social activity, physical activity, or creative/self actualizing activity.
B. Consider alternatives that satisfy the experience desired, (i.e., what specific activities within the chosen area will provide you with the leisure experience desired?).
C. Describe the consequences for each alternative:

1. The amount of enjoyment
2. Whether a partner is required
3. The cost (if any) and affordability of the options
4. Where it takes place and the available transportation
5. The equipment/attire which is required

D. Choose an alternative that satisfies the desired experience.

Participants are exposed to the DML model by way of a picture board portraying the model via symbols and words (See figure 20.2). The picture board is used as a visual aid in the teaching process. The four steps outlined on the picture board are:

Goal–Identify a desired leisure experience
Options–Consider alternatives
If, then–Consequences
Decide–Choose an alternative

Figure 20.2 Picture Board for DML Model (Decision-making in Leisure)

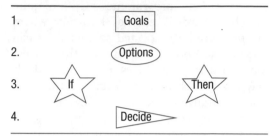

SOURCE: From *The Use of Self-control Techniques to Facilitate Self-Determination Skills During Leisure in Adolescents with Mild and Moderate Mental Retardation,* by M.J. Mahon, 1992. Unpublished Ph.D. dissertation, University of North Carolina at Chapel Hill, Chapel Hill, NC.

These words are displayed in four different colours of felt on a black felt board, approximately 2' by 3'. The teacher/facilitator teaches the participants to utilize these words as a means of 'talking themselves through' a leisure decision.

The self-determination training programme developed by our research team also has a leisure planning and initiation component based on the use of self-control techniques. As was noted earlier, Ward (1988) defines self-determination as the ability to define and carry out one's goals. Within the context of a leisure education programme, this can be translated into the capacity not only to define one's own leisure goals (i.e., make a decision about what to do for leisure), but also to carry out the goal. Once participants have learned to make leisure decisions using the DML model, they are then taught to make a leisure action plan using a leisure action plan card (see figure 20.3). The portfolio and plan is likened to a date book used to remember appointments. Five boxes, 2" by 2", are arranged on the card, each with one of five words representing the components of the plan: what, with whom, where, stuff, when. Once participants have made a leisure action plan, they are then taught to self-monitor using the card as means of helping them to carry out their plan.

Self-regulation (or as it is often referred to, self-control) strategy instruction has been

Figure 20.3 Leisure Action Plan Card

What
With Whom
Where
When
Stuff

Name   Date

proposed as a useful community-based process for facilitating person-centred outcomes for individuals with a disability (Agran and Moore 1987; Martin, Burger, Elias-Burger, and Mithaug 1988). *Self-regulation* has been defined by Martin et al., (1988, p. 157) as "the process of managing one's own behaviour through self-regulation of antecedent or consequent stimuli."

Self-regulation strategies are closely tied philosophically with those of self-determination. Ward (1988, p. 2) suggests that a common element in definitions of self-determination is "the importance of people taking control, without any external influence, over what affects their lives." Wehmeyer and Berkobien (1991) concur, indicating that self-regulation is one of the three critical processes that make up self-determining behaviour. Thus, based upon Ward and Wehmeyer and Berkobien's interpretations, self-control techniques and self-determination are closely aligned. Given this, it makes sense that self-control techniques be used to facilitate some of the central goals of self-determination and leisure: decision making and independent leisure participation. We have already illustrated how self-instruction and self-monitoring can be used within a leisure education programme to support increased decision-making, planning, and initiation. Other cognitive-behavioural strategies that may be useful are self-reinforcement and the use of visual cues.

4 How might the differential ordering of the three domains of the leisure education model influence the nature of the leisure education process and possible outcomes?

THE FUTURE OF LEISURE EDUCATION

During the past decade, a significant body of literature has emerged related to the efficacy of leisure education. Our work is a microcosm of this body of research (Bedini, Driscoll, and Bullock 1991; Bullock and Howe 1991; Mahon and Bullock; 1992b, 1993; Mahon 1994; Mahon and Martens 1996; Mahon and Searle 1994; Searle and Mahon 1991, 1995; Searle et al. 1995). Research has validated leisure education as a process that enhances quality of life in people with disabilities and among older adults by improving life and leisure satisfaction, perceived control and competence, and leisure participation.

Research has also demonstrated that leisure education is a process that can be carried out in traditional and non-traditional settings. For example, Mahon and Bullock (1992b) demonstrated that leisure education could be incorporated into school special education curriculums. They used both small group and one-on-one instruction to introduce leisure education to students with disabilities. Using single subject research design, Mahon and Bullock demonstrated the efficacy of leisure education for enhancing decision-making and leisure initiation. Mahon and Martens (1996) used a similar intervention within a supported employment environment and found similar results. Searle and Mahon et al. 1995) illustrated the utility of delivering leisure education in day hospital programmes for older adults. Later, they also successfully introduced leisure education as a home-based service for older adults (Searle and Mahon, 1991; Searle et al. 1995).

What is evident from this snapshot of current research on leisure education is that, as a process, it has the capacity to improve quality of life for people with a disability, as well as other individuals who tend to experience constraints to leisure (i.e., older adults, youth at risk). It is also clear that leisure education can be incorporated into various environments. One context that is extremely well suited to the incorporation of leisure education is adapted physical activity. Earlier in this text, other authors recognized adapted physical activity to be a process focussed on individual needs and personal growth and development. Our conceptual model for leisure education highlights these same goals.

Leisure education can and should serve as a foundation for the provision of adapted physical education programming. In essence, it can provide an ecological context for the instructor and student. By determining an individual's preferences for leisure, and becoming aware of his or her individual context (e.g., where he or she lives, the resources he or she can access), adapted physical activity instruction can become more ecologically valid. It can provide programming and instruction that is contextualized to the various lives of children and adults with disabilities.

In order to achieve the goal of ecological validity or contextualization, adapted physical activity specialists and regular physical activity specialists must work closely with families, advocates, community recreation specialists, and other related professionals. Coordination with these other groups of individuals will enable programming to achieve the necessary contextualization. For example, in the School-Community Leisure Link Programme (Bullock, Morris, Mahon, and Jones 1992) the leisure education and adapted physical activity specialists within a school district worked with community recreation agencies to help develop more inclusive recreation opportunities within the community. This ensured that the leisure education and adapted physical activity taking place in the school had some connection to the community, and it enabled students to make the transition from school-based physical activity to community-based participation. More specifically, it resulted in the generalization of skills and participation to a number of different settings. This is the ultimate goal of all programming for children and adults with disabilities. The following case example provides a sample of how leisure education can be incorporated into a physical education context.

A Case Example

Samantha is twelve years old. She has an intellectual disability but has attended her neighbourhood school since kindergarten. During her elementary school years she had little difficulty making friends and had a very busy social life. Her mother was quite instrumental in ensuring that Samantha kept in contact with her school friends; she would often invite kids over after school and on weekends. The transition to junior high school has been quite difficult for Samantha. None of her friends from elementary school are in her class, and most of them have become active on school teams. Samantha was not able to make any of the teams. She is getting bored and has begun to become much more sedentary. Thankfully, Samantha has a very perceptive physical education teacher. He and Samantha's mother have decided that action needs to be taken. As a result of some prodding from them, Samantha has decided that she needs to consider some new leisure options. Samantha's mother and the physical education teacher worked with Samantha over the course of a few months to help her identify some new leisure choices. This initially involved trying new things in her physical education classes. Samantha and her mom then investigated which of these activities she could participate in with other kids her age at the local community centre. Samantha has yet to really connect with any new friends, but she and her mom feel that she is moving in the right direction.

Summary

In this chapter we have discussed the role of person-centred leisure education in promoting quality of life for people with disabilities. To be successful, the process of person-centred leisure education must be framed by concepts such as self-determination and interdependence that place the individual with a disability at the centre of the process. Leisure education should be an integral part of adapted physical activity. By connecting leisure education and adapted physical activity, we can ensure that programmes for people with disabilities are contextualized; that they are ecologically valid. This will help to ensure that the overall goal of facilitating quality of life for people with disabilities can be achieved. Future research and practice should explore how the integration of leisure education and more traditional adapted physical activity programming may lead to the enhancement of quality of life for people with a disability.

Study Questions

1. How would a definition of *leisure education* differ from a definition of *person-centred leisure education*?

2. Why is the Chinn and Joswiak definition of *leisure education* so germane to the concept of person-centred leisure education?

3. What is a definition of *quality of life* and how does quality of life relate to person-centred leisure education?

4. Why is self-determination such an important conceptual cornerstone of leisure education?

5. Describe the three key domains of leisure education discussed in this chapter. Which one is most central to the leisure education process?

References

Abery, B.H., Thurlow, M.T., Johnson, D.R., and Bruininks, R.H. (1990, May). *The social networks of adults with developmental disabilities residing in community settings.* Paper presented at the annual meeting of the American Association on Mental Retardation, Washington, DC.

Agran, M., and Moore, S. (1987). Transitional programming: Suggesting an adaptability model. *Advances in Mental Retardation and Developmental Disabilities, 3,* 179–208.

Allen, L.R. (1990). Benefits of leisure attributes to community satisfaction. *Journal of Leisure Research, 22*(2): 183–96.

Bedini, L., Driscoll, L., and Bullock, C.C. (1991). From schools to community: Achieving independence and community integration through leisure education. *Palaestra, 8*(1), 38–43.

Bender, M., Brannon, S.A., and Verhoven, P.J. (Eds.). (1984). *Leisure education for the handicapped: Curriculum goals, activities, and resources.* San Diego, CA: College Hill Press.

Bogdan, R., and Taylor, S. (1987). Toward a sociology of acceptance: The other side of the study of deviance. *Social Policy, 18*(2), 34–39.

Briggs, W. (1977). From isolation to integration in the classroom. *Integrated Education, 16*(5), 20–25.

Brightbill, C.K. (1961). *Man and leisure: a philosophy of recreation.* Englewood Cliffs, NJ: Prentice-Hall.

Brown, P.J. (1988). *Effects of self-advocacy training in leisure on adults with severe physical disabilities.* Unpublished doctoral dissertation, Virginia Polytechnic Institute and State University.

Bullock, C., and Howe, C.Z. (1991). A model therapeutic recreation programme for the reintegration of persons with disabilities into the community. *Theraputic Recreation Journal, 25*(1), 7–17.

Bullock, C., and Luken K. (1994). Reintegration through recreation: A community-based rehabilitation model. In S.E. Iso-Ahola and D.M. Compton (Eds.), *Leisure and Mental Health.* Park City, UT: Family Development Resources.

Bullock, C.C., and Mahon, M.J. (2000). *Introduction to recreation services for people with disabilities: A person centered approach* (2nd ed.) Champaign, IL: Sagamore.

Bullock, C., Morris, L., Mahon, M., and Jones, B. (1992). *School-community leisure link: Leisure education program curriculum guide.* Chapel Hill, NC: The Center for recreation and Disability Studies, Curriculum in Leisure Studies and Recreation Administration at the University of North Carolina at Chapel Hill.

Chinn, K.A., and Joswiak, K.F. (1981). Leisure education and leisure counseling. *Therapeutic Recreation Journal, 15*(4), 4–7.

Coleman, D., and Iso-Ahola, S.E. (1993). Leisure and health: The role of social support and self-determination. *Journal of Leisure Research, 25*(2).

Condeluci, A. (1991). *Interdependence: The route to community.* Orlando, FL: Paul M. Deutsch.

Covey, S. (1989). *The 7 habits of highly effective people.* New York: Simon and Schuster.

Dewey, J. (1917). The need for social psychology. *Psychological Review, 24*(4), 266–77.

Dattilo, J., and Murphy, W. (1991). *Leisure education program planning: A systematic approach.* State College, PA: Venture.

Dattilo, J., and St. Peter, S. (1991). A model for including leisure education in transition services for young adults with mental retardation. *Education and Training in Mental Retardation 26*(4): 420–32.

Fields, S., and Hoffman, A. (1991). *Skills for self-determination.* Paper presented at The Project Directors' Sixth Annual Meeting, Transition Institute at Illinois, Washington, DC.

Godbey, G. (1999). *Leisure in your life* (5th ed.). State College, PA: Venture.

Harris, L., and Associates. (1998). *N.O.D./Harris Survey of Americans with Disabilities*. New York: Author.

Horner, R.H., Dunlop, G., and Koegel, R.L. (Eds.) (1988). *Generalization and maintenance: Lifestyle changes in applied settings*. Baltimore: Paul H. Brookes.

Howe-Murphy, R., and Charboneau, B.G. (1987). *Therapeutic recreation intervention: An ecological perspective*. Englewood Cliffs, NJ: Prentice Hall.

Iso-Ahola, S.E. (1980). *Social psychological perspectives on leisure and recreation*. Springfield. IL: C.C. Thomas.

Kelly, J.R. (1996). *Leisure* (3rd ed.) Boston: Allyn and Bacon.

Kennedy, M., and Killius, P. (1987). Living in the community: Speaking for yourself. In S.J. Taylor, D. Biklen, J. Knoll (Eds.), *Community integration for people with severe disabilities*. New York: Teachers College Press.

Krause, M.S. (1964) Twelve propositions in the semantics of motivation. *Journal of General Psychology, 70*(2), 331–39.

Mahon, M.J. (1992). *The use of self-control techniques to facilitate self-determination skills during leisure in adolescents with mild and moderate mental retardation*. Unpublished Ph.D. dissertation, University of North Carolina at Chapel Hill, Chapel Hill, NC.

Mahon, M.J. (1990). *Facilitation of independent decision-making in leisure with adolescents who are mentally retarded*. Unpublished manuscript, University of North Carolina at Chapel Hill, Division of Special Education, Chapel Hill, NC.

Mahon, M.J. (1994). The use of self-control techniques to facilitate self-determination skills during leisure in adolescents with mild and moderate mental retardation. *Therapeutic Recreation Journal, 28*(2), 58–72.

Mahon, M.J., and Bullock, C.C. (1992a). Decision-making and leisure: Empowerment for people who are mentally retarded. *Journal of Physical Education and Recreation, 63*(8), 36–40.

Mahon, M.J., and Bullock, C.C. (1992b). Teaching adolescents with mental retardation to make decisions in leisure through the use of self-control techniques. *Therapeutic Recreation Journal, 26*(1), 9–26.

Mahon M.J., and Bullock C.C. (1993/94). An investigation of the social validity of a leisure education intervention. *Annual in Therapeutic Recreation, 4*, 82–95.

Mahon, M.J., Bullock, C.C., and Luken, K. (1993). Social validation of a leisure education intervention used with people with severe and persistent mental illness. In C. Cutler Riddick and A. Watson (Eds.) *Abstracts from the 1993 Symposium on Leisure Research*, Arlington, VA: National Recreation and Parks.

Mahon, M.J., Mactavish, J., and Bockstael, E. (2000). Social integration, leisure, and individuals with intellectual disability. *Parks and Recreation, 35*, 25–40.

Mahon, M.J. and Martens, C. (1996). Planning for the future: The impact of leisure education on adults with developmental disabilities in supported employment settings. *Journal of Physical Education Recreation and Dance, 65*(4), 36–41.

Mahon, M.J. and Searle, M.S. (1994). Leisure education: Its effects on older adults. *Journal of Applied Recreation Research, 21*(4), 283–312.

Mannell, R.C. and Kleiber, D.A. (1997). *A social psychology of leisure*. State College, PA: Venture.

Martin, J.E., Burger D.L., Elias-Burger, S. and Mithang, D.E. (1988). Application of self-control strategies to facilitate independence in vocational and instructional settings. *International Review of Research in Mental Retardation, 15*, 155–93.

Mitchell, B. (1988). Who chooses? *National Information Centre for Children and Youth with Handicaps, 5*, 4–5.

Mithaug, D.E., and Martin, J.E. (1987). Adaptability instruction: The goal of transitional programming. *Exceptional Children, 53*(6), 500–505.

Mundy, J. (1998). *Leisure education: Theory and practice* (2nd ed.). Champaign, IL: Sagamore.

Mundy, J., and Odum, L. (1979). *Leisure education: Theory and practice*. New York: Wiley.

Nash, J. (1953). *Philosophy of recreation and leisure*. Dubuque, IA: Brown.

Neulinger, J. (1981). *The psychology of leisure* (2nd ed.). Springfield, IL: Charles C. Thomas.

Nirje, B. (1969). A Scandinavian visitor looks at U.S. institutions. In R. Kugel and W. Wolfensberger (Eds.), *Changing patterns of residential services for the mentally retarded* (pp. 51–57). Washington, DC: President's Committee on Mental Retardation.

Nirje, B. (1985). The basis and logic of the normalization principle. *Australia and New Zealand Journal of Developmental Disabilities, 11*(2), 65–68.

Nirje, B. (1992). *The normalization principle papers*. Uppsala: Centre for Handicap Research, Uppsala University.

Peterson, C.A., and Gunn, S.L. (1984). *Therapeutic recreation program design: Principles and procedures*. Englewood Cliffs, NJ: Prentice Hall.

Peterson, C.A. and Gunn, S.L. (1984). *Therapeutic recreation program design: Recreation in treatment centers*. Englewood Cliffs, NJ: Prentice-Hall.

Rancourt, A.M. (1990). Older adults with developmental disabilities/mental retardation: A research agenda for an emerging sub-population. In M.E. Crawford and J.A. Card (Eds.), *Annual in Therapeutic Recreation: Volume 1* (pp. 48–55). Reston, VA: American Alliance for Health, Physical Education, Recreation, and Dance.

Schalock, R.L. (1996). Reconsidering the conceptualization and measurement of quality of life. In R L. Schalock (Ed.), *Quality of life: Vol. 1: Conceptualization and measurement* (pp.123–39). Washington, DC: American Association on Mental Retardation.

Schoeller, K. (1993/94). Standing together: One family's lessons in self-determination. *Impact, 6*(4).

Searle, M.S., and Mahon, M.J. (1991). *Longitudinal effects of leisure education on selected social-psychological variables.* Paper presented at the 1991 National Recreation and Park Association Leisure Research Symposium, Winnipeg, MB.

Searle, M.S, Mahon, M.J., Iso-Ahola, S., Sdrolias, H., and Dyck, J. (1995). Enhancing a sense of independence and psychological well-being among the elderly: A field experiment. *Journal of Leisure Research 27*(2): 107–24.

Siperstain, G.N., Bak, J.J., and O'Keefe, P. (1988). Relationship between children's attitudes toward their social acceptance of mentally retarded peers. *American Journal on Mental Retardation, 93*(1), 24–27.

Stumbo, N., and Thompson, S.R. (1986). *Leisure education: A manual of activities and resources.* State College, PA: Venture.

Taylor, A.R., Asher, S.R., and Williams, G.A. (1987). The social adaptation of mainstreamed mildly retarded children. *Child Development, 58,* 1321–34.

Taylor, S.J. and Bogdan, R. (1996). Quality of life and the individual's perspective. In R.L. Schalock (Ed.), *Quality of Life Volume I: Conceptualization and measurement* (pp.123–39). Washington, DC: American Association on Mental Retardation.

Ward, M. (1988). The many facets of self-determination. *National Information Centre for Children and Youth with Disabilities. Transition Summary, 5,* 2–3.

Wehmeyer, M.L. (1992). Self-determination and the education of students with mental retardation. *Education and Training in Mental Retardation, 4,* 302–14.

Wehmeyer, M.L., and Berkobien, R. (1991). Self-determination and self-advocacy: A case of mistaken identity. *TASH Newsletter, 17*(7), 4.

Wilson, C.Z., and Alexis, M. (1962). Basic frameworks for decisions. *JAM.* 150–64.

Wolfensberger, W. (1983). Social role valorization: A proposed new term for the principle of normalization. *Mental Retardation, 21*(6), 234–39.

CHAPTER 21

Creating Inclusive Physical Activity Opportunities

An Abilities-based Approach

Patricia E. Longmuir

Learning Objectives

- To understand that all individuals, including those with a disability, have the right to an active living lifestyle.
- To differentiate between inclusive/exclusive and integrated/segregated physical activity opportunities.
- To recognize the impact of attitudes and assumptions on the ability of all individuals to enjoy an active living lifestyle.
- To recognize that providing physical activity opportunities to individuals with a disability is the responsibility of all physical activity professionals, not only those specializing in adapted physical activity.
- To understand and apply the abilities-based approach to enhancing active living for people of all abilities.
- To evaluate activity demands and individual abilities in terms of mobility, object manipulation, cognition, communication and perception, behaviour and social skills, and fitness.

Introduction

A physically active lifestyle is important for all individuals, including those with a disability. However, the availability of appropriate physical activity opportunities often varies, depending on the individual's abilities and interests. Too frequently, the delivery of physical activity opportunities for individuals with a disability is restricted to those with specialist training in fields such as adapted physical activity, therapeutic recreation, or physical therapy. The purpose of this chapter is to focus on the creation of physical activity opportunities that include individuals of all abilities. The philosophy that all physical activity professionals are responsible for the provision of inclusive opportunities is discussed, along with factors such as attitudes and assumptions which may influence successful delivery.

One approach, the abilities-based approach to inclusive physical activity, is discussed in detail as a practical option for the delivery of inclusive physical activity opportunities. It is an approach based on a task-analysis format that may be used by all physical activity professionals. The abilities-based approach identifies the demands of an activity and the abilities of the individual within six categories: mobility, object manipulation, cognition, behaviour and social skills, communication and perception, and fitness. Physical activity professionals can encourage successful participation by developing opportunities that maximize the overlap between the activity demands and the participants' abilities. Several case studies are used to illustrate the use of the abilities-based approach to inclusive physical activity.

Successful Participation in Active Living

All individuals have the right to enjoy an active living lifestyle. Personal interests and preferences should be the basis for activity selection.

This seems such a simple, straightforward statement. How could anyone possibly disagree? The key phrase is **"all individuals."** It means that everyone, regardless of gender, age, cultural background, socioeconomic status, ability, or any other descriptor, has the same rights: the right to choose whether they want to participate in active living opportunities and, if they choose to participate, the right to choose the type of opportunity most suited to their own interests, abilities, resources, and experiences. Given the tremendous psychological, physical, emotional, and spiritual benefits, **all individuals** must have access to a physically active lifestyle.

Recent federal initiatives to increase the proportion of Canadians who enjoy a physically active lifestyle are based on the knowledge that two-thirds of Canadians face increased health risks because of inactive lifestyles and the over 15 percent of Canadians that have a disability are less active than those without a disability (Active Living Alliance for Canadians with a Disability 1999). Active living focusses on enabling people to adopt a way of life that values physical activity so that it becomes part of daily life. The active living approach is particularly appropriate for people

with a disability who have often felt excluded from traditional sport and fitness programmes (Active Living Alliance for Canadians with a Disability 1998).

Adapted physical activity (APA) usually focusses on participants whose skills, experience, or expertise is expected to be substantially below that of participants in 'regular' programmes. Although all professionals use activity adaptations for all participants, APA is most commonly associated with services for people with a disability. Given the range of abilities and interests among all people, with and without a disability, all professionals must be able to adapt or modify the activities that they teach.

INCLUSION OR INTEGRATION

The terms *inclusion* and *integration* are often used interchangeably. However, an examination of the dictionary definitions of these terms suggests that they represent two different concepts. *Include* is to "contain as part of a whole" or "be made up of, comprised or contained." Integrate is to "incorporate, amalgamate, or mix with an existing community" or "absorb into an existing whole" (*Collins English Dictionary* 1990; *The New Lexicon Webster's Dictionary* 1988). When something is included, it is one component of the whole. Integration takes a separate part and adds it to an existing whole. The difference is significant. Integration assumes there is an existing, complete 'whole' to which a new piece is added. Inclusion sees each part as an integral component of the whole. The whole would not exist without **all** of the parts.

In terms of active living and people with a disability, programmes that 'integrate' take existing programmes for people without a disability and 'add' a new piece, the participation of people with a disability. Inclusive programmes are designed so that the participation of people with a disability is one component of the whole programme (see figure 21.1). Thus, inclusion reflects a belief that all potential participants, regardless of ability, are an essential and valuable component to be included in the active living opportunity.

Figure 21.1 Inclusion Considers Each Part to Be One Component of the Whole, Not an Additional Piece

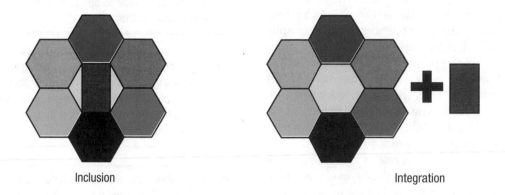

Inclusion   Integration

Figure 21.2 Inclusive or Exclusive Active Living Opportunities Can be Either Integrated or Segregated

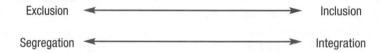

Exclusion ⟷ Inclusion

Segregation ⟷ Integration

Active living can be both integrated and inclusive

One continuum ranges from exclusion (limited or no participation by some interested individuals) to inclusion (designing for all individuals who may wish to participate). A second continuum moves from segregation (limited participation based on individual characteristics) to integration (modifying to permit participation by a variety of participants). Each active living opportunity will fall somewhere on each continuum (see figure 21.2). Inclusive active living opportunities can be provided in both integrated and segregated settings, depending on factors such as the programme goals or available resources. The following examples may help to demonstrate how physical activity opportunities fall on both the inclusion-exclusion and integration-segregation continua:

- A children's learn-to-swim programme. It may be inclusive if it is designed for a variety of children (e.g., males and females, with and without a disability). However, the same programme would also be considered segregated since it provides services only to those needing instruction in basic skills.

- A programme designed to introduce a variety of aquatic activities. This type of programme would also be inclusive if it was designed to serve a variety of children (e.g., males and females, with and without a disability). However, it might use a more integrated model by having participants wear a lifejacket or teaching the activities in shallow water to enable non-swimmers and swimmers to participate together.

Segregated programmes may, at times, be more inclusive because they are designed to serve all members of a particular group. In most cases, membership in the 'group' is based on the demands of the activity rather than characteristics of the individual. Consider a wheelchair basketball league. People with and without a disability are included without modifications to the existing programme, based on their interest and wheelchair mobility skills. Abilities such as manoeuvering a wheelchair, handling the ball, and collaborating with teammates determine membership in the 'group'. Whether the individual does or does not have a disability, and the type of disability that may exist, is not the factor that determines ability to participate. For example, one individual with a behavioural impairment may be able to participate while another may not. Having a behavioural impairment is not a limitation that prevents participation. Rather, it is the impact of the impairment on the individual's ability to meet the demands of the activity that is most important.

The need to 'integrate' a new group only exists if a group was originally 'excluded' from a particular programme. For example, a fitness centre offers aerobics classes. When a person who uses a wheelchair wanted to join, the classes were modified to offer a seated option. The classes were originally exclusive because they were designed in a way that did not allow participation by people who were unable to stand. If the classes had originally been designed to include people of all abilities, seated participants would have been able to join in without the need for programme modifications.

The abilities-based approach defines inclusive active living opportunities as those that are designed on the basis of the abilities required in order to participate successfully. Adaptations that may be required are part of the programme design, so that additional changes are not required for any one individual. Physical activity professionals are challenged to design all of their programmes to include people with and without a disability. It is only through the provision of inclusive programmes that people with a disability will have the same opportunities enjoyed by people without a disability. People without a disability fully expect to use any facility or join any available programme when they choose to do so. People with a disability should expect and receive the same level of service. Consider, for example, how your interest in and motivation for active living might change if the tennis club you decided to join told you that it would be four to six weeks before they could arrange for an instructor who could teach you, or could provide you with access to the courts.

1 Are these definitions of *inclusion* and *integration* similar to others you have heard? If not, how do they differ?

2 Have you ever been denied access, even temporarily, to a physical activity programme or service? If so, what was the reason and how did it affect your interest in or level of physical activity?

3 Think about the physical activity programmes you have been involved in. Can you identify situations in which people with different abilities were, or would have been, denied access to the programme?

AWARENESS OF ASSUMPTIONS, BELIEFS, AND ATTITUDES

Assumptions underlie everything that we think, say, and do. Everyone approaches the delivery of services to people with a disability from a different perspective. Our personal 'ideology' will determine, in large part, the range of opportunities that we naturally consider and the way in which we evaluate the options presented. Physical activity professionals must clearly understand the assumptions, beliefs, and attitudes that they, and others, bring to each active living opportunity before they can critically analyze or evaluate the merits of a particular activity or approach. Each approach to APA, each assessment of an individual's abilities or interests, or the design of each active living opportunity, will be shaped by the assumptions of both professionals and participants.

Historically, it was believed that physical activity was inappropriate for many individuals with a disability. People with a disability were often housed in institutions where physical activity was held to a minimum (Shephard 1990). Time spent on recreation was time 'wasted' or 'stolen' from more important activities, such as education, life skills, or job training. This perception of recreation as a waste of limited energy stores (Shephard 1990) continues even today in the way that our health care systems and community services often do not support active living lifestyles unless there is a scientifically proven, medical benefit. For example, exercise programmes are common for individuals with heart disease. Such programmes focus on enhancing physical capacity for activities of daily living and employment demands. It is much less common for programmes designed to prevent cardiac disease through an active living lifestyle to be supported. Indeed, support for the concept of 'active living', rather than traditional concepts of 'fitness', was only realized after there was scientific evidence to support the benefits of moderate, daily physical activity (Quinney, Gauvin, and Wall 1994).

Ability is defined as "skill or power in sufficient quantity" (*The New Lexicon Webster's Dictionary*, 1988, p. 2). Therefore, the foundation of the abilities-based approach is the consideration of how the individual's skills (e.g., motor skill, knowledge, behaviour) or power (e.g., physical or psychological endurance or strength) match those required by the active living opportunity. It is this author's belief that any evaluation of the individual's "skill or power" (i.e., ability) should be based on the following assumptions:

- All individuals have a right to enjoy the active living lifestyle of their choice.
- Participation in active living opportunities does not have to be 'justified' in terms of the therapeutic benefits that it may provide to people with a disability.
- The interests of the individual, followed by the individual's abilities, should determine the choice of active living opportunities.
- All active living opportunities can be accessed by any individual given sufficient resources and flexibility in programme design.
- An active living lifestyle will be adopted if the experiences are successful and enjoyable.

4 What are your personal beliefs about active living and people with a disability and how might they influence the active living opportunities you provide?

5 Do you agree with these assumptions? What are their strengths and limitations?

6 What assumptions are you making in evaluating these assumptions?

7 How do these assumptions differ from those of other approaches to APA?

APPLYING PROFESSIONAL KNOWLEDGE AND TRAINING

Training as a physical activity professional provides you with virtually all of the knowledge required to provide inclusive active living opportunities to people of all abilities.

If this statement is true, it begs the question "why should I take a course specializing in APA?" Although the statement is true, the existence of knowledge alone is seldom sufficient for the delivery of inclusive active living programmes. Professionals must have experience in applying that knowledge to the creation of inclusive programmes if people with a disability are to have equal access to an active living lifestyle.

What is the knowledge that physical activity professionals possess? Most of the information about disability that traditionally forms the core content of APA courses is based on the fundamental movement sciences, primarily physiology, anatomy, kinesiology, and biomechanics. More recently, recognition of the importance of the social sciences that influence physical activity (e.g., psychology, behaviour change, motivation, and adherence) and their relationship to activity for people with a disability has increased. Knowledge from these core courses is used in all active living settings, including those that provide services to people with a disability. The ability to apply that knowledge to enhance the active living opportunities available to each unique individual is the key area of expertise for specialists in adapted physical activity.

Consider square dancing, for example. Success in square dancing relies on a variety of factors, such as timing, coordination, rhythm, hearing, and physical movement. Knowledge of anatomy identifies the parts of the body involved in a particular movement. For example, the arms and hands must grip the partner, the feet must move quickly, and the vestibular system must adjust to rapid rotation while the partners 'swing'. Greater understanding of the effects of the 'swing' on balance and orientation is created when there is knowledge about the physiology of the semi-circular canals of the inner ear. Knowledge of kinesiology or biomechanics could help to identify alternative positions for each partner so that the effort to swing is minimized or to compensate if one partner had a movement limitation.

To ensure that **all individuals** have access to the active living lifestyle of their choice, **all physical activity professionals** must assume responsibility for providing services to participants with a wide range of abilities and interests, from gifted athletes to those with very limited physical activity experience or skill. How can people with a disability have the same rights as other individuals if only a small select group of specially trained professionals are considered to be 'qualified' to provide services to them? Professionals in areas such as education, recreation, leisure, and fitness commonly experience a wide range of ability and expertise among participants. However, even those in more specialized areas, such as elite sport coaching, should expect and be prepared to work with athletes with a disability.

Professionals often express concern about safety or adverse health consequences for people with a disability who are involved in active living. To address this concern, it is important to recognize the difference between a disability and a health condition that increases the risk for physical activity participation.

Standard physical activity participation screening procedures should be used with all participants, including individuals with a disability, to identify individuals who may have an increased risk of negative health consequences. A disability may or may not influence the safety of physical activity. Professionals wishing to work with 'higher risk' individuals, such as those with cardiac or pulmonary disease, should obtain specialty training and experience in a qualified, supervised setting.

Although all physical activity professionals have the knowledge required to provide inclusive active living opportunities, the comfort level of each professional may vary. Professionals who are uncomfortable providing inclusive services must take responsibility for obtaining additional training and experience. Although professionals have a right to acknowledge their perceived limitations and limit their scope of activities while additional training is obtained, it is inappropriate to refuse services to people with a disability. At the very least, a physical activity professional who is unwilling to provide direct services to a person with a disability must ensure that a willing professional or appropriate programme is identified, and that the person is appropriately connected, introduced, and supported.

Although using your knowledge to create inclusive active living opportunities is a great first step, just being prepared to provide inclusive active living opportunities is not sufficient. Professionals must be pro-active in creating inclusive opportunities and making participants, both current and potential, aware of programmes and facilities. Traditionally, people with a disability have been excluded from physical activities and, therefore, many of them do not expect or seek opportunities. Fortunately, these perceptions are changing. Effective advocacy skills enable physical activity professionals to:

- Convince programme and facility managers to offer inclusive programmes.
- Encourage people with a disability to become involved in active living opportunities.

- Educate people with a disability, their family, friends, and medical professionals about the benefits of active living for individuals of all abilities.

Effective advocacy skills are best developed through actual practice. Until you actually try to advocate for change, it is very difficult to fully appreciate and understand all of the factors which may influence the outcome. The Advocacy Resource Package, developed by the Active Living Alliance for Canadians with a Disability (1990), is a particularly effective resource because it was specifically developed for advocacy efforts to include people with a disability in active living opportunities. For more detailed information on advocacy, please refer to Chapter 6 (McPherson, Wheeler, and Foster) and Chapter 10 (Emes) in this textbook.

8 What are other ways that you can apply your existing knowledge to the understanding of disability and the creation of inclusive active living opportunities?

9 Review Chapter 4 (Squair and Groeneveld) and use your existing knowledge of physiology, anatomy, etc., to consider the potential active living implications of each impairment.

10 Think about an active living opportunity or situation that you would like to change. Can you identify what needs to be changed and one or more potential solutions? What steps would you take to advocate for that change?

11 How comfortable would you be in providing services to someone with limited mobility? Would your level of comfort change if the person had limited cognitive abilities, a chronic medical condition, loss of vision or hearing, or unusual behavioural patterns?

12 If you were unable to provide direct services, what referral options could you provide to the client? How would/did you learn about these referral options?

APPROACHES TO ACTIVE LIVING FOR PEOPLE OF ALL ABILITIES

Providing services to all participants, across the full spectrum of abilities, may seem an impossible challenge. The most effective way to provide services to people with a disability has always been, and continues to be, a major point of discussion for physical activity professionals. A variety of approaches have been suggested, implemented, and evaluated, based on the fundamental beliefs of the professionals involved. Since these beliefs vary greatly, the format, goals, and opportunities available through each approach will also vary. It is not possible to review extensively all of the approaches to providing active living opportunities to people with a disability. However, some discussion of several approaches may be found in Chapter 2 (Reid) and Chapter 13 (Goodwin, Watkinson, and Fitzpatrick).

'Traditional' approaches to APA (e.g., categorical or developmental approach) assume that the participant with a disability is 'different' and therefore the activity must be 'adapted' in order for her or him to participate. In contrast, the abilities-based approach considers each individual to be unique and focusses on the 'match' or degree of overlap between the skills of the individual and the abilities required by the activity (see figure 21.3).

The abilities-based approach uses a task analysis format to analyze both the abilities of the participant and the demands of the activity (Canadian Society for Exercise Physiology 2002; Moving to Inclusion Steering Committee 1994b). It can be used with all active living opportunities and relies on the knowledge and skill of the physical activity professional to create as much overlap as possible between the individual's abilities and the activity's demands, so that

Figure 21.3 Successful Participation Requires Considerable Overlap Between the Abilities of the Individual and the Demands of the Activity

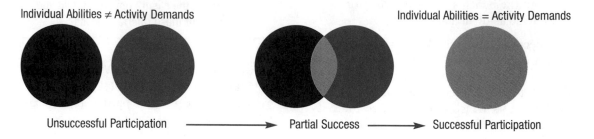

Individual Abilities ≠ Activity Demands   Individual Abilities = Activity Demands

Unsuccessful Participation ——————→ Partial Success ——————→ Successful Participation

successful participation can take place. Each participant's abilities can be influenced by factors such as a disability, prior experience, or motivation. The activity demands depend on the skills required and the activity setting (e.g., instructional, competitive, recreational). Details of this approach are described in the following section, and the pros and cons are summarized in table 21.1.

The abilities-based approach differs from a categorical approach, the most common in APA, which derives from a medical model of sport as therapy for people with a disability and the belief that the disability label primarily determines the active living abilities of an individual. Categorical approaches focus on the impairment rather than its effect on participation. Using this type of approach, appropriate active living opportunities are identified by:

• evaluating or assessing the individual
• 'diagnosing' or identifying the condition
• prescribing the appropriate activity based on the diagnosis

Formal assessments, norm or criterion referenced tests, are usually used to determine participation options using a categorical approach. The taxonomy of impairment provided in Chapter 4 (Squair and Groeneveld) and disability descriptions in many APA texts (e.g., Sherrill 1998; Eichstaedt and Kalakian

1993; Jansma and French 1994) are examples of a categorical approach. Some of the pros and cons of a categorical approach are outlined in table 21.2.

The abilities-based approach also differs from developmental approaches, which are designed to close the gap between the individual's present abilities and a performance target based on 'normal' developmental patterns. The development of the ability to learn, think, or speak can be considered in addition to the individual's movement abilities. Activity choices are designed to maximize the individual's developmental potential. Although a developmental approach can apply across the lifespan, texts and resources often focus on school programmes (Eichstaedt and Kalakian 1993; Seaman and DePauw 1989) since development is a primary concern during childhood. Table 21.3 outlines some of the pros and cons of a developmental approach.

13 Pui-Ying loves to swim and is interested in learning to scuba dive. She has cerebral palsy and has never learned to walk. How would you approach working with Pui-Ying in regards to her active living goal using the abilities-based approach? What would you do if you were using a categorical or developmental approach?

Table 21.1 Pros and Cons of the Abilities-based Approach

Pros	Cons
• Focus on abilities required for success, not disability • Potential active living opportunities not based on the type of disability • Equal consideration to the interests and abilities of the participant • Applicable to all individuals and activities • Holistic approach that considers all aspects of the individual and activity • Relates directly to active living participation	• Relatively new, so texts and resources are somewhat limited at this time • Requires professionals to know each individual's abilities, not just the impairment

Table 21.2 Pros and Cons of the Categorical Approach

Pros	Cons
• Widely known and used, extensive texts and resources • General summary of 'average' abilities within each category • Labels can be effective for communication between professionals • Introduction to a variety of impairments and medical conditions • Does not require in-depth knowledge of each individual's unique abilities	• Focusses on impairment or medical condition • Focus on impairment may limit awareness of each individual's unique abilities • Label is primary determinant of appropriate active living opportunities • General impairment expectations may be inappropriate for any one individual • Less consideration of individual interests

Table 21.3 Pros and Cons of the Developmental Approach

Pros	Cons
• Focus on the individual's level of development • Goal to move the individual towards a more 'normal' developmental level • Programmes based on individual abilities rather than an impairment category • Appropriate for achieving specific therapeutic or educational goals • Evaluates individual abilities and experience	• Activities selected based on developmental goals rather than individual interests • Impairment may preclude a 'normal' developmental level • Focus on improving level of function rather than an enjoyable, active living lifestyle • Developmental activities may not be age-appropriate

The Abilities-based Approach to Inclusive Active Living

The abilities-based approach evaluates the individual's abilities and the demands of the activity in terms of six factors: mobility, object manipulation, cognition, communication and perception, behaviour and social skills, and fitness (see figure 21.4). **All six components are included in all active living opportunities.** However, the relative importance of each component will vary depending on the type of activity or setting. Details of the six components are described in the following sub-sections.

An example may help to illustrate how the importance of each of the six components may vary between activities. Consider the different demands for basketball, weightlifting, and creative dance. Basketball emphasizes mobility (movement on the court), object manipulation (ball handling), communication and perception (with and of teammates), cognition (planning, decision-making), behaviour and social skills (teamwork), and fitness (ability to play an entire game). In contrast, the demands of weightlifting are focussed primarily on object manipulation (control and movement of the weight), cognition (concentration) and fitness (ability to continue as weight increases). Although there are components of mobility (moving to and through the lifting position), communication and perception (seeing the weight), and behavioural and social skills (ensuring safety) in weightlifting, they are usually less important. Creative dance focusses primarily on mobility (movement to music) and communication and perception (hearing the music). Again, object manipulation (dancing with a scarf), behaviour and social skills (interacting with other dancers), cognition (understanding or remembering desired movements), and fitness (dancing for the entire song or class) play a role but they are relatively less important to successful participation than mobility and perception.

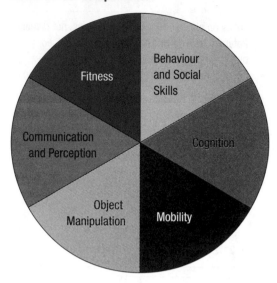

Figure 21.4 Abilities-based Approach Defines Activity Demands and Participant Abilities Based on Six Components.

14 If an individual with limited communication skills wanted to join one of these activities (e.g., basketball, weightlifting, or creative dance), which would you recommend? How could the required communication skills be decreased to enhance the individual's participation in each of these activities?

MOBILITY

Mobility refers to movement of the participant or parts of the participant's body within the active living setting. Through growth and experience, people develop more sophisticated forms of mobility. A toddler may be able to walk, run, or jump on two feet. In contrast, adults usually have sophisticated movement patterns such as skipping, hopping, and dancing. Individuals with mobility limitations may move in different ways or use assistive devices, such as prosthetic limbs, crutches, canes, walkers, manual or power wheelchairs, and scooters. As technology advances, assistive mobility devices are able to provide greater speed, agility, and complexity of movement.

The mobility required for active living varies tremendously. Some activities, soccer or

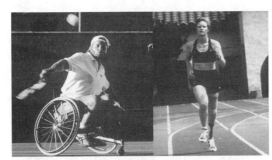

Assistive devices, such as a wheelchair or prosthesis, can be used to enhance mobility.

15 Consider how the mobility requirements differ for the following activities:
- **curling versus ice hockey**
- **volleyball versus basketball**
- **track versus gymnastics**

hockey for example, require a combination of speed and agility. Dance activities may require intricate movement patterns with less emphasis on speed. Sprinting requires more speed but has very consistent movement patterns. Other activities, such as weightlifting, may require very limited mobility. Even activities that are fundamentally very similar may have different mobility requirements. For example, the mobility required for squash or racquetball differs because of differences in ball rebound, racquet size, and the court dimensions between two relatively similar racquet sports. The same activity may also have different mobility requirements depending on the active living setting. For example, consider the differences in mobility required for success in a beginner recreational versus elite competitive synchronized swim programme.

With the almost unlimited variety of active living options available, it is relatively easy to select activities that have mobility demands that match the skills of the individual. For individuals who have limited mobility, try to identify the components of the movement that result in the limitation. Does limited speed result from a lack of training or a disorder that limits muscle contraction? Is limited agility due to a lack of balance or a motor coordination disorder? To enhance active living success, consider modifications to the individual's mobility (e.g., through the use of assistive devices) or the mobility requirements of the activity (e.g., requiring players to remain stationary when in possession of the ball during a basketball game).

OBJECT MANIPULATION

Object manipulation, primarily related to hand or upper limb function (e.g., grasp, strike, catch), is critical to almost all active living activities. However, the control and manipulation of equipment is not just limited to hand grip. Soccer, for example, requires object manipulation skills with the head, trunk, legs, and feet. Activities such as ball sports or gardening rely heavily on object manipulation. Other activities such as walking, jogging, swimming, or dance may require significantly less object-person interaction. The activity setting can also influence the object manipulation skills required. For instance, a person with limited hand grip who wishes to lift weights at the local gym would be able to use straps or tensor bandages to secure the weight in her hands. However, the same person would have to hold the weight without assistance if she was participating in a competitive weightlifting event.

For people with a disability, equipment modifications or assistive devices often play a key role in successful object manipulation. There is a natural tendency to look to sophisticated technology for solutions when object manipulation skills are limited. However, the development of sophisticated technology is extremely time consuming, very expensive, and often has very limited application (i.e., it solves the problem for one particular individual). Physical activity professionals are encouraged to rely primarily on 'low tech' solutions–simple, inexpensive answers that allow people to participate immediately. In many situations, changing the equipment itself, such as using a larger or lighter ball or a racquet with a larger head, will sufficiently improve the participant's control.

There are many resources on equipment modification available to physical activity professionals. Texts on equipment modification

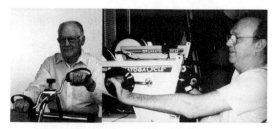

High or low tech solutions can enhance object manipulation.

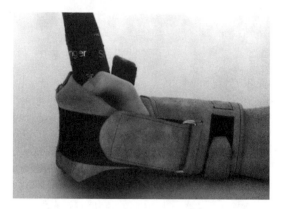

Technology for daily living may enhance active living participation.

(e.g., *Moving to Inclusion* 1994a; Paciorek and Jones 1994), internet resources (e.g., http://www.engr.wisc.edu/news/headlines/1996/Jan22.html>, ABLEDATA <http://www.abledata.com>, Adapt-talk listserv <adapt-talk@lyris.sportime.com>), or inclusive active living magazines (e.g., *Active Living, Sports 'N Spokes, Palaestra*) are just a few potential resources. Some examples of 'low tech' solutions are:

- using straps to maintain static positions (e.g., holding a fishing rod)
- substituting equipment that is easier to manipulate (e.g., a beach ball or balloon has less force and speed than heavier balls; the flexible shape and lack of rebound makes bean bags easier to control than balls)
- using assistive technology for other purposes in the active living setting (e.g., a device to hold a toothbrush or comb may be suitable for holding a fishing rod or table tennis racquet)

16 What 'low tech' solution(s) can you think of that would enable someone with an amputation of the right arm above the elbow to paddle a canoe?

COGNITION

Cognition is "the act or faculty of knowing" (*The New Lexicon Webster's Dictionary* 1988), but how do we 'know'? Although we have very detailed information on a variety of physical functions, our knowledge of the brain remains relatively limited. Acquiring knowledge relies on a variety of cognitive functions, such as perception, recognition, understanding, memory, or attention. An impairment of any one function may result in a cognitive limitation for active living.

Cognitive function is often incorrectly equated with 'intelligence' or 'IQ'. However, individuals may be of 'normal' intelligence and still have limitations related to cognition (e.g., memory, concentration, or attention). Probably the greatest limitation to active living for people with cognitive limitations is the belief by others that they are unable to learn anything. Therefore, physical activity professionals should strive to ensure that they have an accurate understanding of the client's cognitive limitations. The exact extent of an individual's cognitive limitations may be difficult to determine. However, physical activity professionals should seek information about the cognitive limitation from the client and, with the client's permission, from knowledgeable health professionals or individuals familiar with the client's abilities (e.g., family, friends, support worker).

The cognitive skills required for active living participation will differ with the activity and setting. Activities that place consistent, predictable demands on the participants (e.g., walking, jogging, weightlifting) generally require less sophisticated cognitive skills. Group activities require more sophisticated cognitive skills because participants must respond to the activities of others as well as their own efforts. A child may work one-on-one with an APA specialist to learn the motor skills required to use a playground slide (e.g., going up the steps, sitting down, sliding down, standing up). It is much more difficult for that child to use the slide during recess when other children are waiting for a turn, there are many distractions, and others may be climbing up the slide. Competitive activities may also require strategies and planning skills that increase the cognitive demands of the activity. For example, a class on power skating and puck handling skills for hockey will usually have fewer cognitive demands than playing in a game.

To enhance the active living participation of individuals with limited cognitive skills, consider:

- acquiring accurate information about the specific cognitive limitations of the participant
- identifying activities of interest to the individual that have fewer cognitive demands
- modifying activities or using simple progressions to decrease the need for sophisticated cognitive skills

17 What cognitive skills are required for each of the following activities?
- interpretive dance
- personal exercise conditioning programme
- rowing in an eight-person shell

COMMUNICATION AND PERCEPTION

Communication and perception skills are the basis of our interactions with other people and our environment. Through our perceptions we acquire knowledge about what is happening around us, enabling us to respond in an appropriate manner. Our communication skills enable us to convey our thoughts and intentions to others and to receive communications from others.

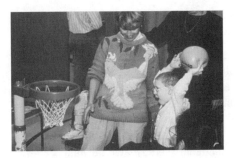

Break tasks into simple steps to decrease the cognitive demands of an activity.

Sensory input is the primary source of perceptual information. Vision and hearing are the most commonly recognized forms of sensory input. However, particularly during physical activity, other forms of sensory information (e.g., kinesthetics, touch) can be equally important. Similarly, both verbal and non-verbal forms of communication are used in a wide variety of activities. Group activities and those performed at high speed require more sophisticated communication and perception skills because participants must quickly and accurately perceive the movements and intentions of others, process sensory input, and effectively communicate thoughts and actions.

In designing activity modifications for people with communication or perception limitations, it is important that the impact of the individual's specific impairment be accurately identified. For example, most individuals with limited hearing or vision have some residual function, a fact that is often overlooked. Active living participation may be enhanced by:

- providing information in more than one format (e.g., verbal description, visual demonstration, tactile assisted movement)
- simplifying communication (e.g., succinct descriptions, a picture may be worth a thousand words)
- providing sufficient indirect lighting to enhance vision and minimize shadows
- using flexible amplification systems positioned to enhance the participants'

ability to hear verbal instructions or auditory cues (e.g., music)

---

18 How do the required communication and perception skills differ for each of the following?
- archery versus dance
- fencing versus wrestling
- gardening versus lawn bowling

BEHAVIOUR AND SOCIAL SKILLS

The way we behave and our knowledge of social skills influence our ability to interact with and respond to other people and our environment. Whether it is a group or individual pursuit, there are very few active living opportunities that do not have specific demands for the types of behaviours that should be performed and the social skills required for successful participation. *Behaviour and social skills* have a significant impact on our interactions, acceptance, perceptions of the experience and, in some situations, the activity outcome. While an individual may be very adept at performing the motor skills required for an activity, perceived success is often based on interpersonal interactions (e.g., Do my teammates like me? Do I make a positive contribution?). Individual pursuits may have fewer demands for behaviour and social skills but physical activities are rarely done in isolation. For example, someone doing an individual fitness programme must still interact with others in the facility, and a lone runner must behave in an appropriate manner (e.g., not unexpectedly darting onto the road in traffic).

Some types of active living opportunities are unsafe for participants who do not possess the required behaviour and social skills. Activities with a risk of injury, such as shooting, archery, rock climbing, or gymnastics, have the highest demand for appropriate behaviour and social skills. The safety of all participants must always be the primary consideration of the physical activity professional.

To enhance active living for individuals with limited behaviour and social skills, consider the following:

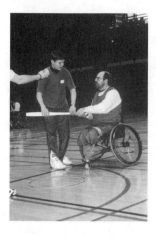

Use a variety of formats (verbal, auditory, tactile, and kinesthetic) to enhance communication and perception.

- Provide opportunities for the individual to learn appropriate behaviour and social skills.
- Focus interaction and reinforcement on positive behaviours and develop support systems to enable behaviour appropriate to the active living setting.
- Focus on the behaviour or social skill as appropriate or inappropriate rather than whether the individual is a 'desirable' participant.
- Establish routines and set consistent limits and expectations.

---

19 Identify three types of physical activity for each of the following activity requirements:
- very specific types of behaviour(s)
- a wide range of acceptable behaviour(s)
- highly developed social skills
- minimal social skills

Fitness

Fitness relates to whether or not the participant is "suited to, healthy enough or in good enough condition" for the activity of choice (*The New Lexicon Webster's Dictionary* 1988). Considerations of 'fitness' often focus on the physical 'fitness' or 'readiness' of the individual. However, the psychological or emotional fitness of the participant must also be considered. Fitness for a particular activity can be considered in terms of many variables, such as endurance, stamina, speed, strength,

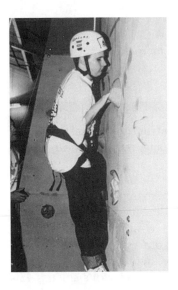

Appropriate behaviour can be critical to participant safety.

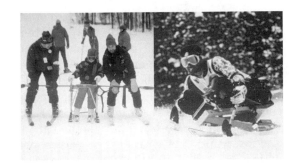

The type of activity, choice of setting, and programme goals can influence the fitness requirements for active living participation.

resiliency, balance, flexibility, or agility. Unlike the other categories (mobility, object manipulation, etc.) which focus on the participant's ability to perform a particular skill, fitness focusses on whether the skill or movement can be performed as often as required by the activity. An individual may be able to run, throw a ball, and behave appropriately, but can he or she continue to perform for the duration of a baseball game?

Fitness requirements may vary between activities or for the same activity in different settings. Running, cycling, and cross-country skiing demand high levels of cardio-respiratory endurance. Shooting and archery require concentration and psychological endurance. Muscular strength and power are critical for weight-lifting, wrestling, or rock-climbing. Activities such as table tennis or billiards rely primarily on coordination. The fitness demands for downhill skiing on a short beginner slope are different from those on a two-kilometre mountain trail with many moguls. Fitness demands also differ between recreational and competitive skiers for the same slope.

Approaches to enhance the participation of individuals with fitness limitations include:

- decreasing the fitness demands of the activity (e.g., slower pace, fewer repetitions)

- increasing skill (e.g., a skilled golfer takes fewer shots and walks a shorter distance)
- enhancing fitness through individualized training programmes
- selecting activities that require lower levels of fitness

20 Think about the physical activities that you enjoy. What components of fitness are required for successful participation in those activities?

21 Using the abilities-based approach, identify the primary components for the following activities and settings:
- **tennis compared to squash**
- **downhill skiing compared to cross-country skiing**
- **figure skating compared to hockey**

The Abilities-based Approach in 'Real Life'

ADRIENNE

Adrienne is five years old and "wants to play with her friends." She has severe cardiac problems and is cyanotic (i.e., her lips and fingernails appear blue due to a lack of oxygen) at rest. Although her doctor does not limit her activity, her parents are afraid that she might over-exert herself. Adrienne has started school and her parents want to know if she should participate in recess.

Using the abilities-based approach to evaluate Adrienne's abilities, we find that her communication and perception, object manipulation, and cognition skills are age-appropriate. Her mobility and behaviour and social skills are limited due to lack of experience. Adrienne's fitness is decreased in all areas, with a severe cardio-respiratory limitation.

Observation of Adrienne's classmates during recess indicates that they play primarily on the playground equipment. The mobility required includes a variety of movement patterns (e.g., walking, jumping, climbing steps), primarily at a self-selected pace. Object manipulation focusses on holding onto the playground equipment. Cognitive skills include knowledge of how the equipment can be used and an understanding of the impact of movement by others. Participation requires the ability to perceive the equipment and others using it and to communicate one's own ideas or intentions. Behaviour and social skills focus primarily on successful interactions with others, but also on behaviour that is appropriate and safe for the equipment. Sufficient fitness is required to participate at a self-selected pace.

How do Adrienne's abilities match the activity demands? Clearly, Adrienne's mobility limitations will have an impact on her participation. Object manipulation, cognition, and communication and perception skills are not a factor. Adrienne's lack of social experience may influence her acceptance. Stamina will always be a major limitation, but other fitness factors can be improved with training.

So, can she participate? Adrienne can probably participate in most recess activities with her friends. However, her chances for success could be enhanced through:

- individualized instruction to develop the required movement patterns and increase her strength before she begins to participate (change in her abilities)
- the provision of support through adult supervision until Adrienne gains experience with social interactions and her peers are supportive of her participation (change in the activity setting)

HECTOR

Hector was born with limited vision. He has moved to a new city for a new job. He wants to join a sports team so he can keep in shape and get to know people. There are adult leagues for darts, soccer, and curling which are recreational, do not keep score, and emphasize enjoyment and equal participation. What team(s) would be most appropriate for Hector?

Let us evaluate the activity options. Darts emphasizes object manipulation and cognition. Soccer requires high levels of mobility, perception and communication, object manipulation, and fitness. Curling focusses on object manipulation and fitness.

Now let us consider Hector's abilities. His limitation relates almost solely to perception, although his object manipulation skills are reduced when contact with the object is not continuous, and his mobility is limited in unfamiliar environments. Cognition, communication, fitness, and behaviour and social skills are not affected.

Given Hector's vision limitation, success in the soccer league would probably require significant modifications. Many physical activity professionals would automatically focus on darts since a beeping sound could be added to the target. However, what has Hector said about his interests and goals? He wants to "keep in shape" as well as "meet people." Since the fitness required for darts is very limited, it would not help him "keep in shape". Although he would probably get to know people, darts would not meet all of his goals. Curling may be a more appropriate activity, particularly since the skip could provide verbal guidance and direction.

MAHMOUD

Mahmoud sustained a traumatic brain injury in a car accident that limits his memory and control of his behaviour. Before his injury, he and his family were avid wilderness canoeists. Since then, Mahmoud has not been involved in outdoor activities. However, he does exercise regularly at the fitness centre near his home. What activities would you recommend so that Mahmoud and his family can return to the outdoor activities they love?

First, consider the wide range of outdoor activities available, such as hiking, canoeing, mountain biking, horseback riding, kayaking, and sailing. What types of mobility, object manipulation, cognition, communication and perception, behaviour and social skills, and fitness are required for each of these activities?

We know that Mahmoud exercises regularly and that his mobility, communication and perception, and object manipulation skills are unaffected. His limitations relate primarily to cognition and behaviour.

Which activities would be suitable? Since Mahmoud will be with his family, they will be able to support him in relation to his memory limitations. Hiking or mountain biking would provide opportunities to get outdoors. Horseback riding may not be appropriate given the potential impact of his unpredictable behaviour on the horse. Similarly, inappropriate behaviour can limit success in canoeing or kayaking because of the instability of these watercraft. Given the family's love of canoeing (i.e., a non-motorized boating activity), sailing may provide the best opportunity. The use of a large, stable sailboat would limit the impact of unpredictable movements and enable Mahmoud's family to be in the same boat to provide any additional support that he may require.

FRANÇOISE

Gardening has been a lifelong passion for Françoise. She has won many awards for the gardens and landscaping around her house. Recently, the effects from her arthritis have increased. It is now difficult for Françoise to bend her knees and standing causes ankle pain. Françoise has asked for your help so that she can continue to work in the garden that she loves.

22 Using the abilities-based approach, identify the activity demands for gardening and the effect(s) of her arthritis on Françoise's abilities.

23 What modifications can you suggest that would enable Françoise to continue working in her garden?

JOSHUA

Joshua and Marika are getting married in February. They will be spending their honeymoon in Belize, since one of Marika's lifelong goals has been to snorkel on tropical reefs. Both Joshua and Marika can swim well, although neither has previously been in the ocean. Joshua is excited about sharing in Marika's dream but is concerned that he will not be able handle the ocean currents and waves since he had both of his legs amputated after a car accident five years ago. Joshua has come to you for suggestions on how he can be more mobile in the water.

24 Use the abilities-based approach to identify the activity demands and the influence of Joshua's disability.

25 What modifications or recommendations would you make to Joshua?

Summary

Active living provides tremendous physical, psychological, emotional, and spiritual benefits to each participant. **All individuals,** regardless of ability, have the right to enjoy an active living lifestyle and the right to choose and participate in activities of interest to them. **All physical activity professionals** must be pro-active in promoting active living opportunities to, and ensuring that the opportunities they provide are inclusive of people of all abilities.

Inclusive programmes, in integrated or segregated settings, are designed to meet the needs of participants with a wide variety of abilities. The design of active living opportunities so that they require modification or the development of alternate programmes for people with different abilities is inappropriate unless the opportunity is designed to be highly segregated (e.g., a pre-Olympic training camp). Physical activity professionals should ensure that all programmes are designed, from the earliest stages, to include people with a variety of abilities. In addition, when programmes that are not inclusive are identified, physical activity professionals should be proactive in making the changes required to move to an inclusive design. The focus on providing inclusive active living opportunities should occur whether or not there are participants with a disability involved, or potentially involved, in the programme.

Lifelong adoption of an active living lifestyle depends on enjoyable and successful participation. Successful participation in active living opportunities depends on matching the individual's abilities with the demands of the activity. It also depends on the availability of activity choices that match the individual's interests, goals, resources, experience, and skills. Individual abilities and activity demands can be described in terms of mobility, object manipulation, cognition, communication and perception, behaviour and social skills, and fitness. Physical activity professionals are responsible for maximizing the overlap between the individual's abilities and the activity demands in order to foster successful active living experiences.

While knowledge of the abilities-based approach is an important first step toward the creation of inclusive physical activity opportunities, it is important for professionals to recognize that knowledge alone is not sufficient. The 'real life' benefits of inclusive active living opportunities will only be realized when professionals apply their knowledge to their own practices. Examine and evaluate your own attitudes and beliefs! Take on an advocacy effort to make a change that you desire! Work to enhance the availability of inclusive active living opportunities! You can make a difference, but only if you take the knowledge you have gained and put it into action.

Study Questions

1. Define and distinguish between *inclusion* and *integration*.
2. Name three approaches to APA and describe the pros and cons of each.
3. How do our personal beliefs, assumptions, and existing knowledge base influence the active living opportunities we create?
4. What are the factors used by the abilities-based approach to evaluate individual abilities and activity demands? Briefly describe each factor.
5. Use the abilities-based approach to identify the general abilities you might anticipate among people with the following conditions (see Chapter 4 by Squair and Groeneveld for details): asthma, osteoporosis, Down's syndrome, schizophrenia, tunnel vision.
6. Use the abilities-based approach to identify the activity demands of each of the following activities in instructional, recreational, and competitive settings: water-skiing, in-line skating, a walking club, badminton, t-ball, tai chi, and ballet.

Acknowledgement

Photographs courtesy of Curtis, Axelson, and Longmuir (1996).

References

Active Living Alliance for Canadians with a Disability. (1990). *Advocacy resource package.* Ottawa: Fitness Canada and the Active Living Alliance for Canadians with a Disability.

Active Living Alliance for Canadians with a Disability, and Health Canada. (1998). *Active Living Alliance for Canadians with a Disability: A blueprint for action.* Ottawa: Author.

Active Living Alliance for Canadians with a Disability. (1999). *Viabilité: A new initiative, a new identity.* Ottawa: Author.

Canadian Society for Exercise Physiology. (2002). *Inclusive fitness and lifestyle services for all disAbilities.* Ottawa: Author.

Collins English Dictionary (2nd ed.). (1990). London: Collins.

Curtis, G. (Producer), Axelson, P.W. (Executive Producer), and Longmuir, P.E. (Associate Producer). (1996). *Tools for Play* [Video]. (Available from Beneficial Designs Inc., 1617 Water Street, Suite B, Minden, NV 89423.) Atlanta, GA: Paralysed Veterans of America.

Eichstaedt, C.B., and Kalakian, L.H. (1993). *Developmental/adapted physical education: Making ability count* (3rd ed.). New York: Macmillan.

Jansma, P.R., and French, R. (1994). *Special physical education: Physical activity, sports, and recreation.* Englewood Cliffs, NJ: Prentice Hall.

Moving to Inclusion Steering Committee. (1994a). *Active living through physical education: Maximizing opportunities for students with a disability.* Ottawa: Active Living Alliance for Canadians with a Disability.

Moving to Inclusion Steering Committee. (1994b). *Active living through physical education: Maximizing opportunities for students with multiple disabilities.* Ottawa: Active Living Alliance for Canadians with a Disability.

The New Lexicon Webster's Dictionary of the English Language. (1988). New York: Lexicon.

Paciorek, M.J., and Jones, J.A. (1994). *Sports and recreation for the disabled* (2nd ed.). Carmel, IN: Cooper.

Quinney, H.A., Gauvin, L., and Wall, A.E.T. (Eds.). (1994). *Toward active living: Proceedings of the International Conference on Physical Activity, Fitness, and Health.* Champaign, IL: Human Kinetics.

Seaman, J.A., and DePauw, K.P. (1989). *The new adapted physical education: A developmental approach* (2nd ed.). Mountain View, CA: Mayfield.

Shepard, R.J. (1990). *Fitness in Special Populations.* Champaign, IL: Human Kinetics.

Sherrill, C. (1998). *Adapted Physical Activity, Recreation and Sport: Crossdisciplinary and Lifespan* (5th ed.). Dubuque, IA: WCB/McGraw.

CHAPTER 22

Inclusive Fitness Appraisal Developments

Christine M. Seidl

Learning Objectives

- To become familiar with the rights of people with disabilities to have equal access to inclusive fitness appraisal services provided by qualified personnel.
- To know that a person with a disability can be 'apparently healthy' and the significance that this has in their participation in the CPAFLA.
- To know the health benefits of regular physical activity for people of all abilities.
- To review terminology (e.g., *health, fitness, exercise, active living,* etc.).
- To understand how the *inclusion* and *active living* philosophies are compatible.
- To learn about the developments in the CPAFLA programme (e.g., emphasis on active living instead of prescriptive exercise, dose-response relationship of physical activity and health benefits, etc.).
- To become aware of some recommendations made by the Canadian Society for Exercise Physiology (CSEP) when providing fitness appraisal services to people with different functional abilities.
- To know the scope of the Supplementary Training Module (STM) for providing training for fitness appraisers and how to access training programmes through CSEP.
- To know which resources and materials for providing inclusive fitness and lifestyle services are available through CSEP and how to access these materials.

Introduction

The second edition of *The Canadian Physical Activity, Fitness and Lifestyle Appraisal* (CPAFLA) was developed and published by the Canadian Society for Exercise Physiology (CSEP) in 1998. The CPAFLA (formerly known as the Canadian Standardized Test of Fitness) has undergone many changes, most importantly, the emphasis on active living as well as the development of counselling and behaviour change applications. This marks an important step forward for fitness appraisal in Canada and broadens its appeal to all Canadians with a variety of fitness profiles and functional abilities. It is an example of inclusive services for the global community. Expanding the use of the CPAFLA to include Canadians of all abilities has been the result of a national initiative for the inclusion of people with a disability (Canadian Society for Exercise Physiology 1998b). It is based on the belief that all 'apparently healthy' Canadians, including those with a disability, should have equal access to fitness appraisal services by trained professionals.

The purpose of this chapter is to provide students in adapted physical activity (APA) with an overview of the CPAFLA programme and how it has become accessible to

Canadians of all abilities. The information should bridge the *inclusion* and *active living* philosophies embedded in CPAFLA's *Supplementary Training Module*, or STM (Canadian Society for Exercise Physiology, 2002). This chapter will briefly examine the historical developments in physical activity practices of people with a disability. The broad category of apparently healthy people with a disability who are eligible for fitness appraisal services under the current CPAFLA standards will be defined. The health benefits of physical activity for people with or without a disability will also be discussed. *Active living*, an approach to healthy living promoted in the CPAFLA, will be discussed in relation to its enhancement of health and its compatibility with the *inclusion* philosophy. A review of the changes in the CPAFLA over the last twenty years will be followed by a description of the more recent initiatives intended to broaden the scope of the programme to better serve people with a disability. Many of the recommendations for fitness appraisal made by CSEP were substantiated by extensive review papers on fitness testing, programming, and counselling considerations for people with a disability (Canadian Society for Exercise Physiology 1998b). Many of these recommendations were used to develop the STM intended to extend the training of certified fitness appraisers. Some of these recommendations, along with practical guidelines for physical activity and fitness appraisal for people with a disability, will conclude this chapter.

ADAPTED PHYSICAL ACTIVITY: A BRIEF HISTORY

It is accepted and documented by APA researchers and practitioners that people with a disability should practice healthy living, participate in physical activity, and have equal opportunities for active living (Canadian Society for Exercise Physiology 1998b). However, people with physical, sensory, or intellectual disabilities often exercise less than people without a disability and demonstrate lower measures of physical fitness (Longmuir 1998; Seidl 1998; Steadward 1998). Exercise

efficiency, or the energy cost at a given workload, can be lower in people with sensory and intellectual disabilities. For example, poor coordination and difficulty in maintaining steady cadences may cause lower efficiency in stair-stepping for women with an intellectual disability (Seidl, Montgomery and Reid 1989). Shephard (1990) reported that the lack of visual information and smaller steps taken by people who are blind can result in lower efficiency during walking exercise. Steadward (1998) stated that physical access and the perception that standardized equipment within a training facility could not be used by people with a physical disability remain a barrier to participation in physical activity. Finally, participation in various physical activities may have been limited in the past, impacting on skill development as well as on physical fitness (Seidl 1998). Overprotection by caregivers and lack of confidence of participants may have as much to do with this as the limited opportunities for sport and leisure offered to past generations of people with a disabilty.

Within the past twenty years, rehabilitation and therapy programmes have given way to a wide range of physical activity programmes, sports, and leisure, with an emphasis on participating in regular activity in inclusive environments. Rehabilitation programmes, however, play a valuable role in the therapeutic realm of living with a disability. In addition, the sport movement for people with a disability has also created activity opportunities that include intense physical training and elite competition.

Over the past two decades, research in APA has examined the health-related fitness components of people with a disability (e.g., Bhambhani, Holland, and Steadward 1993; Montgomery, Reid, and Koziris 1992), identified barriers to their participation in physical activity (e.g., Johnson and Heller 1998), and has helped to understand their exercise performance characteristics and their response to training programmes (e.g., Bhambhani, Eriksson, and Gomes, 1991; Montgomery, Reid, and Seidl 1988). As a result, assessing and improving the health-related fitness of people with a disability has become a realistic priority in the field. Furthermore, the active living movement has helped to create a wider range of physical activity options that are considered beneficial to health. Consequently, Canadians of all abilities will have the opportunity to increase their involvement in physical activity by making it an integral part of their daily lives and by having access to appraisal services.

In a leadership role, a CSEP subcommittee comprised of APA researchers and professionals reviewed fitness appraisal considerations for people with a disability and made recommendations to make appraisal services more accessible to Canadians of all abilities (Canadian Society for Exercise Physiology 1998b). In addition, a supplementary training module, consisting of a manual and delivery system to further the training of certified fitness appraisers to provide inclusive fitness and lifestyle services to individuals with a disability, is currently being field tested in Canada (Canadian Society for Exercise Physiology, 2002).

People With a Disability and Physical Activity

The World Health Organization (1980) refers to *disability* as the restriction in a person's ability to perform a specific activity in a 'normal' manner. That is, *disability* is referred to as a 'difference' in function, and not a 'defect'. More recently, the meaning of *difference* has been taken to a new level by the creation of the International Classification of Function, or ICF (World Health Organization 2001). The ICF classifies the function of all individuals, with and without a disability, in terms of function, activity, participation, and contextual factors. In other words, each individual's ability to be active and participate in activity is a function of unique personal and environmental factors. These factors vary so widely that it is impossible to categorize the performance as 'normal'. Removing the word *normal* from the defining vocabulary of *disability* is welcomed by disability advocates. For the purposes of this chapter, *disability*

refers to any change in activity or participation regardless of the cause.

Depending on whether it was present at birth or acquired during the lifetime, a disability will present a different set of physical activity challenges for each individual. The challenges can range from being highly noticeable in some cases to almost undetectable in others. Fitness appraisers should not generalize the 'abilities' or 'challenges' of one person with a disability to another. They can, however, use their knowledge of active living services to enable a client to maintain an active lifestyle to the greatest extent possible.

It is also important that fitness consultants recognize the distinction between a *disability* and a medical condition, or *illness*. This distinction is often blurred by a lack of understanding and the misconception that all people with a disability have concomitant medical conditions that could place them at risk for physical activity. *Disability* is a change in activity participation and is not necessarily a contraindication to participation in a fitness test or subsequent participation in an exercise regimen or physical activity.

1 How many times have you noticed a person with a disability and *assumed* that there were many things that he or she could *not* do?

2 What tools could be used to identify people with a disability who do not have health restrictions for physical fitness testing?

APPARENTLY HEALTHY PEOPLE WITH A DISABILITY

Currently, fitness appraisers who are certified by the CPAFLA programme are qualified to provide appraisal services to apparently healthy individuals. *Apparently healthy* refers to individuals with no known medical conditions that place them at risk for participation in physical activity. Proper screening measures, such as the Physical Activity Readiness Questionnaire, or PAR-Q (Canadian Society for Exercise Physiology 2002), used in the CPAFLA programme would identify a client in need of medical clearance prior to fitness appraisal. For example, a person with cardiopulmonary disease would be identified by administering the PAR-Q and should consult with his or her physician prior to fitness testing or embarking on a physical activity programme. Currently, excluding people for whom physical activity is appropriate is more common than including people for whom it is contraindicated (Canadian Society for Exercise Physiology 1998A). It is possible, and very common, for people with a disability to participate in physical activity without any medical contraindications. It is also possible that some people with a disability have concomitant medical conditions (e.g., cardiopulmonary disease) that could require further medical clearance. All fitness appraisers (certified fitness consultants, or CFCs, and professional fitness and lifestyle consultants, or PFLCs) should be both qualified and prepared to use basic procedures described in the CPAFLA manual with apparently healthy people who pass the PAR-Q, irrespective of any disability the client may have (Canadian Society for Exercise Physiology 1998b).

Understanding more about 'disabilities' and how to assist persons with a disability effectively should help the appraiser to sort out important misunderstandings and assumptions about their participation in physical activity. Proper training of fitness appraisers should reduce the disability health-status misconception and provide them with the necessary skills and tools to identify apparently healthy people with a disability. However, to assist the client to make active and healthy lifestyle choices, the fitness appraiser must know the potential benefits of physical activity for people with a disability.

HEALTH BENEFITS OF PHYSICAL ACTIVITY
It is important to understand that the benefits of physical activity for people with a disability are essentially the same as those for individuals without a disability. The major causes of death and mortality in Canada are "diseases of lifestyle," that is, diseases that are linked to smoking, poor dietary habits, and lack of physical activity (Paffenbarger, Hyde, Wing, Lee and Kampert 1994). Furthermore, adequate physical activity is essential if good health, quality of life, and longevity are to be preserved.

The major causes of illness and death among people with a disability are essentially the same ones that affect people without disabilities (Shephard 1990). For example, in the 1940s medical complications such as renal failure used to claim the lives of 43 percent of people with spinal cord injuries (SCIs), followed by gastrointestinal complications at 11 percent (Shephard 1990). Cardiovascular disease and respiratory infections followed by claiming the lives of 10 percent and 9 percent of people with SCIs. By the late 1970s Shephard (1990) documented that these types of complications were giving way to "lifestyle diseases" such as chronic cardiovascular or respiratory diseases often associated with unhealthy living, including lack of physical exercise. The fitness appraiser needs to be fully aware that the benefits of physical activity will reduce the risks of coronary heart disease, obesity, osteoporosis, hypertension, and stroke in all people (Canadian Society for Exercise Physiology 1998a). Participating in physical activity can also help people with a disability to manage stress, reduce anxiety, relieve depression, and improve sleep, much as it would for people without a disability (Canadian Society for Exercise Physiology, 2002). Furthermore, physical activity can make a positive contribution to the maintenance of a healthy body weight, psychological well-being, self-esteem, and perceived quality of life for all people. Noreau and Shephard (1995) provide an overview of how physical activity participation may positively influence quality of life of people with a disability, such as improving physiological function, increasing their ability to do activities of daily life, decreasing physical dependence, and improving social integration. Figure 22.1 summarizes the health benefits of physical activity.

Figure 22.1 Health Benefits of Physical Activity

1. Reduces the risk of:
   - coronary heart disease
   - noninsulin dependent diabetes
   - obesity
   - colon cancer
   - osteoporosis
   - hypertension and stroke

2. Helps to:
   - increase resistance to mental fatigue
   - manage stress
   - reduce anxiety
   - relieve depression
   - improve sleep

3. Makes a positive contribution to:
   - maintenance of a healthy body weight
   - psychological well-being
   - self-efficacy and self-esteem
   - perceived quality of life

4. May also help a person with a disability:
   - improve physiological function
   - increase ability to activities of daily life
   - decrease physical dependence
   - improve social integration

NOTE: Columns 1, 2, and 3 identify the health benefits of physical activity for all people (Canadian Society for Exercise Physiology 1998A), while column 4 adds potential benefits for people with a disability (SOURCE: From "Spinal Cord Injury, Exercise and Quality of Life" by L. Noreau and R.J. Shephard, 1995, Sports Medicine, 20(4), pp. 226–50. Adapted with permission.)

PHYSICAL ACTIVITY AND AGING

Paffenbarger et al. (1994) compared the positive benefits of physical activity with the negative consequences of inactivity. A direct link can be drawn between participation in physical activity, a diminished risk of systemic diseases, and longevity. On the other hand, lack of physical activity is associated with an increased risk of systemic diseases and shorter lifespan. These two sequences are illustrated in figure 22.2. Paffenbarger and his colleagues (1994) point out how a change in the downward path of the second sequence can result in a return to the beneficial status of the first. In other words, an inactive person who changes his or her behaviour by becoming more physically active will regain fitness, may avoid cardiovascular diseases, and may expect to live longer.

Although there are limited longitudinal studies looking at reduced risk of diseases and physical activity of people with disabilities, there have been some concerns regarding the poor physical fitness of adults with a disabilty and the decline in fitness levels with aging (Graham and Reid 1998). The thirteen-year follow-up study found a significantly larger decline in health-related fitness components of adults with an intellectual disability compared to what was expected in the general population. Spirduso (1997) emphasized how participation in physical activity has played a significant role in delaying the debilitating effects of aging. Physical activity can serve as a preventative measure for chronic systemic and metabolic diseases and can improve quality of life and physical independence in the older population (Spirduso 1997). The incidence of many disabilities increases with age. For instance, of the 4.2 million Canadians with a disability, 70 percent are over the age of fifty-five (Statistics Canada 1995). One can see the potential health benefits of participating in physical activity throughout the lifespan for all people, with or without a disability.

Health and physical activity professionals need to recognize that people with a disability can enjoy an improved quality of life and, in some cases, increase or maintain their functional independence if they incorporate physical activity into their daily lives. Essentially, they could off-set lifestyle diseases and enjoy healthier and longer lives. Clearly, an appreciation of these advantages makes it worthwhile for fitness appraisers to provide services to people with a disability.

Figure 22. 2 Sequences A and B: A Change in the Downward Path of Sequence B Can Result in a Return to the Beneficial Status of Sequence A.

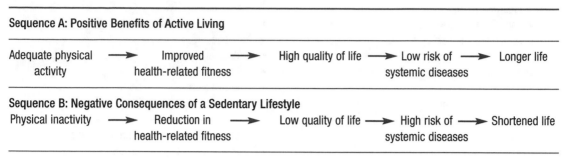

Sequence A: Positive Benefits of Active Living

Adequate physical activity → Improved health-related fitness → High quality of life → Low risk of systemic diseases → Longer life

Sequence B: Negative Consequences of a Sedentary Lifestyle

Physical inactivity → Reduction in health-related fitness → Low quality of life → High risk of systemic diseases → Shortened life

SOURCE: Adapted from Paffenbarger et al. 1994.

---

3 If we believe that all Canadians have the right to enjoy an active lifestyle, and if we accept that appraisal and counselling services are an integral part of increasing their levels of physical activity, then how do we provide this service to *all* Canadians?

The Active Living Philosophy and Inclusion

The Canadian Society for Exercise Physiology has taken the initiative to ensure that the current CPAFLA programme is inclusive by developing guidelines for providing fitness appraisal services geared to people with a disability. The health benefits of living actively throughout the lifespan for people of all abilities is now clear. Prior to describing the progress in this area, a description of the physical activity-health-active living connection will be presented.

THE PHYSICAL ACTIVITY-HEALTH-ACTIVE LIVING CONNECTION

Physical activity, physical fitness, exercise, health and *active living* are all terms used to describe various "processes" or "states of being." However, these terms have specific meanings in the vocabulary of a fitness appraiser. First, let us distinguish between the terms *physical activity, exercise,* and *physical fitness* as they are used and defined in the CPAFLA by CSEP (1998a). *Physical activity* is defined as general body movements (leisure and non-leisure) resulting in an increase in resting energy expenditure. It includes a wide range of activities that may or may not be structured or systematic. *Exercise*, on the other hand, is a form of leisure physical activity that is planned, repetitive, and structured. Type, duration, quantity, and intensity are all variables of exercise that will influence its effect on physical fitness. Furthermore, the intent of most exercise is to improve physical fitness. *Physical fitness* is a set of attributes that are either health- or performance-related. Health-related fitness comprises those components (muscular strength, muscular endurance, flexibility, cardiovascular endurance, body composition) that exhibit a relationship with health status. A favourable state of health-related components of physical fitness will have a favourable effect on health. However, the implications of physical activity and physical fitness are fundamentally different because physical activity is a "process" and physical fitness is a "condition" (Paffenbarger et al. 1994). Although both are capable of favouring health and longevity, Paffenbarger and his colleagues describe *physical activity* as being dynamic, or an on-going concept, and *physical fitness* as being static, or a "cross-sectional" concept. However, they are intertwined because one's physical fitness establishes limits to participating in physical activity, and participating in physical activity modifies the state of one's fitness. Figure 22.3 depicts this relationship.

Figure 22.3 The Inter-relationship Between Physical Activity and Health-related Fitness

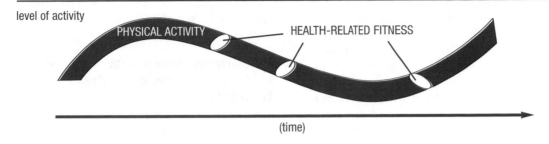

level of activity

PHYSICAL ACTIVITY

HEALTH-RELATED FITNESS

(time)

Health-related fitness is represented as a 'cross-sectional' concept that can establish benchmarks and limitations for physical activity. Physical activity is represented as an 'on-going' concept that modifies a person's health-related fitness from one state to the next, over time. A cross-section of health-related physical fitness at a 'peak' in one's participation in physical activity will differ from the same person's fitness profile during a 'valley'.

SOURCE: Adapted from "Some Interrelations of Physical Activity, Physiological Fitness, Health, and Longevity" by R.S. Paffenbarger Jr., et al., 1994, in C. Bouchard, R.J. Shephard, and T. Stephens (Eds.), *Physical Activity, Fitness and Health.* Champaign, IL: Human Kinetics. Adapted with permission.

People have different physical activity interests and goals. Some may choose competitive activities (e.g., soccer leagues), recreational groups (e.g., outdoors clubs), while others may choose a path of incorporating physical activity into their daily lives (e.g., cutting the grass, walking to work, etc.). In any case, if the activity continues over the lifespan, it will most certainly make a positive impact on health and longevity.

HEALTH AND ACTIVE LIVING

Health is a general term that represents a multidimentional state (physical, social, and psychological dimensions) which both physical activity and physical fitness are capable of favouring. Positive health is associated with a capacity to enjoy life and to withstand challenges. CSEP (1998a) describes health as a "resource" for everyday life and not merely as an absence of disease. By incorporating physical activity into one's daily life, a person has the potential to impact overall health and well-being positively. One way of attaining a state of good health and well-being is through *active living*. Active living includes meaningful and satisfying physical activity as an integral part of daily life. Active living recognizes the social, emotional, physical, intellectual, and

spiritual benefits that result from participation in regular physical activity. In this broad definition of active living, individuals can base their active living involvement on the activities that are most relevant and interesting to them, as well as those that accommodate their individual abilities and differences.

4 What do you think are the most popular physical activities among Canadians?

5 Do you think that activity preferences differ among people of varying abilities?

6 What activity first comes to mind when you think of a person in a wheelchair?

PHYSICAL ACTIVITY PREFERENCES AMONG CANADIANS

Canadian adults with a disability reported that they were most commonly involved in walking, gardening, exercising, cycling, swimming, and dancing (Statistics Canada 1995). In a survey of the general Canadian population aged twelve and over, the most popular form of leisure-time activity was walking, followed by gardening, and home exercising (Health Canada 1999). It is apparent that people with and without a disability participate in similar leisure-time physical activities that can be practiced without considerable equipment, expense, or displacement from the home or local community. Appraisers need to be aware of the many options that are available in the community, and they need to balance these activity options with the personal interests and individual functional characteristics when counselling clients of all abilities. Often, individuals are unaware of opportunities that exist beyond "traditional programmes for the disabled" such as horseback riding for the blind or wheelchair basketball. Clients can be equally uninformed of the potential health benefits derived from everyday leisure and non-leisure activities that are completely accessible.

7 When you think of the word *accessibility*, what comes to mind first? An activity choice? A facility structure? An equipment modification? An inclusive programme? Something else?

THE INCLUSIVE NATURE OF ACTIVE LIVING

Inclusion is the current philosophy that emphasizes the provision of services designed for all potential participants. While *integration* focusses on modifying or altering an activity to be accessible to an individual with a disability, physical activities can be initially designed to be accessible to people of varying abilities. Even among people without a disability, abilities and experiences will differ. Physical activity professionals need to offer a wide range of programmes and opportunities for physical activity, sport, recreation, and fitness that are accessible to people with diverse abilities. This is the core of the inclusion philosophy, and *active living* captures the essence of this inclusive approach to physical activity and fitness. The current CPAFLA programme has evolved to encourage active living and is particularly suited to servicing all

Canadians. Due to the inclusive nature of the active living approach, it is believed that many more people, including those with a disability, will find the CPAFLA programme appealing.

The Canadian Physical Activity, Fitness and Lifestyle Appraisal: The Basics and Its Evolution

In Canada, fitness appraisal has made important progress over the past two decades. The Canadian Standardized Test of Fitness (CSTF) was first published in the 1979 and went through three edition changes over the next seven years (Fitness Canada 1986). It was designed to provide a simple, safe, and standardized approach to assess health-related fitness, with comparative norms for Canadians fifteen to sixty-nine years of age. The underlying philosophy to this approach was prescriptive in nature. Appraisal results were intended to motivate clients to exercise more and develop a healthier lifestyle. The needs of a diverse range of abilities in the population (e.g., people with a disability) were not taken into account in the programme.

In 1987, the publication of the *Canadian Standardized Test of Fitness Interpretation and Counselling Manual* by the Canadian Society for Exercise Physiology was intended to fine-tune the appraisers' counselling skills in order to assist the client with activity choices. A seven-step model was used as a counselling guide and is still used today in the interpretation and guidance of the health-related fitness appraisal component of the CPAFLA. The fourth edition of the CSTF was renamed CPAFLA and is currently published and used in its second edition (Canadian Society for Exercise Physiology 1998a).

The current CPAFLA manual uses a broader perspective and a more contemporary approach to physical activity and fitness appraisal. The "prescriptive" approach which was based on a recommended formula of intensity, frequency, and duration of exercise, has given way to the "healthy and active living" approach, which values all types of physical activity as an integral part of daily life. This evolution is also reflected in the new national health and activity campaign. The ParticipACTION model (based on a more prescriptive approach to activity) has shifted to the more current Vitality model (resembling the values of the active living approach). Vitality uses an integrated approach to healthy living that shifts the focus away from rigid ideals and prescriptive exercise, toward a positive self-image and active living (Canadian Society for Exercise Physiology 1995). The focus today is for Canadians to get active by building physical activity into daily life, and the type and quantity of activity is addressed with a broader perspective.

8 How much physical activity is necessary in order to derive health-related benefits such as reduced risk of diseases and increased quality of life?

THE CHOICE AND VOLUME OF PHYSICAL ACTIVITY

A number of research developments in exercise physiology have helped to define the recommendations for physical activity in the current CPAFLA programme. In the past, vigorous and measureable activities such as running, swimming, and cycling, were emphasized to improve cardiovascular endurance, while weight-training regimens were used to improve muscular strength and endurance. Research now shows the considerable health benefits (e.g., lower blood pressure, decrease in body fat) of moderate-intensity physical activity even in the absence of concrete changes in traditional measures of physical fitness, such as aerobic power (Haskell 1994; Pate et al. 1995). Some health benefits are attainable at lower volumes of physical activity participation, where the 'volume' is the sum of all bouts of activity and can be attained through multiple combinations of frequency, intensity, and duration. This is summarized in the Dose-Response Relationship for Health Benefits and Volume of Physical Activity Participation (Canadian Society for Exercise Physiology 1998a) depicted in figure 22.4.

Figure 22.4 Dose-Response Relationship for Health Benefits and Volume of Physical Activity Participation

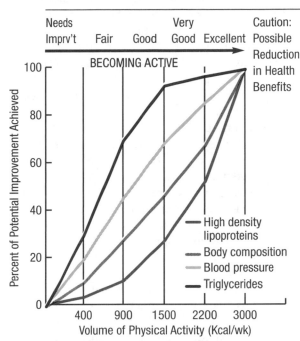

Note: To achieve improvements in many health benefit indicators, the volume of physical activity participation can be attained through any combination of frequency, intensity and duration, but improvements in Aerobic Fitness and Strength can only be achieved by working above a threshold intensity for an appropriate frequency and duration. With increasing exercise volume comes a beneficial blood pressure lowering effect and a decrease in body fat leading to overall healthier body composition, a decrease in blood Tg and an improved HDLP profile, which reduce the risk of cardiovascular disease. Schematic developed by N. Gledhill and V. Jamnik, York University.

SOURCE: From *The Canadian Physical Activity, Fitness and Lifestyle Appraisal Manual: CSEP's Plan for Healthy Active Living* (2nd ed.), 1998, by the Canadian Society for Exercise Physiology, Ottawa, Author. Copyrighted 1998 by the Canadian Society for Exercise Physiology. Reprinted with permission.

The figure shows that a considerable percentage in the potential improvement in health indicators, such as triglycerides and blood pressure, can be achieved at lower levels of physical activity. However, much of the improvement in other health indicators, such as body composition and high-density lipoproteins, requires higher volumes of physical activity. The 'volume' of physical activity is considered the sum of all bouts of activity, regardless of how short the duration. One should realize that the lower intensity, multiple bout, cumulative approach to physical activity will derive a limited number of health benefits. In order to attain measureable 'improvements' in aerobic fitness and muscular strength, one must pursue activities at a more vigorous level and on a continuous basis, such as working above a threshold intensity for an appropriate frequency and duration (Canadian Society for Exercise Physiology 1998a).

To translate this message to all Canadians in a less scientific manner, *Canada's Physical Activity Guide to Healthy Active Living* (Health Canada 1998) uses the catch phrase "Get active your way, every day–for life!" The time needed to acquire health benefits is dependent upon the effort. For example, light effort requires more accumulated time (sixty minutes), daily. For a sedentary individual this could mean incorporating physical activity, such as light housework, casual walking, or easy gardening, in periods of at least ten minutes each. Vigorous effort, on the other hand, requires less time (twenty-thirty minutes) per day. This would involve activities such as high-intensity aerobics, jogging, fast swimming, or even climbing several flights of stairs at a fast pace. Pate et al. (1995) concluded that adults should aim to accumulate a minimum of thirty minutes or more of moderate-intensity physical activity on most days of the week. Activities such as brisk walking or active gardening would constitute a moderate effort. Recall that more Canadians enjoy leisure walking, seconded by gardening, than any other form of exercise (Health Canada 1999). This serves as a strong basis for the active living philosophy. It is also good news to a great majority of Canadians who have not responded in the past to the prescriptive exercise approach, a model which often excluded the participation of people with a disability. Figure 22.5 depicts the time-effort relationship of physical activity and the range recommended to stay healthy.

There is an inverse relationship depicted in figure 22.5. Activities requiring light effort need to be performed over longer periods of time, or more bouts of shorter duration need to be accumulated. Activities requiring a more vigorous effort require less time. Health Canada (1998) recommends that a range in activity levels, types of activity, and duration of practice are needed to stay healthy. These alternatives are captured in the current CPAFLA programme, and the diverse choices in type of activity, intensity, and structure of practice is key to the counselling process.

CHANGING BEHAVIOUR THROUGH COUNSELLING

An important update in the counselling section of the CPAFLA is the extensive information on the stages and processes of change also called the "transtheoretical model." Prochaska and DiClemente (1983), originally described the transtheoretical model as one of the most effective approaches to lifestyle behaviour change. It is one of many behaviour change theories but its value is its practical application to lifestyle change. In practical terms, it helps to establish the motivational level and 'readiness' of the client regarding activity and other lifestyle changes. More specifically, however, the model includes five stages of change (i.e., precontemplation, contemplation, preparation, action, and maintenance) and two processes of change (i.e., ten experiential and behavioural processes). A more detailed list of the stages and processes of change with an example of behaviour change is available in Appendix 22.A. The CPAFLA programme teaches fitness appraisers that people typically cycle through the five stages of change when attempting to modify a behaviour. The processes of change provide

Figure 22.5 Time Needed to Improve Health is Dependent on the Effort

Time-Effort Relationship

Minimal or No Health and Fitness Benefits	Light Effort Accumulate 60 minutes every day	Moderate Effort Accumulate 30–60 minutes 4–7 days/week	Vigorous Effort 20–30 minutes 4–7 days/week	Maximum Effort

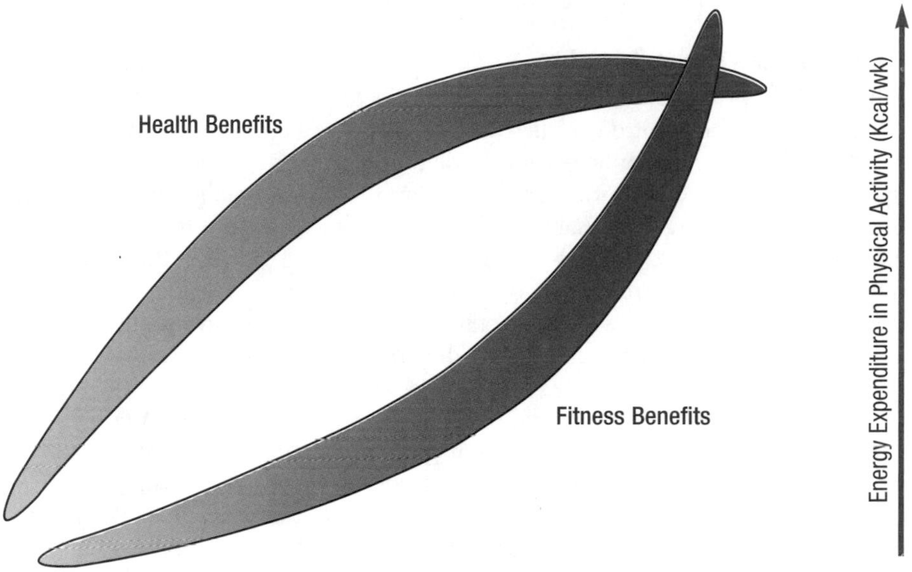

Energy Expenditure in Physical Activity (Kcal/wk)

Health Benefits

Fitness Benefits

	The greatest increase in health benefits occurs when you move from being inactive (little or no activity) to accumulating 60 minutes of light activity daily.	Small increases in fitness occur with light activities. Health benefits may occur without significant changes in body weight.	Additional health and fitness benefits occur when you build up to moderate and vigorous activities.	Too much maximal effort activity may result in health problems.
dusting seated activites	light walking gardening vacuuming Tai Chi	brisk walking biking swimming dancing water aerobics	jogging fast cycling aerobics hockey basketball	sprinting racing training for performance competition

SOURCE: From *Canada's Physical Activity Guide to Healthy Active Living*, 1998, by Health Canada. Ottawa: Author. Copyrighted 1998 by Health Canada. Reprinted with permission.

strategies for the appraiser to help influence a client's feelings about activity and to help people take action. This section draws the link between self-esteem and the crucial role it plays in lifestyle changes. The intention is to provide fitness appraisers with the necessary skills to guide clients in decision making and selecting appropriate alternatives regarding physical activity and other lifestyle behaviours.

The Canadian Commitment to Inclusive Appraisal Services

In 1993, CSEP committed itself to review its existing programmes, policies, and leadership training to better accommodate the needs and interests of people with a disabilty. The society formed a committee entitled the Leadership Development Initiative for People with a Disability (LDI-PWAD), which is still active today. Initially, the primary objective of the LDI-PWAD committee was to review fitness appraisal practices for people with sensory, physical, or intellectual disabilities and to establish physical activity and fitness assessment standards and guidelines for professionals directing programmes for people with a disability. The committee produced a resource document to help make appraisal services more accessible to people with a disability. The Supplementary Training Module (STM) for fitness appraisers already certified by CPAFLA programme standards includes a manual and training workshop available through the CSEP National Office (see Appendix 22.B).

THE RESOURCE DOCUMENT

The recommendations and comprehensive reviews of the scientific literature on physical activity, fitness appraisal, and counselling implications for people with a disability are available in a resource document entitled *Recommendations for the Fitness Assessment, Programming, and Counselling of Persons with a Disability* (Canadian Society for Exercise Physiology 1998b). The publication contributed three important elements to the fitness appraisal process: a) a background section containing fifty recommendations for fitness assessment, programming, and counselling of

people with a disability; b) three review papers encompassing musculoskeletal, neurological, sensory, and intellectual disability implications for fitness appraisal; and c) a list of Canadian organizations relevant to active living programmes for people with a disability. The resource document is available through the CSEP national office. See Appendix 22.B for more information.

THE SUPPLEMENTARY TRAINING MODULE

The Canadian Society for Exercise Physiology (1998b) recommended that fitness appraisers who lack training in APA need theoretical knowledge about disabilities and need more exposure to people with a disability in order to service them adequately. Consequently, the LDI-PWAD committee developed a comprehensive manual that could be used to supplement the training of fitness appraisers within the CPAFLA programme. The companion document to the CPAFLA manual is entitled *INCLUSIVE FITNESS AND LIFESTYLE SERVICES FOR ALL disABILITIES* (Canadian Society for Exercise Physiology, 2002). The purpose of this publication is to provide theoretical knowledge and practical training for fitness appraisers to provide safe and adequate fitness appraisal services to people with a disability. Appraisers with a current certification (CFC or PFLC) and at least one year of experience working as a fitness consultant can apply to attend a training workshop. Experience working with people with a disability is not required in order to attend the inclusion STM. Fitness appraisers can now be trained to provide services to a much broader spectrum of the population. For more information on CPAFLA training workshops, see Appendix 22.B.

Recommendations for Fitness Appraisal for People With a Disability

The Canadian Society for Exercise Physiology (1998b) recognized that fitness appraisers who serve the general population were often reluctant to include individuals with a disability in assessment, programming, and counselling activities. The first recommendation made by

CSEP attempted to address this reluctance and to steer the CPAFLA programme toward more inclusive services for people with a disability.

> RECOMMENDATION 1: The proportion of individuals with a disability who are currently excluded from fitness testing and programmes is excessive. Appropriate programmes and facilities should be provided to allow all individuals to pursue active living. (Canadian Society for Exercise Physiology 1998b, p. 119)

Forty-nine additional recommendations for inclusive fitness appraisal services for people with a disability were divided into the following categories: facilities, training personnel, enhancing communication, screening, informed consent, fitness testing protocols, and counselling. Most of these recommendations have been addressed in the inclusive STM. The following sections will highlight some of the important recommendations made by the LDI-PWAD committee. These recommendations will be substantiated by information outlined in the review papers on physical, sensory, and cognitive disability considerations for fitness appraisal (Canadian Society for Exercise Physiology 1998b) and accompanied by some practical guidelines from the STM (Canadian Society for Exercise Physiology, 2002).

FACILITIES

Inclusive fitness facilities have programmes that are designed to be accessible to people of all abilities. Programme access refers to the use of accessible instructional techniques, the creation of an open and accepting environment, as well as the provision of physical access to the facility. Exercise facilities or sports establishments are the focuses of several recommendations.

In some cases, the physical design of a fitness facility is a barrier to the participation of a person with a disability (Longmuir 1998). The more commonly known modifications that can be made to most existing facilities, such as enlarged washrooms, doorways, access to elevators, wheelchair ramps, and handicapped parking spaces, are largely implemented through municipal by-laws and building codes. Less obvious modifications are aimed to ensure client safety and might include emergency warning systems and procedures for evacuations available in a variety of formats (e.g., flashing lights, loud alarms, etc.) and are not generally implemented. In addition, accessibility to working animals (e.g., seeing eye dogs) must be extended in exercise programmes and facilities.

> RECOMMENDATION 3: High priority should be given to retrofitting existing facilities and programmes to accommodate people with disabilities. (Canadian Society for Exercise Physiology 1998b, p. 121)

However, making sure that new facilities are initially designed to be accessible is most effective and cost efficient.

Often, individuals with a disability can use standard fitness equipment when given the opportunity (Steadward 1998). Fitness appraisers should be aware that when they are unsure about the appropriateness of standard test items or test equipment with respect to their client's disability, the client can be the best resource.

> RECOMMENDATION 4: Fitness appraisers should be encouraged to consult with participants about optimal arrangements for their needs during exercise testing and prescription. (Canadian Society for Exercise Physiology 1998b, p. 121)

TRAINING PERSONNEL AND ENHANCING COMMUNICATION

When training fitness appraisers to provide services to people with a disability using the STM, time is devoted to developing positive attitudes, understanding the functional implications of disability on fitness appraisal, developing resourcefulness, and refining communication skills. CSEP recognized that, in order to encourage active living and lifestyle changes, staff should be comfortable and qualified to work with all people regardless of disability.

RECOMMENDATION 12: Training sessions should examine fitness appraisers' fears and attitudes, provide opportunities to interact with citizens with disabilities, and enable personnel to experience disabilities. Sessions should emphasise the need for sensitivity, so fitness appraisers do not develop patronising attitudes toward people with disablities. (Canadian Society for Exercise Physiology 1998b, p. 122)

Misconceptions also exist about various disabilities. For example, many people equate being blind with seeing 'nothing', when in fact many people who are blind can see some degree of light or shadow. Another common mistake, according to Longmuir (1998), is extending the physical effects of a disability to other senses or functions. For example, speaking louder does not help a blind person understand. In addition to these misconceptions, some people base their knowledge of disabilities on famous portrayals of people with a disability. An example of this is the autistic savant portrayed by Dustin Hoffman in the film *Rainman*. In reality, not all people with autism have highly developed splinter skills such as memory or mathematics.

RECOMMENDATION 13: Training sessions for fitness appraisers should address prevalent myths and misconceptions about disabilities. (Canadian Society for Exercise Physiology 1998b, p. 122)

The STM provides information and training to enable appraisers to focus on individuals rather than disabilities. One of the practical components of the STM is the provision of practice sessions using appraisal techniques with volunteer clients with a disability.

SCREENING PROCESS AND INFORMED CONSENT

The nature of some disabilities may hinder screening and the process of obtaining informed consent. However, using the PAR-Q to screen all clients, including individuals with a disability, is necessary prior to proceeding with the active components of the health-related fitness appraisal. Longmuir

(1998) stated that providing the PAR-Q in other media formats (audio, large print, or Braille) would be helpful to hearing or visually impaired individuals.

RECOMMENDATION 15: All testing and counselling materials must be reviewed for comprehensibility and availability in alternative media formats (audio or large print PAR-Q). In response to this recommendation, the STM has made all screening and information gathering tools in original and alternate formats available on CD-ROM. (Canadian Society for Exercise Physiology, 2002)

It might also be difficult for many people with an intellectual disability to complete the PAR-Q and to communicate accurate information about their medical history (Seidl 1998). In some cases, a primary caregiver or caseworker will need to provide some assistance to clients, such as reading the questions or recording their responses. Interpreting the questions, however, will require a review of the strict policies in place within the CPAFLA programme.

RECOMMENDATION 21: Since current PAR-Q procedures prohibit fitness appraisers from extensively interpreting or clarifying the form, reconsidering procedures is strongly recommended to accommodate people with sensory or cognitive impairments. (Canadian Society for Exercise Physiology 1998b, p. 124)

The original version of the PAR-Q is available in Appendix 22.C. If a person with a disability had difficulty with reading, organizing, or processing information, then understanding the details of the PAR-Q or completing the form could be problematic.

In many cases, there is also a need for gathering additional information about the functional abilities of a client with a disability. The Abilities for Active Living Questionnaire (AAL-Q) or the AAL-Q and You (Canadian Society for Exercise Physiology, 2002) was developed as part of the STM. It was designed to identify conditions that may affect a person's ability to perform certain tasks that are pertinent to the appraisal process or to becoming physically active. It is also helpful to generate information for the fitness appraiser to make appropriate preparations and modifications to the CPAFLA. To view the AAL-Q and You, see Appendix 22.D. The AAL-Q and You is not a substitute for the PAR-Q but should be administered in conjunction with it when servicing a client with a disability. Assisting a client to complete or interpret the AAL-Q is permitted.

Adults with a disability can give legal consent to participate in a fitness test or programme. However, in the case of a person with an intellectual disability, the fitness appraiser may be in doubt as to a client's full understanding of test procedures and expectations for which he or she is expected to give consent. Seidl (1998) suggested that using a combination of instructional videotapes, task simulations, and facility tours may be valuable options to assist in the client's familiarization and understanding of a fitness test. Sometimes, consent forms will be cosigned by caregivers or other support personnel.

RECOMMENDATION 24: Informed consent should be obtained after familiarizing clients with the test setting, staff, procedures, and expectations. (Canadian Society for Exercise Physiology 1998b, p. 124)

FITNESS TESTING PROTOCOL

Personal characteristics of people with a disability (eg., level of intellectual functioning, adaptive skill behaviours, degree of sensory impairment, level of spinal injury, etc.) largely influence which testing methods are useful for fitness testing and counselling. In order to obtain valid and reliable fitness measures for people with a disability, modifying standard test procedures is often necessary.

RECOMMENDATION 27: The standard CPAFLA protocol requires modifications to accommodate people with different disabilities. (Canadian Society for Exercise Physiology 1998b, p. 125)

Steadward (1998) indicated that fitness tests may require systematic equipment and/or procedural modifications. For example, an arm-crank ergometre is often used to test the aerobic fitness of people with spinal cord injuries. Because health and function may relate more closely to submaximal than to maximal aerobic exercise responses, a submaximal test protocol should be included.

RECOMMENDATION 38: Irrespective of methodology, the aerobic test protocol should reflect the body's response to low exercise levels. (Canadian Society for Exercise Physiology 1998b, p. 127)

Some test items in the CPAFLA may require modifications to procedures. Steadward (1998) suggested that anthropometric measurements can be complicated by the level of spinal cord injury.

RECOMMENDATION 35: A general rule of thumb when conducting anthropometric measurements is to evaluate skinfold sites where functional muscle exists. (Canadian Society for Exercise Physiology 1998b, p. 126)

Other CPAFLA test items may require alternative test measures when testing people with a disability. For instance, Steadward (1998) reported that the validity of the flexibility measure can be influenced by lack of innervation in muscle tissue (e.g., spinal cord injuries).

RECOMMENDATION 39: Joint specific flexibility tests will usually be required when assessing individuals with a disability. The Leighton flexometer should be an alternative test method for individuals whose disability precludes a valid sit-and-reach test. (Canadian Society for Exercise Physiology 1998b, p. 127)

Muscular endurance is assessed through the push-up and curl-up protocols of the CPAFLA. For many people with a disability, these exercises can be completed with minor modifications which should not affect interpretation of the results. For example, a visual timing prompt can be used for deaf individuals

(Longmuir 1998). Using equipment such as a leg brace or an inclined surface may enable a person with a low level spinal injury to complete the protocol (Steadward 1998). All test modifications should be recorded clearly to ensure replication during subsequent tests often used to document progress in individuals. In some cases, alternative measures of muscle fitness may be required.

> RECOMMENDATION 41: Alternative measures of muscle strength and endurance should be developed for people with disabilities. For example, a bench press or biceps curl should be investigated as a measure of muscular endurance for individuals whose disability precludes push-ups or curl-ups. (Canadian Society for Exercise Physiology 1998b, p. 127)

The STM includes information on how to use standard equipment and protocols with a client with a disability. It also provides extensive information on alternative protocols and when they should be used with a client with a disability. This includes modified techniques in standard measurements as well as data recording. Appraisers with only standard CFC training must refer clients with a disability to appraisers with more advanced training (PFLC) for the completion of any alternative protocols (Canadian Society for Exercise Physiology, 2002).

FITNESS AND LIFESTYLE COUNSELLING

The specific actions taken or resources and tools used within each step of the the appraisal process may be modified, in accordance with the appraiser's training, depending on the goals and abilities of each client. Fitness testing and counselling aspects of the appraisal process must be done within the consultant's scope of practice. The counselling phase of fitness appraisal for people with a disability aims to do much the same as for people without a disability. Essentially, fitness testing results are reviewed, a needs assessment and overview of current activity and lifestyle habits are conducted, realistic goals are discussed, a programme is recommended, and a means for follow-up and review are generally established.

> RECOMMENDATION 46: Counselling relevant to an individual's needs should include both an interpretation of test results and appropriate activity and lifestyle prescription and outcome measures. (Canadian Society for Exercise Physiology 1998b, p. 129)

Seidl (1998) suggested that people with a disability should be counselled to participate in activities that are meaningful, feasible, generalizable to health and function, community-based, safe, and chosen by the individual. Although they may be unaware of a number of active living opportunities available to them, people with a disability should be encouraged by appraisers to come up with many of their own ideas or solutions for physical activity or lifestyle behaviour changes (Canadian Society for Exercise Physiology, 2002).

In summary, the STM for providing *INCLUSIVE FITNESS AND LIFESTYLE SERVICES FOR ALL DISABILITIES* (Canadian Society for Exercise Physiology, 2002) has included several practical changes to materials and procedures as a supplement to the current CPAFLA. Some highlights found in the STM manual are listed in Appendix 22.E. During an intensive training workshop, fitness appraisers are given an opportunity to practice their practical testing and counselling skills on volunteer participants with a disability.

9 How can the CPAFLA programme continue to improve its accessibility?

10 What would constitute the 'ultimate' inclusive programme?

The CPAFLA and the STM: Broadening the Scope of Accessible Services

By making inclusive fitness appraisal and counselling services accessible to all Canadians, including those with a disability, the CPAFLA could potentially reach an additional 16 percent

Figure 22.6 Cyclical Model of Accessible Services

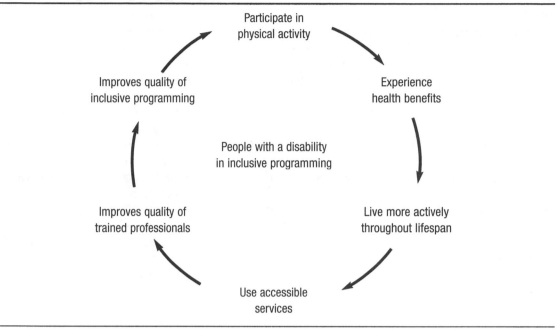

Participate in physical activity

Experience health benefits

People with a disability in inclusive programming

Live more actively throughout lifespan

Use accessible services

Improves quality of trained professionals

Improves quality of inclusive programming

Providing inclusive and accessible services to people with a disability will not only have a positive impact on their health and well-being, but will also serve to improve the fitness appraisal programme.

of the population (Canadian Society for Exercise Physiology 1998b). Trained fitness appraisers have a significant role to play in educating individuals with disabilties about the active living approach and the health benefits of participating in regular activity throughout the lifespan.

Previously, there was no standardized approach to ensuring the professional preparation of fitness appraisers. Sufficient knowledge about people with disabilities and the variety of activity options that remain available to them despite their physical, sensory, or intellectual challenges is critical. The resource document and the STM manual, designed as professional development supplements to the CPAFLA, aim to increase the knowledge base, competency, and confidence of appraisers working with people with a disability. Consequently, fitness appraisers should be able to provide safe and effective testing, programming, and counselling services to individuals with a disability. As more people with

disabilities become aware of inclusive and accessible services that are availabable to them, they will experience the health benefits of physical activity. As people with a disability make a positive impact on their health and well-being, they will be encouraged to live more actively across the lifespan. Finally, as fitness appraisers continue to encounter and service new clients with a variety of abilities and challenges, their experience will broaden, their competency will improve, and this will have a positive impact on inclusive services. This cycle of accessible services, depicted in figure 22.6 illustrates how an active living lifestyle can be promoted through the growth and development of accessible services.

Summary

This chapter outlined the importance of physical activity for all people. For example, the health benefits derived from physical activity are much the same for people with and without a disability. Much information about

Figure 22.7 Summary of the Changes and Developments of the CPAFLA

CSTF (earlier characteristics)	CPAFLA (present characteristics)	STM Manual (added features to current CPAFLA)
• performance-related	• health-related	• health-related
• based on single procedure	• options (client-related)	• additional procedures (e.g., modified protocols, etc.)
• emphasis on fitness	• emphasis on physical activity	• more emphasis on inclusion and active living
• focus on prescribed exercise	• considers broader lifestyle issues	• additional lifestyle issue considerations (e.g., functional ability)
• tests and measures	• information and advice	• additional counselling considerations (e.g., support networks)
• assumed readiness for change	• recognizes/helps 'nonmovers'	• additional lifestyle change considerations (e.g., additional barriers)
• appraisal-reappraisal on client	• various scenarios depending	• increased possibilities and scenarios (client)
		• increased theoretical knowledge (appraiser)
		• increased practical training (appraiser)

Columns 1 and 2 summarize changes in the CPAFLA programme over the past twenty years (Canadian Society for Exercise Physiology 1998a). Column 3 identifies additional characteristics of the STM.

SOURCE: From *INCLUSIVE FITNESS AND LIFESTYLE SERVICES FOR ALL DISABILITIES*, 2002, Canadian Society for Exercise Physiology, Ottawa: Author. Reprinted with permission.

the various physical, psychological, and socio-emotional challenges faced by people with a disability have enabled us to provide better physical activity services and opportunities for them. Yet it has taken several decades for society to embrace the concept of inclusion.

The current CPAFLA has evolved into more than a standardized test battery of health-related fitness and a prescription for increased activity. It emphasizes healthy and active living as well as an understanding of many factors that influence lifestyle change. The development of the STM has made the appraisal programme inclusive for people of all abilities. Figure 22.7 summarizes the many changes that have been incorporated into the CPAFLA and the STM.

All of these changes make fitness appraisal services more appealing and accessible to a broader range of individuals (Canadian Society for Exercise Physiology 1998b). Expanding the CPAFLA to include people with disabilities through its provision of additional training adds several characteristics that make it more inclusive. Canada is taking a leadership role in making appraisal services inclusive and accessible and by promoting active living for all people. The committment to develop and deliver a training module that specifically addresses the testing, programming, and counselling needs of people with a disability has been a major step in achieving that goal. The future of the STM will be largely determined by how extensively it is embraced by the fitness appraisal community and how successful appraisal services are in reaching more Canadians of all abilties.

The LDI-PWAD committee would like to see the future growth of the CPAFLA programme infuse the information and training currently available in the STM. This would help to ensure that the initial training of certified fitness appraisers is inclusive and enables them to provide inclusive fitness and lifestyle services to people of all abilities without seeking supplementary training. Now that would truly define inclusive programming!

Study Questions

1. Why should fitness appraisers provide inclusive fitness and lifestyle counselling for people with a disability?
2. How has the definition of *disability*, changed over the last twenty years?
3. Briefly describe the active living approach and how it is compatible with the inclusion philosophy?
4. What are the main changes in the fitness appraisal programme (CPAFLA) and how has it become more inclusive?
5. What are the current recommendations for physical activity participation and why is this more appealing for people of all abilities?
6. Can you think of two recommendations for inclusive fitness appraisal made by CSEP (1998)? Explain what outcomes have been developed in the STM in response to these recommendations.

References

Bhambhani, Y.N., Eriksson, P., and Gomes, P.S. (1991). Transfer effects of endurance training with arms and legs. *Medicine Science in Sport and Exercise, 23,* 1025–41.

Bhambhani, Y.N., Holland, L.J., and Steadward, R.D. (1993). Maximal aerobic power in cerebral palsied wheelchair athletes: Validity and reliability. *Archives in Physiology, Medicine, and Rehabilitation, 73,* 246–52.

Canadian Society for Exercise Physiology. (2002). *INCLUSIVE FITNESS AND LIFESTYLE SERVICES FOR ALL disABILITIES.* Ottawa. Author.

Canadian Society for Exercise Physiology. (2002). *Physical Activity Readiness Questionnaire: PAR-Q and you.* Ottawa: Author.

Canadian Society for Exercise Physiology. (1998a). *The Canadian physical activity, fitness and lifestyle appraisal manual: CSEP's plan for healthy active living* (2nd ed.). Ottawa: Author.

Canadian Society for Exercise Physiology. (1998b). Recommendations for the fitness assessment, programming, and counselling of persons with a disability. *Canadian Journal of Applied Physiology, 23*(2), 119–30.

Canadian Society for Exercise Physiology. (1995). *Vitality: Update for fitness appraisers.* Ottawa: Author.

Canadian Society for Exercise Physiology. (1987). *Canadian Standardization Test of Fitness Interpretation and Counselling Manual.* Ottawa: Author.

Fitness Canada. (1986). *Canadian Standardized Test of Fitness* (3rd ed.). Ottawa: Fitness and Amateur Sport.

Graham, A., and Reid. G. (1998). *Physical fitness of persons with an intellectual disability: A 13-year follow-up study.* Unpublished master's thesis. Montreal: McGill University.

Haskell, W.L. (1994). Dose-response issues from a biological perspective. In C. Bouchard, R.J. Shephard, and T. Stephens (Eds.), *Physical activity, fitness and health.* Champaign, IL: Human Kinetics.

Health Canada. (1999). *National population health survey highlights: Physical activity of Canadians, cycle 2, 1996/97.* Ottawa: Author.

Health Canada. (1998). *Canada's physical activity guide to healthy active living.* Ottawa: Author.

Johnson, N.A., and Heller, R.F. (1998). Prediction of patient nonadherence with home-based exercise for cardiac rehabilitation: The role of perceived barriers and perceived benefits. *Preventive Medicine, 27*(1), 56–64.

Longmuir, P. (1998). Considerations for fitness appraisal, programming and counselling of individuals with sensory impairments. *Canadian Journal of Applied Physiology, 23*(2), 166–84.

Montgomery, D.L., Reid, G., and Koziris, L.P. (1992). Reliability and validity of three fitness tests for adults with mental handicaps. *Canadian Journal of Sport Sciences, 17,* 309-15.

Montgomery, D.L., Reid, G., and Seidl, C. (1988). The effects of two physical fitness programmes designed for mentally retarded adults. *Canadian Journal of Sport Sciences, 13,* 173–78.

Noreau, L., and Shephard, R.J. (1995). Spinal cord injury, exercise and quality of life. *Sports Medicine, 20*(4), 226–50.

Paffenbarger, R.S. Jr., Hyde, R.T., Wing, A.L., Lee, I.M., and Kampert, J.B. (1994). Some interrelations of physical activity, physiological fitness, health, and longevity. In C. Bouchard, R.J. Shephard, and T. Stephens (Eds.), *Physical Activity, Fitness and Health.* Champaign, IL: Human Kinetics.

Pate, R.R., Pratt, M., Blair, S.N., Haskell, W.L., Macera, C.A., Bouchard, C., Buchner, D., Ettinger, W., Heath, G.W., and King, A.S. (1995). Physical activity and public health: A recommendation from the Centres for Disease Control and Prevention and the American College of Sports Medicine. *Journal of the American Medical Association, 273*(5).

Prochaska, J.O., and DiClemente, C.C. (1983). Stages and processes of self-change in smoking: Towards an integrative model of change. *Journal of Consulting and Clinical Psychology, 51.*

Seidl, C. (1998). Considerations for fitness appraisal, programming and counselling of people with intellectual disabilities. *Canadian Journal of Applied Physiology, 23*(2), 185–211.

Seidl, C., Montgomery, D.L., and Reid, G. (1989). Stair stepping efficiency of mentally handicapped and non-handicapped adult females. *Ergonomics, 32,* 519–26.

Shephard, R.J. (1990). *Fitness in special populations.* Champaign, IL: Human Kinetics.

Statistics Canada. (1995). *A portrait of persons with disabilities.* Ottawa: Author.

Steadward, R. (1998). Musculoskeletal and neurological disabilities: Implications for fitness appraisal, programming and counselling. *Canadian Journal of Applied Physiology, 23*(2), 131–65.

Spirduso, W. (1997). *Human aging: Universal exposure to physical disability.* Paper presented at the meeting of the 11th International Symposium for Adapted Physical Activity. Quebec City, Quebec.

World Health Organization. (2001). *International Classification of Function.* Geneva: Author.

World Health Organization. (1980). *International Classification of Impairments, Disabilities, and Handicaps.* Geneva: Author.

APPENDIX 22.A List of the Stages and Processes of Change in the Transtheoretical Model

Stages of Change	Example Behaviour
1. Pre-contemplation	Client has no intention of making a change (e.g., does not feel the need to be active)
2. Contemplation	Client is considering making changes (e.g., perhaps activity is a good idea)
3. Preparation	Client begins to make small changes (e.g., increases activity patterns a little)
4. Action	Client actively engages in new behaviours (e.g., now doing regular activity)
5. Maintenance	Client sticks with the behaviour change (e.g., remains active through the lifespan)

Processes of Change

1. Experiential	Strategies most often used with client in the first three stages of change
• increasing awareness	e.g., reading articles about exercise
• altering feelings	e.g., reacting emotionally to information
• recognizing alternatives	e.g., awareness of better food choices and activity options
• assessing personal impact	e.g., regular activity will improve health
• assessing environmental impact	e.g., being active will have impact on others by being a positive influence

2. Behavioural	Strategies most often used with client in the last three stages of change
• increasing commitment	e.g., recognizing the power to change
• substituting	e.g., replacing new/positive behaviours for old
• recognizing the barriers	e.g., avoiding people or places that negatively influence old behaviors
• rewarding	e.g., rewarding positive behaviours
• enhancing support	e.g., someone else for support

APPENDIX 22.B Resources available from the Canadian Society for Exercise Physiology

List of Publications:

Recommendations for the Fitness Assessment, Programming, and Counselling of Persons With a Disability. *Canadian Journal of Applied Physiology, (23)*2, April, 1998.

The Canadian Physical Activity, Fitness and Lifestyle Appraisal (CPAFLA): CSEP's Plan for Healthy Active Living, 2nd ed., 2001.

INCLUSIVE FITNESS AND LIFESTYLE SERVICES FOR ALL disABILITIES. (2002).

To obtain copies of these publications or to obtain information about CPAFLA certification courses, contact:

    The Canadian Society for Exercise Physiology
    185 Somerset St. West, Suite 202
    Ottawa, Ontario, Canada K2P 0J2

    E-mail: info@csep.ca
    Phone: (613) 234–3755, Fax: (613) 234-3565, Toll-free: 1–877–651–3755
    Internet: http://www.csep.ca

Physical Activity Readiness
Questionnaire - PAR-Q
(revised 2002)

PAR-Q & YOU

(A Questionnaire for People Aged 15 to 69)

Regular physical activity is fun and healthy, and increasingly more people are starting to become more active every day. Being more active is very safe for most people. However, some people should check with their doctor before they start becoming much more physically active.

If you are planning to become much more physically active than you are now, start by answering the seven questions in the box below. If you are be of 15 and 69, the PAR-Q will tell you if you should check with your doctor before you start. If you are over 69 years of age, and you are not used to be check with your doctor.

Common sense is your best guide when you answer these questions. Please read the questions carefully and answer each one honestly: check Y

YES	NO		
☐	☐	1.	Has your doctor ever said that you have a heart condition <u>and</u> that you should only do physical activity recommended by a doctor?
☐	☐	2.	Do you feel pain in your chest when you do physical activity?
☐	☐	3.	In the past month, have you had chest pain when you were not doing physical activity?
☐	☐	4.	Do you lose your balance because of dizziness or do you ever lose consciousness?
☐	☐	5.	Do you have a bone or joint problem (for example, back, knee or hip) that could be made worse by a change in your physical activity?
☐	☐	6.	Is your doctor currently prescribing drugs (for example, water pills) for your blood pressure or heart condition?
☐	☐	7.	Do you know of <u>any other reason</u> why you should not do physical activity?

If you answered

YES to one or more questions

Talk with your doctor by phone or in person BEFORE you start becoming much more physically active or BEFORE you have a fitness appraisal. Tell your doctor about the PAR-Q and which questions you answered YES.

- You may be able to do any activity you want — as long as you start slowly and build up gradually. Or, you may need to restrict your activities to those which are safe for you. Talk with your doctor about the kinds of activities you wish to participate in and follow his/her advice.
- Find out which community programs are safe and helpful for you.

NO to all questions

If you answered NO honestly to <u>all</u> PAR-Q questions, you can be reasonably sure that you can:
- start becoming much more physically active — begin slowly and build up gradually. This is the safest and easiest way to go.
- take part in a fitness appraisal — this is an excellent way to determine your basic fitness so that you can plan the best way for you to live actively. It is also highly recommended that you have your blood pressure evaluated. If your reading is over 144/94, talk with your doctor before you start becoming much more physically active.

DELAY BECOMING MUCH MORE ACTIVE:
- if you are not feeling well because of a temporary illness such as a cold or a fever — wait until you feel better; or
- if you are or may be pregnant — talk to your doctor before you start becoming more active.

PLEASE NOTE: If your health changes so that you then answer YES to any of the above questions, tell your fitness or health professional. Ask whether you should change your physical activity plan.

<u>Informed Use of the PAR-Q</u>: The Canadian Society for Exercise Physiology, Health Canada, and their agents assume no liability for persons who undertake physical activity, and if in doubt after completing this questionnaire, consult your doctor prior to physical activity.

No changes permitted. You are encouraged to photocopy the PAR-Q but only if you use the entire form.

NOTE: If the PAR-Q is being given to a person before he or she participates in a physical activity program or a fitness appraisal, this section may be used for legal or administrative pu

"I have read, understood and completed this questionnaire. Any questions I had were answered to my full satisfaction."

NAME _____

SIGNATURE _____   DATE _____

SIGNATURE OF PARENT _____   WITNESS _____
or GUARDIAN (for participants under the age of majority)

Note: This physical activity clearance is valid for a maximum of 12 months from the date it is completed and becomes invalid if your condition changes so that you would answer YES to any of the seven questions.

CSEP/SCPE © Canadian Society for Exercise Physiology   Supported by: Health Canada / Santé Canada   continued on other side...

SOURCE: Reprinted from the 2002 revised version of the Physical Activity Readiness Questionnaire (PAR-Q and You). PAR-Q and You is a copyrighted, pre-exercise screen by the Canadian Society for Exercise Physiology.

AAL-Q & YOU
ABILITIES FOR ACTIVE LIVING QUESTIONNAIRE

Do you have a health condition or a disability which may affect the way in which you participate in physical activity and/or a fitness appraisal?

☐ Yes   ☐ No

If you answered yes to the above question, please assist us in providing the best possible service to meet your needs. Read the ten statements below. Indicate by checking "Yes" or "No" whether each statement applies to you. If you check "Yes" to a statement, please use the space provided to tell us more about your abilities or any adaptations that you make. For example, if you check "Yes" for Question #1 please provide information about the difficulty you have in moving from place to place, moving your legs, walking or running.

We encourage you to contact us or have a friend or family member assist you, if you have any questions or require clarification about these questions.

Do you have a condition that affects your ability to:

☐ Yes   ☐ No   1. Move from place to place, move your legs, walk or run?

☐ Yes   ☐ No   2. Grasp objects or move your hands or arms?

☐ Yes   ☐ No   3. Do activities that require a lot of strength?

☐ Yes   ☐ No   4. Move for long periods of time?

☐ Yes   ☐ No   5. Stretch or move your joints?

☐ Yes   ☐ No   6. Cooperate, socialize or interact with others or control your feelings?

☐ Yes   ☐ No   7. Complete tasks in the manner and time expected?

☐ Yes   ☐ No   8. See, hear, speak or feel things?

☐ Yes   ☐ No   9. Think, understand, remember or learn?

☐ Yes   ☐ No   10. Be active in any way not mentioned above?

_____

_____

_____

_____

If you have other information or reports on physical activity which you feel would help us to improve our services to you, please attach them to this form or bring them with you on your next visit.

INCLUSIVE FITNESS SERVICES **TOOL 4**

SOURCE: *INCLUSIVE FITNESS AND LIFESTYLE SERVICES FOR ALL disABILITIES*, 2002. Copyrighted by the Canadian Society for Exercise Physiology. Reprinted with permission.

APPENDIX 22.E Highlights of the Supplementary Training Module

- Definitions and background information on disabilities, health benefits of active living, and the inclusion philosophy
- A functional approach to analyzing physical activity
- Clarification of the definition of "apparently healthy" populations to include people with a disability
- The application of the stages of change theory in counselling people with a disability
- Protocols for alternate measurements of fitness for specific disabilities
- Included, as appendices to the manual, thirty-four tools for counselling people with a disability; questionnaires, forms, and information sheets in original and alternate formats
- Ten case studies on people with various functional ability profiles as alternative examples of test procedures, interpretation, and counselling techniques
- Included, as appendices, an extensive glossary of terms, classifications of disabilities, and fitness jargon, in simple language
- Included, as an appendix, basic sign language for relevant vocabulary
- Included, as an appendix, a list of resources and disability organizations

CHAPTER 23

Community Active Living Programming

Rick Gingras

Learning Objectives

- To differentiate between inclusive, segregated, and specialized active living programming as they relate to a "continuum of choice."
- To understand the need for specialized active living programming for people with a disability.
- To describe the considerations one must make when planning and implementing specialized active living programming.
- To appreciate the diverse needs of this target population and ensure that these needs are met through meticulous planning and input from consumers.

Introduction

The original focus of the fitness and active living movement of the latter quartile of the twentieth century was directed at the able-bodied population. With the movement towards inclusion and inclusive opportunities for persons with disability, it is not surprising that there has been a recent increased focus on provision of fitness and active living opportunities for this population. Up until the 1940s, activity programming for people with disability was unheard of. People were confined to institutions, bedridden, and treated as if they were fragile objects that would break if they attempted anything strenuous. Much has changed in the past couple of decades with the introduction of national strategies to encourage people to become active, such as ParticipACTION in Canada, the implementation of government policy such as the *Americans with a Disability Act* in the United States, the National Integration Strategy in Canada, the active living movement adopted in many countries, and, finally, the worldwide interest in high-performance sport specifically for people with a disability. More than ever before, individuals with disability are including physical activity as part of their lifestyles and are being included in the fitness and active living movement. However, there is still much more to be done to truly make active living a daily part of *everyone's* life—this is just the beginning. Much of what you will read in this textbook focusses on the concept of *inclusion*. In this chapter you will be introduced to the concept of *specialized active living programming for persons with disability*. At first, this might seem a contradiction given the focus of this text. In this chapter, the author challenges you to consider issues of choice in relation to active living programming for persons with disability.

A Matter of Choice?

A number of issues have arisen over the past decade with respect to active living and programme provision for people with disability. The most notable of these issues is whether agencies should provide segregated programming for people with disability, as opposed to providing inclusive programmes.

1 Why would people with disability need an environment where programmes are provided exclusively for people with disability? What assumptions about people with and without disability underlie claims that we need exclusive programmes?

According to the *Concise Oxford Dictionary of Current English* (Thompson 1995), to *segregate* means to "put apart from the rest or to isolate." Back in the days of institutionalization, segregation was rampant, but more to *protect* society from what they feared—people with disability. With increased awareness of the potential of people with disability, as well as high profile accomplishments such as Rick Hansen's Man in Motion World Tour and Terry Fox's Marathon of Hope, the view toward people with disability is changing. The demand and need for segregated programming still exists, but not to isolate people with disability, and not to protect people without

disability. Leading off the new millennium, *segregated programmes* need to refocus with emphasis on *specialized programmes* with the intention of providing choice to those who want a comfortable environment, based on their goals, needs, and abilities, to pursue their active living aspirations.

Specialized, as defined by the *Concise Oxford Dictionary of Current English* (Thompson 1995), is "to make specific or individual." Everyone has specific, or individual, needs. Whether it is lowering the volleyball net from the standard height for grade five students or providing skill instruction in wheelchair basketball, specialization should be viewed as choice in a continuum of active living opportunities. With specialized opportunities, we attempt to offer a wide range of active living opportunities that meet the specific needs of individuals rather than groups. That is, *individuals* make choices to pursue inclusive opportunities, to pursue specific activities that may be specially designed for a small percentage of the population, or to remain in a specialized environment and pursue lifelong active living interests. It is all a matter of choice.

With this 'matter of choice' in mind, this chapter has been created in conjunction with the model below (figure 23.1). Assuming that the person with disability chooses a 'specialized programme', then a series of considerations must be taken into account to provide this individual, or a group, with the best possible programme. This chapter will focus on how to provide specialized active living programming effectively for people with disability.

2 What personal and environmental circumstances might result in the choosing by people with disability to participate in a segregated, an integrated, or an inclusion-oriented active living programme?

The Need for Specialized Active Living Programming

Specialized programming specifically targets people with disability. As the result of a new awareness of the importance of active living,

Figure 23.1 Specialized Programming for Persons with a Disability

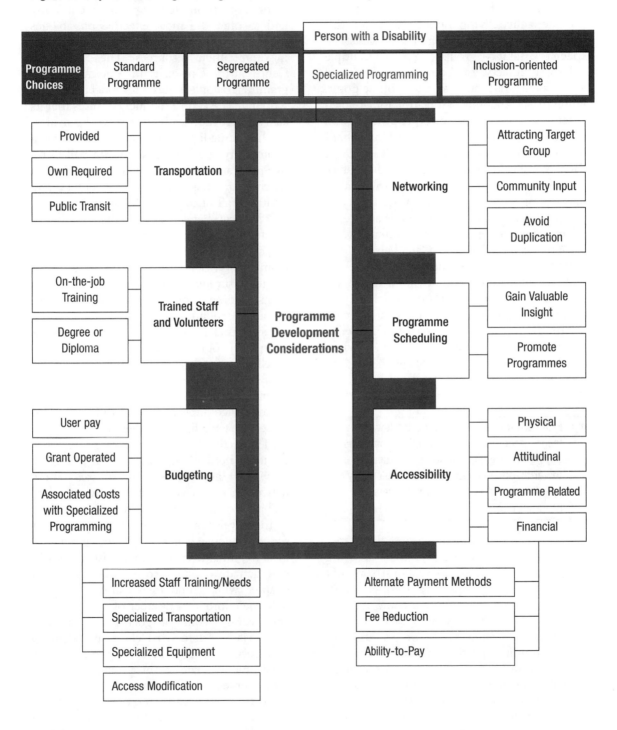

those with disability have, in the past few decades, created the need for new agencies to provide active living opportunities for this market. Many of these agencies focus on a specific disability group (e.g., The Multiple Sclerosis Society of Canada) or focus on activity for a particular segment of the population (e.g., Canadian Association for Disabled Skiers). Many of these organizations and agencies have both provincial and local chapters that offer programmes and services to their members. There are also a number of agencies with no affiliation with provincial or national agencies that offer a wide variety of programmes to meet the demands and needs of members of their own community. A resource created by the Canadian Abilities Foundation provides a central inventory, which includes up-to-date contact information for many of the agencies that provide active living programming in Canada. This nearly seven-hundred-page annual *Directory of Disability Organizations in Canada* (Cohen 1998) is an excellent tool for individuals who need to network with other organizations or to refer their clients effectively to appropriate services.

---

3 From what you have read so far, how do 'segregated' and 'specialized' programmes differ? What beliefs about, or attitudes towards, disability underlie the philosophy of specialized, as opposed to segregated, programmes?

One common thread among these specialized service providers is that most are nonprofit, or charitable, associations. Nonprofit associations are groups organized for a purpose other than to generate income or profit (Garner 1999). Although many of these agencies may be limited by donor contributions and/or nominal participant fees, the variety of services and programmes offered can range from a single activity programme, a local support group, a municipal recreation department, through to a multifaceted facility offering an extensive slate of active living programming.

Networking

In order to promote programmes efficiently and to offer the most effective possibilities within any community, agencies must maximize their resources. The Steadward Centre at the University of Alberta is a programme that illustrates the concept of networking. The centre routinely ensures that its staff actively meet with other service providers in the immediate community. This strong community relationship allows for collaborative programming, which often draws from a much larger base of possible clientele, and informs staff of opportunities in the community that can benefit their clients. One of the most effective local networks used by the Steadward Centre is the City of Edmonton Community Services Department's Interagency Committee. This committee, which exists in some form or another in many communities around the world, brings groups together that provide active living programming for people with a disability. This is an excellent networking opportunity, which could easily be initiated in any community to ensure effective communication and cooperation, to avoid service duplication, and to identify and fill service gaps through collaboration.

The second level of networking is regional. Regional networking can refer to a specific province, state, or geographical area. These networks are typically provincial or state umbrella agencies or committees. Networking at this level can provide a *larger picture,* or scope, for active living programming possibilities. Regional agencies often exist to coordinate activities conducted by their own local chapter, while committees will often coordinate the efforts of a number of agencies who act toward a common goal. For example, a provincial or state wheelchair sports group may exist to coordinate and support numerous local chapters within their zone who offer programmes to their members.

In the past decade, the need to network nationally has become more apparent with the development of groups such as the Active Living Alliance for Canadians with a Disability, a national group focussed on promoting inclusion and active living for Canadians with a disability. This alliance brings people with disability and professionals together nationally, with their annual forum, and locally to collaborate on raising awareness of active living opportunities within their own community. In addition to their annual forum, the alliance also provides publications and a web site for information dissemination.

Designing Accessible Facilities and Programmes

ACCESSIBILITY

Developing an accessible programme and activity environment is paramount to the success of providing specialized programming. *Access*, as defined by the *Concise Oxford Dictionary of Current English* (Thompson 1995), is "a way of approaching or reaching or entering." This definition, specifically the need for **physical** access, is often the only form of access considered when referring to matters surrounding disability. The dictionary extends its definition and refers to *access* as "the right or opportunity to reach, use, or visit." In this sense, accessibility of active living programmes extends to much more than just physical access. It includes what might be called *psychological access* ("Am I welcome in this facility and welcomed by the instructor and the other participants here?"). Specialized active living programming must provide a welcoming and 'comfortable environment', reasonable fees, activities of interest to a target population, and these must be accompanied by a psychological climate that facilitates a sense of belonging or inclusion. All too often inaccessible facilities thwart a person's interest by posing a barrier to participation. At the same time, accessible facilities and programme sites are more than buildings with a ramp, designated parking, and a wheelchair symbol on the door. True accessibility to a programme facility is quite dependent on the ability of the users and their perceptions of their own needs. Keeping this in mind and utilizing guidelines recommended regarding

Figure 23.2

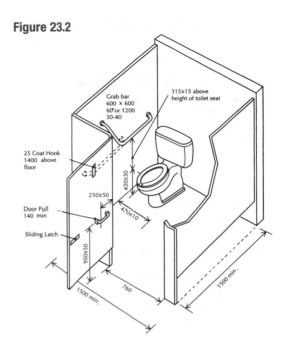

Grab bar
600 × 600
60° or 1200
30–40

315±15 above height of toilet seat

25 Coat Hook 1400 above floor

250±50

430±30

450±10

Door Pull 140 min

Sliding Latch

950±50

1500 min.

760

1500 min.

accessibility, facility administrators should begin with the minimum standards of physical accessibility.

Barrier-free design guides such as the one shown in figure 23.2 (Safety Codes Council 1999) provide facility administrators with recommendations for parking, facility entrance, customer service areas, change rooms and toilets, and even fire alarm systems. These guides are often available through government agencies that deal with architecture or labour standards and typically outline precise accessibility information, often to the millimetre, which include all aspects of the interior and exterior of a facility. These guides often publish 'minimum recommended standards', but following these recommended standards does not mean that the facility will be fully accessible to all. Every person's needs with respect to accessibility are highly personal based on individual ability.

In addition to physical accessibility, other considerations and issues related to the individual's needs will contribute to programme success. Matching the programme's objectives and logistics to the person's needs is foremost to the success of the programme

Figure 23.3 Accessibility Considerations—Facility Related Barrier-free Designs

❑ Is the signage accessible?

Is there adequate contrast between the letters and the background?
Are the letters large enough?
Are the signs in a logical (noticeable) place?

❑ Is the entrance accessible?

Are there exterior walks and ramps?
Are there curb cuts on walks and from the parking area?
Are the doors automatic or have power-assist?
Are there tactile warning signals to notify people with a visual impairment of danger or for way-finding?

❑ Are the washrooms accessible?

Is there an accessible stall?
Are there Braille, or raised letter, signs on entrance doors?
Are there grab bars for toilets and urinals?
Are there raised toilets or toilet seats?
Is the sink accessible with room underneath the sink, or vanity, for a wheelchair user?
Is a person in a wheelchair able to use the soap dispenser, mirror, faucets, and drying systems?

❑ Are the change rooms accessible?

Is there a unisex change room suitable to accommodate an attendant?
Is there an accessible shower stall, or area?
Are there grab bars and shower seats in the shower area?

❑ Do the facility or programme areas provide barrier-free paths of travel?

Are there overhead hazards?
If multilevel, are there elevator, ramp, or passenger elevating devices?
Does the elevator have audio and Braille controls and notification?
Are there stairs with colour-contrasting handrails?

❑ Is the reception/customer service area accessible?

Are there accessible public telephones?
Does the customer service area have a telecommunication device for the deaf (TDD)
for program registration and service inquiries?

❑ Is there accessible spectator seating?

❑ Will the fire safety system notify all participants (hearing, visual, and cognitive impairments)?

❑ Are there accessible parking and passenger loading areas?

and of the individual within it. Figure 23.3 contains further considerations related to programme accessibility.

PROGRAMME OBJECTIVES

The key to success from both a participant's standpoint and a facility standpoint is matching the programme objectives to the goals of the participants (see figure 23.4: Accessibility Considerations–Programming Related). Do the participants want to learn the skills necessary to integrate into other nonspecialized active living programmes, or are they looking for an accessible programme that provides the modifications that they require? Programme leaders and operators need to make the objectives of the programme clear so that the potential participants are clear on what they can expect and what they will actually get out of the programme. If the programme is designed to increase personal fitness or physical skills, this should be stated clearly. If it is designed for a combination of social interaction in a physical activity environment accommodating low skill and minimal levels of fitness and function, this should also be made clear.

TRANSPORTATION REQUIREMENTS

As a programme provider, the first decision to be made is whether or not transportation will be organized and offered to participants as part of the programme, or if the clients are responsible for arranging their own transportation.

Transportation requirements for individuals with disability are dependent on a number of factors. These factors include whether or not they have access to transportation; what transportation options are open to them in the community in which they live; their ability to coordinate, use, and pay for transportation; and whether they require assistance with any of the above.

Whether transportation is included in the programme or not can significantly affect the operation of any programme. People with disability and programme planners must contend with scheduling difficulties. As a programme planner, you must keep in mind that arranging for specialized transportation during peak times (early morning and late afternoon rush hours) may be rather difficult or impossible for your programme participants. For example, there is often a minimum advance-booking requirement to arrange for specialized transportation. Typically this requirement is twenty-four to forty-eight hours in advance of the time of travel. This may make it difficult for spontaneous use of programmes or short notice appointments.

SCHEDULING

Next to transportation scheduling, other issues may arise with respect to scheduling programmes for people with disability. One factor to consider is the population targeted for the programme. For example, Svensson, Gerdle, and Elert (1994) found that individuals with multiple sclerosis typically prefer programmes that are scheduled in the morning due to decreasing energy levels as the day progresses. Another consideration is using consistent times, days, and locations for programming. Individuals with cognitive impairment (e.g., traumatic brain injury, developmental disability) will respond to and adhere better to a structured and regularly scheduled programme since routine is an integral part of many individuals' day. By offering programmes at consistent times and during times conducive to the scheduling requirements of the potential participant, the success of the programme experience will be enhanced.

Involving People with Disability in Programme Planning

One of the most common criticisms with respect to programming for people with disability is that few are involved in the decision-making process. People with disability who intend to participate will provide valuable insight with respect to how they envision the programme proceeding. They can provide feedback on how to improve the programme and make it more enticing for others to participate. Issues such as transportation concerns, and comfort levels with instructors and

Figure 23.4 Accessibility Considerations—Programming Related

❏ Are the programmes scheduled so that people with a disability will be able to attend?

❏ Does any of the programming equipment need modification to accommodate people with disability?

❏ Are the participants expected to provide assistants if necessary?

If so, what is the criteria for them to know when they would be required to bring an assistant?
Are there assistants provided as part of the programme?

❏ Is there a fee reduction programme or method of alternate payment?

❏ Are the staff knowledgeable regarding adaptive programming?

❏ Do your screening measures collect adequate information to effectively provide adequate services?

❏ Did you effectively promote the programme, assuring individuals with disability are aware of your offerings?

❏ Did you network with other facilities, groups, or disability agencies to ensure adequate, efficient, and effective programming?

others can be solved before they become detrimental to the programme. This *buying-in* concept may also increase commitment of the participants as their responsibility for the operation of the programme is increased.

Programme Promotion

Promotion of programmes to people with disability is not too dissimilar to that of any targeted population. Distribution of flyers, posters, ready-to-print newsletter advertisements, mail-out inserts, brochures, and community displays are all effective to a degree, depending on the intended audience (Miller 1995). A number of free advertising alternatives exist as well in the form of public service announcements in print, radio, and television media, and community event bulletins (e.g., community newsletters or community league communications). All of these can reach the intended audience, but are also broad enough to reach individuals who know people who might benefit from a programme. A more focussed approach, which is often effective, is targeting specific groups that provide services to people with disability. Many of these agencies have regular mail-outs, community information guides, bulletin boards, or a newsletter that goes out to their members on a regular basis. Establishing a symbiotic working relationship by offering to reciprocate by promoting programmes and services is an effective means to promote programmes offered and inform your participants of other programmes that might benefit them. One notable addition for effective programme promotion within this target market is the power of 'word-of-mouth'. Although the community of people with disability is much larger than most people would imagine, it is a very cohesive network of individuals and groups. Use it as an inexpensive, effective way to promote your programmes and services.

Registration and Screening

REGISTRATION FORMS AND PREPARTICIPATION SCREENING

Like many other elements of programming for people with disability, the use of registration forms and prescreening procedures is similar to that of programming for any other population. This section will explore the types of registration materials and screening techniques that can be used and unique considerations that may arise when providing programmes for people with disability.

A registration form is a great place to start. This form typically collects information about the prospective member including name, personal contact information, programme interests, and emergency contact information. In addition to this, programme instructors may want to include any of the following items to help with programme organization and to best suit the programme to participants with a disability.

- Transportation requirements (vehicle with a lift, drive own vehicle, dropped-off, etc.)
- Mobility devices used (manual wheelchair, power wheelchair, white cane, etc.)
- Disability specific information (level and nature of disability, level of vision loss, require sign language interpretation)
- Functional level (e.g., able to transfer independently, require an aide to attend, etc.)
- Associated medical concerns (e.g., epilepsy, diabetes, balance impairment, etc.)

It is always a good idea to prescreen your participants to provide as safe an environment as possible for the participant while being responsible as an organization with respect to risk management. By using a few simple, readily available forms, programme instructors and administrators can obtain valuable participant health information as well as fully inform the participants about the activity that they will partake in and the risks involved.

Physical activity readiness questionnaires (PAR-Q), or similar forms used regionally, are useful tools for instructors to have participants complete prior to any physical activity (Canadian Society for Exercise Physiology 2003) (see Appendix 23.A). PAR-Qs screen participants by identifying persons at risk and directing them to seek medical clearance prior to participation in a physical activity programme. If an individual answers "yes" to more than one question on the PAR-Q, then a physical activity readiness medical examination form (PARmed-X) should be used. This PARmed-X (see Appendix 23.B) is a physical activity checklist which is completed by the individual's physician to provide guidance with respect to activity prescription (Canadian Society for Exercise Physiology 2003).

Even though a client may satisfactorily complete the PAR-Q, there may be other disability/impairment-related factors that may affect ability to engage in physical activity or a fitness appraisal. An excellent example of a form which may be used to establish degree of function is one proposed for use in the recently developed *INCLUSIVE FITNESS AND LIFESTYLE SERVICES FOR ALL disABILITIES* (Canadian Society for Exercise Physiology, 2002). In order to gain information of how disability impacts on physical activity, clients are asked to complete the Abilities for Active Living Questionnaire, or the AAL-Q and You. The questionnaire asks clients whether they have a health condition that may affect the way in which the individual participates in physical activity or a fitness appraisal. If the answer is "yes," the client responds to a series of yes/no questions pertaining to conditions that affect mobility, grasping, strength related activities, extended periods of movement, joint mobility, social skills, ability to complete tasks, perception, comprehension, and other factors.

In addition to using a health-screening tool such as the PAR-Q and PARmed-X, programme leaders should also use a waiver and/or informed consent form signed by the client or a guardian. The use of these types of forms is to inform the participants, in clear detail, the nature of the physical activity programme in which they are about to participate (see examples of waivers and informed consent Appendixes 23.C and 23.D).

4 Some participants may have difficulty communicating or even understanding what is typically included in an informed consent. What steps can be taken to ensure that all participants provide informed consent?

FEES

Organizations and programme administrators alike have struggled for years with whether or not people with a disability should pay the 'going rate', a subsidized rate, or not pay at all for programmes in which they participate. This has caused a number of heated debates and remains unresolved. There has yet to be established a consistent view that can be adopted by all organizations and instructors.

Even in the early 1990s, some large public recreation facilities were offering a discounted membership if the participant had a disability. By offering a discounted rate to anyone with a disability, one would assume that everyone with a disability is unable to pay for the programme.

An *ability to pay* method for fee reduction (e.g., a 'means assessment' or sliding scale) may be more appropriate. This method is much more equitable in that it offers a reduction in price to those who are economically disadvantaged. Individuals with and without a disability may fall into this category.

There are a number of alternatives for those with disability who are also economically disadvantaged to participate in the offered programmes. For those unable to pay the advertised price for a facility membership or a programme fee, the opportunity to pay the fee in payments may be helpful (e.g., twelve postdated cheques for the total amount). Facilities may also wish to offer a programme or membership subsidy through a scholarship programme. Through a donation campaign, corporate donations, or a budgetary allotment, programme administrators may be able to subsidize memberships for those who are economically disadvantaged.

Often, individuals organizing specialized programmes for the first time do not realize the extra costs required to operate specialized programmes. Factors that may increase the cost (and fees) for a programme or facility that are specific to this population may include some or all of the following:

- Specialized transportation requirements
- Specialized equipment to operate the programme or facility
- Accessibility upgrades
- Need for increased number of staff to satisfy staff to participant ratios
- Staff training
- Volunteer recruitment

PROGRAMME ATTENDANTS AND AIDES

Individuals with disability may be required to bring an assistant with them to help with mobility, decision making, personal care, transferring, or to make it possible for the participant to enjoy as much of the programme or service offered. The staff-to-participant ratios, the compatibility between the participant's level of ability, and the level of ability required to participate may help to determine whether or not an attendant is required.

An issue arises as to whether an attendant should be charged a fee. This is a controversial area and should be resolved based on specific circumstances including the need for the attendant and whether or not the person with a disability would be able to participate without an attendant. It is very difficult to judge and no formula is available to give advice on what a facility should or should not do. This matter needs to be dealt with dependent on the type of programmes being offered, the level of accessibility of the facility and its programmes, the ability level of the participant, and the necessity of an attendant. A proactive approach is desirable in developing a fair, realistic, and consistent strategy to make it a viable opportunity for both the programme provider and the participant.

CAPITAL AND OPERATIONAL GRANTS

For nonprofit, charitable organizations, grants can be a way of turning a new programme idea into reality. Two main types of grants are typically available. Capital grants, which can be used to renovate facilities or buy new equipment, are the most common forms of a grant. Operational grants, on the other hand, are more difficult to secure and are often used to pay for wages, hire additional staff, or pay for utility costs.

Groups applying for grants can seek these funds through local service organizations (e.g., Rotary Clubs, Lion's Club, etc.), local foundations, regional active living oriented government foundations, and nationally through foundations and government initiatives. Funds that are available may have specific requirements of an applicant (e.g., group providing specialized programming) or may have very general guidelines. The application process, dollar amounts given, and frequency of grant availability is different for each granting agency. The ability to match dollars with a successful grant, as well as a strong partnership effort in both grant applications and ultimate project collaboration, will serve as a tremendous advantage in securing funds.

Volunteer and Staff Roles

Staffing considerations for specialized programming or/for providing inclusive programming opportunities within an existing structure definitely take effort and attention to the needs of the participants. Again, there is no formula for staff-to-participant ratios or other staffing matters, but a number of important issues need to be examined by programme providers to provide adequate and rewarding active living programming for people with disability.

STAFF AND VOLUNTEER TRAINING REQUIREMENTS

Dedicated staff and volunteers are an invaluable resource, especially when offering specialized group activities or services to clients with high needs. Both staff and volunteers can take on a number of roles within a programme environment which will ultimately provide a more positive experience for the participant. Budget conscious programme administrators need to key into the invaluable resource of volunteer support. Volunteers can be comprised of staff who are working extra hours, students receiving credit for hours completed (school age, college, or university), members or programme participants who also assist in other programmes, or a community-minded individual (Scott 1998). A good complement of dedicated and well-trained volunteers can tremendously increase the effectiveness of the services provided. Using volunteers to the full potential can allow facilities to expand services, create closer ties between the facility and community, and perhaps alleviate the need for participants to bring an attendant.

To provide participants with a safe and enjoyable active living experience, facility administrators must ensure that their programme leaders and specialized service providers are qualified to work with people with disability. In addition to the basic training that all active living professionals should possess (e.g., CPR, first aid), staff should also possess postsecondary training that enables them to provide instruction in active living for people with disability. Staff should be aware of the etiology of various disabilities and techniques in adapting active living opportunities and should possess skills related to the programme being offered (e.g., transferring, fitness instruction, behaviour management). Staff should also be professionally prepared to train volunteers.

In Canada, a new programme entitled *INCLUSIVE FITNESS AND LIFESTYLE SERVICES FOR ALL disABILITIES* (Canadian Society for Exercise Physiology, 2002) has been developed which specifically addresses the issue of training health, fitness, and lifestyle appraisal professionals to deliver fitness appraisal and counselling services to persons with disability. You will learn more about this programme in Chapter 22 (Seidl).

Both staff and volunteers should be provided with training opportunities to bring their skills up to the standards necessary for the types of programming being offered. Both staff and volunteers need to be informed about the philosophy of the facility and programmes offered, the emergency procedures, and programme objectives. Staff and volunteers should also have the opportunity to regularly update their skills, not only to make them more effective within the programme environment, but to also motivate them to implement new and innovative ways of providing service to their participants.

Staff- and volunteer-to-participant ratios are quite dependent on the type of programme being offered and the ability level of the participant in relation to the activity. Again, there is no standard formula that outlines exactly how many instructors and assistants there should be for any given programme or activity. It is important for programme planners to anticipate the level of participation required, the environment in which the programme is taking place, and the level of assistance required for both the instructor and the participants. To ensure the safety of both participants and instructors, thought to this matter is paramount to the success of the programme.

Summary

Specialized active living programming should be considered as a programme option within a continuum of programming made available to people with disability. As opposed to segregating people with disability, specialized programming should cater directly to people with disability to meet the specific needs of individuals in active living. Specialized programming offers opportunity to a wide range of potential users, including individuals with severe disabilities who require more support than other programme opportunities can offer, and for those with mild and moderate levels of disability who would prefer to be instructed by staff who have specifically organized a programme or activity for persons with disability.

In adopting a practical approach to specialized programming, issues surrounding accessibility to programmes, the philosophy of the programme provider, as well as appropriateness of services, need to be explored long before the first participant with a disability signs up for programmes. This chapter has provided a practical approach to providing these services. Individual participants will drive much of what one does as a programmer, thus ensuring that the most important concept in this chapter comes true–that active living is for everyone, no matter how one becomes active!

Study Questions

1. Given the current emphasis on inclusion, how can one reconcile the movement to inclusion with the call for specialized physical activity and recreation centres for persons with disabilities?
2. What factors might impact on the decision of a person with a disability to choose a specialized facility or an integrated setting such as a health club environment?
3. Describe the barriers to active living for persons with disability?
4. You are considering developing a specialized exercise facility for persons with disability. What are the main considerations (headings) you would include within your business plan document?

References

Active Living Alliance for Canadians with a Disability. http://www.ala.ca/

Canadian Society for Exercise Physiology. (2002). *Physical Activity Readiness-Questionnaire (PAR-Q)*. Ottawa: Author.

Canadian Society for Exercise Physiology. (2002). *Physical Activity Readiness Medical Examination (PAR-medx)*. Ottawa: Author.

Canadian Society for Exercise Physiology. (2003). *Publications*. Available on-line: http://www.csep.ca/publications.asp

Canadian Society for Exercise Physiology. (2002). *INCLUSIVE FITNESS AND LIFESTYLE SERVICES FOR ALL DISABILITIES*. Ottawa: Author.

Cohen, R.D. (1998). *Directory of disability organizations in Canada*. Toronto: Canadian Abilities Foundation.

Garner, B.A. (Ed.). (1999). *Black's law dictionary* (7th ed.). St. Paul, MN: West Group.

Harvey, W.J. (1997). Some thoughts on physical activity and persons with a disability. *The Canadian Association for Health, Physical Education, Recreation and Dance Journal, 63*(3), 35-36.

Miller, P.D. (Ed.). (1995). *Fitness programming and physical disability*. Champaign, IL: Human Kinetics.

Safety Codes Council. (1999). *Barrier-free design guide*. Edmonton, AB: Safety Codes Council.

Scott, J.T. (1998). *Fundamentals of leisure business success*. New York: Haworth Press.

The Steadward Centre for Personal and Physical Achievement. (2000). *Informed consent form*. Edmonton, AB: Author.

The Steadward Centre for Personal and Physical Achievement. (2000). *Programme waiver*, Edmonton, AB: Author.

The Steadward Centre for Personal and Physical Achievement (2001). *About TSC/History*. Available online: http://www.steadwardcentre.org

Svensson, B., Gerdle, B., and Elert, J. (1994). Endurance training in patients with multiple sclerosis: Five case studies. *Physical Therapy, 74*(11), 1017–26.

Thompson, D., (Ed.). (1995). *The concise Oxford dictionary of current English* (9th ed.). Oxford: Clarendon Press.

Suggested Reading

Harvey, W.J. (1997). Some thoughts on physical activity and persons with a disability. *The Canadian Association for Health, Physical Education, Recreation and Dance Journal, 63*(3), 35–36.

Lyons, R.F. (1991). *Municipal government policy guidelines: Recreation services for persons with a disability*. Ottawa: Canadian Parks and Recreation Association.

Lockette, K.L., and Keyes, A.M. (1994). *Conditioning with physical disabilities*. Champaign, IL: Human Kinetics.

Schleien, S.J., Germ, P.A., and McAvoy, L.H. (1996). Inclusive community leisure service: Recommended professional practices and barriers encountered. *Therapeutic Recreation Journal, 30*(4), 260–73.

YMCA of the USA. (1991). *YMCA program discovery series: Vol. 2(3). Programs for special populations*. Champaign, IL: Human Kinetics.

Physical Activity Readiness
Questionnaire - PAR-Q
(revised 2002)

PAR-Q & YOU

(A Questionnaire for People Aged 15 to 69)

Regular physical activity is fun and healthy, and increasingly more people are starting to become more active every day. Being more active is very safe for most people. However, some people should check with their doctor before they start becoming much more physically active.

If you are planning to become much more physically active than you are now, start by answering the seven questions in the box below. If you are be of 15 and 69, the PAR-Q will tell you if you should check with your doctor before you start. If you are over 69 years of age, and you are not used to b check with your doctor.

Common sense is your best guide when you answer these questions. Please read the questions carefully and answer each one honestly: check YI

YES	NO		
☐	☐	1.	Has your doctor ever said that you have a heart condition **and** that you should only do physical activity recommended by a doctor?
☐	☐	2.	Do you feel pain in your chest when you do physical activity?
☐	☐	3.	In the past month, have you had chest pain when you were not doing physical activity?
☐	☐	4.	Do you lose your balance because of dizziness or do you ever lose consciousness?
☐	☐	5.	Do you have a bone or joint problem (for example, back, knee or hip) that could be made worse by a change in your physical activity?
☐	☐	6.	Is your doctor currently prescribing drugs (for example, water pills) for your blood pressure or heart condition?
☐	☐	7.	Do you know of <u>any other reason</u> why you should not do physical activity?

If

you

answered

YES to one or more questions

Talk with your doctor by phone or in person BEFORE you start becoming much more physically active or BEFORE you have a fitness appraisal. Tell your doctor about the PAR-Q and which questions you answered YES.

- You may be able to do any activity you want — as long as you start slowly and build up gradually. Or, you may need to restrict your activities to those which are safe for you. Talk with your doctor about the kinds of activities you wish to participate in and follow his/her advice.
- Find out which community programs are safe and helpful for you.

NO to all questions

If you answered NO honestly to <u>all</u> PAR-Q questions, you can be reasonably sure that you can:
- start becoming much more physically active — begin slowly and build up gradually. This is the safest and easiest way to go.
- take part in a fitness appraisal — this is an excellent way to determine your basic fitness so that you can plan the best way for you to live actively. It is also highly recommended that you have your blood pressure evaluated. If your reading is over 144/94, talk with your doctor before you start becoming much more physically active.

DELAY BECOMING MUCH MORE ACTIVE:
- if you are not feeling well because of a temporary illness such as a cold or a fever — wait until you feel better; or
- if you are or may be pregnant — talk to your doctor before you start becoming more active.

PLEASE NOTE: If your health changes so that you then answer YES to any of the above questions, tell your fitness or health professional. Ask whether you should change your physical activity plan.

<u>Informed Use of the PAR-Q</u>: The Canadian Society for Exercise Physiology, Health Canada, and their agents assume no liability for persons who undertake physical activity, and if in doubt after completing this questionnaire, consult your doctor prior to physical activity.

No changes permitted. You are encouraged to photocopy the PAR-Q but only if you use the entire form.

NOTE: If the PAR-Q is being given to a person before he or she participates in a physical activity program or a fitness appraisal, this section may be used for legal or administrative pu

"I have read, understood and completed this questionnaire. Any questions I had were answered to my full satisfaction."

NAME _____

SIGNATURE _____ DATE _____

SIGNATURE OF PARENT _____ WITNESS _____
or GUARDIAN (for participants under the age of majority)

> **Note:** This physical activity clearance is valid for a maximum of **12 months** from the date it is completed and becomes invalid if your condition changes so that you would answer YES to any of the seven questions.

CSEP
SCPE © Canadian Society for Exercise Physiology   Supported by: Health Santé
                                                                       Canada Canada   continued on other side...

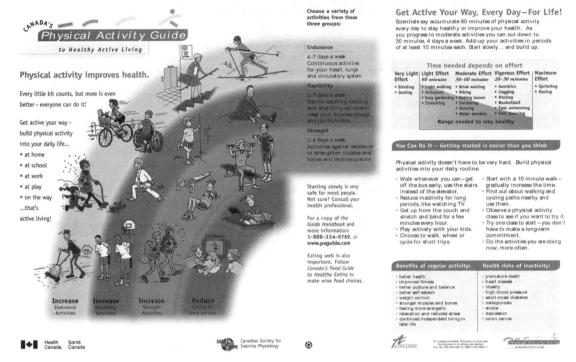

Source: *Canada's Physical Activity Guide to Healthy Active Living*, Health Canada, 1998 *http://www.hc-sc.gc.ca/hppb/paguide/pdf/guideEng.pdf*
© Reproduced with permission from the Minister of Public Works and Government Services Canada, 2002.

FITNESS AND HEALTH PROFESSIONALS MAY BE INTERESTED IN THE INFORMATION BELOW:

The following companion forms are available for doctors' use by contacting the Canadian Society for Exercise Physiology (address below):

The **Physical Activity Readiness Medical Examination (PARmed-X)** – to be used by doctors with people who answer YES to one or more questions on the PAR-Q.

The **Physical Activity Readiness Medical Examination for Pregnancy (PARmed-X for Pregnancy)** – to be used by doctors with pregnant patients who wish to become more active.

References:
Arraix, G.A., Wigle, D.T., Mao, Y. (1992). Risk Assessment of Physical Activity and Physical Fitness in the Canada Health Survey Follow-Up Study. **J. Clin. Epidemiol.** 45:4 419-428.
Mottola, M., Wolfe, L.A. (1994). Active Living and Pregnancy, In: A. Quinney, L. Gauvin, T. Wall (eds.), **Toward Active Living: Proceedings of the International Conference on Physical Activity, Fitness and Health**. Champaign, IL: Human Kinetics.
PAR-Q Validation Report, British Columbia Ministry of Health, 1978.
Thomas, S., Reading, J., Shephard, R.J. (1992). Revision of the Physical Activity Readiness Questionnaire (PAR-Q). **Can. J. Spt. Sci.** 17:4 338-345.

To order multiple printed copies of the PAR-Q, please contact the:

Canadian Society for Exercise Physiology
202-185 Somerset Street West
Ottawa, ON K2P 0J2
Tel. 1-877-651-3755 • FAX (613) 234-3565
Online: www.csep.ca

The original PAR-Q was developed by the British Columbia Ministry of Health. It has been revised by an Expert Advisory Committee of the Canadian Society for Exercise Physiology chaired by Dr. N. Gledhill (2002).

Disponible en français sous le titre «Questionnaire sur l'aptitude à l'activité physique - Q-AAP (revisé 2002)».

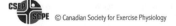 © Canadian Society for Exercise Physiology

Supported by: Health Canada Santé Canada

SOURCE: From Physical Activity Readiness Questionnaire (PAR-Q), © 2002, Canadian Society for Exercise Physiology. Reprinted with permission. Available on-line: http://www.csep.ca/forms.asp (URL on April 30, 2003)

Physical Activity Readiness
Medical Examination
(revised 2002)

PARmed-X PHYSICAL ACTIVITY READINESS
MEDICAL EXAMINATION

**The PARmed-X is a physical activity-specific checklist to be used by a physician with patients
who have had positive responses to the Physical Activity Readiness Questionnaire (PAR-Q). In addition, th
Conveyance/Referral Form in the PARmed-X can be used to convey clearance for physical activity par
or to make a referral to a medically-supervised exercise program.**

Regular physical activity is fun and healthy, and increasingly more people are starting to become more active every day. Being more active is very safe for most people. The PAR-Q by itself provides adequate screening for the majority of people. However, some individua require a medical evaluation and specific advice (exercise prescription) due to one or more positive responses to the PAR-Q.

Following the participant's evaluation by a physician, a physical activity plan should be devised in consultation with a physic professional (CSEP-Professional Fitness & Lifestyle Consultant or CSEP-Exercise Therapist™). To assist in this, the follow instructions are provided:

PAGE 1: • Sections A, B, C, and D should be completed by the participant BEFORE the examination by the physician. The bottom section is to be completed by the examining physician.

PAGES 2 & 3: • A checklist of medical conditions requiring special consideration and management.

PAGE 4: • Physical Activity & Lifestyle Advice for people who do not require specific instructions or prescribed exercise.

• Physical Activity Readiness Conveyance/Referral Form - an optional tear-off tab for the physician to convey clearance for physical activity participation, or to make a referral to a medically-supervised exercise program.

This section to be completed by the participant

A PERSONAL INFORMATION:

NAME _____

ADDRESS _____

_____

TELEPHONE _____

BIRTHDATE _____ GENDER _____

MEDICAL No. _____

B PAR-Q: *Please indicate the PAR-Q questions to which you answered YES*

❑ Q1 Heart condition
❑ Q2 Chest pain during activity
❑ Q3 Chest pain at rest
❑ Q4 Loss of balance, dizziness
❑ Q5 Bone or joint problem
❑ Q6 Blood pressure or heart drugs
❑ Q7 Other reason:

_____

C RISK FACTORS FOR CARDIOVASCULAR DISEASE:
Check all that apply

❑ Less than 30 minutes of moderate physical activity most days of the week.
❑ Currently smoker (tobacco smoking 1 or more times per week).
❑ High blood pressure reported by physician after repeated measurements.
❑ High cholesterol level reported by physician.

❑ Excessive accumulation of fat around waist.
❑ Family history of heart disease.

Please note: Many of these risk factors are modifiable. Please refer to page 4 and discuss with your physician.

D PHYSICAL ACTIVITY INTENTIONS:

What physical activity do you intend to do?

_____

_____

_____

This section to be completed by the examining physician

Physical Exam:

Ht	Wt	BP i)	/
		BP ii)	/

Conditions limiting physical activity:

❑ Cardiovascular ❑ Respiratory ❑ Other
❑ Musculoskeletal ❑ Abdominal

Tests required:

❑ ECG ❑ Exercise Test ❑ X-Ray
❑ Blood ❑ Urinalysis ❑ Other

Physical Activity Readiness Conveyance/Referral:

Based upon a current review of health status, I recommend:

Further Information:
❑ Attached
❑ To be forwarded
❑ Available on request

❑ No physical activity
❑ Only a medically-supervised exercise program until further medical clearance
❑ Progressive physical activity:
　❑ with avoidance of: _____
　❑ with inclusion of: _____
　❑ under the supervision of a CSEP-Professional Fitness & Lifestyle Consultant or CSEP-Exercise Therapist™
❑ Unrestricted physical activity—start slowly and build up gradually

CSEP SCPE © Canadian Society for Exercise Physiology

Supported by: Health Canada Santé Canada

1

PARmed-X
PHYSICAL ACTIVITY READINESS MEDICAL EXAMINATION

Following is a checklist of medical conditions for which a degree of precaution and/or special advice should be considered f⸱ answered "YES" to one or more questions on the PAR-Q, and people over the age of 69. Conditions are grouped by syster categories of precautions are provided. Comments under Advice are general, since details and alternatives require clinical each individual instance.

	Absolute Contraindications	Relative Contraindications	Special Prescriptive Conditions	ADVICE
	Permanent restriction or temporary restriction until condition is treated, stable, and/or past acute phase.	Highly variable. Value of exercise testing and/or program may exceed risk. Activity may be restricted. Desirable to maximize control of condition. Direct or indirect medical supervision of exercise program may be desirable.	Individualized prescriptive advice generally appropriate: • limitations imposed; and/or • special exercises prescribed. May require medical monitoring and/or initial supervision in exercise program.	
Cardiovascular	❑ aortic aneurysm (dissecting) ❑ aortic stenosis (severe) ❑ congestive heart failure ❑ crescendo angina ❑ myocardial infarction (acute) ❑ myocarditis (active or recent) ❑ pulmonary or systemic embolism—acute ❑ thrombophlebitis ❑ ventricular tachycardia and other dangerous dysrhythmias (e.g., multi-focal ventricular activity)	❑ aortic stenosis (moderate) ❑ subaortic stenosis (severe) ❑ marked cardiac enlargement ❑ supraventricular dysrhythmias (uncontrolled or high rate) ❑ ventricular ectopic activity (repetitive or frequent) ❑ ventricular aneurysm ❑ hypertension—untreated or uncontrolled severe (systemic or pulmonary) ❑ hypertrophic cardiomyopathy ❑ compensated congestive heart failure	❑ aortic (or pulmonary) stenosis—mild angina pectoris and other manifestations of coronary insufficiency (e.g., post-acute infarct) ❑ cyanotic heart disease ❑ shunts (intermittent or fixed) ❑ conduction disturbances • complete AV block • left BBB • Wolff-Parkinson-White syndrome ❑ dysrhythmias—controlled ❑ fixed rate pacemakers	• clinical exercise test may be warranted in selected cases, for specific determination of functional capacity and limitations and precautions (if any). • slow progression of exercise to levels based on test performance and individual tolerance. • consider individual need for initial conditioning program under medical supervision (indirect or direct).
			❑ intermittent claudication	progressive exercise to tolerance
			❑ hypertension: systolic 160-180; diastolic 105+	progressive exercise; care with medications (serum electrolytes; post-exercise syncope; etc.)
Infections	❑ acute infectious disease (regardless of etiology)	❑ subacute/chronic/recurrent infectious diseases (e.g., malaria, others)	❑ chronic infections ❑ HIV	variable as to condition
Metabolic		❑ uncontrolled metabolic disorders (diabetes mellitus, thyrotoxicosis, myxedema)	❑ renal, hepatic & other metabolic insufficiency	variable as to status
			❑ obesity ❑ single kidney	dietary moderation, and initial light exercises with slow progression (walking, swimming, cycling)
Pregnancy		❑ complicated pregnancy (e.g., toxemia, hemorrhage, incompetent cervix, etc.)	❑ advanced pregnancy (late 3rd trimester)	refer to the "PARmed-X for PREGNANCY"

References:

Arraix, G.A., Wigle, D.T., Mao, Y. (1992). Risk Assessment of Physical Activity and Physical Fitness in the Canada Health Survey Follow-Up Study. **J. Clin. Epidemiol.** 45:4 419-428.

Mottola, M., Wolfe, L.A. (1994). Active Living and Pregnancy, In: A. Quinney, L. Gauvin, T. Wall (eds.), **Toward Active Living: Proceedings of the International Conference on Physical Activity, Fitness and Health.** Champaign, IL: Human Kinetics.

PAR-Q Validation Report, British Columbia Ministry of Health, 1978.

Thomas, S., Reading, J., Shephard, R.J. (1992). Revision of the Physical Activity Readiness Questionnaire (PAR-Q). **Can. J. Spt. Sci.** 17:4 338-345.

The PAR-Q and PARmed-X were developed by the British Columbia Ministry of Health. They have been revised by an Expert Advisory Committee of the Canadian Society for Exercise Physiology chaired by Dr. N. Gledhill (2002).

No changes permitted. You are encouraged to photocopy the PARmed-X, but only if you use the entire form.

Disponible en français sous le titre
«Évaluation médicale de l'aptitude à l'activité physique (X-AAP)»

Continued on page 3…

2

Physical Activity Readiness
Medical Examination
(revised 2002)

	Special Prescriptive Conditions	ADVICE
Lung	❏ chronic pulmonary disorders	special relaxation and breathing exercises
	❏ obstructive lung disease	breath control during endurance exercises to tolerance; avoid polluted air
	❏ asthma	
	❏ exercise-induced bronchospasm	avoid hyperventilation during exercise; avoid extremely cold conditions; warm up adequately; utilize appropriate medication.
Musculoskeletal	❏ low back conditions (pathological, functional)	avoid or minimize exercise that precipitates or exasperates e.g., forced extreme flexion, extension, and violent twisting; correct posture, proper back exercises
	❏ arthritis—acute (infective, rheumatoid; gout)	treatment, plus judicious blend of rest, splinting and gentle movement
	❏ arthritis—subacute	progressive increase of active exercise therapy
	❏ arthritis—chronic (osteoarthritis and above conditions)	maintenance of mobility and strength; non-weightbearing exercises to minimize joint trauma (e.g., cycling, aquatic activity, etc.)
	❏ orthopaedic	highly variable and individualized
	❏ hernia	minimize straining and isometrics; stregthen abdominal muscles
	❏ osteoporosis or low bone density	avoid exercise with high risk for fracture such as push-ups, curl-ups, vertical jump and trunk forward flexion; engage in low-impact weight-bearing activities and resistance training
CNS	❏ convulsive disorder not completely controlled by medication	minimize or avoid exercise in hazardous environments and/or exercising alone (e.g., swimming, mountainclimbing, etc.)
	❏ recent concussion	thorough examination if history of two concussions; review for discontinuation of contact sport if three concussions, depending on duration of unconsciousness, retrograde amnesia, persistent headaches, and other objective evidence of cerebral damage
Blood	❏ anemia—severe (< 10 Gm/dl)	control preferred; exercise as tolerated
	❏ electrolyte disturbances	
Medications	❏ antianginal ❏ antiarrhythmic ❏ antihypertensive ❏ anticonvulsant ❏ beta-blockers ❏ digitalis preparations ❏ diuretics ❏ ganglionic blockers ❏ others	NOTE: consider underlying condition. Potential for: exertional syncope, electrolyte imbalance, bradycardia, dysrhythmias, impaired coordination and reaction time, heat intolerance. May alter resting and exercise ECG's and exercise test performance.
Other	❏ post-exercise syncope	moderate program
	❏ heat intolerance	prolong cool-down with light activities; avoid exercise in extreme heat
	❏ temporary minor illness	postpone until recovered
	❏ cancer	if potential metastases, test by cycle ergometry, consider non-weight bearing exercises; exercise at lower end of prescriptive range (40-65% of heart rate reserve), depending on condition and recent treatment (radiation, chemotherapy); monitor hemoglobin and lymphocyte counts; add dynamic lifting exercise to strengthen muscles, using machines rather than weights.

*Refer to special publications for elaboration as required

The following companion forms are available by contacting the Canadian Society for Exercise Physiology (address below):

The **Physical Activity Readiness Questionnaire (PAR-Q)** - a questionnaire for people aged 15-69 to complete before becoming much more physically active.

The **Physical Activity Readiness Medical Examination for Pregnancy (PARmed-X for PREGNANCY)** - to be used by physicians with pregnant patients who wish to become more physically active.

To order multiple printed copies of the PARmed-X and/or any of the companion forms (for a nominal charge), please contact the:

Canadian Society for Exercise Physiology
202 - 185 Somerset St. West
Ottawa, ON K2P 0J2
Tel. 1-877-651-3755 • FAX (613) 234-3565 • Online: www.csep.ca

Note to physical activity professionals...

It is a prudent practice to retain the completed Physical Activity Readiness Conveyance/Referral Form in the participant's file.

 © Canadian Society for Exercise Physiology

Supported by: Health Santé
Canada Canada

Continued on page 4...

3

	Special Prescriptive Conditions	**ADVICE**
Lung	❑ chronic pulmonary disorders	special relaxation and breathing exercises
	❑ obstructive lung disease	breath control during endurance exercises to tolerance; avoid polluted air
	❑ asthma	
	❑ exercise-induced bronchospasm	avoid hyperventilation during exercise; avoid extremely cold conditions; warm up adequately; utilize appropriate medication.
Musculoskeletal	❑ low back conditions (pathological, functional)	avoid or minimize exercise that precipitates or exasperates e.g., forced extreme flexion, extension, and violent twisting; correct posture, proper back exercises
	❑ arthritis—acute (infective, rheumatoid; gout)	treatment, plus judicious blend of rest, splinting and gentle movement
	❑ arthritis—subacute	progressive increase of active exercise therapy
	❑ arthritis—chronic (osteoarthritis and above conditions)	maintenance of mobility and strength; non-weightbearing exercises to minimize joint trauma (e.g., cycling, aquatic activity, etc.)
	❑ orthopaedic	highly variable and individualized
	❑ hernia	minimize straining and isometrics; stregthen abdominal muscles
	❑ osteoporosis or low bone density	avoid exercise with high risk for fracture such as push-ups, curl-ups, vertical jump and trunk forward flexion; engage in low-impact weight-bearing activities and resistance training
CNS	❑ convulsive disorder not completely controlled by medication	minimize or avoid exercise in hazardous environments and/or exercising alone (e.g., swimming, mountainclimbing, etc.)
	❑ recent concussion	thorough examination if history of two concussions; review for discontinuation of contact sport if three concussions, depending on duration of unconsciousness, retrograde amnesia, persistent headaches, and other objective evidence of cerebral damage
Blood	❑ anemia—severe (< 10 Gm/dl)	control preferred; exercise as tolerated
	❑ electrolyte disturbances	
Medications	❑ antianginal ❑ antiarrhythmic ❑ antihypertensive ❑ anticonvulsant ❑ beta-blockers ❑ digitalis preparations ❑ diuretics ❑ ganglionic blockers ❑ others	NOTE: consider underlying condition. Potential for: exertional syncope, electrolyte imbalance, bradycardia, dysrhythmias, impaired coordination and reaction time, heat intolerance. May alter resting and exercise ECG's and exercise test performance.
Other	❑ post-exercise syncope	moderate program
	❑ heat intolerance	prolong cool-down with light activities; avoid exercise in extreme heat
	❑ temporary minor illness	postpone until recovered
	❑ cancer	if potential metastases, test by cycle ergometry, consider non-weight bearing exercises; exercise at lower end of prescriptive range (40-65% of heart rate reserve), depending on condition and recent treatment (radiation, chemotherapy); monitor hemoglobin and lymphocyte counts; add dynamic lifting exercise to strengthen muscles, using machines rather than weights.

Refer to special publications for elaboration as required

The following companion forms are available by contacting the Canadian Society for Exercise Physiology (address below):

The **Physical Activity Readiness Questionnaire (PAR-Q)** - a questionnaire for people aged 15-69 to complete before becoming much more physically active.

The **Physical Activity Readiness Medical Examination for Pregnancy (PARmed-X for PREGNANCY)** - to be used by physicians with pregnant patients who wish to become more physically active.

To order multiple printed copies of the PARmed-X and/or any of the companion forms (for a nominal charge), please contact the:

Canadian Society for Exercise Physiology
202 - 185 Somerset St. West
Ottawa, ON K2P 0J2
Tel. 1-877-651-3755 • FAX (613) 234-3565 • Online: www.csep.ca

Note to physical activity professionals...

It is a prudent practice to retain the completed Physical Activity Readiness Conveyance/Referral Form in the participant's file.

 © Canadian Society for Exercise Physiology

Supported by: Health Canada   Santé Canada

Continued on page 4...

3

PARmed-X
PHYSICAL ACTIVITY READINESS MEDICAL EXAMINATION

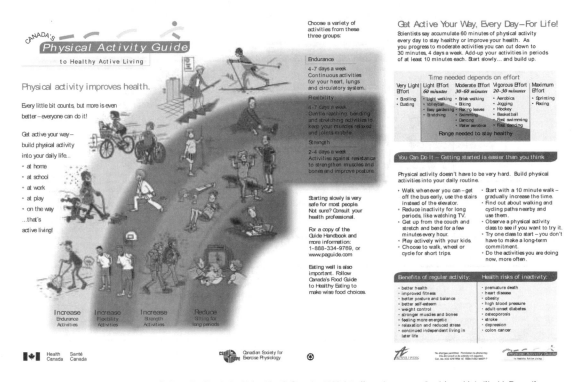

CANADA'S
Physical Activity Guide
to Healthy Active Living

Physical activity improves health.

Every little bit counts, but more is even better – everyone can do it!

Get active your way –
build physical activity
into your daily life...
· at home
· at school
· at work
· at play
· on the way
...that's
active living!

Increase
Endurance
Activities

Increase
Flexibility
Activities

Increase
Strength
Activities

Reduce
Sitting for
long periods

Choose a variety of
activities from these
three groups:

Endurance
4-7 days a week
Continuous activities
for your heart, lungs
and circulatory system.

Flexibility
4-7 days a week
Gentle reaching, bending
and stretching activities to
keep your muscles relaxed
and joints mobile.

Strength
2-4 days a week
Activities against resistance
to strengthen muscles and
bones and improve posture.

Starting slowly is very
safe for most people.
Not sure? Consult your
health professional.

For a copy of the
Guide Handbook and
more information:
1-888-334-9769, or
www.paguide.com

Eating well is also
important. Follow
Canada's Food Guide
to Healthy Eating to
make wise food choices.

Get Active Your Way, Every Day–For Life!
Scientists say accumulate 60 minutes of physical activity
every day to stay healthy or improve your health. As
you progress to moderate activities you can cut down to
30 minutes, 4 days a week. Add-up your activities in periods
of at least 10 minutes each. Start slowly... and build up.

Time needed depends on effort

Very Light Effort	Light Effort 60 minutes	Moderate Effort 30-60 minutes	Vigorous Effort 20-30 minutes	Maximum Effort
· Strolling · Dusting	· Light walking · Volleyball · Easy gardening · Stretching	· Brisk walking · Biking · Raking leaves · Swimming · Dancing · Water aerobics	· Aerobics · Jogging · Hockey · Basketball · Fast swimming · Fast dancing	· Sprinting · Racing

Range needed to stay healthy

You Can Do It – Getting started is easier than you think
Physical activity doesn't have to be very hard. Build physical
activities into your daily routine.

· Walk whenever you can – get
off the bus early, use the stairs
instead of the elevator.
· Reduce inactivity for long
periods, like watching TV.
· Get up from the couch and
stretch and bend for a few
minutes every hour.
· Play actively with your kids.
· Choose to walk, wheel or
cycle for short trips.

· Start with a 10 minute walk –
gradually increase the time.
· Find out about walking and
cycling paths nearby and
use them.
· Observe a physical activity
class to see if you want to try it.
· Try one class to start – you don't
have to make a long-term
commitment.
· Do the activities you are doing
now, more often.

Benefits of regular activity:	Health risks of inactivity:
· better health · improved fitness · better posture and balance · better self-esteem · weight control · stronger muscles and bones · feeling more energetic · relaxation and reduced stress · continued independent living in later life	· premature death · heart disease · obesity · high blood pressure · adult-onset diabetes · osteoporosis · stroke · depression · colon cancer

Health Canada / Santé Canada

Canadian Society for Exercise Physiology

Source: *Canada's Physical Activity Guide to Healthy Active Living*, Health Canada, 1998 *http://www.hc-sc.gc.ca/hppb/paguide/pdf/guideEng.pdf*
© Reproduced with permission from the Minister of Public Works and Government Services Canada, 2002.

✂ . . . .

PARmed-X Physical Activity Readiness Conveyance/Referral Form

Based upon a current review of the health status of _____, I recommend:

❏ No physical activity

❏ Only a medically-supervised exercise program until further medical clearance

❏ Progressive physical activity

   ❏ with avoidance of: _____

   ❏ with inclusion of: _____

   ❏ under the supervision of a CSEP-Professional Fitness &

   Lifestyle Consultant or CSEP-Exercise Therapist™

❏ Unrestricted physical activity — start slowly and build up gradually

Further Information:
❏ Attached
❏ To be forwarded
❏ Available on request

Physician/clinic stamp:

_____ M.D.

_____ 20 _____
(date)

**NOTE: This physical activity clearance is
valid for a maximum of six months from the
date it is completed and becomes invalid if
your medical condition becomes worse.**

4

SOURCE: From Physical Activity Readiness Medical Examination (PARmed-X), © 2002, Canadian Society for Exercise
Physiology. Reprinted with permission. Available on-line: http://www.csep.ca/forms.asp (URL on April 30, 2003)

Appendix 23.C The Steadward Centre for Personal and Physical Achievement Programme Waiver (The Steadward Centre for Personal and Physical Achievement 2001)

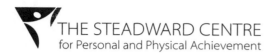
THE STEADWARD CENTRE
for Personal and Physical Achievement

W1-67 Van Vliet Centre
University of Alberta
Edmonton, Alberta
Canada T6G 2H9
Phone 1-780-492-7298
Fax 1-780-492-7161
www.steadwardcentre.org

PROGRAM WAIVER / RELEASE FORM

I, _____, have committed to participating in a physical activity program conducted by The Steadward Centre, University of Alberta.

I understand that there are potential risks of injury to myself involved with the physical activity program that I will participate in. These risks have been explained to me and I have had full opportunity for discussion of them and have a full appreciation of them.

In consideration of participating in a physical activity program, I do hereby for myself, successors and assigns, release, forever discharge and waive The Steadward Centre and the University of Alberta or the employees or agents of these from any and all action, causes of action, claims and demands for upon or by reason of any damage, loss or injury to person and property which hereafter may be sustained in consequence of my participation in a physical activity program at The Steadward Centre.

Date: _____   Participant: _____

Witness: _____

Appendix 23.D The Steadward Centre for Personal and Physical Achievement Informed Consent Form (The Steadward Centre for Personal and Physical Achievement 2001)

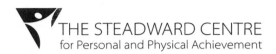

THE STEADWARD CENTRE
for Personal and Physical Achievement

W1-67 Van Vliet Centre

University of Alberta

Edmonton, Alberta

Canada T6G 2H9

Informed Consent Form

Phone 1-780-492-7298

Fax 1-780-492-7161

www.steadwardcentre.org

I, _____, authorize The Steadward Centre and the University of Alberta to administer and conduct tests and/or training programs to increase my physical work capacity.

I understand that my level of physical fitness will be assessed and that, based on the results, an individualized training program may be prescribed. I realize that I will be requested to perform exercises to evaluate and/or improve one or more of the following: a. Muscular Fitness, b. Cardiovascular Fitness, c. Body Shape and Build, d. Flexibility, and that the data may be used for educational and/or promotional purposes.

I understand that there are potential risks of injury to myself involved with any exercise and performance testing or training program. These risked have been explained to me and I have had full opportunity for discussion of them and have a full appreciation of them. I also understand that at any time during the testing or training sessions that I experience unusual discomfort I may choose to discontinue the exercise.

In consideration of being allowed to utilize The Steadward Centre for testing and/or training purposes, I do hereby for myself, my heirs, executors, administrators, successors and assigns, release, forever discharge and waive The Steadward Centre and the University of Alberta or the employees or agents of either from any and all action, causes of action, claims and demands for upon or by reason of any damage, loss or injury to person and property which hereafter may be sustained in consequences of my utilization of and participation in testing or training conducted by The Steadward Centre, University of Alberta.

I have read this form and understand the testing and training program in which I will be engaged. I consent to participate in this testing or training session(s).

Date: dd_____/mm_____/yy_____   **Participant:** _____

Parent or Guardian: (if under 18 years) _____

Witness: _____

The information on this form is collected under the general authority of the *University Act* (R.S.A. 1980, c. U-5). It is directly related to and needed by The Steadward Centre for recording personal and research information about its clients. The information will be used for research purposes including research data collection, obtaining informed consent, and identifying candidates for future research and/or for activity programming including creating tables of fitness norms, identifying candidates for research projects, contacting someone in an emergency, and developing a fitness program. If you have any questions about the collection and use of this information, please contact: Ewen Nelson; Information Systems; Rick Hansen Centre; Phone: (780) 492-7091; Fax: (780) 492-7161; E-mail: ewen.nelson@ualberta.ca

ADAPTED PHYSICAL ACTIVITY

CHAPTER 24

Disabling Aspects of Aging

*The Role of Active Living in
Promoting Life Span Autonomy*

Sandra O'Brien Cousins

Learning Objectives
- To better appreciate the myths and realities of age declines.
- To gain an understanding of how age declines that lead to disablement are socialized, and how each of us contribute to disabling processes.
- To increase awareness of the role of active living strategies in preventing and reversing disablement processes.

Introduction

Chronological aging has long been blamed as the cause of "a disablement process" (Verbrugge and Jette 1994). Disability in late life is conspicuous, but it is not the norm. While age, gender, educational level, social support, number of chronic conditions, and cognitive status are important predictors of functional status (Mendes de Leon, Seeman, Baker, Richardson, and Tinetti 1996), it is noteworthy that a majority (62 percent) of older adults aged eighty-five and older have no chronic condition, cognitive problem, or requirement for assistance that would place them at risk for institutionalization (National Advisory Council on Aging [NACA] 1996). Although disability rates rise steeply after age seventy-five, only 2 percent of adults sixty-five years and older, and only 10 percent of adults eighty-five years and older, are actually at risk of being institutionalized. But even more noteworthy is the statistic that only a minority of these same individuals would actually consider themselves with a disability; the overwhelming evidence is that the vast majority of seniors are not frail or disabled (NACA 1996).

New evidence is accumulating that age declines are accelerated and exacerbated by social policies and ageist stereotypes that encourage older people 'to take it easy' once they reach retirement (Health Canada 1999b; O'Brien Cousins 1998). This link between inactivity and health was proposed more than thirty years ago when Kraus and Raab (1961) first coined the term *hypokinetic disease*. As we enter the new millennium, the poor health and disability outcomes of being a sedentary individual are receiving a good deal of research attention. While there are no guarantees that aging adults can avoid all medical afflictions with an optimally active lifestyle, there is a good deal of evidence to suggest that, on average, sedentary living shortens life span by as much as two years (Paffenbarger, Hyde, Wing and Hsied 1986).

More serious though, in terms of suffering and burden, are the postural deformity, brittle bones, muscle weakness, social isolation, dementia, and general apathy for living among many older people. Sadly, many of our current veterans who fought for freedom in World War II have given up the fight (Morrison 2001). By succumbing to the lethargy of growing old and spending their last few years in institutional care, the freedom our heroes won seems to have been stolen by Father Time. Or was it all of 'us' (society at large) who have given up on these old bodies? What could possibly be the role that you have played in disabling the elders you know? What would you do if your grandmother asked you to help her go sky-diving? What would you say if your great-grandfather had drowned while fishing alone in a river? Should not old people just take it easy, reduce adventure, and ride out their late years on slow speed?

Simply by thinking that passive forms of growing old are more appropriate for retired people, Canadians of all ages unwittingly promote age stereotypes. While biological aging, by itself, does take a toll on our health and well-being, we all must take responsibility for promoting processes of disablement among our elders and ourselves. By thinking of aging as a disease, or a time to withdraw, our society expects cautious behaviour. Treating people differently simply based on their age is a type of socialization called *ageism* and insures older people do slow down. By cooperating with these social expectations, most people significantly reduce their potential health span and quality of life (Shephard 1997). And that is how many of our aging veterans, once fit enough to fight and win a world war, have ended up in wheelchairs. Sadly, their apparent apathy for life now is formed out of our deep respect for them to age without interference; we have not encouraged them to fight the ravages of aging.

Fortunately, there are veterans in our midst who offer positive challenges to age stereotyping. One example is Stan Dyer, born in Edmonton in 1921, who repaired radios in World War II. At twenty-four he was near the front lines maintaining communication links from his tool truck. At night he put his tool boxes under his truck and slept between them to avoid enemy fire. He claims those tools saved his life many times. On his return to Canadian life, Stan was a successful businessman with Snap-on Tools. He travelled all over Alberta, gaining weight and smoking for twenty-seven years. Heart symptoms surfaced, and the doctor told him to get exercising. Taking up running (which he did not enjoy at all) was Stan's next 'tool' (figure 24.1). He survived the war, survived those decades of smoking, survived a quadruple bypass, and since age fifty-seven, detected and avoided health problems by conditioning his body to an optimum. In the 1970s, he joined the U of Agers, a men's gymnastics group who train alongside the varsity team. Within a few years, Stan was doing giant swings on the high bar and the iron cross on rings. Physical activity was now in Stan's tool box and, accordingly, this too saved his life. He is one veteran over age eighty whom you won't find in a wheelchair, one older Canadian who trained the last thirty years of his life instead of just the first thirty.

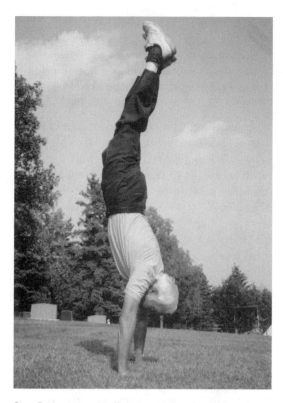

Stan Dyer, at age 78, flaunting his handstand in a cemetery.

Why is it so important to stay active in later life? New evidence is being published in over two hundred scientific journals (O'Brien Cousins and Horne 1999), that a physically active lifestyle adds years to life by reducing all-cause mortality (Paffenbarger, Hyde, Wing, and Hsied 1986), extending health-span, detecting disease early, and providing rapid healing and recovery. Changing disability outcomes has been a more challenging task for researchers to prove (Keysor and Jette 2001). While weak research designs are often blamed, "the theoretical basis of interventions aimed at reducing disability may need to extend beyond exercise and address other behavioural and social factors" (Keysor and Jette 2001, p. M412). Thus, while strong scientific evidence is mounting that even small increases in daily physical activity can significantly improve both quality and quantity of life for elderly adults (Health Canada 1999a),

the actual collective of research showing that disability is significantly benefitted by exercise is limited. The explanation may be, in part, the unique features of the person experiencing the physical disability; that is, physical disability may be moderated or exacerbated by others, or interpreted differently by individuals—a mind over matter issue (Keysor and Jette 2001).

We know that reversals of age declines are possible to a point (O'Brien Cousins and Burgess 1998). Eventually the improvements in physiological function plateau, and the age decline resumes, albeit from a more optimal functional point. For example, progressive strength training can double muscle strength in people over age ninety (Fiatarone et al. 1994). Bone loss can be temporarily halted with certain kinds of exercise and bones can be partially remineralized over a year of progressive resistance training (Nelson et al. 1994; Hatori et al. 1993). But prevention is the preferred route to healthy aging, because physical age declines can be virtually cut in half with more active living throughout the adult years (Shephard 1997).

Age disability is not as prevalent among older adults as most people think. Virtually everyone can expect to experience some kind of chronic or temporary illness by late life, but only 10 percent of Canadians between the ages of sixty-five and sixty-nine have multiple disabilities (Canada 1996). Therefore, most elderly people are *not* disabled. Though chronological aging is inevitable, the rate of biological aging and the extent of disability related to disease processes are somewhat manageable. To some degree, disability may be preventable altogether (Verbrugge and Jette 1994). Even as our population ages, disability rates are dropping. Disability rises to 25 percent only among persons eighty and older (1996) but only 10-15 percent of older people are institutionalized at any point in time. Current thinking is that care institutions (such as nursing homes) should not be 'the end of the line' to people's lives. As many as 29 percent of those people in nursing homes are high functioning and, once stable, should be returned to the community (Buttar, Blaum, and Fries 2001). Thus, with very elderly cohorts exhibiting the fastest population growth, preventing disability and restoring abililty among elders is an important issue.

The purpose of this chapter is to explore biological, social, and psychological forces that act as disabling factors to lifelong vitality and autonomy. My aim, as author, is to "disentangle the process of disablement" (Jette 1999) from those of biological decline, but to also highlight how social stereotyping, environmental constraints, and psychological adaptations can exacerbate, or compensate, for biological declines. In addition, I hope to highlight the potent enabling role of active living processes, of regular involvement in fitness activities such as sport, active recreation, dancing, and outdoor pursuits such as hiking, gardening, skating, and skiing. While age changes *do* bring declines that lead to vulnerability and increased risk for disability, active living is a powerful human resource that provides social, physical, and emotional sustenance. Even in very late life, active living can make a significant contribution, not just to slowing the disablement process, but to the restoration and maintenance of capabilities to enjoy life to its fullest (Langley and Knight 1999).

1 Is disability an inevitable feature of growing old? How much of aging is preventable?

2 How does society contribute to disability in older people?

3 When is someone too old to be a beneficiary of a physically active lifestyle?

The Aging-disablement Process

Disability has been defined as "difficulty doing activities in any domain of life (from hygiene to hobbies, errands to sleep) due to a health or physical problem" (Verbrugge and Jette 1994, p. 3).

"Disablement" refers to impacts that chronic and acute conditions have on the functioning of specific body systems and on people's abilities to act in necessary, usual, expected and personally desired ways in their society. (Verbrugge and Jette 1994, p. 3)

Verbrugge and Jette (1994) claim that intrinsic disability (without using personal or technical aids) is distinguished from actual disability (with such aids or assistance). Thus, mobility disability is not a personal characteristic, but it is a gap between personal capability and environmental demand (Patla and Shumway-Cook 1999). As such, disability becomes the third level of a process that includes the onset of impairments (abnormalities of organ structures or body systems), which lead to functional limitations (restrictions in physical and mental actions), and ultimately lead to disability, or the difficulty in performing social roles. Such definitions are important to clarify, because "the fundamental absence of a uniform definition of disablement" undermines a researcher's ability to categorize his or her findings (Verbrugge and Jette 1994).

The aging-disablement process, as explained by Verbrugge and Jette (1994), organizes potential disablement risk factors into three categories: 1) *predisposing risk factors* (background risk factors that existed before the onset of the disablement process); 2) *intra-individual factors* (psychosocial attributes, lifestyle, and behaviour changes that exacerbate the disablement process; and, 3) *extra-individual factors* (physical and social environments that intervene in the disablement process). Gerontologists are attempting to trace trajectories of disabilities over time to understand the pathways that provoke, exacerbate or propel, and even slow, disability's pace (Verbrugge 1995). Conceptual schemes are being advanced by Verbrugge and Jette (Verbrigge 1995; Verbrugge and Jette 1994) that link pathology, impairments, functional limitations, disability, and social disadvantage. They also have identified predisposing risk factors, interventions, and exacerbators that alter the pace of the pathway.

Notably, Verbrugge (1995) has compared the disabling impact of seven disease conditions: three nonfatal and four fatal health conditions. Arthritis, visual impairment, and hearing impairment were the three nonfatal conditions, while ischaemic heart disease (IHD), chronic obstructive pulmonary disease (COPD), diabetes mellitus, and malignant cancers represented fatal conditions. In asking 'how disabling' a condition is, Verbrugge studied both aggregate rates, or prevalence in a population, and also examined disabling impact, or the chance of actually being limited with the condition. Using those criteria, arthritis becomes the leading disabler from middle-age on due to its high prevalence and moderate chance of causing disability. Interestingly, for all four fatal conditions, disabling impact peaks in mid-life, plateaus or falls off in later ages. Meanwhile, the impact of nonfatal conditions generally rises with age, especially for arthritis and visual impairment. "At older ages, fatal and non-fatal health problems have an approximately equal impact; this is a telling illustration of the importance of non-killers in late life." (Verbrugge 1995, p. 23)

Often people accept disease-related declines as 'normal' aging, and thereby become too accepting of their problems. Self-rehabilitation and self-care can be too easily exchanged for passivity and dependency. Verbrugge (1995) notes that efforts to overcome and adjust to disability are often "silent, private, and even unconscious." One way Verbrugge recommends that we study the effects of disability is to assess how chronic conditions affect time use: the activities that a person does, the procedures undertaken, and the frequency and duration.

For example, researchers at the Baltimore Longitudinal Study on Aging (BLSA) studied changes in how people spent their time as they got older. Time spent on obligatory activities (personal care, errands, chores, and sleep) and passive leisure increased as people got older, while time on work and other responsibilities (employment, optional shopping, and errands) and discretionary activities (visiting, entertainment, public service, sports and active recreation, religion, and hobbies) decreased with age (Verbrugge 1995). Longitudinal studies show that older people tend to respond more intensely to their chronic conditions by reducing their committed and discretionary activities more so than younger people with the same impairment.

Thus older people do react differently to disability, as if they assume they will never get better; they tend to use swift and enduring ways to overcome dysfunctions. Older people do not attempt for very long to restore function to what it used to be, but rather, they modify steps and bathrooms, use a cane, hire help for heavy chores, and relax their standards of performance. Such relaxed standards, it could be argued, lead to permanent and irrevocable functional decline. In contrast, younger people tend to work very hard at restoring functional losses after being afflicted with a disabling condition. Thus, Verbrugge advocates for more emphasis and social recognition of nonfatal conditions such as arthritis, urinary incontinence, lower back pain, and vision problems. Such chronic issues in older people, while equivalent to fatal conditions with their prevalence and disability, do not have to be accepted as a permanent burden in the older population. Some of these conditions can be prevented or healed, if aging adults were not so quick to simply blame their problems on age and be so permanently accepting of what may be temporary health conditions.

Baltes (1996) has described three variations of dependency in his book, *The Many Faces of Dependency in Old Age*. Learned helplessness and learned dependency are both outcomes of previous and ongoing person-environment transactions as well as of life events. But a third style of life adaptation is presented as "successful aging" in which dependency is managed as "selective optimization with compensation" (p. 145). This third paradigm of behavioural dependency is explained as a self-regulated model in which forms of performance reduction have "positive adaptive value." With this strategy, the individual does acknowledge losses in reserves and strengths, but considers compensatory options, persists in recovery efforts longer, and makes adjustments accordingly. Which activities to give up, which to maintain, which to become dependent on will vary from person to person, reflecting inter-individual differences in preferences, motivations, skills, and so on. In the model of selective optimization with compensation, Baltes argues that effective coordination of the three processes of selection, compensation, and optimization will ensure successful aging despite many losses and the diminuation in reserve capacities. In this next section, losses are presented in three facets of aging: processes of biological decline, influential processes of socialization, and psychologically adaptive processes.

4 Briefly explain the meaning of *disablement*.

5 How do younger people generally differ from older people in handling new physical limitations?

6 Name three types of factors creating risk for future disablement.

THE DISABLING ASPECTS OF AGING: BIOLOGICAL DECLINE

Aging, considering only its physical form, is mainly a process of biological decline. The nature of this decline is complex, however, as noted by Roy Shephard in his book *Aging, Physical Activity and Health* (1997). Although the nature and rate of physical decline is measurable across all major physiological systems, the actual role of biological aging in the decline process is under debate. Shephard (1997) notes that interpreting the role of aging in physical declines that lead to disability is problematic; he reports that interpretations are difficult because of an incomplete sampling of populations under study, age-related changes in habitual physical activity, dietary patterns and body build,

secular changes in lifestyle, and an age-related increase in the prevalence of chronic disease. Thus, while it is unclear just how much of these declines that lead to disability can be blamed on biological aging, and how much can be blamed on disease, genetics, or on social stereotypes and social policies such as mandatory retirement, there is no doubt that aging is accompanied by declines in physical function and performance. The rate of decline after the age of thirty is at a rate of a 10 percent per decade in most functions, such that serious disablement can occur by mid- to later life when function has dropped to 50 percent or more (Shephard 1997). However, these declines are only typical of sedentary adults: more active people can cut these biological declines virtually in half and prolong functional fitness into very advanced age.

The notion that disabling processes are very much the result of not meeting the needs and demands of the surrounding environment is prevalent. Patla and Shumway-Cook (1999) have conceptualized eight dimensions of mobility related to community ambulation: walking distance, time constraints, ambient conditions, terrain characteristics, external physical load, attentional demands, postural transition, and traffic level. Thus their premise that "the environment and the individual conjointly determine mobility disability" (p. 7) has an ecological perspective.

Other perspectives differ from the ecological perspective. Autonomy in activities of daily living (ADL) is thought to be mainly dependent on individuals maintaining an appropriate level of muscular and joint fitness (more so than aerobic fitness) (Phillips and Haskell 1995). But discerning the pathways from disease to disability is a challenge. Certain diseases can lead to rapid declines in function, but not consistently. Individual self-care, attitude, and willingness to 'fight' disease seems to make a difference in the outcomes of people who have the very same disease in the very same environment. In this way,

the pathway from disease to disability is obscured by the influence of many non-disease factors, such as depression, social support, and health behaviours. (Patla and Shumway-Cook 1999, p. 8)

Critics of population health promotion contend that healthier lifestyles by many individuals may actually increase morbidity or disease (and health expenditures) late in life by prolonging the number of years people live with chronic illness, suffering, and disability (Warner 1992). Countering that argument are large population studies that show disability rates are dropping rapidly in the last two years (Health Canada 1999b). Disability rates for men dropped from 13 percent in 1994–1995 to 12 percent in 1996–1997 while women dropped from 17 percent in 1994–1995 to 14 percent in 1996–1997. Activity limitations dropped over the same time period from 20 percent to 15 percent for men and from 21 percent to 17 percent for women. Higher income groups have about half of the disability rates of low-income groups, but it is not clear whether disabilities lead to lower income, or if low income status leads to disablement. Similar data are reported for the United States:

> We have indications that those now entering their senior years are healthier and more fit than previous groups at the same point in their lives. In a fairly recent U.S. study, researchers at Duke University (Manton, Corder, and Stallard, quoted 1993) reported that the total prevalence of disability actually declined from 1984 to 1989. If the apparent gains in health and illness underlying these changes stand up, we may encounter disability rates below past levels among young seniors. (NACA 1996)

Even if it were true that prolonged disability did accompany longer life spans, a wellness/fitness approach would be the preferred alternative to ignoring the problems of hypokinesis and then advising the taking of medications (Senior's Advisory Council for Alberta 1992).

7 What are four other factors besides chronological aging that contribute to disability among some elders?

8 If physically active older people cut typical declines in half, what is the average decline they could expect on an annual basis?

9 If it is true that disability rates are dropping, what could be the explanation(s)?

SOCIAL PROCESSES AND STEREOTYPES THAT LEAD TO DISABILITY

The social interpretations of aging that vary from one culture to the next and from one generation to another are just as noteworthy and conceptually problematic as biological age declines. Although the pace of disablement is linked to some aspects of chronological aging, other factors such as socialized expectations related to gender and age may accelerate the process (Verbrugge 1995, Verbrugge and Jette 1994).

Gender

Lifelong gender disparity in leisure lifestyles has been assessed, with far more males pursuing vigorous forms of physical activity at every life stage (Stephens and Craig 1990). So disparate are men and women in vigorous forms of physical activity that older women are tempted to attribute the shorter longevity of men to their higher levels of physical activity in sports and active recreation. In reality, moderately active males can expect to gain about two years of life (Paffenbarger et al. 1986), but the illusion to many older people is that exercise is too risky and even harmful (O'Brien Cousins 2000). Women's lower activity levels are unfortunate given the fact that by age ninety, women outnumber men by almost three to one (Statistics Canada 1990) and their prospects for aging well are undermined by their less active living (Laukkanen, Sakari-Rantala, Kauppinen, and Heikkinen 1997). As a consequence of their more sedentary aging, women encounter chronic diseases earlier than men, and these chronic conditions are often used as reasons excusing older women from exerting themselves. Old age, for women in particular, seems to be so strongly socially constructed that the older that people become, the more they use their chronological age to judge how they should look after themselves, regardless of their actual health and capability (Vertinsky 1998).

Continued medicalization of the female body and the perpetuation of disempowering stereotypes in old age create a substantial obligation for women to 'age gracefully' even if it means surrendering to institutionalization by eighty-five (Vertinsky 1998). Thus, older women are generally less physically fit than men, have slower reaction times, walk and climb stairs more slowly, and are significantly weaker in muscle strength (Era and Rantanen 1997). While some older men find themselves as caregivers, and endure similar challenges to female caregivers, generally the large majority of caregivers are women, and some are of very advanced age.

Sadly, the generous care-giving effort by aging women for their older parents and relatives can translate into their own demise for health; in catering to the needs of family members and friends, an older woman may neglect her own needs for healthy, active recreation (O'Brien Cousins and Vertinsky 1991). As a caregiver's stress levels rise, she may never think to cope with her own problems with healthy, active recreation. Though her volunteer achievements in caring for others are magnanimous and good-intentioned, this self-sacrifice of older women to look after others leads to a sad irony; the caregiver may choose to ignore her own self-care needs and thus increases prospects for becoming dependent on others too. Thus, late life for older women is too often experienced as a "bitter fruit" (Vertinsky 1998).

Vertinsky (1998) has argued that there remain formidable challenges to achieving social equity in opportunities for healthy physical activity. She noted,

Women's voices are conspicuously absent in helping policy makers understand how the uncritical pursuit of body training, ultra-fitness, and unattainable slimness and beauty compromises the health of some women, while lack of regular physical activity and nonparticipation in active leisure remain all too often the norm for adolescent girls, working women, mothers, poor women, women from ethnic minorities and aging females. (Vertinsky 1998, p. 85)

Even though discouraging stereotypes about the aging female body and its unproven physical liabilities in sport settings do not fit the typical experience of contemporary older women, they do linger (Vertinsky 1998). The self-perception of baby boomer women who are well settled into mid-life careers and families is of interest to exercise gerontologists. Will these women try to defy the ultimate forces of aging by doing things differently than their parents and grandparents? If they are so empowered, how will they try to age better? Will a physically active lifestyle be part of their aging strategy? What will be the outcomes for disability within the next generation?

Age

Evidence is mounting that a compression of morbidity is occurring such that more people are living closer to optimal maximum life span and are delaying the onset of disease process until later in life (Fries 1980, 1989). Extending better health and longevity to more people has been visualized as a "rectangularization" of the mortality curve (Fries 1989) and is likely attributed to improvements in the broader determinants of health. Indeed, persons with higher socioeconomic status (House et al. 1990), higher educational levels (Leigh and Fries 1994), and those who engage in regular aerobic activity (Fries et al. 1994) have substantially better health. These kinds of studies provide support for the hypothesis that,

persons with lower health risks (at mid-life) will have disability later in life, will have less disability at any given age, and will have less cumulative disability than persons with greater health risks. (Vita, Terry, Hubert, and Fries 1998, p. 1035)

10 Why are older women reluctant to participate in the more vigorous forms of physical activity and sport?

11 How do women's roles as primary caregivers add to their health risk in late life?

12 People who are leading healthy lifestyles through their middle years are less likely to experience disability. True or false?

PSYCHOLOGICAL LINKS TO DISABILITY IN OLDER ADULTS

Associations between psychological factors and functional attributes are receiving attention in contemporary gerontological literature. The stress and coping paradigm of Lazarus and Folkman (1984) suggested that high levels of psychological resources may protect against the progression of disability over time. Indeed, aging (the chronological number) on its own may be considered a chronic stressor that can induce stress responses such as anxiety, depression, and demoralization. People may think they are simply running out of time. In addition, older people can experience various senses of loss as they age: social losses such as widowhood, deaths of friends and family members; productivity and wage losses related to an abrupt retirement experience; leaving the familiarity of their neighbourhoods for smaller accommodations; physical losses accompanying functional changes; and, memory changes, hearing and vision losses, as well as acute and chronic diseases processes which sap emotional strength and energy.

There is a good deal of evidence that age self-stereotyping also demoralizes older people (Vertinsky, O'Brien Cousins and Tan, in review). They learn that younger people do not like them or value their life experience. Depressive responses to these changes may result in higher levels of associated disability (Prince, Harwood, Blizard, Thomas, and Mann 1997). Some older people have learned how to make a psychological adaptation and develop a resilience that seems to reduce distress and protect against further declines (Ormel et al. 1998).

Older people who feel more in control seem to be better at avoiding disabling conditions. Perceived control, or mastery, a concept related to self-efficacy, indicates the extent to which one regards one's life changes as being under one's control rather than be due to fate, chance, or luck. Thus higher levels of perceived mastery are hypothesized to predict higher levels of functional ability (Kempen, van Sonderen, and Ormel 1999). People who perceive a strong sense of life control and self-efficacy were observed to have better physical function and fewer limitations (Kempen et al. 1999). For example, overall levels of disability among low-functioning elderly persons (average age of seventy-two with at least four physical limitations) who were living in the community did increase over a two-year period, although those who showed high levels of self-perceived mastery did not have appreciable declines (Kempen et al. 1999). Indeed, associations between psychological attributes (such as self-efficacy and mastery) on the one hand, and self-management of disability on the other hand, have been widely studied in patients suffering from rheumatoid arthritis (Krol et al. 1998). Longitudinal studies are rare, but a study by Mendes de Leon et al. (1996) provided support for the buffering effect of ADL-related self-efficacy on functional decline in community-living elders.

It should be no surprise that active living is positively linked to beliefs about personal competence, locus of control, and physical capability—even into late life (O'Brien Cousins 1997a). Older people in physical training may have a lot in common with any athlete who is training with special physical challenges such as disability. Both seniors and disabled athletes have learned that sport can be a vehicle to be seen as normal (Martin 1999) as well as being "beyond normal" (Wheeler, Malone, VanVlack, Nelson, and Steadward 1996). An elevated sense of physical efficacy is an attribute among active elderly women, and the origins of such beliefs may stem from situations and mastery experiences as far back as childhood (O'Brien Cousins 1997a). Moreover, self-efficacy and sense of life control do seem to be readily enhanced when less active older adults first engage in physical activities which they enjoy and from which they experience quite rapid social and health benefits (O'Brien Cousins 1998).

Other work suggests that the association between perceived control and health status in older persons is mediated by exercising (Menec and Chipperfield 1997). Kempen et al. (1999) assessed the amount of time spent on physical activities, and an index was constructed to estimate the number of hours per month regularly spent on nine physical activities: swimming, playing tennis, gardening, bowling, dancing, shopping, walking, cycling, and gymnastics (van Eijk 1997). Significant associations were found between level of physical activity and concurrent level of disability (-.346) (p<.05). However, causation is not clear in this correlation study that tells us only that increased levels of physical activity are statistically linked to lower disability rates. However, other work has been published that does suggest causation. (See forthcoming section, Aging Better, Preventing Disability).

Within the MacArthur Studies of Successful Aging (Seeman, Unger, McAvay, and Mendes de Leon 1999), longitudinal data tested the hypothesis that stronger self-efficacy beliefs would protect against the onset of perceived functional disabilities over a 2.5-year follow-up, independent of underlying physical ability. Standard self-report scales were used to assess perceived functional disabilities, ranging from mild performance difficulties (Nagi scale) to more severe disabilities (Katz ADL scale). Gender-specific multiple regression models revealed that weaker self-efficacy beliefs predicted declines in reported functional status among both men and women.

> These findings suggest that self-efficacy beliefs have significant impacts on perceptions of functional disability, independent of actual underlying physical abilities. Through such influences on perceptions of disability, self-efficacy beliefs may importantly affect lifestyles and quality of life at older ages. (Seeman et al. 1999, p. P214)

However, psychological factors can also be altered by the events of people's lives, the seasons, and chronological time, and thus the correlates of individual well-being, while easy to identify, are not simple to understand. A fear of falling on icy walks and streets can lead to immediate reductions in community mobility and rapid deterioration in older adult health. A 'downward spiral' in health can be provoked by a number of negative events that happen to coincide in time (Burgess and O'Brien Cousins 1998); the older adult reduces physical activity as a form of coping and thus becomes vulnerable to rapid age declines. All hope of recovery is soon lost, and disability and acute problems accelerate.

Reversing a downward spiral in physical health and psychological well-being is very difficult once it starts, and such reversals are time and labour-intensive, not to mention very professionally challenging (Burgess and O'Brien Cousins 1998). But there is some evidence it can be done. Physiotherapists note that one of the key ingredients in making reversals possible is the will and motivation of the individual to try. One case study has been documented in the physical activity profession. Dr. Art Burgess, campus fitness and lifestyle director at the University of Alberta during the 1980s and 1990s, has presented his learnings with an eighty-year-old woman experiencing multiple health problems. She seemed to have exhausted all forms of medical intervention, her therapy was no longer helping, and as a last resort, she turned to Dr. Burgess for a simple walking and gentle stretching programme (Burgess and O'Brien Cousins 1998).

Once a powerful voice as a former CBC radio broadcaster, Ethyl Marliss had become a timorous, breathless, and weak old woman with multiple and severe health concerns. With daily physical activity, ongoing personal supervision and support, she was gradually able to restore herself and regain her identity. After about a year of almost daily persistence in walking, strengthening, and stretching, she was able to develop enough strength, mobility, and respiratory fitness to do away with her walking cane, strengthen her heart, reduce her breathlessness, and renew her social vitality to the point of socially entertaining at her home. When I last saw her, she made an impromptu speech before one hundred people at a retirement party for Dr. Burgess, and without microphone, cracked jokes, and 'roasted' the retiree. Then she talked about her indebtedness to Dr. Burgess, and swung her leg up both sides of the dinner table to show everyone how high she could kick. It was the 'old' Ethyl, now restored, with her booming vocal chords and sense of humour. She lived five years more with much improved quality of life, and passed away rather quickly without spiralling again into chronic disablement.

13 Why are older people vulnerable to depression?

14 What psychological attribute enhances the self-management of disability?

15 Is the 'downward spiral' a physical or psychological phenomenon?

AGING BETTER, PREVENTING DISABILITY

Contemporary research provides convincing evidence that pursuing healthy lifestyles will not only extend life, but will also extend healthspan and lead to economic savings and independent living (Furman 1995). Long-term data from the Chicago Heart Association Study showed that middle-age health factors predicted later life health bills. Daviglus et al. (1998) found that people with favourable cardiovascular risk profiles in middle age had lower average annual Medicare charges in older age. The total annual health care charges (in US dollars) for the men at low risk were less than two-thirds of the charges for the men at higher risk ($1615 less); for the women at low risk, the charges were less than one half of those for the women at higher risk ($1885 less). In other words, people at initially high risk for heart problems cost the health care

system virtually double than those who were at low risk. Thus, by these estimates, middle-aged people who have one or more heart health risk factors (sedentary living, smoking, hypertension, high LDL cholesterol) had accelerated their possibilities for future cardiovascular (and other) disease.

Fries (1980) and others have attacked the stereotype of old age as a time of disability and helplessness. His hypothesis was that societies can age better. In the ideal case, the citizens of modern society would survive to an advanced age with their vigour and functional independence maintained, and their morbidity and disability compressed into a relatively short period before death (Campion 1998). Indeed, the survival curve *is* becoming increasingly compressed and rectangular, with most deaths occurring after age seventy-five (Nusselder and Mackenbach 1996).

Longitudinal data lends strong support for the idea that disability can be prevented. Vita et al. (1998) studied health risks of smoking, body mass index, and exercise patterns in 1741 middle-aged university alumni from 1962 to 1994 for cumulative disability. By 1994, the average age of the survivors was seventy-five years. Persons with high health risks in 1962 or 1986 had twice the cumulative disability of those with low health risks (disability index 1.02 vs. .49; p <0.001). The results were consistent among survivors, subjects who died, men and women, and for both the last year and the last two years of observation. Overall, the onset of disability was postponed by more than five years in the low-risk group as compared with the high-risk group. Thus Vita and colleagues concluded,

> Smoking, body-mass index, and exercise patterns in midlife and late adulthood are predictors of subsequent disability. Not only do persons with better health habits survive longer, but in such persons, disability is postponed and compressed into fewer years at the end of life. (1998, p. 1035)

Peel, Utsey, and MacGregor (1999) are among a few researchers who have conducted exercise training targeted at older adults to have known limitations in physical function. Within eight weeks, patients randomly assigned to a three-times per week exercise group had significantly improved their scores in cardiovascular fitness, muscle force production, and reduced time taken to complete physical performance tasks. Still, exercising regularly is far from even being contemplated among most elderly, according to Nigg's research team (1999). Most older individuals are not even thinking about losing weight and exercising, "making these behaviours a priority for intervention research" (p. 473).

16 Why is higher risk for heart disease often linked to higher risks for other disease?

17 What factors at mid-life predict later disability?

A NEW GENERATION OF DISABILITY?
The new millennium brings new demographic challenges as Canadian society ages. The baby boomers are at the new cusp of middle age. They are entering their fifties and by 2030 to 2040 most of them will still be alive and entering their eighties. Governments at all levels, and the health care community in particular, are extremely concerned, since by current aging standards, virtually all of these elderly boomers will be impacting in unprecedented ways on the major social systems (pensions, social security, health care, and community resources). By 2040, the surviving boomers will be turning ninety, an age when disability rates are the highest, and nursing home requirements are expected to triple (American Association of Retired Persons 1998). At the same time, there will be a shrinking pool of middle-aged caregivers:

> As the number of persons either disabled or in nursing homes continues to grow due to greater longevity, the pool of available caregivers relative to age groups with the greatest need of care will shrink over time

because of the smaller size of boomer families. (AARP 1998, p. 51)

In 1990, the ratio of the caregiving population (usually aged fifty to sixty-four) compared to those likely to need care (eighty-five and over) was eleven to one. In 2030, the ratio will be six to one and, by 2050, four to one. With activity limitations tripling at the same time that the caregiver pool diminishes by two-thirds, it is projected that disability will be the 'norm.' There are simply so many people in the baby boomer generation that they have experienced shortages most of their lives–from lack of school classrooms to educate them, to lack of employers to hire them. Therefore, boomers' confidence in their future health care benefits is as shaky as their confidence in public pensions, and many middle-aged adults are not confident that future health benefits will be even equal to those received by current retirees. Almost 70 percent of boomers lack confidence that public medicare benefits will be maintained, even though, as long-time adult taxpayers, they have been heavy investors in supporting a health system hungry for advanced technology, universality, and rapid service.

Yet, many adults in this huge generation of middle-aged people will ignore effective, enjoyable, low-cost, and low technology ways of improving health and preventing disability. For example, we know that even low intensity general physical training in older subjects can lead to significant improvements in fitness factors that promote heart health and reduce risk factors for other diseases (De Vito, Hernandez, Gonzalez, Felici, and Figura 1997). But as with everything else affected by the baby boom, even a small proportion of this huge bulge in the population could overwhelm the health care system.

Boomers do seem to be different in some important ways. They are a highly educated generation, even physically educated (remember the hoola hoop), and most of them will find a way to make the most of their retirement. Many do not trust medical advice, are suspicious of new drugs, and a good number are in professional roles that have forced them to become adept at using Web sites. If the boomers prove to be wiser than previous generations, they will recognize that 98 percent of health dollars are invested in trying to fix people once they are sick. With this kind of health care economics, boomers would certainly overwhelm a tertiary care system in sheer volume of illness. There are some early signs that many boomers are going to try to age better and put more effort into self-care. They only want to live long if they can live well, and one aging goal that is telling is depicted in the expression, "Club Med, not Club Bed."

Investing in primary prevention makes more sense because it aims to avert the onset of pathology altogether; and secondary prevention could play a stronger role in the early detection and medical management of pathology. Tertiary care is meant to cover all disease impacts, functional limitations, disability, life-sustaining care, and then even death itself (Verbrugge 1995). The boomers are generally on the right track because current economic downsizing in health care suggests that tertiary care strategies are already in trouble.

Economically and ethically, traditional medicine has much to learn about aging and disablement; the contemporary determinants of lifelong health are no longer attributed to the successful diagnoses of heart disease, nor to the detection power of newer technologies such as breast cancer screening. Such diagnoses and technologies can even lead to increased risks, physical harm, and even mortality in the very diseases they are meant to prevent (Watmough et al. 1997). For example, breast biopsies can spread cancer by dragging the biopsy needle through mammary tissues. Unwittingly causing harm (making people worse) works against the Hippocratic Oath of medicine to "do no harm" and is labelled as *iatrogenesis*. So, although medicine receives and deserves many accolades for good practice, health promotion studies reveal that social, ecological, and psychological factors are surfacing as key determinants of health. Poverty, fear, food distribution, and material deprivation (Bernard and Smith 1998) and issues

related to education, adequate employment, and cultural issues related to race and gender are considered better explanations for the strong health gradients found in populations (Sakari-Rantala, Heikkinen, and Ruoppila 1995; Tannahill 1998). Thus, disablement is linked to social status such that people in less power and control of their lives are more likely to experience a disability.

18 Why is disability predicted to be the 'norm' in the next few decades?

19 Are baby boomers likely to age better than previous generations? Explain.

20 What, outside of medicine, contributes to health?

THE ROLE OF MEDICAL AND REHABILITATIVE PROFESSIONALS

How do doctors feel about the role of aging in producing disability? How do they feel about partnering with physical educators to help people age better? Little information exists as to the role and interests of physicians in affiliating with the physical activity community, but we do know that the medical curriculum is full, and there is apparently no room for developing skills in physical activity counselling. Moreover, physicians bill by the patient, so there is little incentive to sit down with an older person and prescribe a detailed active living plan. Rather, we in the active living community must take a lead and develop medical and therapeutic links to our services. Doctors will support high-quality programmes by making patient referrals to them, once they trust the expertise in the community. One study that shed some light on this issue found that physicians have generally *not* advocated exercise for adults over age seventy-five (Damush, Stewart, Mills, King, and Ritter 1999). Only 48 percent of older adults had ever received advice to exercise, while adults who were younger, sedentary, and had a higher body mass index were more likely to get medical advice to exercise. Both the most sedentary and the most active adults apparently were unlikely to be asked about exercise by their physician.

Programmes for older adults should be sensitive to the special needs of certain elderly participants, most of whom will not be seriously physically limited. But many so-called healthy seniors do have a joint problem or vulnerability, such as low bone density, that should be kept in mind. Generally, however, physical educators tend to grossly underestimate what older people can do. Just because one shoulder has a torn biceps tendon does not mean that both arms are compromised in movement.

Older participants should be empowered to exercise at a personally comfortable pace and not compete with others (MYOB: mind your own business!). Previous muscle and joint injury should be part of the initial assessment process so that exercise supervisors can customize programmes to individuals who may have special physical concerns. Physical educators should also use perceived exertion scales and encourage older people to 'listen to their bodies.' By age sixty-five, older people know a lot about their bodies and how they work. They should be considered the experts in that regard. Findings from a rare study on older adult injury in exercise programmes are worth noting. Ready and colleagues (1999) found that 12 percent of adults walking sixty minutes five days a week reported injuries serious enough to necessitate programme withdrawal, while 18 percent reported minor injuries, and 26 percent reported injuries requiring medical treatment. Yet age, weight, previous fitness level, and walking volume were not significantly related to injuries. The researchers concluded that women with prior musculo-skeletal problems were more likely to sustain injuries requiring medical treatment. The initial progression may have been too rapid, suggesting that "musculo-skeletal screening and gradual progression guided by

staff is important for moderate as well as intense activity programmes" (Ready et al. 1999, p. 91).

Recently, the World Health Organization issued a set of *Guidelines For Promoting Physical Activity Among Older Persons* (Chodzko-Zajko 1997) to "provide guidelines for facilitating the development of strategies, policies, and both population and community-based interventions aimed at maintaining and/or increasing the level of physical activity for all older adults" (p. 1). As gatekeepers of health information, physicians are recognized as *essential players* in advocacy for more active living among older adults. Dozens of studies now confirm the importance of maintaining muscle strength among older adults in order to prevent chronic bone loss and reduce the risks for falling and the injuries caused by falls (Smith and Tommerup, 1995). In addition, an active lifestyle is important if one hopes to avoid functional dependence and institutionalization in late life (Mihalko and McAuley 1996; Nichols et al. 1995; Shephard 1997). In controlled laboratory settings, increases in strength (in excess of 100 percent improvement) have lead to remarkable reversals in functional frailty of people in their nineties (Fiatarone et al. 1994)! Given the amount of accumulating evidence linking regular exercise to health promotion and disease prevention, some scientists have suggested that regular *physical activity is the most important public health concern* among the very old (Miller, Haskell, Berra, and DeBusk 1984; Nelson et al. 1993; O'Brien Cousins and Horne 1999).

21 What is a typical error made by new exercise leaders of older adults?

22 At what age do the benefits of strength training diminish?

23 Who is the expert of the older person's exercise pace?

A GLOBAL PROBLEM NEEDING GLOBAL SOLUTIONS

This chapter has summarized a good deal of evidence showing that population health promotion, primary prevention, and individual self-care have significant roles to play in reducing later life disability. Self-care in the form of daily physical activity is increasingly becoming an essential health resource for improved quality of life for aging adults (O'Brien Cousins 1998). Active living among older adults is supported by hundreds of studies in over two hundred journals that collectively have linked various kinds of exercise interventions to disease prevention (coronary heart disease, osteoporosis, colon cancer, improved immune response); to improved disease management (arthritis, diabetes, dementia); to functional fitness and physical performance benefits (muscle strength, flexibility, aerobic capacity, and balance); to increased indicators of psychological and social well-being (less depression and social isolation); and to short and long-term cognitive benefits (memory, reaction time, alertness) (O'Brien Cousins, and Horne 1999).

The overall contribution of physical activity to health and quality of life is so widely accepted that, in Canada, the non-profit Active Living Coalition for Older Adults (ALCOA) (www.alcoa.ca) has been created to meet demand for more information; it operates as a national network agency and communication centre for over thirty health/community organizations. Working within Health Canada with the Canadian Society of Exercise Physiology, ALCOA celebrated 1999, the International Year of the Older Person, with the introduction of the first *Canada's Physical Activity Guide to Healthy, Active Living for Older Adults*. In the US, interest is building around older adult fitness at the American College of Sports Medicine (ACSM), and a new international body, the International Society for Aging and Physical Activity (ISAPA) formed in January 1999 with links to Human Kinetics and their *Journal of Aging and Physical Activity*.

At the University of Western Ontario, The Centre for Activity and Aging has had an international role in biological and medical research on aging and physical activity with applications to community leadership and home care programmes. Since the mid-1980s, Alberta seemed to be taking the lead in Western Canada, and by 1997 the Alberta Centre For Well-Being refocussed its energy on older adult physical activity as one of its research themes and administrative units. Guided by the astute vision of Dr. Art Burgess, Project: Alive and Well was initiated in the mid-1980s—a series of sports and fitness programmes for adults fifty-five and up. The Faculty of Physical Education at the University of Alberta has had a tradition in promoting national initiatives related to health promotion, and established an exercise gerontology research lab in 1997 with the main focus on the motivational barriers (social psychology) of older adult physical activity.

EMPOWERING ABLENESS

To help Albertans understand how physical activity links to independence and quality of life, the word and acronym, ABLE, has been used to describe the notion of **A**ging **B**etter with a **L**ittle **E**xercise. The question that is asked of middle-aged people is, "Will you be ABLE?" and of older people, "Are you ABLE?" Recreation and physical therapists, physical educators, and public health clinicians are promoting the concept that people can age better with a little exercise. Four abilities deserve regular attention in everyone's lives: having adequate joint flexibility to tie shoes and reach zippers (flexABLE), being able to lift, carry and move objects (liftABLE), having stamina to get things done (endurABLE), and being capable of moving around without risk of falls (stABLE). The phrase "a little exercise" is used to impress on low-active adults that even a little bit of physical activity can help them do better. The four abilities remind people that a variety of physical activity is important to reap a variety of benefits; that is, walking is not enough to maintain arm strength and joint mobility, and Tai Chi will help with mobility and balance but not with optimal strength and endurance. Avoiding any one of these ABLE components is a liability that cannot be ignored if lifelong independence is the goal.

Assessing the impact of an ABLE intervention in a community or facility is crucial. Planning for the implementation of physical activity programmes for seniors should include planning for programme, process, and health outcome evaluations. Without formal evaluations, the impact of programmes will never be known, and the strengths and weaknesses of active living interventions can only be guessed. Dr. Anita Myers, at the University of Waterloo, has published supportive material in vitality indicators, balance confidence, and quality of life assessments (Myers et al. 1999) and has also published an in-depth easy-to-read guide to programme evaluation for activity professionals to use (Myers 1999). Many of the ratings that are useful are easy to obtain using surveys or guided interviews. Recent research supports the value of simple self-ratings of health and self-assessment of functional ability (Bernard et al. 1997). In a US national sample of older adults, Bernard and colleagues found that three-year mortality outcomes were predicted by a global self-measure of perceived ability to function independently. Individuals who rated themselves as 0 or "not at all able" to care for themselves incurred a tenfold increase in their risk of death during the 2.5 year follow-up period compared with those who rated themselves as 10 or "completely able" to care for themselves. O'Brien Cousins (1997b) found that over a four-week period, older people can reliably report their age (r = .99) and weight (r = .99), number of prescription medications (r = .86), and illness symptoms (r = .67). Adequate reliability and validity among older adults for reporting weekly exercise has also been established (O'Brien Cousins 1997c). Among those who are experiencing physical limitations, assessments should focus on the assessment of ability, rather than on disability, especially when disability is in the eye of the beholder.

This chapter aimed to bring attention to the disabling aspects of sedentary living that often accompany and add confusion to the actual aging process. Without denying the biological changes that lead to real age declines, the reader can appreciate that there are important social and behavioural adjustments that exacerbate that biological decline. Aging is not a natural process of disablement leading to dependency. Old people are not intended to become frail, bent over, weak, off balance, and breathless. These abnormal characteristics accompany hypokinetic disease or the disuse of the body. Such frailty seems 'normal' because so many people are not optimally active. If we were to imprison a body on a chair for many years in a four-foot-high space, and not allow the body to stretch, push, pull, and run about, this is what the body would become—stiff, bent, and weak. Disablement in old age is sometimes a process of disease, but in many cases, it is a process of unnatural immobilization. While disablement in elders seems untreatable, it is largely preventable, and new evidence suggests that quite substantial reversals in function are possible. Even when arthritis and osteoporosis are present, old adults who have neglected their bodies can improve their quality of life by restoring more active lifestyles. They can become more flexible, build strength, improve posture, and breathe better. It is never too late, you are never too old, and thus 'being able-bodied' is a healthy mind-set. The disabling aspect of aging has more to do with 'hardening of the attitudes' than with the physical challenges that old age may bring.

24 Why is physical activity so important to older adult health and wellness?

25 What did Health Canada offer older adults, in celebration of 1999, the International Year of the Older Person?

26 Is walking the 'best exercise?' Why or why not?

Study Questions

1. What is the role of physical activity in the experience of aging?
2. What is the role of aging in the experience of physical activity?

References

American Association of Retired Persons. (1998). *Boomers approaching midlife: How secure a future?* Washington, DC: Author.

Baltes, M.M. (1996). *The many faces of dependency in old age.* Cambridge, NY: Cambridge University Press.

Bernard, S.L., Kincade, J.E., Konrad, T.R., Arcury, T.A., Rabiner, D.J., Woomert, A., DeFriese, G.H., and Ory, M.G. (1997). Predicting mortality from community surveys of older adults: The importance of self-rated functional ability. *Journal of Gerontology: Social Sciences, 52b,* s155–63.

Bernard, S., and Smith, L.K. (1998). Emergency admissions of older people to hospital: A link with material deprivation. *Journal of Public Health Medicine, 20*(1), 97–100.

Burgess, A.C., and O'Brien Cousins, S. (1998). "Reversing the downward spiral." In *Exercise, aging and health: Overcoming barriers to an active old age.* Philadelphia, PA: Taylor and Francis.

Buttar, A., Blaum, C., and Fries, B. (2001). Clinical characteristics and six-month outcomes of nursing home residents with low activities of daily living dependency. *Journal of Gerontology: Medical Sciences, 56a,* 5, m292–97.

Campion, E.W. (1998). Aging better. *The New England Journal of Medicine, April 9,* 1064–66.

Canada. National Advisory Council on Aging. (1996). Age and disability. *Info-age, 16,* 4.

Chodzko-Zajko, W.J. (1997). The World Health Organization issues guidelines for promoting physical activity among older persons. *Journal of Aging and Physical Activity, 5*(10), 1–8.

Daley, M.J., and Spinks, W.L. (2000). Exercise, mobility and aging. *Sports Medicine, 29*(1), 1–12.

Damush, T.M., Stewart, A.L., Mills, K.M., King, A.C., and Ritter, P.L. (1999). Prevalence and correlates of physician recommendations to exercise among older adults. *Journal of Gerontology: Medical Sciences, 54a,*(8), m423–27.

Daviglus, M., Liu, K., Greenland, P., Dyer, A., Garride, D., Manheim, L., Lowe, L., Rodin, M., Lubitz, J., and Stamler, J. (1998). Benefit of a favorable cardiovascular risk factor profile in middle age with respect to medicare costs. *New England Journal of Medicine, 339*(16), 1122–28.

De Vito, G., Hernandez, R., Gonzalez, V., Felici, F., and Figura, F. (1997). Low intensity physical training in older subjects. *Journal of Sports Medicine and Physical Fitness, 37,* 22–27.

Era, P., and Rantanen, T. (1997). Changes in physical capacity and sensory/psychomotor functions from 75 to 80 years of age and from 80 to 85 years of age: A longitudinal study. *Scandinavian Journal of Social Medicine, 53* (suppl.), 25–43.

Fiatarone, M.A., O'Neill, E.F., Doyle, R.N., Clements, K.M., Solares, G.R., Nelson, M.E., Roberts, S.B., Kahayian, J.J., Lipstiz, L.A., and Evans, W.J. (1994). Exercise training and nutritional supplementation for physical frailty in very elderly people. *New England Journal of Medicine, 25,* 1765–75.

Fries, J.F. (1980). Aging, natural death, and the compression of morbidity. *New England Journal of Medicine, 303,* 130–35.

Fries, J.F. (1989). The compression of morbidity: Near or far? *Millbank Quarterly, 67,* 208–32.

Fries, J.F., Singh, G., Morfeld, D., Hubert, H.B., Lane, N.E., and Brown, B.W., Jr. (1994). Running and the development of disability with age. *Annals of Internal Medicine, 121,* 502–9.

Furman, C.S. (1995). "Survival of the fittest." In *Turning point: The myths and realities of menopause.* New York: Oxford University Press.

Hatori, M., Hasegawa, A., Adachi, H., Shinozaki, A., Hayashi, S., Okano, H., Mizunuma, H. and Murata, K. (1993). The effects of walking at the anaerobic threshold level on vertebral bone loss in postmenopausal women. *Calcified Tissue International, 52,* 411–14.

Health Canada. (1999a). *Canada's physical activity guide to healthy, active living for older adults.* Ottawa: Active Living Coalition for Older Adults.

Health Canada. (1999b). *The health status of Canadians.* Ottawa: Health Services and Programmes Branch.

House, J.S., Kessler, R.C., Herzog, A.R., Mero, R.P., Kinney, A.M., and Breslow, M.J. (1990). Age, socioeconomic status and health. *Millbank Quarterly, 68,* 383–411.

Jette, A.M. (1999). Disentangling the process of disablement. *Social Science and Medicine, 48,* 471–72.

Kempen, G.I., van Sonderen, E., and Ormel, J. (1999). The impact of psychological attributes on changes in disability among low-functioning older persons. *Journal of Gerontology: Psychological Sciences, 54b,* 1, p23–p29.

Keysor, J.J., and Jette, A.M. (2001). Have we oversold the benefit of late-life exercise? *Journal of Gerontology: Medical Sciences, 56a*(7), m412–23.

Kraus, H., and Raab, W. (1961). *Hypokinetic disease.* Springfield, IL: C.C. Thomas.

Krol, B., Sanderman, R., Suurmeijer, T.P.B.M., Doeglas, D., Van Sonderen, E., Van Rijswijk, M., Van Leeuwen, M., and Van den Heuvel, W.J.A. (1998). Early rheumatoid arthritis personality and psychological status: A follow-up study. *Psychology and Health, 13,* 35–48.

Langley, D.J., and Knight, S.M. (1999). Continuity in sport participation as an adaptive strategy in the aging process: A lifespan narrative. *Journal of Aging and Physical Activity, 7*(1), 32–54.

Laukkanen, P., Sakari-Rantala, R., Kauppinen, M., and Heikkinen, E. (1997). Morbidity and disability in 75- and 80-year-old men and women: A five-year follow-up. *Scandinavian Journal of Social Medicine, 53*(Suppl.), 79–106.

Lazarus, R.S., and Folkman, S. (1984). *Stress, appraisal and coping*. New York: Springer.

Leigh, J.P., and Fries, J.F. (1994). Education, gender, and the compression of morbidity. *International Journal on Aging and Human Development, 39*, 233–46.

Martin, J.J. (1999). A personal development model of sport psychology for athletes with disabilities. *Journal of Applied Sport Psychology, 11*, 181–93.

Mendes de Leon, C.F., Seeman, T.E., Baker, D.I., Richardson, E.D., and Tinetti, M.E. (1996). Self-efficacy, physical decline, and change in functioning in community elders: A prospective study. *Journal of Gerontology: Social Sciences, 51b*, s183–90.

Menec, V.H., and Chipperfield, J.G. (1997). Remaining active in later life: The role of locus of control in senior's leisure activity participation, health, and life satisfaction. *Journal of Aging and Health, 9*, 105–25.

Mihalko, S., and McAuley, E. (1996). Strength training effects on subjective well-being and physical function in the elderly. *Journal of Aging and Physical Activity, 4*, 56–65.

Miller, N.H., Haskell, W.L., Berra, K., and DeBusk, R.F. (1984). Home versus group exercise training for increasing functional capacity after myocardial infarction. *Circulation, 70*(4), 645–59.

Morrison, B., and Lilford, R. (2001). How can action research apply to health services? *Qualitative Health Research, 11* (4), 436–49.

Myers, A.M. (1999). *Program evaluation for exercise leaders*. Champaign, IL: Human Kinetics.

Myers, A.M., Malott, O.W., Gray, E., Tudor-Locke, C., Ecclestone, N.A., O'Brien Cousins, S., and Petrella, R. (1999). Measuring accumulated health-related benefits of exercise participation for older adults: The Vitality Plus Scale. *Journal of Gerontology: Medical Sciences, 54a*(9), m456–66.

National Advisory Council on Aging. (1996). Age and disability. *Info-Age, 16*, 4.

Nelson, M.E., Fiatarone, M.A., Morganti, C.M., Trice, I., Greenberg, R.A. and Evans, W.J. (1994). Effect of high-intensity strength training on multiple risk factors for osteoporotoc fracture. *Journal of the American Medical Association, 272*(24), 1909–14.

Nelson, M.E., Bortz, S.S., Crawford, B., Economos, G., Fiatarone, M.A., Trice, I., and Evans, W.J. (1993). Strength training in postmenopausal women: Effects on bone and body composition. *Medicine and Science in Sports and Exercise, 25*(suppl.), s1–2.

Nichols, J.F., Hitselberger, L.M., Sherman, J.G., and Patterson, P. (1995). Effects of resistance training on muscular strength and functional abilities of community-dwelling older adults. *Journal of Aging and Physical Activity, 3*, 238–50.

Nigg, C.R., Burbank, P.M., Padula, C., Dufresne, R., Rossi, J.S., Velicer, W.F., Laforge, R.G., and Prochaska, J.O. (1999). Stages of change across ten health risk behaviours for older adults. *The Gerontologist, 39*(4), 473–82.

Nourhashemi, F., Andrieu, S., Gillette-Guyonnet, S., Vellas, B., Albarede, J.L., and Grandjean, H. (2001). Instrumental activities of daily living as a potential marker of frailty: A study of 7364 community-dwelling elderly women (The epidos study). *Journal of Gerontology: Medical Sciences, 56a*(7), m448–53.

Nusselder, W.J., and Mackenbach, J.P. (1996). Rectangularization of the survival curve in The Netherlands, 1950–1992. *The Gerontologist, 36*, 773–82.

O'Brien Cousins, S. (1996). Exercise cognition among elderly women. *Journal of Applied Sport Psychology, 8*(2), 131–45.

O'Brien Cousins, S. (1997a). Elderly tomboys? Sources of self-efficacy for physical activity in late life. *Journal of Physical Activity and Aging, 5*, 229–43.

O'Brien Cousins, S. (1997b). An older adult exercise inventory: Reliability and validity in women over age 70. *Journal of Sport Behaviour, 19*(4), 288–306.

O'Brien Cousins, S. (1997c). Validity and reliability of self-reported health of persons aged 70 and over. *Health Care for Women International, 18*, 165–74.

O'Brien Cousins, S. (1998). *Exercise, aging and health: Overcoming barriers to an active old age*. Philadelphia: Taylor and Francis.

O'Brien Cousins, S. (2000). "My heart couldn't take it": Older women's beliefs about exercise benefits and risks. *Journal of Gerontology: Psychological Sciences, 55b*(5), p283–94.

O'Brien Cousins, S., and Burgess, A.C. (1998). "Reversing the downward spiral." In *Exercise, aging and health: Overcoming barriers to an active old age*. Philadelphia: Taylor and Francis.

O'Brien Cousins, S. and Horne, T. (1999). *Active living among older adults: Health benefits and outcomes*. Philadelphia, PA: Taylor and Francis.

O'Brien Cousins, S. and Vertinsky, P.A. (1991). Unfit survivors: Exercise as a resource for aging women. *The Gerontologist, 31*, 347–58.

Ormel, J., Kempen, G.I.J.M., Penninx, B.W.J.H., Brilman, E.I., Van Sonderen, E., and Relyveld, J. (1998). Functioning, well-being and health perception in late middle-aged and older people: Comparing the effects of depressive symptoms and chronic medical conditions. *Journal of the American Geriatrics Society, 46*, 39–48.

Paffenbarger, R.S., Jr., Hyde, R.T., Wing, A.L., and Hsied, C.C. (1986). Physical activity, all-cause mortality, and longevity of college alumni. *New England Journal of Medicine, 314*(10), 605–13.

Patla, A.E., and Shumway-Cook, A. (1999). Dimensions of mobility: Defining the complexity and difficulty associated with community mobility. *Journal of Aging and Physical Activity, 7,* 7–19.

Peel, C., Utsey, C., and MacGregor, J. (1999). Exercise training for older adults with limitations in physical function. *Journal of Aging and Physical Activity, 7,* 62–75.

Phillips, W.T. and Haskell, W.L. (1995). "Muscular fitness": Easing the burden of disability for elderly adults. *Journal of Aging and Physical Activity, 3,* 261–89.

Prince, M.J., Harwood, R.H., Blizard, R.A., Thomas, A., and Mann, A.H. (1997). Impairment, disability and handicap as risk factors for depression in old age: The Gospel Oak Project V. *Psychological Medicine, 27,* 311–21.

Ready, A.E., Bergeron, G., Boreskie, S.L., Naimark, B., Ducas, J., Sawatzky, J.V., and Drinkwater, D.T. (1999). Incidence and determination of injuries sustained by older women during a walking programme. *Journal of Aging and Physical Activity, 7,* 91–104.

Sakari-Rantala, R., Heikkinen, E., and Ruoppila, I. (1995). Difficulties in mobility among elderly people and their association with socioeconomic factors, dwelling environment and use of services. *Aging, 7*(6), 433–40.

Seeman, T.E., Unger, J.B., McAvay, F., and Mendes de Leon, C.F. (1999). Self-efficacy beliefs and perceived declines in functional ability: MacArthur Studies of Successful Aging. *Journal of Gerontology: Psychological Sciences, 54b*(4), p214–24.

Seniors Advisory Council for Alberta. (1992). *Older Albertans, 1992.* Edmonton: Author. (Available from Seniors Advisory Council for Alberta, #610, 10405 Jasper Avenue, Edmonton, AB T5J 3N4.)

Shephard, R.J. (1997). *Aging, physical activity and health.* Champaign, IL: Human Kinetics.

Smith, E.L., and Tommerup, L. (1995). Exercise: A prevention and treatment for osteoporosis and injurious falls in the older adult. *Journal of Aging and Physical Activity, 3,* 178–92.

Statistics Canada. (1990). *Women in Canada: A statistical report.* Ottawa: Minister of Supply and Services.

Stephens, T., and Craig, C.L. (1990). *The well-being of Canadians: Highlights of the 1988 Campbell's Survey.* Ottawa: Fitness Canada.

Tannahill, A, (1998). *The Scottish Green Paper: Beyond a healthy mind in a healthy body.* New York: Oxford University Press.

van Eijk, L.M. (1997). *Activity and well-being in the elderly.* Unpublished doctoral dissertation, University of Groningen, The Netherlands.

Verbrugge, L.M. (1995). New thinking and science on disability in mid- and late life. *European Journal of Public Health, 5,* 20–28.

Verbrugge, L.M., and Jette, A.M. (1994). The disablement process. *Social Science and Medicine, 38,* 1–14.

Vertinsky, P. (1998). "Run, Jane, Run": Central tensions in the current debate about enhancing women's health through exercise. *Women and Health, 27,* 4, 81–111.

Vertinsky, P.A., O'Brien Cousins, S., and Tan, M. *Physical activity, aging and stereotypes.* Manuscript submitted for publication.

Vita, A.J., Terry, R.B., Hubert, H.B., and Fries, J.F. (1998). Aging, health risks, and cumulative disability. *New England Journal of Medicine, 338,* 1035–41.

Warner, K.E. (1992). Effects of workplace health promotion not demonstrated. *American Journal of Public Health, 82,* 126–27.

Watmough, D.J., Bhargava, S., Memon, A., Syed, F., Roy, S., and Sharma, P. (1997). Does breast cancer screening depend on a wobbly hypothesis? *Journal of Public Health Medicine, 19,* 4, 375–79.

Wheeler, G., Malone, L.A., VanVlack, S., Nelson, E.R., and Steadward, R. (1996). Retirement from disability sport: A pilot study. *Adapted Physical Activity Quarterly, 13,* 382–99.

CHAPTER 25

Fitness and Physical Activity for Older Adults

Arthur C. (Art) Burgess
John C. Hudec

Learning Objectives

- To develop an understanding of how social forces shaped the attitudes of the members of today's older adults and, in turn, how older adults of the future will have attitudes shaped by such forces.
- To understand the barriers, both physical and psychological, that prevent many older adults from being physically active at a time in their lives when physical activity would benefit them significantly.
- To understand a method of presenting organized physical activity to older adults, keeping in mind their health and viability and their unique attitude base.

Introduction

Much of this chapter is based on field experience in programming fitness activities for older adults. Many of the concepts and practices described here were derived in pioneer fitness programmes at the University of Alberta. One of the earliest fitness courses, Fitness for Seniors, was initiated by the University of Alberta's Faculty of Extension in 1983. It explored the practicality of leading retired adults in basic fitness activities. This was an initiative without precedence that produced huge enthusiasm among older adults in Edmonton. The obvious success of that initiative resulted in the development of Project: Alive and Well. This was the first reported fitness programme for older adults that challenged them to work to their limit, whatever that was. Project: Alive and Well commenced in 1988 and continues to this day, operated by the University of Alberta's Campus Recreation. At its inception, there were virtually no fitness programmes for older adults. Many of the concepts and practices in these pioneer programmes were developed on the spot, based on fundamental principles of physical education and common sense.

Most of us have relatives, friends, or acquaintances who are older than we are. They may have been born into a generation that lived through different experiences. The environment that surrounds us affects our reactions to physical activity and recreational activities. Some older adults experienced the most turbulent times of the twentieth century. The Great Depression of the 1930s, World War II of the early 1940s, and the twenty-year economic boom of the post-World War II era shaped their attitudes and their way of life, predisposing them to behaviours which ultimately affect the way they are living out their retirement years. In much the same way, those who experienced the destruction of the World Trade Center in New York City in 2001 will react differently to their environment than those who did not. In short, the times in which we develop affect our lives and our lifestyles.

From an era when infectious diseases ended lives long before the wear and tear of living, medical science has increased the life expectancy of Canadians to over seventy-five years. Society has moved from promoting physical activity as a way to increase longevity, to promoting such activity as a way to improve quality of life, to promoting it as a part of our normal activity from when we are young until we die. Too often the years of retirement are characterized by inactivity and declining health. Free from the busy schedule of their working lives, without a home full of active young people to care for, many older adults drift into a low energy lifestyle. They mistakenly avoid physical exertion. A passive, low activity lifestyle leads them into hypokinetic diseases such as obesity, adult-onset diabetes, hypertension, coronary artery disease, osteoarthritis, and osteoporosis. All of these conditions are improved (not cured) by regular physical activity. There are strong reasons to promote regular physical activity among older adults, but there are strong influences of misinformation, cultural bias, and lethargy that prevent its general adoption as a health maintenance strategy. This chapter will review some of these influences and propose an approach to presenting group exercise to older adults.

Describing the Clientele

Some readers of this chapter will be in their early twenties with a limited experience with older people. Others may be twenty-five or forty-four and may be experiencing life with older parents. Our interaction with older generations is somewhat dependent on our own situation. For example, a younger person may only interact with an older neighbour or their own grandparents. In contrast, those in 'sandwich' situations may be responsible for caring for their own children and, at the same time, feel responsible for some degree of care of their aging parents. While both of these scenarios may provide some experience, each may not give an accurate picture of older age groups. In Canada it is common to categorize those fifty-five years of age and above as older adults and compare their level of activity to those in the previous stage of life, where individuals range from forty-five to fifty-four years of age (Torrance 1991). In reality, there is a great amount of diversity in those fifty-five years of age or older. The group may consist of healthy, vibrant individuals of any age. In other cases, aging has effects derived from previous lifestyle, degeneration, or disease. It is important to recognize and accommodate this diversity when programming for older adults.

There are a number of terms commonly used for people of advanced years. Some are more acceptable than others, not because of political correctness but out of respect. It is prudent to address both individuals and groups in a way with which they are comfortable. Just as you may find that some people are more comfortable with formal names rather than first names, you may find individuals who prefer specific terms in reference to their age group. In general, it is best to avoid such categorization when possible. In programming for older groups, remember the issue of respect and temper it with humour and fun. Some of the common terms used to

Table 25.1 Terms Used to Describe Older Individuals

Terminology	Connotations
Old people or old folks	Suggestion of institutionalization, frailness, infirmity
Aged	Expectations of frailty; suggestion of a lesser version of people in their prime
Elderly	Hints of infirmity; implies frailty brought on by advancing years
Golden Ager	Patronizing; not commonly used by older people when they describe their stage of life
Senior or senior citizen	Suggests retirement or collection of pension, which may not be the case
Older adult	Indicates a state of life without quantifying the degree of aging; over used; patronizing; begs the question: older than what?

represent older groups of participants are presented in table 25.1. Each of these terms has connotations and presents issues.

We all have biases and preferences that influence the terminology we use and who we think of as old. A child may think of parents as old while the parents look at those of their parents' generation as old. In many ways it is best to avoid categorization whenever possible; sometimes it is best just to recognize your bias. The writer discloses his bias in this small catalogue of terms by listing them in order of acceptability. The term *older adult* is the preference of the list since it avoids a specific age definition while leaving no doubt that the person described is of advanced years.

Socio-economic Influences on Older Adults

A number of factors determine our attitudes. According to the theory of planned behaviour (Ajzen 1991), our attitude toward a behaviour is a product of what we perceive as the costs and benefits of an activity and the amount of enjoyment we expect from an activity. Today's older adults have passed through times that influence their current attitudes. They are subject to approval or disapproval from their peers as well as from others in their environment. These factors influence their intention to participate in physical activity and, in turn,

their eventual behaviour. Here is a review of some of the historical influences on older adults.

THE HUNGRY THIRTIES

People seventy years and older in the year 2000 were born at the end of the 1920s which had been characterized by a decade-long post-war economic boom. That decade was called the Roaring Twenties. It ended with the stock market crash of 1929. This signalled the start of a decade-long depression, which crippled the world economy. It has shaped attitudes and influenced lives right to this day (Broadfoot 1973).

The deprivations of the 1930s resulting from the Great Depression were pervasive. Many youth of those years left school and travelled across the country to find work, mostly in menial jobs. Away from school, youth did not have the associations that led to games and activities. They lacked equipment and the facilities. At that time only a few major cities in Canada, and practically no towns, had community indoor swimming pools, gymnasiums, and indoor skating rinks. In the schools and in the communities at large, the depression created a ten-year deficit of facilities, equipment, and programmes. This was followed by five years of war, which completely focussed public energies in aid of the war effort. Sports and games were generally regarded as frivolous diversions from the serious business of job-seeking or working to fight a war.

Schools in the 1930s coped with the lack of resources, but the physical education concepts just emerging from universities and normal schools of that era were dampened by the economic hardship. The subsequent war, which ended the depression, devoured resources and conscripted able-bodied male teachers to train the largest military force in the history of Canada. This national preoccupation produced a generation that was unaccustomed to organized physical education.

SEPTEMBER 1939—WORLD WAR II

With the coming of World War II in September 1939, the loss of able-bodied men into the armed forces decimated the male teaching staffs in the schools. Many schools abandoned any attempt at formal physical education. Sports promotion organizations became moribund through lack of personnel and the distractions of the war effort. With the urgency of the war as the daily focus of the whole society, fitness and physical education were given a token recognition at best.

Many young men, conscripted into the armed forces, were thoroughly disenchanted by the forced activity demanded of them through military training. This shaped their attitudes for life. At home, young women continued to be acculturated to passivity in physical activity (Gee and Kimball 1987). As a result of the depression and World War II, this generation left school with very few physical activity skills. As a result, the positive effects from a life full of active recreations were lost to them. Later, as they grew into adulthood, they were dismissive of physical activity as an enhancer of their lives.

One of the powerful influences of World War II was the shortage of food. This was more acute in Europe, but even in North America the use of sugar, butter, coffee, meat, and alcohol was controlled and rationed. This made life less enjoyable and left many people longing for a full meal. Gasoline was rationed, as were tires for automobiles and trucks. As a result, people walked to all their short distance destinations.

Following the war, the returned service people became preoccupied with resuming their interrupted lives. Job training, marriage, raising a family, and building a home were their central focusses. For many, the opportunity for sport and physical activity was lost in the pursuit of these 'real life' issues, made more intense by their wartime postponement. Thus, at a point in their lives where physical activity was particularly necessary for its health benefits, it was lost in a myriad of negative attitudes and conflicting priorities.

1945—THE POST WAR

The post war decade saw unprecedented technological growth. A backlog of scientific and technological wonders, nearly a decade long, was rushed into the production of labour-saving home appliances. Home heating with gas or petroleum replaced coal or wood. Elevators, escalators, and low cost public transportation made getting around easier. The automobile became generally affordable, producing drive-in conveniences: theatres, restaurants, banks, and the growth of automobile travel as entertainment. The unprecedented affluence of the general public resulted in a consumerism that troubled community leaders.

After the hard depression years, people were free to eat the expensive food that they could now well afford. Food in a wide variety was available at a relatively low cost. The Hungry Thirties were hard years that burned deprivation into the collective psyche of this generation. In their post-war affluence they denied themselves very little. In a decade, western society lost the lean and hungry look of the thirties.

The combined effects of low energy output in the daily work regimen in the 1950s and 1960s were profound. A manual worker in the 1920s used 3500 to 4500 calories per day. This was in an era of relatively simple diets. The post-World War II generation, working in physical energy-reduced occupations, utilized about 2200 calories per day. The inevitable result was an epidemic of obesity and hypo-kinetic diseases. People overate, spent less energy in their low energy lifestyles, and grew hypoactive and obese. These are some of the historical influences on the generation now living out their lives in retirement.

---

1 If for five years you had been deprived of anything more than basic food and had been forced to work on a project that totally involved you but paid you little, what would be your reaction to a return to a normal lifestyle? Relate your reaction to the returned veterans of World War II.

---

2 Consider the socio-economic conditions that surround you. What effects will your surroundings have on your attitudes toward physical activity as you age?

Common Assumptions

Before discussing how to work with older adults, it would be useful to confront the common stereotypes that exist about them.

Older adults are fragile and seden-tary. It has been reported that as many as 35 percent of adults over the age of sixty-five indicate a significant decrease in their ability to do their everyday tasks (Canadian Fitness and Lifestyle Research Institute (CFLRI) 1995, 1998). In contrast, many older adults are remaining active. Inspiring case studies include race-walkers, yoga instructors, sprinters, and tennis players in their seventies or perhaps eighties (Scott and Couzens 1996). While some older adults experience stiff joints, weak muscles, or a lack of energy, others are in a compromised state and could be considered fragile due to disease or the effects of long-term inactivity. A greater pro-portion of older adults are becoming moti-vated to maintain their independence. More than 75 percent of adults fifty-five years and older would prefer to live in their own home as long as possible (National Advisory Counsel on Aging (NACA) 1993), indicating they are active enough to live autonomously.

While it is true that osteoporosis, the prin-cipal cause of fragility, afflicts some older women and fewer older men, these people are the eldest of the cohort. Individuals from all ranges of ability or disability can benefit from appropriate regular exercise. Even much older adults or those who are frail can benefit from physical activity participation. A new set of training goals replaces those of prevention of cardiovascular disease, cancer, or diabetes or increasing life expectancy (Mazzeo et al. 1998). Goals such as minimizing the biolog-ical changes of aging, reversing symptoms of disuse, control and rehabilitation of chronic conditions, maximizing psychological health, increasing mobility and function now become paramount.

Older adults are very much alike. Older adults have few things in common beyond their advanced years. It is the result of the age effect. The longer one stays alive, the more different one becomes from peers. Their health, their income, their education, their vast array of previous experiences, all com-bine with their genetic predisposition to indi-vidualize them. A fundamental error of workers with older adults is to assume homo-geneity. Each one is different in many ways (Nelson and Dannefer 1992).

Most older people are in poor health. Most older people are in good health! Of older persons aged seventy years and older, 70 percent state that their health is good, very good, or excellent, while 30 percent reported activity limitations (Torrance 1991). Most are in such good health that they are not even recognized as older. They are on the golf course, in the skating rinks, the swimming pools, and on the hiking trails. They are in the supermarkets buying and carrying their own groceries. They are the older couples strolling in the shopping malls. They popu-late the ski slopes on week-day mornings. They are the daytime clientele in many YMCAs and public fitness centres. Because they do not reflect the stereotype, they become invis-ible to the casual watcher. In some older people infirmity is observable. They limp with a cane in the malls. Many of those in wheelchairs or walkers are older adults. They are seen sitting patiently in doctors' waiting rooms. They stroll about between services at church. They occupy the front row reserved seats on the buses. Because they express the stereotype, they may be disproportionately remembered. Although long-term illness and injury are more prominent in older adults, not all can be considered in poor health (CFLRI 1995).

Older adults are resistant to change. A commonly held belief about older adults is that they are resistant to new ideas. This stereotype is too general to be accurate. It is true that some older adults are suspicious of change but so are some young people. In fact more than 68 percent of Canadians over sixty-five hold a very positive attitude toward the benefits of physical activity. Much like other Canadians, fewer change their behaviours to incorporate physical activity into their lifestyle (CFLRI 1998). The adoption of a new idea or innovation has been studied by Rogers and Shoemaker (1971). They describe a set of adopter characteristics that are related to the speed with which an individual adopts a new idea. Early adopters, also called innovators, are better educated, more affluent, younger, and derive their ideas from outside their community. Late adopters, also called laggards, tend to be of low income and education. They receive their ideas from family, similar others, and tradition. The mass of the population falls between these two extremes.

Rogers and Shoemakers' concept of adopter categories cuts across age divisions. There are young laggards and elderly innovators. Resistance to change is dependent on a set of characteristics of which advanced years are but one. Older adults are not by definition change resistant.

---

3 Of the listed stereotypes of older adults, which do you find to be the most accurate? Which is the most off the mark? Describe any stereotypical older adult you have met in your own experience.

Barriers to Participation in Regular Physical Activity

CUMULATIVE DISABILITY
Through years of deprivation or careless personal habits, disability gradually accumulates and leaves older persons unable to take action to alleviate their problems (Vita, Terry, Hubert, and Fries 1998). Hypokinetic conditions such as obesity, Type II diabetes, hypertension, angina, osteoarthritis, osteoporosis, as well as psychological disorders such as depression and Alzheimer's disease are common among older adults. While regular, gentle physical activity is a standard prescription for these conditions, many of the very elderly are so debilitated, so under motivated in their ennui, that it is difficult to break the cycle of debilitation. They are in a circular dilemma. As their disability accumulates, they can do less. The less they do, the less they can do—until they have lost the capacity to do anything without help. This is the downward spiral, which ends in their demise. Although not stereotypical of all older adults, long-term illness or injury and the fear of such injury are far more prominent barriers to physical activity among older populations. Older adults report two barriers more commonly than long-term illness. As with the general population, lack of energy and lack of motivation stand as greater barriers to participation (CFLRI 1995).

LOW FITNESS LEVEL
Deconditioning in many older adults may be the result of years of sedentary living. Their working life may have been physically unchallenging. They may not participate in active recreation or leisure pursuits. As a result, they have become deconditioned to well below the healthy optimum for their age group. While still untouched by illness, they are headed inevitably towards hypokinetic disease. This group is usually those adults ranging in age from fifty-five to sixty-five. Since most hypokinetic disease becomes evident with increased age, the urgency to take action is greatest with this younger cohort where prevention is still a great possibility. Perceptions of discomfort

and misconceptions strengthen the inertia which maintains some older adults' inactivity (Dunlap and Barry 1999). Being in poor fitness heightens the fear of looking silly. These barriers can possibly be countered by education and active role models. What they need most is the vision of themselves as healthy, vibrant people able to take control of their own well-being. Many from this group are unaware of what they should do to change their circumstances. Low fitness and lack of information prevent them from taking action.

FEAR OF INJURY FROM PARTICIPATION IN EXERCISE

A common reason that older adults avoid physical exercise is the fear of being injured. The actual risk is low. Burgess (1996) reported seventeen small injuries requiring the injured person to cease exercising on the day of occurrence. These happened over a nine-year period of 680,000 participant hours. In this programme, participants were led through an exercise routine comprised of static stretching, aerobic walking, balance drills, muscular strength, and endurance exercises. The rate of injury is similar for younger and older populations. The locations of injury and the form of activity vary, but the prevalence of injury was only minimally elevated in older populations (Matheson, Macintyre, Taunton, Clement, and Lloyd-Smith 1989). Although the actual risk of injury is low, the perception of risk can set a barrier to activity participation. Promoting benefits such as increased mobility and independence, along with a realistic picture of the actual risks, will tip the balance in favour of active living.

The misperception that exercise injury is a significant hazard is one of the challenges facing fitness programmers in motivating older people. Adults between fifty and eighty may be susceptible to overuse injuries aggravated by arthritis or to conditions such as bursitis and tendonitis (Scott and Couzens 1996). Allowing older adults to be active with lowered resulting pain improves the likelihood that individuals will continue to be active. If fear of injury blocks their involvement (NACA

1993), O'Brien Cousins (1997) suggests low-impact, shorter distances, and sub-maximal efforts such as walking to keep the benefits of physical activity with minimal risk of injury. With such modification and education about both the realistic risks and how to prevent injury, participation in physical activity within this population is more likely.

---

4 In talking with older adults to induce them to join a fitness group you are helping to organize, what would be your strategy to dispel their concerns?

LACK OF SKILLS

Many of today's older people lack the basic skills necessary to take up a physical activity as a form of recreation or leisure. This is particularly true for many women who early in their lives were not involved in sport activities or physical leisure (McPherson, Curtis, and Loy 1989). It should be stated immediately that women of the retired generation were by no means inactive. They worked at home, did much of their housework by hand, tended a garden, raised large families, and participated in community and social activities. They were always very busy but seldom in health-maintaining physical activity or in sport. To a lesser extent, the same was true for men. As they grew older, their priorities systems pointed them away from direct participation in physical activity. A general lack of resources and opportunity combined with preoccupation with other life issues resulted in a lack of fitness and training skills across society.

Two examples illustrate this. In 1960 the Canadian Red Cross Water Safety Service reported that only one in ten Canadian adults could pass a simple beginner's swimming test. In 1972 ParticipACTION Canada reported that only 2 percent of the adult Canadian population was physically active and this only once a week. The point of citing these ancient statistics is to illustrate the degree of inactivity prevalent among today's older adults who were then in their early forties. National preoccupation with survival through the depression years and the years following World War II resulted in lost opportunities to learn the basic skills and attitudes that would have produced a fit and active older generation at the millennium. As reported earlier in this chapter, attitudes toward physical activity benefits are positive with close to 70 percent of those over sixty-five years of age feeling that such activity is very beneficial (CFLRI 1998). Although this attitude is a start, extra effort may be needed to master the skills required to enjoy a variety of physical activities.

FEAR OF RIDICULE

People of the retired generation have reached a place in their lives where there are social expectations as to how they should conduct themselves. There are broad norms in society as to what is appropriate behaviour for people of their advanced years. Peers are quite ruthless in their condemnation of those who depart from the norm. Brooks reported that 55 percent of older men experienced social pressure to avoid strenuous activities (Brooks 1993). Such pressure may be due to concerns for health risk or may be only due to a lack of social support or social norm. Statements such as "Animals sweat, men perspire, women do neither" were common advice in the 1930s to 1950s (Dunlap and Barry 1999). More recently, during a research interview, a man resistant to partaking in regular exercise stated that "exercise is not a strange activity but a lot of strange people are active" (Hudec 1999).

Older adults are well aware of the expectations placed on them by their peers and their young adult family. An excursion into martial arts or ballet dancing gives pause for comment and a speculation about their sensibility. The possibility of exposing themselves to these criticisms blocks the participation of many. When this is combined with chronic health problems, a low fitness level, and a lack of the essential training skills, the older person quickly dismisses the idea of regular physical activity as a health improvement strategy. On top of the perceived health risk is the profound risk of looking foolish. Isolation from active peers may limit role modelling which could ease the fear that limits active leisure participation.

5 Of the reasons stated by older adults for nonparticipation in physical activity, which seems the most plausible to you? Which seems the least? Give reasons based on your own readings and suggest strategies for fitness and lifestyle promoters to overcome those reasons for nonparticipation.

6 What physical activities or leisure pursuits do you perceive as odd or unusual for a person of your age? Do you see yourself doing such activities when you are a bit older?

Guidelines for the Operation of Older Adult Group Fitness Activities

FULL DISCLOSURE OF MEDICAL CONDITION

Information may be disclosed through the use of the PAR-Q (modified) questionnaire (Thomas, Reading, and Shephard 1992). The 1992 revisions were conducted to reduce the excessive number of healthy older adults who were being screened out by the tool. The use of the PAR-Q places the onus on the participant to disclose any condition that would make participation in physical activity risky for them. Persons responding "yes" to any of the seven questions are given a medical follow-up form–the PARmed-x that must be completed by their physician before they are cleared for exercise. This leaves the medical examination question with the physician who can order tests if he or she sees fit. The PARmed-x must be signed by the physician and returned to the programme operator. Such screening devices provide a good review of conditions that are of concern for older adults who wish to begin regular activity.

The current thought on screening for participation in group physical activity has loosened the requirements for full medical screening prior to exercise training or testing (Gill, DiPietro, and Krumholz 2000). For example, it is now common for individuals recovering from serious surgery to be up and moving soon afterwards. Complete bed rest is less common than in previous years. The contraindications to exercise training or testing are similar for younger or older participants. Major absolute contraindications include recent electrocardiogram changes, or myocardial infarctions, unstable angina, uncontrolled arrhythmias, third-degree heart blocks, and acute congestive heart failure. Other relative contraindications should raise attention. More care should be taken when conditions such as elevated blood pressure, cardiomyopathies, valveular disease, complex ventricular ectopy, and uncontrolled metabolic diseases are disclosed (Mazzeo et al. 1998). The question of pre-exercise screening continues to concern the medical and fitness communities. Liability issues around charges of negligence from allowing unscreened persons to exert themselves are a continuing dilemma for all. What protection does a medical examination provide? It provides very little. A medical examination is like a snapshot. It shows the person as he or she was at the time of the examination. It does not make predictions. Apparently healthy persons who die while exercising, although they have had a full medical screening, are a continuing tragic reality.

For the physician, the question of how far to test is troubling. Should he or she merely take a resting blood pressure and heart rate, ask the usual questions, and give clearance? Will this give a false sense of security, which might later turn into a nightmare of litigation? Or should he or she insist on a full battery of tests, including a treadmill test with its attendant risk and additional cost? Sometimes these things are necessary, but minimal screening using well-established questionnaires is often the appropriate option.

For the older person, the prospect of a medical examination and tests, with all they entail, is more than many of them are prepared to accept. This is particularly so when all they get is a bill for a third-party medical and the right to exert themselves.

For the programmers, the problem of inducing this population of Great Depression survivors and World War II veterans to take up exercise is complicated. The task is to motivate them while many perceived barriers stand in their way. Demotivation must be counteracted and replaced by motivation. A number of sources of demotivation were discussed earlier in this chapter. But a powerful source of demotivation is the medicalization of fitness activities and with it the implied danger of being physically active. This is a serious dilemma for programmers: how to maintain reasonable safety standards that are cost effective without driving away the clientele by treating them as if they were sick.

From the perspective of a programmer, the less medical involvement, the better. A medical examination needlessly confuses the issue because fitness is a health matter (Rosenstock, Stretcher, and Becker 1988). The medicalization of physical activities for older adults is a demotivating, costly procedure of questionable benefit. A medical examination is an expensive snapshot and one that provides an illusion of security.

THE WAIVER OF LIABILITY AND INFORMED CONSENT

It is important to inform participants in group activity programmes of the inherent risks. Informed consent forms provide participants with a review of risks so they can make informed decisions to participate if they feel secure doing so. Some agencies, in an attempt to protect themselves from legal action stemming from an injury to a participant, will have them waive any claims of liability. A waiver says in effect, "If you act negligently and cause me injury, I agree not to take legal action for damages." This is a fallacy. It will not stand up in court because a legal principle states that you cannot contract out of negligence. Regardless of whatever document is signed by the participant, the fact remains that if you are negligent you are liable. Waivers may place a negative cast on the whole process of being involved in a fitness class and this is counterproductive to creating a positive class situation. Informed consent may be somewhat more positive and can heighten the understanding of participants, and perhaps even acting to prevent possible injuries or emergencies. Informing participants can add to their learning. Neither waivers nor informed consent tools should be used at the expense of personal contact. An experienced leader can go miles in providing a positive learning experience, while screening a potential participant to ensure contraindications to physical activity are addressed.

ONGOING SCREENING OF ALL PARTICIPANTS

If we accept that a medical examination of candidates for a fitness class is of limited effectiveness, we are faced with the risk of operating blindly, with no way of checking their capacity for the activities. For some agencies, this is an unacceptable risk, but one that is more apparent than real.

In a pioneering older adult fitness programme at the University of Alberta, prospective clients were screened using the Physical Activity Readiness Questionnaire (PAR-Q Revised) (Thomas, Reading, and Shephard 1992). Thirteen percent of the participants fifty-five to seventy-five years of age gave a positive response and were referred to their family physician for a medical clearance. Of these, 2 percent were advised by their doctor to have medical tests before starting to exercise (Burgess 1990). A fitness agency must identify those who could be at risk from exercise, but screening at registration should be part of an ongoing process, not a one-time occurrence.

Conducting activities in a positive atmosphere makes possible a safe experience for all. In this atmosphere, self-screening is ongoing. The important feature of a class operating within this philosophy is that everyone feels free to modify the workload to suit their own needs. They are self-paced. They don't have to 'keep up' because there is no 'up' to keep.

7 What effect would you expect from establishing strict medical standards as a means of screening older adult participants in a fitness class? Would you be more assured that all participants were equally able to participate? For how long do you think a medical screening would have application to an individual?

GRADUATED LEVELS OF INTENSITY

Training a deconditioned older person from a state of inactivity to optimal fitness requires time and motivation. Starting at too high an intensity level is demotivating and possibly hazardous (Kavanagh and Shephard 1978). Canada's older adult physical activity guide recommends a starting load of ten-minute activity segments that will total thirty to sixty minutes per day of light activity (Health Canada, 1999b). The guide is directed at individual fitness initiatives by older adults. At some point in a personal rehabilitation programme, the older person may wish to learn more about training methods and to collaborate with other kindred spirits in their quest for personal fitness. Enrollment in an older adult fitness programme is an inexpensive option compared to engaging a personal trainer. Regardless of the option, the concept of graduated intensity is paramount in successful retraining. In simple terms, anyone who begins a new activity needs to start at a moderate intensity and progress from there. The process is not much different for an older adult or a younger one. Rates of progress vary with each individual, but for older adults the rate of progress is slower.

Older adults respond to training in much the same way as young adults. The major difference lies in the length of time required for results to appear (Klingman, Hewett, and Crowell 1999). An accompanying risk in older adults retraining is the increased incidence of muscle and tendon injuries. At the earliest stage of retraining, the risk of injury from seemingly low-intensive activities is a concern (Kavanagh and Shephard 1978).

A thorough warm up and a concerted effort to make the early lessons gentle can largely prevent exercise injuries. Very often, older adults do not understand the value of a gentle warm up before the main activity begins. It is important to have well-directed preparatory activities, which include gentle locomotion, and a full range of static stretches before starting the main part of the training. This warm up should be performed in a leisurely fashion and could take as long as twenty minutes.

After several weeks, adaptation to the workload begins to occur in regular participants. They become more able to accept an increased workload. This is the essence of training. The notion of continuity is an important training concept and must be imparted to the participants early in the course. If their attendance is sporadic, the training effect will be minimized.

Scheduling three lessons a week will produce the greatest improvement with a minimum of over-use injury. An exercise class once every seven days produces a low level of improvement. Additionally, a once-a-week lesson missed becomes once every fourteen days, and the hazards of restarting the training cycle increase with the time between lessons. The economics of three times a week, both in financial terms and in terms of conflicting personal commitments, may prevent some older adults from participating that often. This calls for the participants' individual initiative in getting the ideal third workout per week on their own. This need not be a formalized, gymnasium-based, exercise session. Rather, there are a vast array of backyard maintenance tasks and light recreations such as skating, swimming, cycling, and hiking, to name a few—all of which can be aggregated to produce a fitness effect. *Canada's Physical Activity Guide to Healthy Active Living for Older Adults* suggests that physical activity be built into a daily routine of thirty to sixty minutes. This will improve health and fitness.

As the class becomes more able to accept an increased workload they should be challenged regularly to accept a bit more. This is the method by which reconditioning occurs. But the challenge must be open-ended. For example, an open-ended challenge would ask, "Do you think you could do a few more?" (repetitions of an exercise) as contrasted with a demand "Okay, ten more" which has failure built in. The point of this is that the participants have control of their workload and are never left in an evaluative situation should they decide to not accept the challenge or fall short of it.

It is through this chain of realizable challenges that people come to know their own capacity. When the challenges are small, the danger of over-load is slight. When the participants know that their performance is always acceptable, they have the confidence to stop before it hurts them. The participants should always be able to rise to a challenge saying to themselves, "I can do that."

---

8 In counselling an older adult (or a class of older adults) in achieving an ideal training frequency, what options could you suggest to them? What principal safety guideline should be part of your advice?

SAFETY OF ALL PARTICIPANTS IS THE FIRST PRIORITY

While the risk of injury to older adults in a well-conducted fitness programme is small, some risk does exist as in any fitness class. Anticipating situations or activities that are potentially hazardous can minimize it. Injuries in older adult fitness activities occur when participants are insufficiently prepared for the activity or progress too quickly. It may be that they are not properly warmed up. It could be that they are misdirected and are attempting workloads that are excessive for them. Or, the activity is unsuitable for a person of their age and fitness level. Situations such as these often occur in the early lessons of a fitness course (Kavanagh and Shephard 1978). The participants are still learning how to participate. Bear in mind that some older individuals have never been in an organized activity class. This may be true of some older men, but there are some men of this generation who still carry vestiges of their military "be fit or die" philosophy. They enter the exercise experience "unwisely and too well" and become casualties (O'Brien-Cousins and Burgess 1992). It is in the context of safety for all that the following set of principles for safe practice of group exercise is proposed.

The Safety Attitude

Class safety comes about from a variety of factors, which interact to eliminate high-risk situations. It is based on an attitude that arises in the participants as they discover the class belongs to them. It is their class, their experience, and it is their fitness level that we are helping them to change. The class does not belong to the instructor. The primary goal of older adult fitness classes is to empower the participants. If the individual is controlled by the class, it makes them subject to injury from working to other people's workloads. When they realize their fitness class is a venue for their own physical expression, they become able to take charge of their own training. This is the ultimate goal of all older adult instruction. Not only does this add to the safety but it increases the level of commitment to a programme when goals are set and then pursued by the individual. Individuality should be promoted within an atmosphere with both instructor responsibility and participant safety.

Long, Continuous, Gentle, Warm up

When we begin physical activity it takes some time for our body to adapt to the increased demands placed on the heart and lungs. Our heart rate is increased along with our respiration. Older adults may take more time to adapt to this exertion. Of course this is dependent on both their age and physical condition. Additionally, some older adults have subclinical osteoarthritis or other restrictions. Older adults stand to benefit from an extended warm up that improves mobility, reduces risk and minimizes discomfort.

The warm up should include locomotion and static stretches, all of which start at a submaximal level and gradually increase in intensity, leaving the participant(s) perspiring slightly prior to starting the main body of the workout. The period devoted to stretching in a standard class will be about ten minutes.

Uninterrupted Breathing

Many inexperienced exercisers will hold their breath while exercising due to concentration on the activity. Breath-holding while straining at an exercise creates a Val Salva effect, which can cause a marked increase in blood pressure and in the work of the heart. It also restricts the return circulation to the heart and the flow through the coronary arteries. This occurs at a point where the heart needs more oxygen, and yet it receives less, which is dangerous for older deconditioned people.

Holding one's breath during locomotion ensures that the activities will become anaerobic. While trained athletes have formidable anaerobic capacities, deconditioned older adults may no longer have this to any extent and do not require it in their early training. In fact, going into oxygen debt resulting from anaerobic training is undesirable for older adults since it leaves them breathless and sometimes apprehensive. Anaerobic respiration is accompanied by rapid heart rates, which is stressful and perhaps dangerous for deconditioned older adults. A safe practice is the Talk Test, which states that participants should work no harder than at a pace that will allow them to carry on a conversation (Goode, Sharpe, and Shaiman 1993). Since fat metabolism occurs best in an oxygen-rich environment, keeping the workload in the aerobic range has the added advantage of metabolizing body fat.

9 Explain why uninterrupted breathing prevents the Val Salva effect.

An Erect Head Position

Apart from the aesthetics of an erect posture, an upright position of the head during exercise has several safety features. Lowering the head below the level of the heart, as in forward flexion of the trunk, can cause dizziness when the older person straightens up. This occurs particularly in those who have poor blood pressure compensatory responses. Dizziness and falls can result.

The balance centres in the middle ear normally are only moved through a limited range in deconditioned older persons. They are often unaccustomed to head positions that are away from the normal standing, sitting, and lying.

In fact, the head position in each of those three postures is quite similar through the use of back supports or a pillow. When an inexperienced exerciser tilts sideways, bends forward, or turns the trunk laterally, he or she may experience dizziness and loss of balance. "Stand straight, keep smiling" is the catch line.

Low Impact Activities

A significant part of a fitness routine is directed at improving aerobic capacity. To be most productive, aerobic exercisers should strive for fifteen minutes without interruption. The intensity level must be such that heart rate increases to between 60 and 70 percent of maximal heart rate (Van Camp and Boyer 1989). Older adults if previously sedentary will tolerate low intensity longer duration programmes of exercise better than higher intensity shorter duration programmes. With appropriate intensity, duration, and frequency, a training effect will occur.

BASIC LOCOMOTIONS—STROLLING, WALKING, MARCHING

Locomotions are moving around on the feet using one's own power, from strolling to sprinting. The basic locomotions can be performed safely by older persons (fifty-five to eighty years) provided they do not have a condition that contraindicates sub-maximal exercise. Older adults starting in a beginner-level fitness programme should be taught to walk safely so they can continue to walk for aerobic exercise on their own. Most participants come to a beginner's fitness class in a deconditioned state–they are unfit. It is important that they are not over-stressed by activities that are too difficult. This is particularly true in their early training.

At the start of their training, the locomotions of older adults should be as free of impact as possible. Impact occurs when the body, which is lifted off the ground by the action of sprinting, running, or mis-jogging, lands on the lead foot with an impact that is absorbed by the ankle, knee, and hip joints. This is the basis of much of the stress injury that afflicts beginning joggers and runners. It is recommended that jogging, running, and sprinting be avoided by older adults until they are able to walk vigorously for an extended period. The process of becoming an older adult runner is based on having learned to jog safely and to practice it in training for at least a year.

JUMPING, HOPPING, SKIPPING

Each of these movements has in it the feature of leaving the ground momentarily from one foot or two. These movements have inherent acceleration and shock absorption problems. The higher and faster the movement, the greater the problem.

Accompanying the stress of shock absorption is the problem of incontinence, which is common in some older individuals. As a matter of principle, classes that include any hopping, skipping, and jumping should be offered carefully and with a clear understanding of the group's capability and condition. As a matter of good practice, it is strategic to mention a trip to the washroom as a standard procedure before the class starts. This can be included in orientation material.

---

10 Describe the mechanics of stress injury to the lower rear part of the leg.

BALLISTIC MOVEMENTS

Ballistic movements are those involving swinging of the limbs, the trunk, or the head. The part involved is swung through its normal movement trajectory and acquires momentum that is added to by the mass of the limb and by gravity. What starts out to be a controlled swing quickly develops its own momentum and, instead of the natural slowing that occurs at the end of the range, the part continues to accelerate until it reaches the limits of movement and sometimes over-stresses the joint(s) involved. Ballistic movements are a continuing source of injury. To avoid creating ballistic injuries, exercise leaders have to avoid fast training rhythms either from the musical accompaniment or from over-enthusiasm. A safer procedure is to demonstrate the exercise, stress the cautions, and allow the participants to set their own rate. When a well-taught class is meeting regularly, it is not too long before the participants are aware of these cautions. This is much to be desired.

Risky Activities

There are so-called 'risky activities' that are common in fitness classes offered to young and middle-aged adults. They pose no special hazard to vigorous people, but present an unacceptable risk to deconditioned older adults. With risky activities, the circumstances in which they are performed may play a significant part in creating that risk. While the age and health of the participants is a factor, the overall fitness and the presentation of the so-called risky activities may eliminate or significantly reduce the hazard. It would be unfortunate to eliminate risky activities totally for all participants if they are fit and capable of them. Here are a number of activities that could be risky for older adults:

- paired exercises involving partners straining against each other, e.g., pushing or pulling a resisting partner
- resisting muscle movement of a partner thus creating an isometric contraction
- power stretches using leverage
- muscular strength and endurance exercises against partner resistance, e.g., resistance push-ups

All of the above can be appropriate exercises with proper precautions. Since all require a near maximum output, it is essential that correct breathing techniques be used. None of these activities should be done until the last third of the workout when the effects of the warm up are at a maximum. None of them are appropriate for older adults starting a reconditioning programme.

LOCOMOTIONS THAT DISRUPT BALANCE AND CONTROL

In the process of maturation, there is an increasing disinclination among older people to attempt activities that challenge their ability to control direction and balance. Most cannot remember the last time they ran backwards or scurried sideways. Two factors seem to be involved: one is increased body fat and the other is decreasing strength of the legs. Both of these contribute to the loss of acuity in their balance. Since this is a multifaceted problem, it is safer for older adult fitness classes to avoid walking or running backwards. Similarly, travelling sideways by sliding one foot to the side and then sliding the other up to it should be taught carefully, ensuring that the participants do not step on their own feet, which usually causes a fall. Spinning or pirouetting also challenges balance and should not be suggested as a group activity due to the increased likelihood of falling. Hands-in-a-circle, a common folk dance manoeuvre, should never go round more than sixteen counts before reversing direction. Many manoeuvres common in square or folk dances are done with great gusto by older adults. These activities are within the capacity of some older adults if they are introduced with caution and performed with restraint.

Accelerated or accelerating movements should be avoided. All exercise movements should be within the normal range of motion for the body parts involved. The use of fast counting should be avoided. This includes accompanying music that is too fast, or erratic. The participants should not be dragged along into movements that are too fast for their safety. The same is true of movement patterns that have a tendency to speed up. An alert instructor should intercept an exercise tempo that is getting out of hand. Music selection is crucial to avoiding this problem (*cf* [orig. p. 465–66]).

POTENTIALLY DANGEROUS EXERCISE APPLICATIONS

These are movements that may compromise the structural integrity of the various joint systems involved. It is important to remember that the most innocuous exercise can cause injury if it is performed vigorously without a warm up. Similarly, if an exercise is too difficult for the participant who is urged to keep trying, an injury may occur. Injuries can also result from an overload situation where the participant is unable to perform the number of repetitions demanded. All these situations involve participants doing exercises that are common and basically safe. The injury comes from misapplication.

A number of exercises by definition are thought to be dangerous and so are called contraindicated. This means that they should not be done at all. Examples of contraindicated exercises are:

- straight-legged sit-ups
- full deep knee bends
- two arm lateral swings
- circumduction of the head
- trunk hyperextension
- lateral bending of the trunk with arms overhead
- continuous running up and down stairs
- high kicks forward
- the hurdler's hamstring stretch

Each of these has inherent a potential for structural injury. They should not be included in any exercise routine for older adults.

EARLY EMPOWERMENT OF CLASS MEMBERS

Empowerment is vesting the individual with the power to make decisions on her own behalf. Empowerment of individual members of a fitness class comes from having confidence that they are an accepted member of the group. They know by name a number of people in the group, who know them by name. They are familiar with a number of others whom they recognize. This familiarity is the coinage of group membership and is the basis for much of the interaction, which creates a sense of belonging.

A starting objective of a fitness leader should be to learn as many names as possible. While learning names is important, 'trafficking' in names is essential. Trafficking is using people's names audibly so the others can hear them. This process gradually grows acquaintances, friendships, and a sense of belonging, which is the underpinning of empowerment.

Empowerment is also derived from knowing what will go on in the class. It comes from

familiarity with the location. The class knows where the washrooms are, they are aware of what to do and where to go if they feel unwell. They know what behavioural latitude they have. In short, they are comfortable and confident with the situation they have entered.

A class will become more empowered as they learn the activities. Knowing the specifics of the activities removes the unknown factors on which uncertainty hangs. As the class becomes familiar with each other, with all aspects of the experience, they become confident. When the setting or the atmosphere is friendly and accepting, when they know what to do or how to deal with that which they cannot do, they are put at ease, and it is this confidence that gives them power to take control of their own physical fitness. They are empowered.

11 If you were teaching an older adult fitness class, what would be your first action in attempting to create a sense of empowerment in the class?

PERSONAL RESPONSIBILITY FOR THE WELL-BEING OF THE CLASS

Responsibility for class well-being grows out of the empowerment of the individual participant. It is derived quite naturally from the life experiences of class members, a majority of whom are women (Burgess 1990). They are experienced in the role of caregiver and homemaker so are predisposed to help one another. Because of this, it is easy to mobilize older women to care for each other.

Class well-being may be as simple as making sure that everyone has a partner in a partner routine or that each one has an exercise implement as needed. Class well-being is expressed when a newcomer shows up or when someone, long away, returns and is greeted warmly. Individual responsibility is expressed when a situation occurs that requires an action unspecified in the flow of the activity. Someone sees a need to act and does it because it is the right thing to do.

The well-being of all is the responsibility of everyone. This creates a culture of caring which enriches the experience of the class. Older adult fitness is not a competitive sport. It is a process of self-improvement, which occurs best in a caring environment. Empowerment makes class members party to their own improvement but, more importantly, also to the well-being and improvement of their fellow participants.

DEVELOPING PARTICIPANT INDEPENDENCE

A prime objective of older adult fitness programmes should be to teach the participants how to conduct their own exercise. With the growing number of retirees (Torrance 1991) and their increasing longevity, it is becoming increasingly difficult to meet the increasing need. (Burgess 1990: O'Brien-Cousins and Burgess 1992).

Do-it-yourself fitness activities are a natural outcome of the increasing number of older adults who are regularly active. (Health Canada 1999b). While a small risk of inappropriate activity may occur, this will be alleviated through information and practice under the direction of a qualified instructor before they graduate to freelance fitness. It is misprogramming to retain participants beyond the point where they can become autonomous exercisers. Fitness class graduates should move on to make room for those needing a safe start under supervision. Autonomous exercisers should be able to carry out their own personal exercise programme and will be well enough versed in fitness information to exercise alone. With their experience, they will be able to find help and information if needed. It should not usurp the leadership of trained professionals; rather, it places the onus on the professional to teach how to exercise, rather than merely to conduct a workout. Participants should learn safe exercise technique, proper warm up and cool down, appropriate loading, and a safe system to challenge them. When a successful course is completed, the participants should be well enough informed to continue training on their own. The availability of printed handouts provides take-home information. Most important, they should be motivated to continue either as a solo exerciser or as part of another exercise group. It is the greatest complement to an instructor if their clients begin to train on their own. Even more rewarding is to see older adults gain the confidence to help their peers or exercisers younger than themselves.

---

12 In dealing with a group of older adult fitness class participants, how could you create conditions that would make your own role as instructor redundant in the long term?

CONSIDERATIONS WHEN PROGRAMMING FOR OLDER ADULTS

It is difficult in a single chapter to present the wide range of activities that could be used in a fitness class for older adults. These activities can be found in a number of fitness leadership manuals. The goal of any programme should be to influence five components of fitness, including cardiovascular fitness, muscular strength and endurance, flexibility, body composition, and balance (Klingman, Hewitt, and Crowell 1999).

The purpose here is to present a philosophical approach to engaging older people in activities that will hold their interest. It deals with the attitude of the fitness leader and a special approach to involving older people in the activities. The focus is on the presentation, not the content. To this end, a methodology will be described for presenting organized activity that will be safe, effective, and enjoyable.

At the start, fitness in older adults improves slowly, so it is important to keep them regularly involved. Merely attending a class is of value regardless of the degree of participation. Even low intensity activity (less than 50 percent maximum heart rate) has value for a beginner (Health Canada 1999a). The generalized activity of a fitness class increases circulation. Additionally, the respiratory system, the endocrine system, and the muscles involved are positively affected by the increased activity. At low levels of exertion, these generalized effects are of minor intensity and of short duration, but they do occur (*Fitness and Aging* 1982). They account for the subjective good feelings experienced by low intensity exercisers in the early stages of training. More importantly, they calm the apprehension of inexperienced exercisers. These mildly pleasant feelings are the first positive reinforcement of participation in an exercise class.

When older adults participate regularly, the benefits start to happen. In addition to the positive somatic feelings that come from fitness activities, there are enjoyable moments that occur in a well-run class. These create a happy scene that contributes to making the class a pleasant experience. There are many opportunities for spontaneity and humorous comments.

As a matter of class safety, it is useful to have people talking and interacting as part of the class. As long as people keep chatting, they are likely not over-stressed. The first sign of overexertion is accelerated breathing which causes them to stop talking. A talking person is a breathing person. Active breathing keeps the exercise aerobic. Talking also provides a sound check for the instructor—as the level of exertion increases, the level of conversation decreases (Goode 1998). This is a practical approach to appraising exertion without stopping for a heart rate count, which some older adults do poorly.

A central intent of leading an older adult fitness class is to make the time spent enjoyable. An older adult fitness class is an exercise in existentialism; it places the greatest importance on just being there. The fitness experience must be centred in the now. Older adults are less concerned about their long-term future than they are about their present. While young adults are more easily convinced to train hard for future benefit, older people tend to be concerned about how they feel now. The fitness experience has an immediacy for them. Thus, each class should include pleasant,

funny moments that soften what can otherwise be an exercise of authority and control.

13 In your mind, which is more important, a strong level of class control or a loose, informal situation? Which do you think will be most effective with older adult participants?

MUSIC FOR OLDER ADULT GROUP EXERCISE

Certain assumptions are made in utilizing music in an exercise class. First of all, the class must be able to hear it. Music should accompany the activity, not dominate it. Well-chosen music provides an engaging sound 'fill' so participants do not become too self-absorbed. The external stimulation of well-chosen music leads people out of introspection and draws them into a group, sharing rhythm, melody, and good feelings.

It is nearly impossible to select music that will appeal to everyone, all the time. Since music is peripheral to the focus of a class, it is possible to mis-choose a selection without causing a revolution. The principle of infrequent insult states that a violation of someone's musical sensibilities will be overlooked provided it is of short duration and infrequent occurrence. Using common sense and calling upon the taste of participants can go a long way in selecting music that heightens enjoyment and motivation of all participants. Here are some working guidelines for the selection of exercise music for older adults:

- Avoid music that is faster than 140 met (metronome).
- Avoid music without a clear rhythm or music with an irregular beat.
- Avoid loud, extended percussion and strident high-pitched brass.
- Avoid discordant or atonal music.
- Avoid vocal music in a foreign language except if it expresses the class.
- Avoid soft, gushy, sentimental sounds.
- Avoid music with distasteful lyrics.

Variety is the spice of music selection. Use instrumental music in preference to vocals. A working rule is five instrumentals to one vocal. Vocals very often carry with them an emotive quality, which can create a mismatch when several vocals are played in sequence. Also, a vocal may be out of character with the mood of the class thus creating a dissonance. Classical music of the right tempo works, provided it is not too long–three to four minutes maximum. Quartets, small ensembles, popular organ, or electronic music works well. Military or circus bands play engagingly and can be adapted well to group exercise. Avoid lush, pompous presentations of symphony orchestras. They tend to overpower. Well-known rock music or rhythm and blues are well received, provided they meet the tempo/volume criteria.

The crucial factors in using music successfully in an exercise class have to do with the tempo and the volume at which it is played. Fast music can be a frustration. It negates all the positives that justify the use of music. Fast music is a contributor to injury (Kaplan, Siscovick, and Goldbaum 1983) as exercisers attempt to stay with a tempo and become casualties as a result. While each exercise has its own inherent rhythm, the right music can make the movements more sure, more elegant. Properly timed, music transforms mere movement into a kind of art. The enjoyment of this is elevated when the music is appropriate.

A general range of tempos for exercise is from 100-144 metronome. Metronome (met) is the counting system to determine the speed of music (138 met is 138 beats per minute). For comparison, military bands will play at 120 met for marching in a parade. Large movements of the limbs are done easily to 120 met, more difficulty to 138, and dangerously above 144. Rock music will speed along impossibly at 168 met.

The volume of music is like a hammer. At high volume levels, the rhythmic patterns are driven into the consciousness of the listeners. Even a selection usually enjoyed becomes a burden at high volume. Loud music intimidates the listeners. They cannot hear them-selves think. They cannot hear anyone speak. Many instructors in studios where loud music is common suffer hearing disorders. Older adult participants under these conditions complain of feelings of claustrophobia. They become very uneasy because it is impossible to communicate with the leader or anyone else due to the loud sound.

Accompanying the disturbing volume level is the problem of the instructor who, in order to be heard, resorts to a microphone and amplifier. This utterly removes any control of the class from the participants who cannot be heard should they try to speak. The one-way microphone is the antithesis of the situation desired in an older adult exercise class. Older adults should always be able to talk with the instructor and with other class members.

14 If you were going to use music in teaching an older adult fitness class, where would you find appropriate music? What guidelines would direct you in your choice of music and how would you present it?

CONDUCTING AN EXERCISE CLASS FOR OLDER ADULTS

A general exercise class for older adults is designed to meet the needs of a broad uniform group of about thirty exercisers age fifty-five to eighty. The starting premise is that all the participants are in normal health for their age and have no conditions that would be aggravated by exercise. Screening with a PAR-Q or a medical referral provide a satisfactory level of confidence of their capacity for beginner level exercise. A fitness class for novice older adult exercisers should take sixty minutes. It is comprised of six components, which are offered in sequence without interruption.

Warm up and stretching (10–12 minutes)

This is designed to raise core body temperature to the point where light perspiration occurs. A warm up is comprised of light aerobic locomotions interspersed with static stretching of all the major muscle-tendon groups. The two elements are complementary. The aerobic locomotions increase circulation and raise core temperature allowing the static stretches to be performed with a minimum risk of injury.

Aerobic activity (12–15 minutes)

This is designed to raise the heart rate and to increase the uptake of oxygen. Aerobic activity can be accomplished in a variety of ways. A stationary bicycle or treadmill is common for individual use. Group aerobic activity can be any of the following locomotions: slow walking (43m/min) to brisk walking (120m/min) as the group fitness level will allow. Shuffle jogging (maintaining one foot in contact with the ground throughout), low intensity folk dances, and rhythmic step routines with low impact are a challenge. All these forms of locomotion are accompanied with concerted breathing. Locomotions should be sustained through the twelve to fifteen minutes to have a training effect.

In order to accommodate the variety of capabilities in an older adult fitness class, it is important to structure the aerobic locomotions so that each participant can work to her or his own capacity. A circular walking course around a volleyball court is nearly seventy yards around, as walkers will swing wide. The traffic flow should allow fast walkers room to pass. A circular walking pattern can be reversed every few minutes so as to relocate the fast walkers at the back of the pack. Dances and step routines can be danced on the volleyball court with mixed intensity levels. This allows the less vigorous to have time to catch their breath. The imperative to stay in the 'action' must be replaced by a culture of common sense that applauds people who know when to slow down (not stop!). Aerobic activity is continuous for those who are capable. A slow walk after a brisk folk dance is still sustaining the motion and has value in aiding recovery. To ensure that participants see application of the common sense culture, a chair for sitting at each corner allows for a sitting recovery for those who need it.

Balance activities (4 minutes)

Balance is improved by systematic challenges to the neuromuscular mechanisms and effecter muscles in the legs and feet. This is done by isolating one leg in a balance situation: standing on one foot while holding lightly to a support with the fingers, the individual gradually releases the finger hold and tries to maintain balance without that contact. At any point, if the balance is lost, the hand/finger hold is resecured and the process goes on. Balances on one foot at a time, simultaneously on the toes of two feet, on the toes of alternate feet, are challenges of ascending order of difficulty. As participants improve, these balances can be done with the eyes closed. Various postures and arm positions can be added for an increased challenge. With continued practice, the hand support can be abandoned. Participants should be encouraged to practice daily at home. In older adults, it is recommended that balance drills be performed while wearing good-fitting exercise shoes. Balance improvement is dependant on regular frequent practice. It also improves with general improvements in physical fitness (Hu and Woollacott 1994; Petrella 1999).

---

15 What do you think causes older people to become less steady on their feet? What fitness component seems most likely to effect balance improvement?

Muscular endurance from free-standing calisthenics (15 minutes)

Free-standing calisthenics are movements that involve contractions of the limbs, the abdominal muscles, the shoulders, and back. The movements use the weight of various body parts as sources of resistance. Improved muscle tone and endurance results from regular training. At the start of a training regimen, some improvement in strength will occur due to the training stimulus, but improvement in strength ceases once the muscles become accustomed to the training stimulus. Improvements in endurance continues, however. To avoid injury, these exercises require a thorough warm up and so are more safely placed in the latter half of the workout.

Muscular strength exercises (14 minutes)

These are resistance exercises using hand weights, elastics, or rubber tubing as resistance. The intent is to improve the strength of the various muscle groups involved. With a mixed group of thirty novice older adults, it is time-consuming to test each participant individually to determine individual workload for as many as ten different resistance exercises. This is group activity, after all. For a start, it is prudent to have everyone working at a submaximal workload, which can be established by consensus. Assuming that the largest proportion of the class will never have tried resistance training, it is safe to aim low in setting loads for the initial classes. As the group becomes more experienced, they should be encouraged to select more resistance, bearing in mind that an operational load will be that with which they can correctly perform eight repetitions without holding their breath or with facial distortion from straining. To avoid a Val Salva effect, concerted exhalations with all lifts are essential for safety.

Here is a strength training system: determine the maximum load with which an individual can complete eight repetitions of an exercise in good form. This is the training load for that particular exercise. The individual trains on alternate days attempting to increase the number of repetitions completed. The objective is twelve repetitions. When this occurs, a new increased maximum weight for eight repetitions is determined and the process is repeated, starting at eight repetitions with the increased load and so on. The warm up and breathing protocols prevail.

16 What do you think would happen to members of a class if the muscular strength segment of the workout were scheduled at the beginning?

Cool-down

This workout plan is designed to have a maximum level of cardio-respiratory activity in approximately the first half of the sixty-minute exercise period. The most intensive part of the workout occurs from the tenth to the twenty-second minute. From the balance drills at twenty-two minutes until the end, the workout continues to decline in intensity. The muscular endurance and the strength activities are in the last half of the class. This allows a peaking of energy output at about twenty minutes. While the muscular endurance and strength sections are a challenge, they do not demand the same heart rate response as the aerobic activities. Thus in the last fourteen minutes there is a natural slowing of heart and metabolic rates. The cool-down, which should occur in the last five minutes, fits naturally into the slowing of the metabolism from the exercise peak at about twenty minutes. Activities at the end should facilitate the cool-down process. The core body temperature is at the highest so that static stretches for improved flexibility are most effective then. Various muscle groups might be affected by increased lactic acid production that has resulted from the accumulated exercise effects. This is an ideal point at which to do a number of static stretches to offset any possibility of spontaneous muscle cramps. At the end of the workout, effort should be made to promote circulation by continuous shakes and swings of the limbs. Breathing should be accelerated with an emphasis on exhaling forcefully. Elevating the limbs and continuous movement stimulate circulation and metabolize lactic acid. Relaxation is central.

SPECIAL CONSIDERATIONS FOR VERY OLD OR FRAIL ADULTS

Physical activity can enhance the quality of life for those who are very old or who are frail as a result of aging if modifications take place in the programming of activity. The frail and very old are trainable. The principles of training that apply to younger populations apply to them as well (Mazzeo et al. 1998). Focussing on proven strategies is wise in older populations. Strength training has been supported in maintaining functional independence, morale, quality of sleep, and appetite, while reducing pain in this target population. The benefits of lower intensity aerobic activities have been associated with modest improvements in cardiovascular efficiency and mobility (Mazzeo et al. 1998). A multidisciplinary approach to counselling the frail or very old is helpful. Physiotherapists can aid in accommodating for previous disability; pharmacists can outline medical interactions that may hinder exercise; family and friends can play a motivating role and often can provide many opportunities for enjoyable activity.

The benefits associated with lower intensity aerobic activity, strength training, and balance work to influence the quality of life of older adults whether they are living in their own homes or residing in an institution. Removing barriers for this group and promoting activity can add to quality of life while preventing new disability and aiding in rehabilitation from chronic conditions.

Summary

Older adults are living out their lives steeped in the influences and attitudes that they have developed in over sixty or more years of living. Their current behaviours are influenced by these attitudes. After a lifetime of hard work, many of this generation are disinclined to continue to be active. They see their retirement as the reward for the unremitting years of holding a job, but scientific research points to a physically active retirement as an important means of enhancing their declining years (Mazzeo et al. 1998). As a result of this misunderstanding, many older persons retreat from activity and so enter a cycle of debilitation. The accumulation of their disability results in an extended period of morbidity that is a burden on themselves, their families, and the health care system.

Regular physical activity can play a significant part in postponing or shortening the period of morbidity, provided these older people could be motivated to be active. The motivation to be active comes from a positive perception of the activity, the instructor, the class circumstances, and a recognition of their own ability to cope and even flourish. This aura of positiveness results from a sense of empowerment in these older adult participants. Empowerment results from the presentation by the instructor, which must be focussed on the process of being part of a class rather than on the content of the activities. The involvement of older adults in organized fitness activities must be done light-heartedly with humour and good grace. The safety of these late-life exercisers is paramount.

Study Questions

1. Consider the barriers to participation in regular physical activity by older adults and outline how you would present activities that would engage their early interest. Describe how you would sustain this interest so that they could receive a maximum benefit from their participation.
2. Describe a strategy that could be used to encourage older adults to become involved in regular physical activity.
3. Outline the societal distractions imposed on the now-retired generation that predispose them to be resistant to involvement in regular physical activity.
4. When presenting organized fitness activities to older adults, how would you order the various components of a fitness exercise routine? Describe the duration and safeguards of each.
5. You are presenting a class fitness activity to music. What are the most important features of music accompanying physical exercise? Discuss some of the considerations of musical taste and the effect of appropriate music on the class environment.

References

Ajzen, I. (1991). The theory of planned behaviour. *Organisational Behaviour and Human Decision Processes, 50,* 179–211.

Broadfoot, B. (1973). *Ten lost years, 1929–1939: Memories of Canadians who survived the depression.* Toronto: Doubleday.

Brooks, J.D. (1993). Exercise: It adds life to our years so why don't more people do it. Poster presentation at the Gerontological Society of America Annual Scientific

Meeting, New Orleans. Social Pressure Against Exercise, p. 10.

Burgess, A.C. (1988). *A fitness class description: Project Alive and Well*. Edmonton: University of Alberta, Department of Athletics, Campus Fitness and Lifestyle Programme.

Burgess, A.C. (1990). *Project Alive and Well report*. Edmonton: University of Alberta, Department of Athletics, Campus Fitness and Lifestyle Programme.

Burgess, A.C. (1991) Project Alive and Well: Physical activity programmes for well-being. In C. Blais (Ed.), *Aging into the twenty-first century* (pp. 173–85). North York, ON: Captus University.

Burgess, A.C. (1996). *Project Alive and Well report*. Edmonton: University of Alberta, Department of Athletics, Campus Fitness and Lifestyle Programme, Campus Recreation.

Canadian Fitness and Lifestyle Research Institute. (1995, 1998). *Physical activity monitor benchmarks*. Available online: http://cflri.ca/cflri/pa/profcorner/index.php

Christmas, C., and Anderson, R.A. (2000). Exercise and older patients: Guidelines for the clinician. *Journal of the American Geriatric Society, 48*(3), 318–24.

Dunlap, J., and Barry, H.C. (1999). Overcoming exercise barriers in older adults. *The Physician and Sports Medicine, 27*(11), 1–11.

Fitness and aging. (1982). Ottawa: Fitness and Amateur Sport and Canada Fitness Survey.

Gee, E., and Kimball, M. (1987) *Women and aging*. Vancouver: Butterworth.

Gill, T.M., DiPietro, L., and Krumholz, H.M. (2000). Role of exercise and stress testing and safety monitoring for older persons starting an exercise programme. *JAMA, 284*(3), 342–49.

Goode, R.C. (1998). Voice, breathing and control of exercise intensity. *Advances in Experimental Medicine and Biology,* (450), 223.9.

Goode, R.C., Sharpe A., and Shaiman S. (1993). Speech, breathlessness and monitoring exercise intensity. *Canadian Journal of Physiology and Pharmacology, 71*(2): AVI.

Health Canada. (1999a). *Canada's physical activity guide to healthy active living*. Ottawa: Author.

Health Canada. (1999b). *Canada's physical activity guide to healthy active living for older adults*. Ottawa: Author.

Hu, M.H., and Woollacott, M.H. (1994). Multisensory training in older adults. *Journal of Gerontology, 49*, m52-m71.

Hudec, J.C. (1999). *Individual counseling to promote physical activity*. Unpublished doctoral dissertation, University of Alberta, Edmonton.

Kaplan, J.P., Siscovick, D.S., and Goldbaum, G.M. (1983). The risks of exercise: A public health view of injuries and hazards. *Public Health Reports, 100*, 189–95.

Kavanagh, T, and Shephard, R.J. (1978). The effects of continued training on the aging process, *Annals of the New York Academy of Sciences, 301*, 656–70.

Kligman, E.W., Hewitt, M.J., and Crowell, D.L. (1999). Recommending exercise to healthy older adults, *The Physician and Sports Medicine, 27*(11), 1–16.

Matheson, G.O., Macintyre, J.G., Taunton, J.E., Clement, D.B., and Lloyd-Smith, R. (1989). Musculoskeletal injuries associated with physical activity in older adults, *Medicine and Science in Sports and Exercise, 21*(4), 379–85.

Mazzeo, R.S., Cazanaugh, P., Evans, W.J., Fiatarone, M., Hagberg, P., McAuley, E., and Startzell, J. (1998). ACSM position stand on exercise and physical activity for older adults. *Medicine and Science in Sports and Exercise, 30*(6), 992–1008.

McPherson, B.D., Curtis, J.E., and Loy, J.W. (1989) *The social significance of sport*. Champaign, IL: Human Kinetics.

National Advisory Council on Aging. (1993). *Aging Vignette Nos. 2, 4, 12, 13, 14, 15, 16, 17. Re: Frequency of Exercise*.

Nelson, E.A., and Dannefer, D. (1992). Aged hetrogeneity: Fact or fiction? The fate of diversity in gerontological research. *The Gerontologist, 32*(1), 17–23.

O'Brien Cousins, S. (1997). Elderly tomboys? Sources of self-efficacy for physical activity in late life. *Journal of Physical Activity and Aging, 5*, 229–43.

O'Brien Cousins, S., Burgess, A.C. (1992). Perspectives on Older Adults in Sport and Physical Activity. In *Educational Gerontology in Canada, 18*, 461–81.

Petrella, R.J. (1999). Exercise for older patients with chronic disease. *The Physician and Sports Medicine, 27*(11), 79–110.

Rogers, E.M., and F.F. Shoemaker.(1971). *Communication of innovations: A cross-cultural approach*. New York: The Free Press.

Rosenstock, I.M., Stretcher, V.J., and Becker, M.H. (1988). Social learning theory and the health belief model. *Health Education Quarterly, 15*(2), 175–183.

Scott, W.A., and Couzens, G.S. (1996). Treating injuries in active seniors. *The Physician and Sports Medicine, 24*(5), 1–9.

Thomas, S., Reading, J., and Shephard, R.J., (1992). Revision of the Physical Activity Readiness Questionnaire. *Canadian Journal of Sport Science, 17*(4), 338–45.

Torrance, G.M. (1991). Campbell survey results for older Canadians. Ottawa: Fitness Development Unit, Fitness Canada

Van Camp, S.P., and Boyer, J.L. (1989). Exercise guidelines for the elderly. *The Physician and Sports Medicine, 17*(5), 83–88.

Vita, A.J., Terry, R.B., Hubert, H.B., Fries, J.F. (1998). Aging, health risks and cumulative disability. *New England Journal of Medicine 338*(15), 1035–41.

VII ■ THE REALM OF SPORT

CHAPTER 26

History of Disability Sport

From Rehabilitation to Athletic Excellence

Robert D. Steadward
Sheri L. Foster

Learning Objectives
- To understand the evolution of sport for athletes who are hearing impaired.
- To learn about Sir Ludwig Guttmann's rehabilitative efforts among World War II veterans with a spinal cord injury.
- To learn about the growth of the Paralympic movement and the Paralympic Games.
- To learn about the evolution of the International Sport Organizations for the Disabled.
- To learn about the development of the International Paralympic Committee and its role in governing disability sport.

Introduction

Sport for athletes with a disability dates back over a century, whereas many of the organizations developed for the purpose of disability sport governance are only in their infancy, especially when one considers the relative new evolution of an umbrella committee called the International Paralympic Committee (IPC) which was founded in 1989. Today, six existing organizations, with the exception of the Comité International des Sport des Sourds (CISS), are all members of the IPC. These organizations include: Cerebral Palsy International Sport and Recreation Association (CP-ISRA), International Blind Sports Federation (IBSA), International Sports Federation for Persons with an Intellectual Disability (INAS-FID), International Stoke Mandeville Wheelchair Sports Federation (ISMWSF), and the International Sports Organization for the Disabled (ISOD).

The road to international acceptance for many of these organizations has been a challenging path, a path similar to the one individuals with a disability have been travelling along to be included into the larger society.

The purpose of this chapter is to present an account of the historical emergence of international sport for athletes with a disability, with an emphasis on the growth of today's major sport organizations and the evolution of the Paralympic movement.

Before examining the history of disability sport, however, one may wish to become more familiar with the evolving terminology that is used in the area. For example, for individuals involved in sport who have a disability, various terms have emerged, such as *adapted sport, sport for athletes with a disability, deaf sport, disabled sport, disability sport, handicapped sports, sport for the disabled,* and *wheelchair sport.* These terms generally imply a sport context designed for individuals with a disability and, in some instances, the type of disability. DePauw and Gavron (1995) suggest that these terms do not adequately describe the broader existence of sport in which athletes with a disability can be found: sport for athletes with a disability specifically, and sport that includes both athletes with a disability and athletes without a disability.

Terms such as *disabled sport* or *sport for the disabled* have and continue to be used to describe that which we will refer to as *disability sport.* As DePauw and Gavron (1995) point out, *disability sport* is preferred, as sport can not be 'disabled' and 'sport for the disabled' does not utilize *person first* language. This chapter will focus on sport for athletes with a disability—*disability sport.* This term has been adopted to refer to sport that has been designed for, or specifically practised by, athletes with a disability. Disability sport includes sports that have been designed for a selected disability group (e.g., boccia played by athletes with cerebral palsy, sledge hockey for athletes with a physical disability, and goalball for athletes who are visually impaired). Disability sport also includes those sports, practised by able-bodied individuals, that have been modified or adapted to include athletes with a disability (e.g., tandem cycling), as well as those that require little or no modification to allow individuals with a disability to participate (e.g., swimming).

The Early Days (1870–1940)

SCHOOLS

The 1870s provided the stage for the earliest documented sport participation by individuals with a disability in the United States. During that time, schools for the deaf participated in sporting events including baseball, and in 1885 football was introduced and became a major sport in many schools for the deaf. In 1906, basketball was introduced at the Wisconsin School for the Deaf (Gannon 1981). At approximately the same time, schools for the blind were also participating in sport in the United States. In 1907, a track meet took place between the Overbrook and Baltimore schools for the blind via telegraphic communications—which recorded the results to determine placings. Such schools have continued to compete against each other and against athletes in 'regular' schools (Winnick 1990). With the growth of competitive sport for these athletes in the early 1900s, it was not long before the arrival of international competition opportunities.

COMITÉ INTERNATIONAL DES SPORT DES SOURDS (CISS)

Prior to 1924, opportunities for deaf people to participate in sporting competitions at the international level appeared to be nonexistent. In 1924, two important milestones were reached which would generate sporting opportunities for individuals with a disability in years to come. The first occurred due to the leadership of Eugene Rubens-Alcais (see table 26.1 for a listing of CISS presidents and secretary-generals). He successfully convinced the six existing national sport federations at the time (Belgium, Czechoslovakia, France, Great Britain, the Netherlands, and Poland) and competitors from three other countries (Hungary, Italy, and Romania) to compete in the first International Silent Games, held in Paris, France (Dresse, Jordan, and CISS n.d.). This international sporting competition was the first event to be organized for competitors with a disability and included 133 athletes from nine nations (International Committee of Sports for the Deaf 1999; Winnick 1990). Events

Table 26.1 CISS Presidents and Secretary-generals

CISS Presidents	CISS Secretary-generals
Eugene Rubens-Alcais (1924–1953)	Antoine Dresse (1924–1967)
Oscar Ryden (1953–1955)	Jens Peter (J.P.) Nielsen (1955–1961)
Pierre Bernhard (1961–1971)	Osvald Dahlgren (1967–1973)
Jerald M. Jordan (1971–1995)	Knud Sodergaard (1973–1997)
John M. Lovett (1995–current)	Donalda K. Ammons (1997–current)

included athletics, cycling, football, shooting, and swimming. The success of these games led to the decision by deaf sporting leaders that the International Silent Games should be held every four years (Dresse et al. n.d.).

As the first International Silent Games approached completion, another milestone was reached in which the deaf international sporting organization was established and named the International Committee of Silent Sports (Lovett 1988). Under its first president, Eugene Rubens-Alcais, these games, and the organization itself, were modelled after the Olympic Games and governed by the International Olympic Committee (IOC). In 1939, an agreement was made to institute technical commissions (technical delegates) responsible for each of the sporting branches within the organization. The same year marked the beginning of what was to be a lengthy ten-year hiatus from international competitions due to World War II. In 1949, the first International Silent Winter Games took place in Seefeld, Austria. The first winter quadrennial event would have a humble beginning with only thirty-three competitors from five nations (Dresse et al. n.d.). After originally scheduling the International Silent Summer and Winter Games to take place every four years during the same year, the third International Silent Winter Games were held in 1955, so that the Summer and Winter Games would alternate every two years (International Committee of Sports for the Deaf 1999). Today, the Olympic and Paralympic Games precede the Silent Games by one year.

In 1955, the IOC announced its unanimous recognition of CISS as an "International Federation with Olympic standing" (Lovett 1988). In 1966, the IOC awarded the Olympic Cup, or Coubertin Cup (created by Baron Pierre de Coubertin in 1906, who was the father of the modern Olympic Games), in recognition of CISS's strict adherence to the Olympic ideal and its service to international sport (Dresse, et al. n.d.). The following year, the name International Silent Games was officially changed to the World Silent Games to recognize their worldwide nature (Lovett 1988).

American Jerald Jordan assumed the position of CISS president in 1971. In 1975, the name of the games was changed to the World Games for the Deaf. In 1979, just prior to the ninth Winter World Games for the Deaf, the Congress decided to change the title of its organization to Comité International des Sport des Sourds (in English this translates to the International Committee of Sports for the Deaf, today known as CISS). In 1981, a large majority of delegates decided to use only the English language (instead of both French and English). However, the title of the organization was retained in French in remembrance of the organization's origin (Dresse et al. n.d.).

In 1985, the president of the IOC, Juan Antonio Samaranch, requested that CISS join the International Coordinating Committee for the World Organizations of Sports for the Disabled (ICC) (this organization will be discussed in more detail in the Growth of the Paralympic Movement section of this chapter) to provide an organizational structure that would allow CISS to retain its autonomy and continue with its own games. CISS agreed to join the ICC and was admitted in 1986. Furthermore, when the IPC replaced the ICC in 1989, CISS became a founding member (Dresse et al. n.d.).

CISS had many concerns about participating in the Paralympic Games, these included:

1. How many deaf athletes would be allowed to participate in the Paralympics?
2. What events would be permitted?
3. To what extent would the IPC fund expenses for interpreters that would be incurred to allow athletes who were deaf to communicate with other athletes and officials?
4. To what degree would CISS retain control over their own sport technical decisions?
5. Would the IPC make available the latest technology, such as visual devices to parallel auditory devices?
   (Dresse et al. n.d.)

In 1990, CISS participated in the IPC General Assembly. An agreement between both organizations was met, with the following major points:

1. CISS was to be recognized as the supreme authority of sports for the deaf.
2. The World Games for the Deaf would have the same status as the Paralympic Games.
3. Autonomy and independence of all national deaf sports federations were to be encouraged and respected.
4. Funding for athletes with a disability were to be shared with CISS on a proportional basis.
   (Dresse et al. n.d.)

However, the articles in the agreement were not fully met between CISS and the IPC. In 1993, the CISS Congress was filled with considerable debate over their continuation of membership with the IPC. CISS decided that the only way to resolve the confusion created between the Paralympics and the World Games for the Deaf was either to participate in the Paralympic Games or to resign its membership from the IPC.

In 1995, CISS withdrew its membership from the IPC and once again resumed its independence. In response, the IOC accepted this decision and indicated that they would continue to recognize and support CISS and its games (Dresse et al. n.d.). That same year, Jordan retired and received the Olympic Order (International Committee of Sports for the Deaf 1999).

In 1997, the games organized by CISS were renamed to the Deaf World Games (Dresse et al. n.d.). In 2001, the IOC approved the name change to Deaflympics (Ammons 2001; see table 26.2 for a listing of all the games). To avoid potential confusion of the various title changes, all CISS games will be referred to as the Deaflympics. In 2002, CISS had a membership of eighty-four countries (International Committee of Sports for the Deaf (n.d.)).

David Stewart (1990), director of the Deaf Education Program at Michigan State University, illustrates CISS's spirit well:

> World Games for the Deaf are a source of leadership and cultural awareness for deaf communities around the world…. Lacking big bucks sponsorship and glitter of their hearing counterpart, the Olympics, these Games may well be one of the only remaining international sport competitions that upholds the original Olympic ideals of what being an amateur is all about. (p. 32)

WHY DO ATHLETES WHO ARE DEAF PARTICIPATE IN THEIR OWN GAMES?

Many individuals question why athletes who are deaf compete in their own games and do not participate in the Olympic and/or Paralympic Games. Jordan, past president of CISS, has addressed this concern, noting that people who are deaf do not consider themselves disabled–particularly in physical ability, as they are able to compete without significant restrictions, with the exception of communication barriers (Jordan n.d.). The deaf athletic community believes that their limits are not physical, but rather that their limitations are in the social realm of communication. These restrictions are nonexistent in the Deaflympics, where sports and rules are identical to those of able-bodied athletes, with the only adaptation made so that auditory cues

Table 26.2 Deaflympics

Summer Games	Winter Games
1924 Paris, France	
1928 Amsterdam, Netherlands	
1931 Nuremberg, West Germany	
1935 London, England	
1939 Stockholm, Sweden	
1949 Copenhagen, Denmark	1949 Seefeld, Austria
1953 Brussels, Belgium	1953 Oslo, Norway
1957 Milan, Italy	1955 Oberammergau, West Germany
1961 Helsinki, Finland	1959 Montana, Switzerland
1965 Washington, DC, USA	1963 Are, Sweden
1969 Belgrade, Yugoslavia	1967 Berchtesgaden, West Germany
1973 Malmo, Sweden	1971 Abelboden, Switzerland
1977 Bucharest, Rumania	1975 Lake Placid, USA
1981 Cologne, West Germany	1979 Meribel, France
1985 Los Angeles, USA	1983 Madonna di Campiglio, Italy
1989 Christchurch, New Zealand	1987 Oslo, Norway
1993 Sofia, Bulgaria	1991 Banff, Canada
1997 Copenhagen, Denmark	1995 Ylass, Finland
2001 Rome, Italy	1999 Davos, Switzerland
2005 Melbourne, Australia	2003 Sundsvall, Sweden

are visible (e.g., strobe lights for starting signals). A distinction exists, however, in that individuals who are deaf consider themselves to be part of a linguistic and cultural minority.

Furthermore, those who compete in the Deaflympics are all in the same classification. In the Paralympic Games there are many more competitions due to the classification system. If athletes who are deaf were to compete in the Paralympic Games, there would continue to be another 'mini-Games', with one significant difference being that the deaf athletes would continue to be segregated from all other athletes due to their communication difference (Jordan n.d.).

Jordan points out that the athlete who is deaf views an athlete with a disability as being a *hearing* person first and disabled second. When athletes congregate at any event, hearing people, regardless of their physical limitations, are able to communicate freely as long as there is a common language. The athlete who is deaf is excluded, invisible, and unserved from the group's interaction. Conversely, in the Deaflympics the athletes interact and compete with other athletes without sign language interpreters, except when needed for officials. Moreover, while sign language interpreters reduce the communication/cultural barrier, they do not provide individuals who are deaf the barrier-free environment of their own community–in which they flourish (Jordan n.d.).

Another concern is the number of athletes permitted to compete in the Paralympic Games, as these games are faced with restrictions on the number of competitors. The Paralympics would not be able to host the additional forty-five hundred athletes who compete in the Deaflympics today (Ammons 2001; Jordan n.d.). Some athletes with other disabilities, therefore, may not be able to compete in order to allow for a limited number of athletes who are deaf to participate. Consequently, all athletes would suffer (Jordan n.d.).

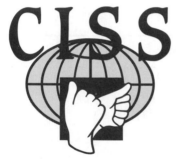

Figure 26.1 CISS logo

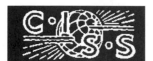

Figure 26.2 Original CISS logo

CISS Logo and Motto

In 1988, CISS ran a worldwide competition for a new logo, which culminated in an exhibit at the Deaflympics in New Zealand. CISS decided on two winning designs that were incorporated into one logo and adopted in 1989 (figure 26.1). Prior to 1989, CISS's logo was the same as their flag, which was adopted in 1937 (figure 26.2). Today's logo illustrates the international sign for sport, which is superimposed on the world to indicate Deaf Sports of the World. In 1983, CISS established a motto, Equal through Sport (Lovett 1988; International Committee of Sports for the Deaf n.d.).

> **1** CISS wishes to retain its own identity as an athletic organization. Comment on the potential for this to perpetuate segregation of persons with a disability in sport and in society at large. Comment on the impact of the maintenance of separate disability-specific organizational identities on the movement to inclusion.

Medical Rehabilitation and the Introduction of Wheelchair Sport— The Guttmann Era (1940s)

At the end of World War II, a relatively large segment of the world's population found itself unable to participate in society's mainstream.

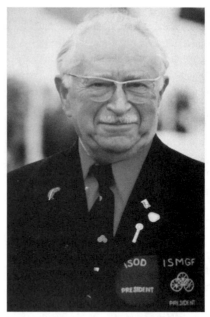

Figure 26.3 Sir Ludwig Guttmann (1899–1980)

As a result, a number of rehabilitative hospitals were developed throughout Europe and North America that served to reintegrate these individuals into society.

In particular, one rehabilitative hospital in England, Stoke Mandeville, played an instrumental role in rapidly advancing rehabilitative efforts for veterans with a spinal cord injury. The enthusiastic and determined Dr. Ludwig Guttmann, a distinguished neurologist and neurosurgeon, took command of this revolutionary hospital (figure 26.3) (Guttmann was later knighted in 1966 for his work and will be referred to as Sir Guttmann throughout). A German of the Jewish faith, he was forced to flee Germany in 1939 to escape Nazi persecution. Shortly after his arrival in England, he was appointed to the National Spinal Cord Injury Centre at the Stoke Mandeville Hospital, in Aylesbury, Buckinghamshire, England, where he began practising in 1944.

Sir Guttmann's work was viewed by many as futile, as the average life expectancy of a person with a spinal cord injury at that time was six weeks (with the primary causes of death due to pressure sores and urinary infections leading to renal failure). Guttmann,

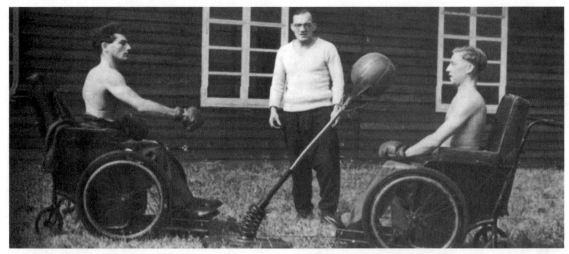

Figure 26.4 Punchball exercises during hospital treatment. From *Textbook of Sport for the Disabled* by L. Guttmann, 1976, Aylesbury, UK: HM+M Publishers. Reprinted by permission.

however, was convinced that if he abandoned the old methods of treatment (i.e., a passive approach, which was mostly gentle massage) and trained his staff in new ideas of "purposeful, dynamic physical management," he could succeed in making life, and a future, possible for his patients (figure 26.4; Goodman 1986).

Sir Ludwig Guttmann, never losing sight of his true objective–to return the majority of his patients to the community as self-sufficient citizens–insisted that work be part of every patient's therapy. Prevocational workshops were created in the hospital where patients could do woodwork, make instruments, and repair clocks and watches (Goodman 1986). Through his years of experience working with veterans, Poppa, as he had come to be known at Stoke, became convinced that work and recreation of all kinds improved the mental and physical well-being for those with a spinal cord injury (figure 26.5). The development of recreation, which evolved to include sport, was a logical outcome of his strongly-held convictions and his competitive nature.

Determined to find ways to encourage patients back into a meaningful life, Sir Guttmann investigated the possibilities of sport. Simple ball games were followed by

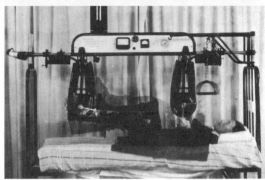

Figure 26.5 The Stoke Mandeville Pedal Bed Cycle. From *Textbook of Sport for the Disabled* by L. Guttmann, 1976, Aylesbury, UK: HM+M Publishers. Reprinted by permission.

archery, netball, and table tennis. With the mandatory work already established and now sport, plus the non-stop treatment by the physiotherapists constantly trying out new exercises, Stoke Mandeville's Spinal Injuries Unit became known for its ceaseless activity. One legendary story was about a paralyzed boxer on the ward who was heard to complain one day, "There's no bloody time to be ill in this bloody place" (Goodman 1986, p. 129).

To Sir Guttmann, the benefits of sport were obvious:

> The great advantage of sport over formal remedial exercise lies in its recreational value...by restoring that passion for playful activity–the desire to experience joy and

pleasure in life–so deeply inherent in any human being. The aims of sport for the disabled as well as the able-bodied are to develop mental activity, self-confidence, self-discipline, a competitive spirit and comradeship (Goodman 1986, p. 156).

Sir Guttmann's pioneering methods helped towards the current thinking that people with spinal injuries should live as part of, and not apart from, the community (Goodman 1986). This new rehabilitative approach introduced sport as a paramount part of the total rehabilitation package. Rehabilitation sport evolved rather quickly to recreational sport, with the next step–competitive sport–only being a matter of time.

Growth of the Paralympic Movement (1948–Present)

On July 28, 1948, after four years of pioneering efforts, Sir Guttmann founded the Stoke Mandeville Games, which were held on the Stoke Mandeville Hospital grounds. It was no coincidence that the Olympic Games were opening in London, England, on the same day. The initial games included archery, with fourteen male and two female athletes participating (figure 26.6; Goodman 1986). Sir Guttmann described the games as a demonstration to the public that competitive sport was not the prerogative of the non-disabled, but that even those with severe disability could become sportsmen and sportswomen in their own right (Scruton 1998a). From this humble beginning grew one of the most prestigious international events available for wheelchair competitors.

Sir Guttmann helped germinate the seeds he planted into other activities such as table tennis, bowling, punchball, darts, and snooker. In an effort to create events that would make sport more specific to the enhancement of wheelchair manoeuverability, Stoke Mandeville contests began to include the use of the wheelchair. For example, slalom and obstacle races against time were introduced (Shephard 1990). Competition soon blossomed into more demanding sports such as wheelchair polo, badminton, and netball. In addition, with

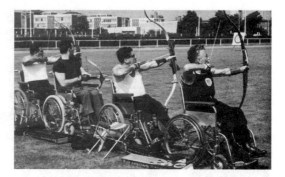

Figure 26.6 Archery competition during Stoke Mandeville Games. From *Textbook of Sport for the Disabled* by L. Guttmann, 1976, Aylesbury, UK: HM+M Publishers. Reprinted by permission.

the building of a specially heated indoor pool and an outdoor green at Stoke, swimming and lawn bowling were added (Goodman 1986).

Understandably proud of the sports movement he was building, Sir Guttmann recalled,

> At the prize-giving ceremony in 1949, I was somewhat carried away by the success of the Games that year and I dared to express the hope that the time might come when this event would be truly international and the Stoke Mandeville Games would achieve world fame as the disabled men and women's equivalent of the Olympic Games (Goodman 1986, p. 150).

Following its birth in 1948, the Stoke Mandeville Games continued on a yearly basis. The number of events began to increase, as did the number of participants through to 1952 when a contingent of Dutch ex-servicemen from the Netherlands arrived to take part in what was to become the first International Stoke Mandeville Games. The competition saw 130 participants converge at Stoke Mandeville for this historical moment, competing in events such as snooker, darts, archery, and table tennis.

With the overwhelming success of the first International Stoke Mandeville Games in 1952, and the determination of Sir Guttmann to realize his vision of an international sporting festival for wheelchair athletes comparable to that of the Olympic Games, additional countries joined the following year including Canada, Finland, France, Israel, and the Netherlands (Goodman 1986). A few years later, in 1956, the IOC awarded the Fearnley Cup to the organization of the International Stoke Mandeville Games for their "outstanding achievement in the service of Olympic ideals" (Goodman 1986).

In 1960 the International Stoke Mandeville Games left British soil for the first time and unfolded in Rome, Italy. It was at these games–the first of the present day Paralympic Games–that the dreams of Sir Guttmann for an Olympic festival were realized. Indeed, with the event being staged in the same city where only weeks before the 1960 Olympic Summer Games transpired, all athletes, coaches, and administrators alike would surely become part of a significant international experience.

That same year the International Stoke Mandeville Games Committee (ISMG Committee) was constituted, under the leadership of Sir Guttmann, to promote and sanction international sport for wheelchair athletes. The organization changed its name in 1972 to the International Stoke Mandeville Games Federation (ISMGF). Under this organization, the yearly International Stoke Mandeville Games continued to develop through to the present, with another name change occurring in 1990 to the International Stoke Mandeville Wheelchair Sports Federation (ISMWSF) (Scruton 1998b). To avoid potential confusion, ISMWSF will be used throughout the rest of this section.

The ISMWSF initially limited competitive participation to those athletes with a spinal cord injury. It was recognized that, although international sport for spinal cord paraplegic and tetraplegic athletes had been established for some years through the ISMWSF, there was an urgent need to organize international sports for other disability groups (apart from deaf athletes who participated under the governing body of CISS) and to set up an international organization for this purpose (Scruton 1998b). In 1960, under the aegis of the World

Veterans Federation (WVF), the International Working Group on Sports for the Disabled was established to study the problems of sport for persons with a disability. This led to the creation in 1964 of an international sport federation called the International Sport Organization for the Disabled (ISOD), with Norman Acton, secretary-general of the WVF, elected as president. Two years later, Sir Guttmann became president of ISOD (Scruton 1998b). ISOD offered opportunities for those athletes who could not affiliate to ISMWSF– amputees, the blind, and those with cerebral palsy.

The British Sports Association for the Disabled (BSAD), a founding member of ISOD, organized two world games at Stoke Mandeville. The first event, called the First World Festival of Sport, took place in 1974, with amputee, blind, and paraplegic athletes participating. This festival was a forum for establishing rules of sport for amputee and blind athletes in preparation for the 1976 Paralympic Games in Toronto, Canada (called the Torontolympiad), which, for the first time, were to include these two categories of disability. The 1976 Paralympic Summer Games incorporated this historic event into their logo, whereby the disabilities were represented by three intertwined rings with a triumphant person above (figure 26.7; Scruton 1998b). In 1979, following the success of the First World Festival of Sport, the BSAD organized its second world games termed the International Multi-Disabled Games of ISOD, which included athletes who were amputees, blind, or who had cerebral palsy. This event was a trial run for the 1980 Paralympics in Arnhem, The Netherlands, where for the first time, athletes with cerebral palsy participated (Scruton 1998b).

While the ISMWSF had established the Paralympic Summer Games and they were becoming a thriving event by 1976, the first Paralympic Winter Games, called the Winter Olympic Games for the Disabled, were just beginning in Örnsköldvik, Sweden (figure 26.8). Athletic disability groups included amputees, the blind, and individuals

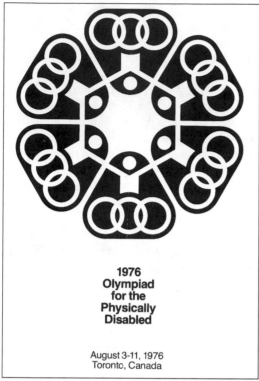

Figure 26.7 1976 Paralympic Summer Games Motto and Logo.

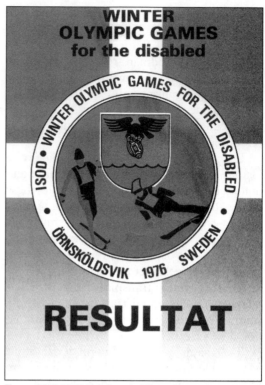

Figure 26.8 1976 Paralympic Winter Games Logo.

with a spinal cord injury. The development of the Paralympic Winter Games was initiated by individuals with a sports background and, therefore, the games were operated on the basis of functional classification. The Paralympic Winter Games were organized according to the athletes' physical ability to participate in a particular sport, rather than classified according to their medical diagnosis.

Even though ISOD joined ISMWSF in patronage of the Paralympic Games in 1976 and 1980, individual disability groups wanted to be in charge of their own affairs and form their own international organizations. This led to the establishment of two new international sport bodies: the Cerebral Palsy International Sport and Recreation Association (CP-ISRA), which was founded in 1978 under the chairmanship of founding president Commander Archie Cameron, and the International Blind Sport Association (IBSA), which was formed in

1981 under the chairmanship of founding president Dr. Helmut Pielasch (Scruton 1998b).

With the existence of four international sport organizations for athletes with a disability, pressure arose "to establish a committee with equal representation from each [organization] to provide for the conduct of multi-disabled games [i.e., Paralympic Games] in each Olympic year at a common site and a unified voice for responding to all IOC injunctions" (Labanowich 1987, p. 42). Furthermore, with ISMWSF's large international recognition, groups such as CP-ISRA, IBSA, and ISOD pushed for the ISMWSF to give them equivalent power with respect to the governance of world sport for athletes with a disability. This pressure was intensified by the IOC's expressed desire for a single organization with which it could communicate. Such pressures prompted the ISMWSF to agree with the recommendation generated in the ISOD General Assembly in 1981, that a committee be created to represent each of the four international sport organizations (Steadward and Walsh 1984).

Dr. Robert Jackson assumed the task of developing a written constitution for this new organization, whereby giving responsibility and authority to this cooperative committee in the making (Labanowich 1987). At the time, Jackson was the president of the ISMWSF (after serving as vice-president for four years and initiating the Canadian wheelchair sport movement in 1967), and had began this position when Sir Ludwig Guttmann died on March 18, 1980 (Scruton 1998b).

In 1982, in Lausanne, Switzerland, the ICC was established by CP-ISRA, IBSA, ISMWSF, and ISOD, agreeing that chairmanship of meetings would rotate among the four presidents of these international organizations (see figure 26.9 for ICC logo; Scruton 1998b). Each of these organizations had three representatives participate in ICC assemblies. The development of the ICC was of great significance for those involved in the disability sport movement. Increased communication between different disability groups would carry with it more cooperation and less overlapping when scheduling national and international events. As well, recognition, subsequent funding, and increased cooperation with the IOC would all prove beneficial for the campaign towards the inclusion of athletes with a disability into the Olympics.

Two more disability-specific sport associations were granted membership into the ICC in 1986, bringing its member count to six International Organizations of Sport for the Disabled (IOSDs) (Scruton 1998b). One of the new affiliates was the well-established CISS. Under encouragement of IOC President Juan Antonio Samaranch, CISS joined the ICC with the understanding that the autonomy of their organization, as well as the exclusiveness of their Deaflympics would remain intact (Ammons 1990). CISS, by choice, did not participate in the Paralympic Games. However, the Deaflympics were recognized by the ICC as having the same sports level as the Paralympic Games (Scruton 1998b).

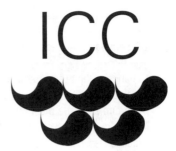

Figure 26.9 ICC logo

A second partner joined with an understanding similar to that of CISS. This new federation was to govern sport on an international level for those athletes with an intellectual disability. The name of the organization at that time was the International Sports Federation for Persons with Mental Handicap (INAS-FMH). The organization changed its name in 1999 to the International Sports Federation for Persons with an Intellectual Disability (INAS-FID). (To avoid potential confusion, the acronym INAS-FID will be used.)

The ICC delivered a noble effort in the infancy of disability sport; however, problems arose. For example, the IOSD's refused to allow inclusion of their categorically-defined athletes into each other's events. As a result, the ICC was quickly challenged and plans were initiated to develop a new world organization. In 1987, in Arnhem, 106 voting delegates present at the ICC seminar voted to change the structure of the ICC (Lindstrom 1990). During the Arnhem meeting, each country and federation was given the opportunity to make formal presentations on the future directions of sport for athletes with a disability, and after two days of discussion and debate, the assembly received twenty-three motions to consider. Of these, there were seven key recommendations (table 26.3), laying the foundation for the subsequent creation of the IPC (refer to the appendix to review all of the recommendations).

An ad hoc committee was elected at this meeting in order to develop a constitution for a new world organization. Discussions, debates, and much compromising took place

Table 26.3 Key Recommendations from the ICC Seminar

Number	ICC Seminar: Key Recommendations out of 23	For	Against
1	A change in the present structure of ICC.	106	0
2	The future structure must recognize national representation.	104	2
5	The future structure must recognize representation from the athletes.	82	24
15	To produce common rule books for summer and winter sports.	97	9
16	Reduced classes.	93	11
22	Increased participation of disabled athletes in able-bodied competition, e.g., Olympic Games, World Championships and others, always safeguarding their own identity.	103	0
23	The structure must allow for the development of organizations according to sport rather than to categorical disability.	82	7

Table 26.4 Founding members of the IPC—International Organizations of Sport for the Disabled

Acronym	International Organizations of Sport for the Disabled (IOSDs)	Web site
CISS*	Comité International des Sport des Sourds	
CP-ISRA	Cerebral Palsy International Sport and Recreation Association	
IBSA	International Blind Sports Federation	
INAS-FID	International Federation of Sports for Persons with Intellectual Disability	http://www.inas-fid.org
ISMWSF	International Stoke Mandeville Wheelchair Sports Federation	http://www.wsw.org.uk
ISOD	International Sports Organization for the Disabled	

* CISS withdrew from IPC in 1995.

between March 1987 and September 1989, when the inaugural general assembly finally decided on a draft and founded the IPC in Düsseldorf, Germany, on September 22, 1989. Dr. Robert Steadward, a Canadian, was elected as the founding president of the IPC and served three terms (the constitution's maximum time limit) until December 2001.

The six founding IOSDs of the IPC were CISS, CP-ISRA, IBSA, INAS-FID, ISMWSF, and ISOD (table 26.4). The IPC took over responsibilities from the ICC immediately after the 1992 Paralympic Summer Games in Barcelona and Madrid (i.e., the Madrid Games were organized for individuals with an intellectual disability), with the Lillehammer Paralympic Winter Games in 1994 being the first Paralympic Games to take place under the auspices of the IPC. The IPC's foundation began a new chapter in the history of disability sport: whereas most other international sports organizations represent one disability group or one specific sport, the IPC is the sole umbrella organization, representing all sports and disabilities.

The IPC would seek to provide five essential components involving the organizational structure for sport governance–some of which were not previously available in the ICC. These included:

1. national representation
2. elective representation
3. representation by athletes
4. an organizational structure based on sport rather than disability
5. a decrease in the current number of competition classes prevalent in sport for athletes with a disability

Table 26.5 Olympic and Paralympic Games (1960 to present)

Year	Season	Olympic Games	Paralympic Games	Same Venues
1960	Winter	Squaw Valley, US	n/a	
	Summer	Rome, Italy	Rome, Italy	Yes
1964	Winter	Innsbruck, Austria	n/a	
	Summer	Tokyo, Japan	Tokyo, Japan	Yes
1968	Winter	Grenoble, France	n/a	
	Summer	Mexico City, Mexico	Tel Aviv, Israel	No
1972	Winter	Sapporo, Japan	n/a	
	Summer	Munich, Germany	Heidelburg, Germany	No
1976	Winter	Innsbruck, Austria	Örnsköldvik, Sweden	No
	Summer	Montreal, Canada	Toronto, Canada	No
1980	Winter	Lake Placid, US	Geilo, Norway	No
	Summer	Moscow, USSR	Arnhem, The Netherlands	No
1984	Winter	Sarajevo, Yugoslavia	Innsbruck, Austria	No
	Summer	Los Angeles, US	Stoke Mandeville, England, and New York, US	No
1988	Winter	Calgary, Canada	Innsbruck, Austria	No
	Summer	Seoul, Korea	Seoul, Korea	Yes
1992	Winter	Tignes-Albertville, France	Tignes-Albertville, France	Yes
	Summer	Barcelona, Spain	Barcelona, Spain	Yes
1994	Winter	Lillehammer, Norway	Lillehammer, Norway	Yes
1996	Summer	Atlanta, US	Atlanta, US	Yes
1998	Winter	Nagano, Japan	Nagano, Japan	Yes
2000	Summer	Sydney, Australia	Sydney, Australia	Yes
2002	Winter	Salt Lake City, US	Salt Lake City, US	Yes
2004	Summer	Athens, Greece	Athens, Greece	Yes
2006	Winter	Turin, Italy	Turin, Italy	Yes
2008	Summer	Beijing, China	Beijing, China	Yes

The IOSDS are also called international federations and are made up of national members. Each federation has a written constitution and works on democratic principles. The national members, recognized in their own countries as the authorized sports body, decide on the policies of the IOSDS.

Today, the Paralympic Games, similar to the Olympics, take place every two years, alternating between summer and winter sports (table 26.5). However, it was not until 1994 that the Olympic and Paralympic games followed this format, whereas previous games were held every four years, with both the summer and winter games taking place in the same year. Today, the country hosting the Olympic Games also hosts the Paralympics, which immediately follow the Olympics. In June 2001, the IOC and IPC presidents signed an agreement that the Paralympic Games will take place shortly after the Olympic Games, using the same sporting venues and facilities (International Paralympic Committee n.d).

The Paralympics have become the equivalent to the Olympics in recognizing athletes' achievements and abilities, rather than focussing on their disabilities. The only difference between the two games is that the Paralympics provide an elite competition opportunity to athletes with a disability, which often precludes their involvement in the Olympic Games. All Paralympic athletes are highly trained sportsmen and sportswomen who have ambitions to be the best that they can be in their particular discipline. The Paralympic athletes who compete for their country are elite athletes and must meet strict qualifying standards to be eligible to compete. The Paralympics are not a participatory event in which everyone who enters receives a medal for involvement.

The word *Paralympic* was first introduced by the Japanese in preparation for the thirteenth International Stoke Mandeville Games in Tokyo, Japan (figure 26.10 and figure 26.11) (Japanese Organizing Committee of the XIII International Stoke Mandeville Games 1964). It was not until 1985, however, when negotiations between the ICC and IOC presidents

that the term *Paralympic* was officially adopted to be used by the ICC and the national disability sport organizations. This development was the result of the IOC stipulating in 1983 that the ICC and disability sport organizations must refrain from using the word Olympics—as some of the Paralympic Games had been in the past referred to as the Olympic Games for the Disabled (DePauw and Gavon 1995).

The word *Paralympic* has different connotations. It comes from the Latin word *para* meaning "with" and from the word *Olympic*. In the past, however, many individuals have associated the word with the first part of *paraplegia*, which stands for a spinal injury (International Paralympic Committee 1999). There was some opposition against the naming of what is now called the International Paralympic Committee, as many viewed this new name not inclusive of all of the disability groups (i.e., it was suggested that *para* was referring to individuals with a spinal injury). However, the word *Paralympic* within the acronym IPC reflects a sports movement in 'parallel' to the Olympic Games and the IOC.

The IPC's philosophy on classification is 'sports specific' and not 'disability orientated'. This is the reason why classification is becoming increasingly based on functional rather than medical categories. In order to provide a level playing field where athletes can compete fairly with their peers, each Paralympic athlete is classified according to his or her functional ability. Functional classification implies that athletes with similar capabilities, and not necessarily similar impairments, are in the same class. This type of classification has been around for sometime and was initiated within the international wheelchair sport movement before the establishment of the IPC.

Most Paralympic sports and events are modifications of Olympic sports, and sporting events implement classification rules which allow for the functional ability of their respective athletes. In some sports, athletes from all disability groups participate, whereas in other sports, athletes from only one type of disability participate, such as athletes who are visually

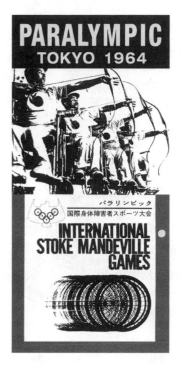

Figure 26.10 First historical reference to the term *Paralympic*

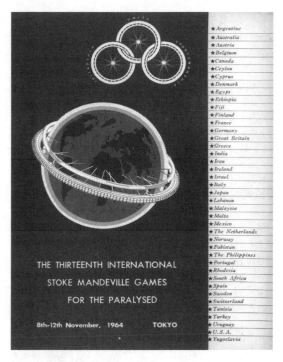

Figure 26.11 Sports programme for the 1976 International Stoke Mandeville Games

impaired competing in judo and goalball, and athletes with cerebral palsy competing in boccia and soccer (International Paralympic Committee 1999). In 2000, the IPC coordinated the following twenty summer sports at the Sydney Paralympic Games: archery, athletics, basketball-id (intellectual disability), basketball (wheelchair), boccia, cycling, equestrian, fencing, goalball, judo, powerlifting, rugby (wheelchair), sailing, shooting, soccer, swimming, table tennis, tennis (wheelchair), and volleyball (sitting and standing). The IPC coordinated the following three winter sports at the Salt Lake City 2002 Paralympic Games: alpine skiing (downhill, super G, giant slalom, slalom), nordic skiing (crosscountry skiing, biathlon), and ice sledge hockey (International Paralympic Committee n.d.).

RELATIONSHIP BETWEEN THE IPC AND THE IOSDs

As members of the IPC, the IOSDs have direct representation on the executive committee and support the IPC as the body responsible for the Paralympic Games and multi-federational World Regional Championships (International Paralympic Committee n.d.). Notwithstanding, the IPC equally recognizes the importance of the IOSDs whose function is much more than just being members of the IPC—they continue their autonomous roles within the international disability sport movement which is evolving under their jurisdictions. The IOSDs additionally complement and support the Paralympic movement and the IPC, by virtue of the activities and programmes that they undertake (Strange 2001).

2 Imagine that Sir Ludwig Guttmann had not initiated the concept of disability sport. Based on your knowledge of other historical influences impacting on persons with a disability, how might this have influenced opportunities for active living for persons with a disability today?

Table 26.6 ISMWSF Presidents and Secretary-generals

ISMWSF Presidents	ISMWSF Secretary-generals
Ludwig Guttmann (1960–1980)	Joan Scruton (1960–1993)
Robert W. Jackson (1980–1984)	John M. F. Grant (1984–1993)
Donald Royer (1993–1997)	Maura Strange (1993–current)
Robert McCullough (1997–2001)	Paul DePace (2001–current)

International Organizations of Sport for the Disabled (IOSDs)

INTERNATIONAL STOKE MANDEVILLE WHEELCHAIR SPORTS FEDERATION (ISMWSF)

This organization commenced life in 1952 with the first International Stoke Mandeville Games. ISMWSF was inaugurated in 1960 with Sir Ludwig Guttmann as president, and that same year it established the first of the present-day Paralympic Games (see table 26.6 for a listing of ISMWSF presidents and secretary-generals). Today it is a multidisability federation encompassing wheelchair athletes (Scruton 1998b; Strange 2001).

ISMWSF has a fifty-year history, some of which has been detailed within this chapter. This federation has welcomed tens of thousands of wheelchair athletes into its programmes and has been the main instigator of sport-specific development, encouraging independent growth and operation. Two independent wheelchair sports federations have emerged out of ISMWSF sport section committees–the International Wheelchair Basketball Federation (IWBF) and the International Wheelchair Tennis Federation (IWTF). These federations have established themselves to the degree of independence and the right to govern and administer their own sport. A close working relationship exists between these federations and ISMWSF, and they continue to be involved in the annual ISMWSF World Wheelchair Games (Strange 2001; Wheelchair Sports Worldwide n.d.).

Sport-specific rules, regulations, and classifications governing a wide range of wheelchair sport continue to be refined by the ISMWSF. In fact, it was ISMWSF that paved the way for the

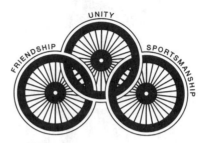

Figure 26.12 ISMWSF logo

universal adoption of the functional classification systems in the 1980s through promotion and application of new sport specific procedures. Current endeavours of ISMWSF focus on the promotion of sport-specific competitive opportunities and the maintenance of the World Wheelchair Games programme, with future plans in the latter area to include regional and youth games for wheelchair athletes (Strange 2001).

ISMWSF sees the importance of training and education programmes as a cornerstone to the ongoing development of the disability sport movement on a global scale. Today, access to information on global wheelchair sport events via the Internet can be found through the Wheelchair Sports Worldwide Web site–a wholly-operated foundation of the ISMWSF. In 2002, ISMWSF had a membership of fifty-nine countries (Wheelchair Sports Worldwide n.d.).

ISMWSF's Logo and Motto

The ISMWSF logo represents Sir Ludwig Guttmann's belief that sport is of even greater significance for the well-being of individuals with a disability. The logo–three intertwined wheels (with ISMWSF's motto written above each)–represents friendship, unity, and sportsmanship (figure 26.12; Goodman 1986).

Table 26.7 ISOD Presidents and Secretary-generals

ISOD Presidents	ISOD Secretary-generals
Norman Acton (1964–1966)	Edgar Joubert (1964–1966)
Ludwig Guttmann (1966–1980)	Charles Dunham (1966–1973)
Marcel Avronsart (1980–1982)	Joan Scruton (1973–1981)
Guillermo Cabezas (1982–1992)	Hans Lindström (1981–1989)
	Hugh Glynn (1989–1991)
Juan Palau Francas (1992–current)	Alan Dean (1991–current)

Their logo and motto embodies their mission statement: "To foster and encourage the development and self-determination of athletes in wheelchair sport internationally from grass roots to elite level in a spirit of friendship, unity and sportsmanship."

INTERNATIONAL SPORT ORGANIZATION FOR THE DISABLED (ISOD)

As a result of the World Veterans Federation, a number of countries met in Paris in 1960 to discuss how to organize international sports for athletes who were amputees and visually impaired. This led to the creation of ISOD in 1964, with twelve national members. When ISOD's first president, Norman Acton, resigned in 1966, Sir Ludwig Guttmann was elected and the ISOD's headquarters were transferred from Paris to Stoke Mandeville (see table 26.7 for a listing of the ISOD presidents and secretary-generals). Originally, ISOD was established to offer opportunities for those athletes not eligible in the ISMWSF.

Rule and classification development began on a disability specific basis for athletes with an amputation in the late 1960s and for blind athletes in the 1970s (Strange 2001). In 1976, these athletes were included at the first Winter Olympic Games for the Disabled and the Paralympic Summer Games called the Torontolympiad. Athletes with cerebral palsy first competed at the 1980 Paralympic Summer Games. In the late 1970s and early 1980s additional disability-orientated international organizations, CP-ISRA and IBSA, were established (see following sections for information on these organizations). ISOD was a founding member of both the ICC and IPC.

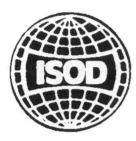

Figure 26.13 ISOD logo

Today, ISOD represents many outstanding athletes who do not fall into any of the categories covered by other international federations (i.e., CISS, CP-ISRA, IBSA, INAS-FID, ISMWSF), whereby ensuring that these athletes can compete at the international level (Doll-Tepper and Scoretz 1997). Such athletes include people with amputations and *les autres* athletes–those who are affected by a range of conditions resulting in locomotor disorders which do not fit into the above mentioned categories covered by the other international federations (e.g., dwarfism and multiple sclerosis) (International Paralympic Committee 1999). In 1998 and 1999, there were forty-two and thirty-one member countries in ISOD, respectively. A working group with the task of achieving amalgamation between ISMWSF and ISOD has not accomplished its goal. Further information on this amalgamation will be available after the ISMWSF General Assembly of Nations in Paris, France, April 2002.

ISOD's Logo and Motto

There is no information available on the development of ISOD's logo (figure 26.13). ISOD does not have a motto.

Table 26.8 CP-ISRA Presidents and Secretary-generals

CP-ISRA Presidents	CP-ISRA Secretary-generals
Archibald Cameron (1978–1985)	Ton Hessels (1978–1985)
Arie Klapwijk (1985–1988)	André van Schaveren (1985–1990)
Jack Weinstein (1988–1993)	Jaap Brouwer (1990–1994)
Elizabeth Dendy (1993–1997)	Rob Arbouw (1994–1995)
Lina Faria Galinha (1997–1999)	Alan Dickson (1995–1998)
Colin E. Rains (1999–current)	Margret Kellner (1998–current)

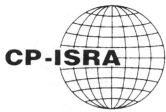

Figure 26.14 CP-ISRA logo

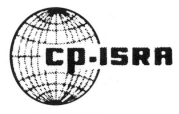

Figure 26.15 original CP-ISRA logo

CEREBRAL PALSY INTERNATIONAL SPORTS AND RECREATION ASSOCIATION (CP-ISRA)

CP-ISRA was founded in 1978 with Archibald Cameron as president (see table 26.8 for a listing of CP-ISRA presidents and secretary-generals). Prior to this date, sport activities for people with cerebral palsy were organized by the sports and leisure subcommittee of the International Cerebral Palsy Society. This subcommittee sponsored the first international athletic competition in France in 1968 for athletes with cerebral palsy (DePauw and Gavron 1995). Today, CP-ISRA is the international authority on sports matters for persons with cerebral palsy and related neurological conditions. CP-ISRA is the only international disability sports organization that actively promotes recreation.

CP-ISRA was a founding member of both the ICC and IPC, competing in the Paralympic Games since 1980 (Doll-Tepper and Scoretz 1997). Over the past twenty years there has been a growing movement in the world for increasing sports opportunities for all persons with cerebral palsy. Today, CP-ISRA places a special emphasis on the sports in which women and individuals with a more severe disability participate. These individuals have been identified by CP-ISRA as being under-represented and at times discriminated against.

Since 1989, CP-ISRA has held its own World Games in Nottingham, England, called the Robin Hood Games. These games are held one year after the Paralympic Summer Games. In 2000, there were forty-five countries holding membership in CP-ISRA (Cerebral Palsy International Sport and Recreation Association n.d.).

CP-ISRA's Logo and Motto

In 1991, CP-ISRA changed its logo. This change was the result of CP-ISRA believing it would be more appropriate for the word CP-ISRA to move into the world, rather then move out from the world (figure 26.14 and figure 26.15). This change in logo was to reflect CP-ISRA's developmental role and its mission to go into various regions of the world that had not recognized individuals with cerebral palsy, let alone given them sporting opportunities. In 1999, CP-ISRA changed its motto from CP-ISRA On the Move to CP-ISRA Moving Forward (Cerebral Palsy International Sport and Recreation Association n.d.).

ADAPTED PHYSICAL ACTIVITY

Table 26.9 IBSA Presidents and Secretary-generals

IBSA Presidents	IBSA Secretary-generals
Helmut Pielasch (1981–1985)	Jan Molberg (1981–1985)
Jens Bromann (1985–1993)	Björn Eklund (1985–1989)
	Fernando García (1989–1991)
	Enrique Sanz (1991–1993)
Enrique Sanz (1993–2001)	Michel Berthèzéne (1993–2001)
Enrique Pérez (2001–current)	Alberto Bravo (2001–current)

INTERNATIONAL BLIND SPORTS FEDERATION (IBSA)

IBSA was founded in 1981. Its athletes have competed in the Paralympic Games (see table 26.9 for a listing of presidents and secretary-generals). In 1997, IBSA changed the last word of its name from Association to Federation, as IBSA defines itself as "an association of associations"; however IBSA maintains its original acronym (International Blind Sports Federation 1997, p. 10). IBSA serves athletes with visual impairments, and often incorporates three different levels of classification (i.e., B1, B2 and B3). IBSA was the last disability-specific sport organization to attain recognition by ISOD and compete under its sanction (DePauw and Gavron 1995).

IBSA was a founding member of both the ICC and IPC (Doll-Tepper and Scoretz 1997). IBSA's activities are based on the principles of the International Physical Education and Sports Charter, adopted by the United Nations Educational, Scientific, and Cultural Organization (UNESCO) in 1978. In 1999, sixteen visually impaired athletes participated in two demonstration events (i.e., 100 m for women; 200 m for men) in the World Athletics Championships in Seville, Spain. This was the first time that blind athletes participated in such a prominent able-bodied championship. As of the year 2002, there were 102 countries holding membership in IBSA (International Blind Sports Federation n.d.).

IBSA's Logo and Motto

In 1994, IBSA unveiled their new logo to the world which was to have "a personality more in tune with the modern world" (figure 26.16).

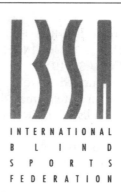

Figure 26.16 IBSA logo

Given that IBSA encompasses a wide range of activities, they decided that the logo should be very general and focus on the type of lettering and colour. The vertical, upwards-oriented nature of the typeface "symbolizes the effort made and spirit of self-improvement that imbues paralympic sport." Likewise, the colours chosen came from the world of sport, rather from the world of logos, ensuring that the "logo would not go unnoticed in a world like ours, saturated with brand names, logos and trade marks." The design of IBSA's new logo was to take another step towards reaching two of their goals: the normalization and universalization of Paralympic sport (International Blind Sports Federation 1994, p. 16).

Capable of Everything is IBSA's motto and is a reflection of its approach. IBSA is driven by the belief that athletes who are visually impaired are capable of achieving athletic goals they set for themselves. IBSA's athletes are capable of flying, fighting, entertaining, being the best, working hard, dreaming, striving to the maximum and, of course, excelling themselves (International Blind Sports Federation n.d.).

Table 26.10 INAS-FID Presidents and Secretary-generals

INAS-FID Presidents	INAS-FID Secretary-generals
Joseph Kieboom (1986–1988)	Loek van Hal (1986–1989)
Fernando Martín Vicente (1988–1993)	Mats Hamberg (1989–1995)
Bernard Atha (1993–1997)	Roger Biggs (1995–1997)
Fernando Martín Vicente (1997–2000)	Jos Mulder (1997–1999)
	Zenon Jaszczur (1999–2000)
Jos Mulder (2000–current)	vacant

INTERNATIONAL SPORTS FEDERATION FOR PERSONS WITH AN INTELLECTUAL DISABILITY (INAS-FID)

INAS-FID was founded in 1986 to work with athletes with an intellectual disability (see table 26.10 for a listing of INAS-FID presidents and secretary generals). Once established, INAS-FID joined the ICC and became a founding member of the IPC. Before 1999, this organization was originally called the International Sport Federation for Persons with Mental Handicap (INAS-FMH). At its outset there were fourteen countries affiliated to INAS-FID. In 1992, there were fifty-one member countries, and as of 2002, INAS-FID had a membership of eighty-six countries (International Sports Federation for Persons with an Intellectual Disability n.d.).

In 1992, athletes with an intellectual disability participated in the Paralympic Winter Games for the first time in Tignes-Albertville, France. These athletes participated in alpine and crosscountry skiing demonstration events only. When INAS-FID was informed by the Barcelona Olympic Organizing Committee that their athletes could take part only in demonstration events in the 1992 Paralympic Summer Games, INAS-FID sought sanction from ICC to host separate Paralympic Games. In 1990, the ICC agreed that INAS-FID could hold games in 1992, under the auspices of the ICC and the flag of the Paralympic Games in a different venue and at a different time from the Paralympics in Barcelona (Scruton 1998b). In September 1992, approximately twenty-five hundred athletes and team officials from seventy-three countries participated in the first Paralympic Summer Games for persons with an intellectual disability. The sports included in these games were athletics, basketball, indoor soccer, swimming, and table tennis.

In 1994, the Lillehammer Paralympic Winter Games included demonstration events for INAS-FID athletes. These events included a 5-km nordic ski race for ten sportsmen and ten sportswomen. In 1996, INAS-FID athletes took part for the first time in full medal events in the Paralympic Summer Games in Atlanta. In athletics, men and women (twenty-three in total) from thirteen countries participated in the long jump and 200m events. Whereas, men and women swimmers (thirty-three in total) from ten countries participated in the 50 m and 100 m freestyle events (DePauw and Gavron 1995; Doll-Tepper and Scoretz 1997; International Sports Federation for Persons with an Intellectual Disability 1999).

In January 2001, the IPC suspended INAS-FID from its membership. This decision was based on findings that the process of assessment and certification of athletes with an intellectual disability at the Sydney 2000 Paralympic Summer Games had not been properly carried out (International Paralympic Committee 2001, No. 1). The IPC Investigation Commission was established in December 2000, when it became evident that several Spanish athletes had competed in events for athletes with an intellectual disability at the Sydney 2000 Paralympic Games without being eligible (International Paralympic Committee 2001, No. 2).

In December 2001, the suspension of INAS-FID from membership in the IPC was lifted by

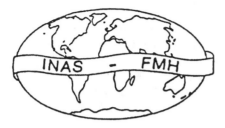

Figure 26.17 INAS-FMH logo

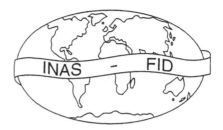

Figure 26.18 INAS-FID logo

the IPC General Assembly. This decision was the result of the new eligibility verification procedures developed by new leadership in INAS-FID. The effective development and application of these procedures will be monitored by the IPC, and only if the IPC is completely satisfied, will athletes with an intellectual disability be able to compete in IPC events. INAS-FID athletes were not permitted to compete in the 2002 Paralympic Winter Games and the 2002 World Championships as the event programmes, schedules, and standards had already been established and distributed before INAS-FID's reinstatement (International Paralympic Committee n.d.).

Another organization, Special Olympics Incorporated (SOI), was founded in 1968 and also serves persons with an intellectual disability. However, SOI has different missions and goals than INAS-FID (see also Chapter 30 (Mactavish and Dowds)). SOI is not a member of IPC and does not participate in Paralympic events and activities. Notwithstanding, SOI was formally recognized by the IOC and given permission to use the word *Olympics* in their title in 1988. This permission was granted under the condition that the word *Olympics* only be used in conjunction with *Special* (DePauw and Gavron 1995).

INAS-FID's Logo and Motto
The INAS-FID logo has existed since 1986. A minor change was made to the logo in 1999, when the federation changed its name (figures 26.17 and 26.18). Currently, INAS-FID does not have a motto.

3 INAS-FID was suspended from IPC membership pending investigations regarding cheating at the 2000 Paralympic Summer Games. As a coach of an athlete with an intellectual disability, and recognizing the potential impact on the athlete with an intellectual disability regarding future competition, should the cheating behaviour of a few individuals impact on the athletic careers and opportunities of many?

THE INTERNATIONAL PARALYMPIC COMMITTEE (IPC)
The IPC is one of the largest sport organizations in the world whose key focus is on organizing, supervising, and co-ordinating the Paralympic Summer and Winter Games and other multifederational world and regional championships at the elite sports level (see table 26.11 for a listing of IPC presidents and secretary-generals). In 2001, the IPC had a membership of 159 national Paralympic committees (NPCs). The highest IPC body is the General Assembly comprised of the national Paralympic committees, the five IOSDs, and the Paralympic sport committees. Members have full voting rights to govern the organization democratically and are entitled to participate in all IPC events (see table 26.12 for a listing of IPC's objectives and principles) (International Paralympic Committee 1999; International Paralympic Committee n.d.).

The growth of the IPC created the need for a permanent worldwide headquarters. Bonn, the former German capital, was selected in 1999. The movement's growth is best

Table 26.11 IPC President and Secretary-generals

IPC President	IPC Secretary-general
Robert D. Steadward (1989–2001)	André Raes (1989–1997)
Philip Craven (2001–current)	Miguel Sagarra (1997– current)

Table 26.12 IPC Objectives and Principles

IPC's Objectives and Principles

According to its constitution, the **IPC** shall have the following objectives and principles:

1. To form and be the international representative organization of sports for athletes with disabilities at Paralympic standards.
2 a. To award, supervise, and coordinate the summer and winter Paralympic Games.
2 b. Where the sport is in full membership of IPC's Sports Council, to award, sanction, and where appropriate assist in the co-ordination and supervising of world and regional multidisability games and championships as the sole international multidisability organization with the right to do so.
3. To coordinate the sports competition schedule of international and regional competitions for athletes with disabilities whilst guaranteeing to respect the sports technical needs of each individual disability group.
4. To seek the integration of sports for athletes with disabilities into the international sports movement for able-bodied athletes, whilst safeguarding and preserving the identity of sports for disabled athletes.
5. To liaise in pursuance of these objectives and principles with the International Olympic Committee and all other relevant international sports bodies.
6. To assist and encourage educational and rehabilitation programmes, research, and promotional activities to achieve these objects and principles.
7. To promote sports for athletes with disabilities without discrimination for political, religious, economic, disability, sex, or racial reasons.
8. To seek expansion of the opportunities for persons with disabilities to participate in sports and of their access to training programmes designed to improve their proficiency.
9. To promote the inclusion in the summer and winter Paralympic programmes of sports and events for athletes with a more severe disability and female athletes.
10. To do all things necessary or convenient to achieve or further any of these objects and principles.

SOURCE: From *International Paralympic Committee Handbook*, n.d., International Paralympic Committee, http//www.para-lympic.org (URL on December 2, 2002. Web site).

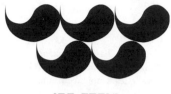

Figure 26.19 1988 Paralympic Summer Games logo

Figure 26.20 IPC logo

exemplified through the phenomenal rise of the Paralympic Games—more nations competed at the Sydney 2000 Paralympic Summer Games (122 nations) than in the Munich 1972 Summer Olympic Games (121 nations) (International Paralympic Committee 1999; International Paralympic Committee n.d.; International Olympic Committee 2000).

IPC's Logo and Motto

The IPC logo evolved from the one that was developed for the 1988 Paralympics Summer Games in Seoul, Korea, which incorporated five *tae-geuks* (which look like teardrops) based on the symbol of yin and yang (figure 26.19). The configuration of the five *tae-geuks* were in the same pattern and colours as the Olympic rings which were also used at the Albertville, Barcelona, and Lillehammer Paralympic Games.

When the IPC was created in 1989, the five *tae-geuks* logo was adopted by the IPC to be used as their logo. However, in 1991 the IOC objected, saying it was too similar to the five Olympic rings and would adversely affect their marketing. In the interest of creating harmony between the two organizations, the IPC changed its logo to a new configuration of three *tae-geuks*, to match the words of their motto: Mind, Body, Spirit—the most significant components of any human being (figure 26.20; International Paralympic Committee 1999; Steadward and Peterson 1997).

Summary

While sport has value in anyone's life, it may be even more important in the life of a person with a disability. This is due to sport's rehabilitative influence and because sport may be a

means to include an individual into society. Sir Ludwig Guttmann recognized this and began a new approach to rehabilitating individuals with a spinal cord injury. Rehabilitation sport evolved rather quickly to recreational sport, which led to competitive sport. Participation at the international competitive level requires the same attributes required by all athletes: dedication, determination, mastery, sacrifice, and a will to win. Giving individuals with disability an equal opportunity or fair chance to excel in sport often means a complete transformation of lifestyle and attitude.

Guttmann envisioned an international sporting festival of great magnitude, one that would be equivalent to that of the Olympic Games themselves. Indeed his dream has become reality in reference to the international presence that the Paralympic Games command in the world of sport. The Paralympic Games continue to develop into a sporting sphere for competitors of all disabilities. Guttmann, however, originally felt that the games he spearheaded should be restricted to participation by athletes with a spinal cord injury. Thus, when a need was echoed for the inclusion of athletes with other disabilities (such as amputee, blind, and *les autres*) he instituted ISOD with the intention of creating separate games and/or events within which athletes with a disability, other than that of spinal paralysis, could participate. This action prompted other groups to act in an analogous manner, whereby the eventual existence of the six separate, international sporting federations have evolved.

Today, the inclusion of athletes with a disability within one competitive arena and, at times, within the same event, has also taken a closer step towards the inclusion concept as a whole. Furthermore, athletes with a disability are slowly receiving recognition and acceptance into the Olympic family. Since 1984, athletes with a disability have participated in demonstration events at the international level including the Winter and Summer Olympics. Efforts are under way to secure the right for selected athletes with a disability to compete in full medal events in the Olympics.

The Paralympic Games have a tradition of bringing elite athletic competition to the forefront of public consciousness. Competitive sports have proven to be an effective vehicle to promote accessibility, equality, inclusion, and awareness about the capabilities of those with a disability. Competitive sports dispel the stigma surrounding disability and illuminate the realm of the possible–they emphasize an athlete's ability, rather than disability. The Paralympics promote the realm of possibility.

Study Questions

1. Why does CISS have its own separate games (i.e., Deaflympics) and why does it not participate in the Paraylmpics?

2. Who played an influential role in revolutionizing hospital care for World War II veterans with a spinal cord injury? What was the name of this hospital where this work was completed? Which country was this hospital in?

3. Which year is considered the first year that the now-termed Paralympics took place? At that time, what were the games called? Which athletes participated in these games? Who coined the word *Paralympic*?

4. How often are the Paralympic Games held? Do the Paralympic Games take place before or after the Olympics? Where were the 2000 Paralympic Summer Games and 2002 Paralympic Winter Games? Since the 2002 Paralympic Games, where and when (over the next six years) will the following Paralympic Summer and Winter Games take place?

5. Name (spell out completely and as an acronym) the six disability specific sport federations. What year was each federation founded? Which athletes do they serve?

6. What year was the IPC founded? What umbrella organization preceded it?

References

Ammons, D.K. (1990). Unique identity of the world games for the deaf. *Palaestra, 6*(2), 40–43.

Ammons, D.K. (2001). *Deaflympics website, www.deaflympics.com, to launch today!* [On-line]. Available: www.deaflympics.com (URL on December 2, 2002).

Cerebral Palsy International Sport and Recreation Association. (n.d.). [On-line]. Available: www.cpisra.org (URL on December 2, 2002). [Web site].

DePauw, K.P., and Gavron, S.J. (1995). *Disability and sport.* Champaign, IL: Human Kinetics.

Doll-Tepper, G., and Scoretz, D. (1997). *Database for disability sport organizations.* Berlin: Freie Universität Berlin.

Dresse, A., Jordan, J., and CISS *Bulletin.* [n.d.]. *Full version.* [On-line]. Available: (URL on December 2, 2002).

Gannon, J.R. (1981). *Deaf heritage: A narrative history of deaf America.* Silver Spring, MD: National Association for the Deaf.

Goodman, S. (1986). *Spirit of Stoke Mandeville: The story of Sir Ludwig Guttmann.* London: Collins.

Guttmann, L. (1976). *Textbook of Sport for the Disabled.* Aylesbury, UK: HM + M Publishers.

International Blind Sports Federation. (n.d.). [On-line]. Available: www.ibsa.es/ (URL December 2, 2002). [Web site].

International Blind Sports Federation. (1994, January). *Blind sports international* (5th ed.). Madrid: Author.

International Blind Sports Federation. (1997, July). *Blind sports international* (13th ed.). Madrid: Author.

International Committee of Sports for the Deaf. (n.d.). [On-line]. Available: www.ciss.org (URL December 2, 2002). [Web site].

International Committee of Sports for the Deaf. (1999). *Comité International des Sport des Sourds: International Committee of Sports for the Deaf, 1924–1999: Celebrating 75 years of service to international deaf sports.* Frederick, MD: Author. [Brochure].

International Olympic Committee. (2000). *Olympic movement directory 1999.* Lausanne: Author.

International Paralympic Committee. (n.d.). [On-line]. Available: www.paralympic.org (URL on December 2, 2002). [Web site].

International Paralympic Committee. (1999). *International Paralympic Committee: Mind, body, spirit.* Bonn: Author. [Brochure].

International Paralympic Committee. (2001). INAS-FID suspended from membership. *The Paralympian: Newsletter of the International Paralympic Committee, 1.*

International Paralympic Committee. (2001). Suspension of INAS-FID reaffirmed. *The Paralympian: Newsletter of the International Paralympic Committee, 2.*

International Sports Federation for Persons with an Intellectual Disability. (1999). *Official programme for the INAS-FID World Athletics Championships–Seville.* [Brochure].

International Sports Federation for Persons with an Intellectual Disability. (n.d.) [On-line]. Available: www.inas-fid.org (URL on December 2, 2002). [Web site].

Japanese Organizing Committee of the XIII International Stoke Mandeville Games. (1964). [brochure].

Jordan, J. (n.d.). *The World Games for the Deaf and the Paralympic Games.* [On-line]. Available: www.ciss.org/about/news/jj.html (URL on December 2, 2002).

Labanowich, S. (1987). The physically disabled in sports. *Sports'n Spokes, 12*(6), 33–38, 40, 42.

Lindstrom, H. (1990). The dramatic birth of a new international sports body for the disabled. *Palaestra, 6*(2), 12–15.

Lovett, J.M. (1988). History of the world games for the deaf. *New Zealand Journal of Sports Medicine, 16*(4), 80–82.

Scruton, J. (1998a). The legacy of Sir Ludwig Guttmann. *Palaestra, 14*(2), 24–27, 44–47.

Scruton, J. (1998b). *Stoke Mandeville: Road to the Paralympics.* Aylesbury, England: Peterhouse Press.

Shepard, R.J. (1990). *Fitness in special populations.* Champaign, IL: Human Kinetics.

Steadward, R.D., and Peterson, C. (1997). *Paralympics: Where heroes come.* Edmonton: One Shot Holdings.

Steadward, R., and Walsh, C. (1984). Training and fitness programmes for disabled athletes: Past, present, and future. In C. Sherrill (Ed.), *Sport and disabled athletes* (pp. 3–17). Champaign, IL: Human Kinetics.

Stewart, D.A. (1990). Global dimensions of world games for the deaf. *Palaestra, 6*(2), 32–35, 43.

Strange, M. (2001). Personal communication.

Wheelchair Sports Worldwide. (n.d.). [On-line]. Available: www.wsw.org.uk/ (URL on December 2, 2002). [Web site].

Winnick, J.P. (1990). *Adapted physical education and sport.* Champaign, IL: Human Kinetics.

Appendix
Recommendations brought forward for voting at the ICC Seminar in Arnhem, The Netherlands (March 13–14, 1987)

#	Recommendation (23 in total)	For	Against
1.	Do you want a change in the present structure of ICC?	106	0
2.	The future structure must recognize national representation.	104	2
3.	The future structure must recognize representation from the existing international federations sports for disabled with the continuation of the existing international federations.	62	38
4.	The future structure must recognize regional representation.	100	5
5.	The future structure must recognize representation from the athletes.	82	24
6.	Do you want the future structure to deal only with the Paralympics and elite sports?	25	81
7.	Do you agree with the appointment of an ad-hoc committee?	106	0
8.a.	Composition of the ad-hoc committee: • six (6) representatives of the international sports organizations for the disabled appointed by them • six (6) national representatives nominated from the floor • one (1) athlete nominated from the floor • one (1) observer from the International Fund Sports Disabled	25	60
b.	Recommendation from the British Sports Association for the Disabled, which is the British Member of ISOD: That an ad-hoc Working Group be created with • six (6) International Federation representatives • six (6) Continental representatives from the nations • three (3) current or former athletes • one (1) representative of the International Fund Sports Disabled	55	45

#	Recommendation (23 in total)	For	Against
9.	Mandate and purpose of the ad-hoc committee:		
a.	to formulate a constitution of the new organization that will replace the ICC		
b.	to consider the financial implications subsequent to the work of this ad-hoc committee	99	1
c.	to report back to ICC Bureau	95	2
10.	The draft constitution will then be circulated to the member organizations of ICC and their member nations.	105	0
11.	Within an approved period, a constitutional assembly will be called to ratify the new constitution.	105	1
12.	Olympic programme to be limited to elite athletes.	89	11
13.	Competition programme to be established as follows: Year 1. Regional Championships Year 2. World Championships (joint or combined) Year 3. Regional Championships Year 4. Olympic Games	36	48
14.	Competition programme proposed by ICC Technical Sub-Committee and supported by the ICC Executive Committee:	Accepted without vote	

Summer Sports
Year 1. Invitational Tournaments
Year 2. Regional Championships
Year 3. World Championships
Year 4. Olympic Games

Winter Sports
Year 1. World Championships
Year 2. Olympic Games
Year 3. Invitational Tournaments
Year 4. Regional Championships

#	Recommendation (23 in total)	For	Against
15.	To produce common rule books for summer and winter sports.	97	9
16.	We recommend to reduce classes.	93	11
17.	We recommend that all international organizations for sports for the disabled look upon how they can reduce classes. (This also applies to IBSA.)	104	2
18.	We recommend to continue to make experiments with integrated classifications in order to achieve a reduction of classes and improve the sports.	101	5
19.	We recommend that integrated classification can only be accepted when a clear and adequate system has been developed on scientific knowledge and research.	99	3
20.	The ICC shall continue to function under the existing agreement until a new structure has been determined and accepted.	102	1
21.	We recommend to work towards signing an agreement with international sports federations for able-bodied.	104	2
22.	We seek increased participation of disabled athletes in able-bodied competition, e.g., Olympic Games, World Championships, and others, always safeguarding their own identity.	103	0
23.	The structure must allow for the development of organizations according to sport rather than to categorical disability.	82	7

CHAPTER 27

Sport Medicine

Joan Matthews White
Robert Burnham

Learning Objectives
- To define the field of sport medical care for athletes with disabilities and state key reasons for providing sport medical care for athletes.
- To explain the meaning of *sport epidemiology* in disability sport and describe the strengths and limitations of this type of research.
- To describe the common sport injuries for athletes with disabilities.
- To identify the disability-specific medical problems of athletes with disabilities.
- To state at least five different medical conditions related to physical activity.
- To identify injury prevention techniques to minimize sport injury for athletes with disabilities.

Introduction

As athletes with disabilities moved from a rehabilitation model where sport was used as a valuable tool for therapy, education, and socialization, to a sport model where activity is embraced for the challenge of personal excellence, thrill of competition, and a profession for some elite, so too has the sport medicine field evolved. Sport medicine is a field that adopts a holistic, comprehensive, and multidisciplinary approach to health care for those involved in sporting or recreational activities. This field of medicine deals with aspects of sport that have beneficial (therapeutic) or detrimental (sport injury) medical implications.

Sport injury occurs as a result of participation in a practice or game. Acute injuries are caused by trauma; chronic injuries can result from overuse as would occur with the repetitive dynamics of throwing, running, or wheeling.

Sport medicine consists of a growing list of professionals, including but not limited to, sport medicine physicians, athletic therapists, physical therapists, coaches, nutritionists, exercise physiologists, sport psychologists, biomechanists, equipment design technicians, sport technical delegates, doping officers, scientists, and researchers. They are making major contributions to athletic preparation in training, competition, and sport injury management and prevention for athletes participating in disability sport. While sport medicine has its roots in able-bodied sport, the expectations of excellent athletic training and medical care are no different for the athlete with a disability.

Sport medicine for athletes with disabilities is an evolving discipline. There is a further need to explore the sport injury experiences and medical needs of athletes with disabilities in order to fully understand their needs. Today, athletes in disability sport look to the sport medicine team to help manage and prevent injuries and conditions associated with physical activity, manage aspects of their medical condition(s) that adversely impact on sport participation, and ethical strategies to enhance performance. The intention of this chapter is to address medical issues confronting athletes with disabilities in sport at the recreational, competitive, and elite levels and to help students appreciate the breadth and scope of the sports health care required by these athletes.

The Evolution of Sport Medicine

Sport has value in everyone's life; it is just as important in the life of a person with a disability (Noreau and Shephard 1995). Beneficial effects on physical fitness, stabilization of health, and social and vocational rehabilitation have been attributed to disability sport involvement (Shephard 1990; Guttmann 1976). Historically, medical and allied health care professionals focussed on the medical needs of individuals with disabilities. This medical model was illness-focussed and primarily physician-driven, with little involvement of other health care professionals. The benefits of remedial exercise or specialized corrective programmes were recognized; facilities were created specifically for the restoration of body function and correction of physical defects and deformities, but not for sport. This medical perspective imposed restrictions for individuals with a disability and provided a basis for their exclusion from sport, games, or recreational activities.

As veterans returned home from wars with physical impairments, the value of therapeutic exercise and physical medicine was increasingly recognized (Wheeler and Hooley 1969). For example, at the request of the British government, Sir Ludwig Guttmann, an English neurosurgeon at Stoke Mandeville Hospital in Aylesbury, England, began the treatment of soldiers during World War II at the National Spinal Injury Centre. With his intuitive understanding of rehabilitation and his passion for care of individuals with disabilities, he advanced the concept of health for this population. He recognized the value of sport, games, and other forms of recreation as a tool for the rehabilitation, education, and motivation for patients in maintaining health and personal welfare, and he applied these principles by utilizing an array of professionals in a coordinated multidisciplinary team. He reported that exercise through sporting activities improved balance in the wheelchair under various conditions, strengthened muscles faster, and improved the condition of the entire body (Guttmann 1976). In 1948, he organized the first Stoke Mandeville Games, which opened on July 28, 1948, with the participation of sixteen World War II veterans. The opening of the games was deliberately timed to coincide with the XIV Games of the Olympiad, as a symbolic gesture to bring attention to sport for persons with disabilities. Sir Guttmann's work became well known, as the athletic abilities of persons with disabilities grew to encompass international competition. Many credit him with being instrumental in initiating the disability sport movement. Sir Guttmann's contribution is also discussed in Chapter 3 (Wall) and Chapter 26 (Steadward and Foster).

With the incorporation of sport and competition into the rehabilitation model, remarkable changes were seen in the external qualities, structure, and values of sport for people with disabilities. The transition from the rehabilitation model into the sport model became evident as training volumes increased and participation outcomes became performance oriented. As sport evolved, so did the demand for more sophisticated medical support, coaching, and technological advances in equipment design. Athletes incurred injuries as a result of their sport participation which affected their performance and ability to compete. As a result, athletes demanded the appropriate medical care and treatment to return to sport participation.

Sport Epidemiology

When the sport medicine literature is surveyed for able-bodied sport, we see an evolution in:

a. describing the extent of the problem
b. establishing the cause and injury mechanism
c. proceeding to determine how to manage and care for these injuries
d. identifying preventive measures based on this injury data
e. assessing the effectiveness of intervention programmes (Van Mechelen, Hlobil and Kemper, 1992)

1 If *epidemiology* is the study of the distribution and determinants of disease frequency, what is *sport epidemiology*?

Sport epidemiology research is a method of information gathering to help us understand sport injuries and risk of injury in sport participation. The majority of research in disability sport medicine as it relates to injury is presently in the first stage—identifying and describing the types, locations, and risks of injury. There is a larger body of research that examines the physiological gains experienced through benefits of sport participation among athletes with disabilities. Research on disability sport related injuries has only been reported since the early 1980s. Curtis (1981) first described the types and locations of sport injuries for athletes during wheelchair sport participation. This study reported that

athletes who participated in road racing, basketball, and track were most frequently injured and that soft tissue injuries (muscle strains, sprains, bursitis, and tendonitis), blisters, and skin lacerations or abrasion involving the upper extremity were the most common injury type. Subsequent epidemiological research has included more sophisticated injury recording systems and registries involving a larger number of athletes, disability types, and sports. Such information has been invaluable in guiding sport medicine research and treatment priorities, rule changes, and sport policy modifications.

2 What accounts for our limited information about sport injuries in disability sport research?

Sport Injuries

Sport injury profiles suggest that both type of sport and type of disability are factors in the location of injuries (Burnham, Newell, and Steadward 1991; Ferrara and Peterson 2000). Upper extremity injuries are most prevalent in sports that use the upper body predominantly, such as wheelchair track, wheelchair basketball, and swimming. Thus, by virtue of the ambulation limitations imposed by their disability, athletes with spinal cord injury are predisposed to upper extremity injuries. Conversely, athletes involved in ambulatory sports (standup events) are more prone to develop injuries of the lower extremity. Athletes with visual impairments commonly fall into this category. An overview of this research is presented in the following sections for summer and winter sports.

SUMMER SPORTS

Many studies have reported a consistent pattern of injuries among the repetitive wheelchair sports of track, basketball, road racing, and rugby (Burnham, Higgins, and Steadward 1994; Burnham, Newell, and Steadward 1991; Curtis and Black 1999; Curtis and Dillon 1985; Ferrara and Davis, 1990; Ferrara, Buckley, Messner and Benedict, 1992; Ferrara, Palutsis,

Snouse, and Davis, 2000; McCormack, Reid, Steadward, and Syrotuik 1991). Hand injuries such as blisters, skin abrasions, and lacerations are most common. Blisters and abrasions are often related to repetitive friction at the hand-wheel interface and can be compounded by inadequate use of protective hand gear, debris on the wheel, and early season competition before the skin of the hands has had a chance to toughen up. Wheelchair athletes with hand blisters rarely limit sport involvement or seek medical attention as a result of their injury. Other hand injuries such as sprains, strains, fractures, or dislocations are more commonly caused by direct impact with the floor, wheelchairs, or basketballs. Elbow and shoulder injuries follow in terms of incidence but are more serious (Burnham, Higgins, and Steadward 1994; Ferrara and Davis 1990). A high percentage of these injuries are severe enough to cause the athlete to stop sport participation for more than three weeks and to seek sport medical attention. Most commonly repetitive stress in nature, these injuries are associated with multisport involvement and an increased number of training hours per week (Burnham, Higgins, and Steadward 1994; Curtis and Dillon 1985).

Ferrara and Buckley (1996) developed a crossdisability epidemiological project called the Athletes with Disabilities Injury Registry that followed 319 athletes over three years. The information from this study allowed an injury rate to be calculated, which is the number of injuries a participant incurs for every 1,000 times the athlete participates in his or her sport. An overall injury rate of 9.45 injuries per 1,000 athlete-exposures was reported. This injury rate was comparable with those reported for able-bodied athletic populations, but the injury site (shoulder, hands, and fingers) and protracted time lost from sport participation due to injury were distinct among athletes with disabilities. The researchers concluded that these findings necessitated further research and emphasized the importance of continual monitoring of injury patterns. It has been hypothesized that

reasons for the slow return to sport following injury may be due to a delayed healing process or a conservative treatment approach (Ferrara and Davis 1990). For example, athletes who use a wheelchair may never get a chance to rest a shoulder or hand injury as the upper extremities are used for most of the activities of daily living, particularly weight bearing during wheelchair transfers and excessive demands of wheelchair propulsion. Therefore, athletes must pay attention to early signs and symptoms of injury, such as pain or swelling, and treat the condition early and aggressively before it becomes chronic and interferes not only with sport participation but with activities of daily living. Wilson and Washington (1993) found that 97 percent of young athletes who use a wheelchair to participate incurred a sport injury. A wide variety of injuries were reported, ranging from soft tissue injuries such as blisters, wheelburns, abrasions, and bruising to overheating. The authors expressed concern that children may be more susceptible to certain types of injuries such as those involving the bone growth plates (epiphyses), articulating joints, and tendon apophyses during their growth and development phase. Physical development and growth spurt activity should be followed, and adjustments made to training schedules when appropriate.

Repetitive pinching of the tendons of the rotator cuff and subacromial bursa of the shoulder results in inflammation, pain, and weakness of these structures, a condition called *impingement syndrome*. Impingement syndrome is the most common cause of shoulder pain in wheelchair athletes. Predisposing factors include repetitive shoulder use, frequent overhead arm positioning, weight bearing through the arms, relative weakness of the muscles that pull the humeral head down and away from the rotator cuff tendons and bursa (shoulder adductors and rotators) compared to those muscles that pull the humeral head upward (shoulder abductors), tightness of the anterior shoulder (scapular protractor) muscles, and weakness of the posterior (scapular retractor) muscles (Burnham, May, Nelson, and Steadward 1993). Early treatment of shoulder problems in athletes using wheel-chairs includes adequate rest and recovery time, inflammation reduction, minimizing shoulder impingement positions, strengthening the musculature in the posterior shoulder complex such as scapular retractors, rotator cuff and shoulder adductor muscles, and stretching the anterior shoulder musculature (Burnham, Curtis, and Reid 1995). The posi-tive effect of this intervention to address the above postural changes and related muscular imbalance has been documented by one efficacy study (Curtis et al. 1999).

Numbness and tingling of the hands may signify nerve entrapment. One study found that 23 percent of wheelchair athletes pre-sented with symptoms and signs compatible with upper extremity peripheral nerve entrap-ment. When evaluated electrophysiologically, using nerve conduction studies, the prevalence of peripheral nerve entrapment of the upper extremities was 61 percent. Carpal tunnel syn-drome (entrapment of the median nerve at the wrist/hand) made up the majority of these cases. Less commonly, entrapment of the ulnar nerve at the hand (Guyon's canal) or elbow was identified (Burnham and Steadward 1994). Carpal tunnel syndrome typically pres-ents as numbness and tingling involving the thumb, index, and middle digits, often worse at night time or with repetitive hand activity. Hand pain and weakness can also occur. The repetitive pounding of the heel of the hand against the wheelchair push rim and frequent wrist extension positions are thought to be predisposing factors for its development. Additionally, repetitive compression over Guyon's canal, which lies between the hook of the hamate and pisiform bones of the hand, is thought to predispose athletes who use wheelchairs to ulnar nerve compression there. Ulnar nerve entrapment usually presents as numbess and tingling of the ring and small fingers. The use of hand protection, such as gloves with padding over the base of the palm, may minimize the risk of developing nerve entrapments of the hand.

Infrequent utilization of the sport medi-cine services postinjury has also been reported.

Athletes have been self-treating their injuries and not seeking professional assistance (Ferrara and Davis 1990). A Canadian study by a recall questionnaire profiled ninety athletes using wheelchairs. They found that 346 injuries were reported in eighteen different wheelchair sports with less than one-third of all athletes seeking professional medical assistance or care for their injuries (McCormack, Reid, Steadward, and Syrotuik 1991). Authors have speculated that possible reasons may include a loss of independence by seeking help, fear of being told to stop activities, previous nega-tive experiences during treatment, or a lack of familiarity on the part of the medical profes-sionals with the sport and/or disability (Burnham, Curtis, and Reid 1995). In a study by Matthews White (2001), athletes were self-treating the majority of their sport injuries by peer consultations and previous experience.

---

3 What might lead athletes with disabilities to continue training with an injury in spite of risk to health?

Athletes continued to participate in sport with chronic injuries and pain by avoiding actions or activities that created the pain. Perceived internal and external barriers deterred athletes in accessing and utilizing medical assistance.

---

4 How might chronic injuries acquired through sport impact on athletes in life after sport? What obligations does this imply for the institutions of sport?

Sport injuries have also been reported in athletes with visual impairment, cerebral palsy, or limb amputation. Typically involved in stand-up sports, lower extremity injuries were most frequently reported, with the knee, leg, and ankle the most common locations (Ferrara, Buckley, Messner, and Benedict 1992). One study found a disproportionately high number of back injuries among athletes with cerebral palsy (Burnham, Newell, and Steadward 1991). Baseline information on injury occurrence in amputees playing soccer was documented by

Kegel and Malchow (1994). This preliminary study showed that injuries were minor, sustained to the knee, ankle, face, and shoulder, similar to those reported for able-bodied soccer players. While the sport of soccer was identified as low-injury risk, more extensive injury documentation over a longer period is required to confirm these results.

WINTER SPORTS

Only a few articles have described sport injuries for athletes in winter disability activities. In a study by McCormick (1985a), sixty-eight skiers at a regional US skiing championship were surveyed. The results indicated that 70 percent of the skiers had never been injured while skiing. Of the 30 percent who reported injuries, the knee was the most commonly injured body part. An overall injury rate of two injuries per 1,000-skier days was calculated which was reported to be within the same range as that for skiers without disabilities. The data for skiers with disabilities, gathered from instructional programmes at multiple sites, suggested that the skier with a disability is at no greater risk of injury, in terms of actual incidence rate and severity, than skiers without disabilities (Laskowski and Murtaugh 1992). The authors concluded that the learning or noncompetitive skier with a disability is at less risk for serious injury and more likely to sustain only minor bruises. Major sports injuries, such as fractures or trauma leading to further permanent disability, were rare. McCormick (1985b) surveyed twenty-three sit-ski racers and calculated a rate of sixteen injuries per 1,000-skier days. This injury rate was eight times higher than the skier with a disability who did not use a sit-ski. Also, the sit-skier's type of disability appeared to be related to the likelihood of injury. Skiers with high-lesion spinal cord injuries (above thoracic level eight) incurred more injuries than those with low spinal cord injuries (below thoracic level eight).

An increase in injuries in skiers with spinal cord injuries above thoracic level six was also reported by Ferrara, Buckley, Messner, and Benedict (1992). They identified the training

and injury experiences of the competitive skier with a disability by surveying sixty-eight US national skiers. The number of chronic injuries reported was greater than the number of acute injuries to the shoulder, thigh/knee, arm/elbow, and neck/spine. Only 40 percent of those reporting an injury sought professional medical treatment, which was deemed unacceptable by these authors for this level of sport participation.

One study in the literature profiles the sledge hockey athlete (Matthews White 2001). This study examined the type and locations of injuries sustained by Canadian ice sledge hockey players. Injuries were sport-related, not disability-related, with injuries to the fingers, hand, shoulder, and spine caused by physical contact with other players, the boards, the puck, pic, or sledge, resulting in a moderate time loss to participation. It was recommended that protective equipment, including adequate material for hockey gloves to protect the hand and fingers from the blade of the sledge, be explored.

Management and Prevention of Sport Injuries

Despite the fact that sport epidemiology research has shown that a significant number of athletes do get injured during participation and their recovery and return to activity may be protracted when compared to able-bodied athletes, a minority of athletes with a disability seek professional medical care. Ideally, an aggressive, early intervention, multidisciplinary approach should be taken by the sport medicine team for the management and treatment of these injuries. The principles and practices that have been developed and used for sports and athletics in general are equally applicable to athletes involved in disability sports. This approach involves a thorough understanding of the athlete that includes his or her sport, sport equipment, sport-specific injuries, and the disability-related conditions.

5 What are the physiological demands of sport? How do they impact on athletes of different disabilities?

For example, the athlete's disability as well as the injury predisposition may dictate his or her position on the team, such as wheelchair basketball centres whose shooting and rebounding roles require repetitive overhead arm postures that require them to sit high in their chairs and possess excellent trunk balance. Accordingly, they have to be neuromuscularly intact above the knees. Often, athletes with lower limb amputations are best suited to play centre, whereas paraplegic athletes have to sit low in their chairs due to impaired trunk control and will often play the guard position, with primary responsibilities of bringing the ball up the court, passing, and setting screens. Research has documented a four times greater risk of shoulder injuries among wheelchair basketball centres—likely attributable to their frequent overhead arm (rotator cuff impingement) position (Burnham, Higgins, and Steadward 1994). Conversely, in winter sports very little information has been published.

---

6 Given what is known in wheelchair basketball, what sports injuries could be predicted in ice sledge hockey? What is unique about the athletes who play sledge hockey? What injuries would be expected?

How can a specific sport injury be prevented? To prevent sport injuries, the environment, sport equipment, and the disability need to be considered. This phase of sport medicine is just beginning to develop for disability sport. Prevention is specifically intended to assist athletes with disabilities to better perform their sport activity with a reduced risk of injury. There are a few studies on prevention implications that suggest methods for improvement (Bloomquist 1986; Curtis 1996; Ferrara, Buckley, McCann, et al. 1992; Laskowski 1994; Mangus 1987; Shephard 1988), but there is a need for more injury prevention programmes and research. Authors have recognized that several components of fitness were particular risk elements affecting the rate and severity of injury. Therefore, a prevention programme designed to reduce

the rate and severity of injury would need to address flexibility and weight training for athletes in disability sport. Documenting injuries and time away from participation will educate athletes and sport medicine researchers on the effectiveness of any injury prevention measures.

General Medical Conditions: A Disability-specific Perspective
The health care needs of athletes with disabilities pose unique sport medicine challenges due to their unique physiology, psychology, sports, and adaptive sport equipment. While many of the same sport-related injuries such as soft tissue injuries (sprains, muscular strains) and general medical conditions (colds, flu) arise in this population as in athletes without disabilities, the underlying impairment of the athlete with a disability is a further important concern. These athletes are vulnerable to specific medical conditions related to their disability. Such disability-specific conditions have been described in the literature (Curtis and Gailey 1996; Davis and Ferrara 1995; Hoeberigs, Debets-Eggen, and Debets 1990; Mangus 1987; Martinez 1989; Wilson, and Washington 1993) and some will be summarized in the following pages.

SPINAL CORD INJURY
The spinal cord is comprised of a series of nerve projections (axons) some of which extend down from the brain, giving messages to the body below it, and some project upward, taking messages from the limbs and torso back to the brain. Axons with similar functions are closely grouped together into spinal cord *tracts*. When the spinal cord is injured, some or all of the tracts are damaged at the level of injury and result in predictable impairments. Although traumatic spinal fracture or dislocation is the most common cause of spinal cord injury, disease processes such as multiple sclerosis, transverse myelitis, or spinal tumor may also result in similar spinal cord tract damage. Three tracts are particularly relevant when considering an athlete's physiologic response to exercise stress and

disability-specific medical conditions. Damage to the tracts that carry movement messages from the brain down to the skeletal muscles of the body (corticospinal tracts) result in paralysis below the level of spinal injury. Damage to the tracts that carry pain and temperature sensation (spinothalamic tracts) and touch, vibration, and position sense sensation (dorsal column tracts) result in loss of sensation below the level of the spinal cord lesion. The portion of the spinal cord housed within the thoracic spine (first through twelfth thoracic) also contains the cell bodies of the nerves that carry sympathetic nervous system output to the body (intermediolateral columns). Under normal circumstances, the sympathetic nervous system output is balanced by descending impulses from the base of the brain where the parasympathetic nervous system is largely housed. However, an injury at or above the sixth thoracic level (between the shoulder blades) disconnects the major portion of the sympathetic nervous system from the parasympathetic nervous system, resulting in partial autonomy of these two arms of the autonomic nervous system. This predisposes the quadriplegic or high-paraplegic athlete to certain disability specific medical conditions.

Hypothermia

Under normal circumstances, body temperature information is relayed to the body's thermostat in the brain (hypothalmus). If the core body temperature becomes too low, messages from the hypothalmus travel down the corticospinal tracts causing the skeletal muscles to contract rhythmically (shivering). The sympathetic nervous system cell bodies of the intermediolateral columns are also stimulated, resulting in constriction of the skin blood vessels, thus shunting blood from the periphery to the body's core. Both phenomena serve to increase core body temperature. With spinal cord injury, the tracts carrying messages for shivering and vasoconstriction are disrupted, rendering the spinal cord injured athlete susceptible to hypothermia. Additionally, the amount of skeletal muscle under voluntary

control is reduced. Spinal cord injured athletes can develop hypothermia when exercising in ambient temperatures as high as ten degrees Celsius. Preventative measures include wearing appropriate multilayered clothing, adequate hydration, and replacing wet clothing with dry after training or competition. The hypothermic athlete may appear clumsy, apathetic, or confused. More severe cases can lead to coma, cardiac, or respiratory failure. Treatment starts with anticipating the possibility of hypothermia and having the athlete make the diagnosis by recording core body temperature (tympanic or rectal). Triage includes replacing wet clothing with dry, covering the athlete with insulated blankets, and applying hot water bottles or heating pads (wrapped to avoid causing skin burns) adjacent to the hypothermic athlete. Severe cases require emergency transfer to a medical facility.

Hyperthermia

In neurologically intact individuals, the body's response to hyperthermia is to shunt blood from the core to the periphery by constriction of splanchnic circulation and dilatation of the skin circulation. Additionally, sweating is stimulated. All of these events are triggered through the sympathetic nervous system. With spinal cord injury, the tracts carrying the message from the thermostat in the brain to the sympathetic cell bodies are interrupted. Medications sometimes used for bladder, pain, or spasticity control in persons with spinal cord injury can also contribute to problems dissipating heat. Therefore, the spinal cord injured athlete who is exercising vigorously in a hot ambient environment is at increased risk of developing hyperthermia. Minimizing exposure to the heat, such as planning training and competition times during early morning or evening hours, adequate hydration, acclimatization, and using cooling towels or spraying water over the body surfaces, can help prevent hyperthermia. Athletes with hyperthermia may present with fatigue, weakness, lightheadedness, headache, muscle pains, nausea, vomiting, and, in severe cases, an altered state of consciousness.

Figure 27.1 Proposed Mechanism of Autonomic Dysreflexia

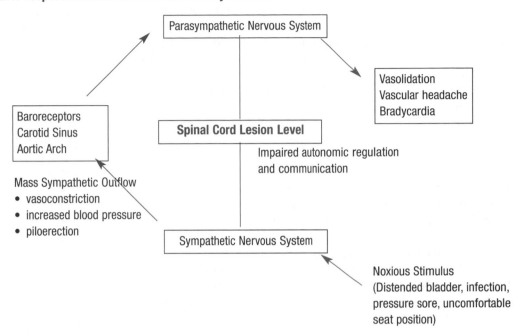

Measurement of core body temperature (tympanic or rectal) confirms the diagnosis. Triage includes removal of the athlete's clothing, external cooling, and fluid replacement. Oral fluids should not be given if the athlete's state of consciousness is impaired. Intravenous fluids and emergency transfer to a medical facility are warranted in such circumstances.

Autonomic Dysreflexia

This phenomenon consists of an exaggerated response to a mass sympathetic nervous system discharge induced by a pain source below the level of the spinal cord lesion (figure 27.1). Common pain sources include bladder over-distension, urinary infection, bowel or bladder obstruction, pressure sores, blood clots, unrecognized muscle or bone injury, and sunburn. Autonomic dysreflexia can have disastrous medical complications due to sudden extreme elevations of blood pressure and heart rhythm disturbances resulting in seizure, brain or eye haemorrhage, or even death. Any athlete who presents with signs of sweating, shivering or goose bumps (above the level of the spinal cord lesion), high blood pressure and slow heart rate, or symptoms of throbbing headache, blurred vision, or excessive anxiety should be suspected of having autonomic dysreflexia. Sometimes athletes try to induce this dysreflexic response intentionally for the adrenalin/noradrenalin rush ('boosting') for performance enhancement purposes during competition (Burnham et al. 1994). They commonly employ techniques such as bladder over-distention by high fluid intake or clamping the catheter, excessively tight leg straps, or skin electrical stimulation. These practices are dangerous and should be discouraged. If an athlete presents with signs or symptoms suggestive of autonomic dysreflexia, blood pressure and heart rate recordings should be made immediately. If the blood pressure is elevated (with or without bradycardia), the pain source triggering the sympathetic discharge must be identified and relieved (empty bladder, loosen restricting clothing or straps, check for skin problems in insensate areas, etc). If the blood pressure does not rapidly return to normal, emergency transfer of the athlete to a medical facility is warranted.

Pressure Sores

These occur most commonly over the ishial tuberocities and sacrum. The spinal cord injured athlete is predisposed to pressure sore development because skin sensation is impaired, muscle mass overlying areas of bony prominence is reduced, extended periods of time are spent sitting, and sport wheelchairs are often designed to have the knees higher than the buttocks which results in the increased buttock pressure. Athletes must pay attention to proper cushions, periodic weight shifts, limiting the duration of training sessions, and proper nutrition and should frequently inspect insensitive skin areas to detect pressure sores early. Anytime there is redness of the skin, the area should be kept clean and be relieved of weight until normal skin colour returns. It may be necessary to protect the area with Second Skin or Duoderm. Athletes with open pressure sores should not participate in competition or training until the area is completely healed.

Urinary Tract Infections

Normal bladder function depends on a well-coordinated interaction between sympathetic and parasympathetic messages to the bladder muscle and internal sphincter and voluntary brain messages to the external sphincter. With spinal cord injury, the tracts carrying these messages are disrupted, resulting in *neurogenic bladder*. Many athletes empty their bladders by intermittently catheterizing, sometimes dehydrating themselves to decrease the need for catheterization as often. Sometimes the bladder does not completely empty and renders the spinal cord injured athlete susceptible to developing urinary infection. Fever, chills, increased spasticity, or unusual incontinence suggest the diagnosis and urine culture confirms it. Antibiotic treatment is usually curative. Coaches and athletes need to be aware of the signs of urinary infection and ensure that athletes have access to adequate fluid intake and bathroom facilities.

Altered Exercise Response

Athletes with spinal cord injuries have a blunted cardiovascular response to exercise for several reasons. Their disrupted autonomic reflexes result in decreased sympathetic innervation to the heart which impairs cardiac output by reducing stroke volume and heart rate responses. Autonomic dysfunction also reduces the redistribution of blood flow to exercising muscle during exercise and of venous blood from the legs to the heart. Additionally, spinal cord injured athletes have a reduced mass of voluntary exercising muscles. As a result, maximum oxygen uptake rates for elite wheelchair athletes are approximately half of their able-bodied counterparts.

AMPUTATION

Stump problems are unique to athletes with amputation. Malfitting prostheses, soft tissue overuse injury, and skin irritations and infections are common. A prosthetist can be an invaluable member of the sport medicine team in these circumstances.

CEREBRAL PALSY AND TRAUMATIC BRAIN INJURY

Cerebral palsy and traumatic brain injury can be associated with seizure disorders. Having a precompetition medical history from each athlete helps alert the sport medicine team to the possibility of dealing with seizure. It is wise for the medical team to have a stock of antiseizure drugs, as it is not unusual for athletes to forget their medications before competitions. Although seizures rarely occur during sport competition because the state of metabolic acidosis associated with high-intensity exercise stabilizes nerve membranes, seizures are more typically seen during travel and other times of stress, dehydration, and temperature extremes. If a seizure occurs, protecting the head, airway, and rest of the body during the fit is important. Following the seizure, the sport medicine team physician should review the athlete's neurologic status regularly to insure there has been no sustained deterioration. Hospitalization is usually unnecessary unless there is neurologic deterioration or the seizure activity is new or different than that typically experienced by the athlete.

Future Research Directions

Sport epidemiology and interventional research in the area of disability sport medicine has contributed greatly to our present knowledge. However, this population of athletes is challenging to study. The number of potential study subjects is small. Classification systems, created to ensure equitable competition, further fragment the number of subjects. It may seem unrealistic to profile injuries and injury risks for a group of athletes who participate in downhill skiing under twelve different disability classifications. Additionally, quantitative research assumes homogeneity, yet disability is heterogeneous. There is not only heterogeneity between athletes with the same diagnosis or functional classification, but heterogeneity *within* the individual athlete. An individual athlete can experience rapid fluctuations in physiological parameters often measured in quantitative sport medicine research. For example, an athlete with multiple sclerosis can experience extreme generalized fatigue and weakness with even slight elevations in core body temperature. By definition, athletes with exacerbating-remitting forms of multiple sclerosis will have variations in the severity and location of physical impairment, depending on disease activity. Athletes with high spinal cord injury can experience autonomic dysreflexia within seconds of a painful stimulus below their spinal cord lesion level that can profoundly affect heart rate, blood pressure, and sport performance (Burnham et al. 1994). Quantitative research has continued to contribute greatly to advances in medical science, but other research models such as case studies, single-subject designs, and qualitative research may have continuing relevance.

Summary

A historical review of the interaction of athletes with disabilities with medical professionals and physical educators reveals a pattern of progressive inclusion and acceptance.

Individuals with a disability have continually tried to enter the highly visible arena of sport, as athletes. Though decreasing, barriers to full and unrestricted sport participation for persons with a disability still exist. Some medical professionals with whom persons with a disability have a significant amount of contact maintain a medical model perspective and do not recommend sport or fitness opportunities. Some possible reasons include lack of awareness of the opportunities available, lack of understanding of the sport or the person's capabilities, or overprotectiveness.

The development and design of new adapted sport equipment, improved and accessible facilities, coupled with the growth of recreation and sport organizations for athletes with disabilities have supported and encouraged an increase in participation. Consequently, sports medicine now faces a number of challenging problems and issues. Some include a shortage of qualified sport-oriented medical specialists; educating the athletes on the importance of proper injury management; lack of qualified coaches, training guidelines, protective equipment; and evidence-based research on sport injuries prevention and treatment. As sport medicine evolves, the roles and responsibilities of the medical professionals will also change to concentrate their efforts to enhance healthy athletic performance by:

a. providing expertise and counsel in the area of sports science and medical matters
b. providing expertise and recommendations in matters of doping control
c. bringing issues from the sports science and medical area of operations to committees, administrators, and researchers (International Paralympic Committee Task Force Report 1996)

Yet, many countries continue to have a disability or rehabilitative approach to sport excellence with the medical professions controlling the rules and regulations of athlete participation.

The intention of this review is to encourage students and practitioners in the health care disciplines and disability sports organizations to consider both medical and situational factors in assessing the impact of disability in sport at recreational, competitive, and elite levels. It is the intent of these authors to address issues confronting athletes in disability sport and to help students and researchers appreciate the breadth and scope of the sports health care required by these athletes.

SUMMARY OF SPORTS MEDICINE RESEARCH

- Sport specific injuries include lower extremity musculotendinous strains or stress fractures in running athletes and hand or shoulder injuries in wheelchair athletes.
- The most common injuries sustained by wheelchair athletes involve the hands; however, the most serious in terms of time lost from activity and medical care required involve the shoulders.
- Common hand injuries include jammed or sprained digits, skin abrasions, and nerve entrapment, the most common of which is carpal tunnel syndrome.
- Carpal tunnel syndrome needs to be detected and treated early in this group of athletes to prevent additional disability. It usually presents with nocturnal hand numbness and pain and occasionally hand weakness.
- The most common shoulder condition among wheelchair athletes is rotator cuff impingement syndrome. Predisposing factors for rotator cuff impingement syndrome include overuse, recurrent placement of the shoulder into rotator cuff impingement positions (overhead and upper extremity weight bearing), strength imbalance (scapular retractor, shoulder rotator and adductor weakness in relation to the deltoid muscle), and rounded shoulder posture with tight anterior shoulder muscles.
- Injury locations are sport-dependent and disability-dependent.
- Injury prevention requires training guidelines, expert coaching, technological advances, and equipment rules.

- Medical conditions are disability-specific, (examples include problems with thermo-regulation, pressure sores, autonomic dysreflexia, urinary tract infections, seizures, and stumps).

Study Questions

1. Which one of the following is not a contributing factor in the development of shoulder rotator cuff impingement syndrome in athletes using wheelchairs?
   a) overuse
   b) inadequate deltoid strength
   c) frequent overhead arm position and weight-bearing transfers
   d) rounded shoulder posture due to tight anterior shoulder structures

2. You are supervising an athlete with quadriplegia while he works out on an arm-crank ergometer. You notice his face is flushed, he has goosebumps on his arms and legs, and he complains of a throbbing headache and blurred vision. You should:
   a) reduce the ergometer resistance
   b) allow him to warm up in a blanket
   c) get him something to drink in order to rehydrate
   d) check his blood pressure and pulse

3. The athlete who uses a wheelchair and has carpal tunnel syndrome:
   a) usually complains of hand numbness at night-time
   b) should tape his index and middle fingers together when wheeling
   c) has pinching of the ulnar nerve at the wrist
   d) needs an operation urgently

1.b; 2.d; 3.a

Give an example of each of the following conditions you would likely see while training a multidisability group of athletes:

General medical condition:

Disability-specific medical condition:

Sport-specific injury:

References

Arnheim D, and Prentice W. (2000). *Principles of Athletic Training* (10th ed.). St. Louis, MO: C.V. Mosby.

Bloomquist, L.E. (1986). Injuries to athletes with physical disabilities: Prevention implications. *Physician and Sports Medicine, 14,* 97–105.

Burnham R., Curtis K., and Reid D. (1995). Shoulder problems in the wheelchair athlete. In F.A. Pettrone (Ed.), *Athletic injuries of the shoulder.* New York: McGraw-Hill.

Burnham R., Higgins J., and Steadward R. (1994). Wheelchair basketball injuries. *Palaestra,* Winter, 43–49.

Burnham R., May L., Nelson E., and Steadward R. (1993). Shoulder pain in wheelchair athletes: The role of muscle imbalance. *American Journal of Sports Medicine, 21*(2), 238–42.

Burnham R., Newell E., and Steadward R. (1991). Sports medicine for the physically disabled: The Canadian team experience at the 1988 Seoul Paralympic Games. *Clinical Journal of Sport Medicine, 1,* 193–96.

Burnham R., and Steadward R. (1994). Upper extremity peripheral nerve entrapments among wheelchair athletes: Prevalence, location and risk factors. *Archives of Physical Medicine and Rehabilitation, 75,* 519–24.

Burnham R., Wheeler G., Bhambhani Y., Belanger M., Eriksson P., and Steadward R. (1994). Intentional induction of autonomic dysreflexia among quadriplegic athletes for performance enhancement. *Clinical Journal of Sports Medicine, 4,* 1–10.

Curtis, K.A. (1981). Wheelchair sports medicine: Part 4: Athletic injuries. *Sports 'n Spokes,* January/February, 20–24.

Curtis, K.A. (1996). Health smarts: Strategies and solutions for wheelchair athletes. *Sports 'n Spokes,* January/February, 25–31; March/April, 13–19; May/June, 21–28.

Curtis, K.A., Black, K. (1999). Shoulder pain in female wheelchair basketball players. *Journal of Orthopaedic and Sports Physical Therapy, 29*(4), 225–31.

Curtis, K.A., and Dillon, D.A. (1985). Survey of wheelchair athletic injuries: Common patterns and prevention. *Paraplegia, 23,* 170–75.

Curtis, K.A, and Gailey, R.S. (1996). The athlete with a disability. In James E. Zachazewski, David J. Magee, and William S. Quillen (Eds.), *Athletic injuries and rehabilitation.* Philadelphia: W.B. Saunders.

Curtis, K.A, Tyner, T.M., Zachary, L., Lentell, G., Brink, D., Didyk, T., Gean, K., Hall, J., Hooper, M., Klos, J., Lesina, S., and Pacillas, B. (1999). Effect of a standard exercise protocol on shoulder pain in long-term wheelchair users. *Spinal Cord, 37,* 421–29.

Davis, R., and Ferrara, M. (1995). Sports medicine and athletes with disabilities. In K. Depauw and Gavron, S. (Eds.), *Sport and Disability.* Champaign, IL: Human Kinetics.

Ferrara, M.S., and Buckley, W.E. (1996). Athletes with disabilities injury registry. *Adapted Physical Activity Quarterly, 13*(1), 50–60.

Ferrara, M.S., and Buckley, W.E., McCann, B.C., Limbird, T.J., Powell, J.W., Robl, R. (1992). The injury experience of the competitive athlete with a disability: Prevention implications. *Medicine and Science in Sports and Exercise, 24*(2), 184–88.

Ferrara, M.S., and Buckley, W.E., Messner, D.G., Benedict, J. (1992). The injury experience and training history of the competitive skier with a disability. *The American Journal of Sports Medicine, 20*(1), 55–60.

Ferrara, M.S., and Davis R. (1990). Injuries to elite wheelchair athletes. *Paraplegia, 28,* 335–41.

Ferrara, M.S., Palutsis, G.R., Snouse, S., Davis, R.W. (2000). A longitudinal study of injuries to athletes with disabilities. *International Journal of Sports Medicine, 21,* 221–24.

Ferrara, M.S., and Peterson, C.L. (2000). Injuries to athletes with disabilities. *Sports Medicine, 30*(2), 137–43.

Guttmann, Sir L. (1976). *Textbook of sport for the disabled.* Aylesbury, UK: HM+M Publishers.

Hoeberigs, J.H., Debets-Eggen, H.B., Debets, P.M. (1990). Sports medical experiences from the International Flower Marathon for disabled wheelers. *The American Journal of Sports Medicine, 18*(4), 418–21.

International Paralympic Committee. (1996, August 16). *International Paralympic Committee Task Force report: Partnership and unity towards the twenty-first century.* Atlanta: Author.

Kegel, B., and Malchow, D. (1994). Incidence of injury in amputees playing soccer. *Palaestra,* Winter, 50–54.

Laskowski, E.R. (1994). Rehabilitation of the physically challenged athlete. *Sports Medicine, 5*(1), 215–32.

Laskowski, E.R., and Murtaugh, P.A. (1992). Snow skiing injuries in physically disabled skiers. *The American Journal of Sports Medicine, 20*(5), 553–57.

Mangus B. (1987). Sports injuries, the disabled athlete, and the athletic trainer. *Athletic Training, 22*(4), 305–10.

Martinez, S. (1989). Medical concerns among wheelchair road racers. *The Physician and Sports Medicine, 17*(2), 63–66.

Matthews White, J.M. (2001). *Sport medical care for athletes with disabilities.* Unpublished doctoral dissertation, University of Alberta, Edmonton.

McCormack, D.A., Reid, D.C., Steadward, R.D., and Syrotuik, D.G. (1991). Injury profiles in wheelchair athletes: Results of a retrospective survey. *Clinical Journal of Sport Medicine, 1,* 35–40.

McCormick, D. (1985a). Injuries in handicapped alpine ski racers. *The Physician and Sports Medicine, 13*(12), 93–97.

McCormick, D. (1985b). Skiing injuries among sit-skiers. *Sports 'n Spokes,* March/April, 20–21.

Noreau, L., and Shephard, R. (1995). Spinal cord injury, exercise and quality of life. *Sports Medicine, 20*(4), 226–50.

Shephard, R.J. (1988). Sports medicine and the wheelchair athlete. *Sports Medicine, 4,* 226–47.

Shephard, R.J. (1990). *Fitness in special populations.* Champaign, IL: Human Kinetics.

Van Mechelen, W., Hlobil, H., and Kemper, H. (1992). Incidence, severity, aetiology and prevention of sports injuries: A review of concepts. *Sports Medicine, 14,* 82–9.

Wheeler, R.H., and Hooley, A.M. (1969). *Physical education for the handicapped.* Philadelphia: Lea and Febiger.

Wilson, P.E., and Washington, R.L. (1993). Pediatric wheelchair athletics: Sports injuries and prevention. *Paraplegia, 31,* 330–37.

CHAPTER 28

Principles of Fitness Assessment and Training for Wheelchair Athletes

Yagesh Bhambhani

Learning Objectives

- To provide the adapted physical activity professional with an overview of metabolic and cardiorespiratory responses pertinent to wheelchair racing in athletes with a disability.
- To learn methods of assessing anaerobic and aerobic fitness in wheelchair athletes.
- To understand the relationship between wheelchair racing performance and measures of anaerobic and aerobic fitness.
- To learn how to design physical training programmes for wheelchair athletes with a disability.
- To learn about the adaptations resulting from anaerobic and aerobic fitness training in wheelchair athletes with a disability.
- To review pertinent research studies on athletes with spinal cord injury and cerebral palsy so that a firm foundation for the development of athletes with disabilities can be established.

Competitive Sport for Individuals With Disabilities

Competitive sport for individuals with disabilities has experienced an unprecedented growth since the First International Wheelchair Games were held in Aylesbury, England, in 1948. During the XI Paralympic Games in Sydney, Australia, in 2000, more than three thousand athletes with a variety of disabilities competed in eighteen individual and team events (International Paralympic Committee 2000a). Wheelchair athletics, particularly wheelchair racing, was most frequently participated in among the individual sports. In international competitions, athletes with different disabilities (e.g., spinal cord injury, cerebral palsy) are classified according to their individual functional capabilities so that they can compete on an equitable basis. This implies that athletes with similar capabilities and not necessarily similar medical disabilities can compete in the same class for a given event (International Paralympic Committee 2000b; Jones 1988; Shephard 1990).

From a physiological perspective, there are some unique differences between athletes with spinal cord injury and cerebral palsy that could affect their competitive performance. It is important, therefore, that physical training programmes designed to improve the fitness of athletes with disabilities be developed on the basis of sound physiological principles specific to the disability (Chow and Mindock 1999). Unfortunately, this area of research has not kept pace with the unprecedented growth in Paralympic sport during the last five decades. An international study (Liow and Hopkins 1996) that examined the training practices of competitive athletes with disabilities (wheelchair racers, swimmers and throwers) indicated that one third of the athletes did not have a coach. Comparisons between the subgroups indicated that most of the swimmers were coached regularly, while the racers and throwers received minimal coaching.

Many professionals who work with athletes with disabilities develop their training programmes on the basis of principles that are derived on able-bodied individuals. The validity of some of these training techniques for athletes with disabilities can be questioned because of the unique physiological changes that occur in some of the disabilities (e.g., spinal cord injury). It is important, therefore, that a specific body of knowledge pertaining to disability sport training be developed so that these athletes continue to improve their performance.

Energy Systems Specific to Wheelchair Racing Performance

Wheelchair races for persons with disabilities range from short sprints, such as the 100-metre dash, to the traditional marathon. The energy requirements for such races will vary depending upon the intensity and duration of the performance. It is generally accepted that the chemical energy for muscular work is derived from three main sources: *(a) immediate, (b) short-term,* and *(c) long-term* (Astrand and Rodahl 1986; McArdle, Katch and Katch 1996).

The *immediate* source of energy is stored in the muscle in the form of adenosine triphosphate (ATP) and creatine phosphate (CP). This energy is available for rapid use in the muscle and is considered to be anaerobic in nature because it does not require the utilization of oxygen. It is also referred to as the *alactacid energy source* because it does not result in the formation of lactic acid, which is the end product of anaerobic metabolism via the glycolytic pathway. The amount of energy available from this source is very limited and is usually sufficient for approximately ten to fifteen seconds of high-intensity work in the able-bodied individual. Because ATP is located in close proximity to the contractile elements (myofibrils), the energy is available almost instantly for muscle contraction.

The *short-term* energy source is utilized during high-intensity muscular work when the immediate source of energy is in short supply or depleted. Energy is metabolized in the exercising muscle from a carbohydrate store, primarily intramuscular glycogen (a glucose polymer), without the utilization of oxygen. This metabolic pathway, which is referred to as *anaerobic glycolysis*, also results in a limited amount of energy for muscular work, but the overall capacity exceeds that available from the immediate energy source. Energy is derived under these conditions from a series of chemical reactions that result in the production of lactic acid in the muscle. This metabolite, when present at high concentrations, has been associated with muscular fatigue under aerobic and anaerobic conditions (Wenger and Reed 1973). The accumulation of lactate in the blood is usually used as a biological marker for anaerobic metabolism.

The *long-term* energy sources are utilized during continuous submaximal exercise that lasts from several minutes to hours. Under these conditions, energy is derived primarily from the breakdown of carbohydrates and fats with the utilization of oxygen; hence the term *aerobic metabolism*. The carbohydrates metabolized include intramuscular glycogen and blood glucose, while the fats metabolized include intramuscular fat, as well as free fatty acids that are derived from the breakdown of subcutaneous fat. Proteins contribute only

3 to 5 percent of the total energy requirement during prolonged work. Under fully aerobic conditions, (i.e., when oxygen supply by the perfusing blood is sufficient to meet the demands of the exercising muscle), large quantities of ATP are produced in the mitochondria so that the muscle can continue working for a prolonged duration. End products of aerobic metabolism include carbon dioxide, a gaseous substance that is released in the expired air, and water, which facilitates cooling of the body during prolonged work.

Several important points pertaining to energy metabolism must be noted. Firstly, these energy sources form a continuum (i.e., there is no definite line of demarcation between the immediate, short- and long-term energy sources). This implies that the energy to perform a given task is not derived entirely from one source but is dependent upon a combination of these sources. Secondly, the relative contribution of the anaerobic and aerobic sources is dependent upon the intensity and duration of the exercise bout. Short-term, high-intensity exercise will be dependent primarily upon the anaerobic (immediate and short-term) energy sources. In contrast, prolonged submaximal exercise will rely primarily upon aerobic sources of energy production. From a practical point of view, a 100-metre wheelchair race, which usually lasts between fifteen to twenty seconds, is dependent primarily upon the immediate source of energy with a limited contribution from the short-term source. Races of longer durations, such as the 200- to 400-metre events, which usually last between thirty seconds to ninety seconds, are dependent upon both the immediate and short-term energy sources. Generally, the contribution from the short-term source increases with the duration of the race. It is generally accepted that the energy requirements of high-intensity physical work that lasts approximately two minutes are derived equally from anaerobic and aerobic sources of energy production (Astrand and Rodahl 1986). Wheelchair races ranging from the 1500 metres to the marathon (time duration ranging from approximately five minutes to two hours,

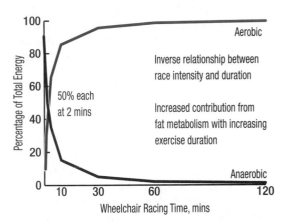

Figure 28.1 Theoretical Relationship Between Wheelchair Racing Time and Energy Utilization

fifteen minutes) are dependent primarily upon aerobic sources of energy production. Usually, as the duration of the race increases, the proportion of energy derived from free fatty acids also increases, with a proportional decrease in the contribution from carbohydrates. The theoretical relationship between wheelchair racing time and energy utilization is illustrated in figure 28.1.

There is limited research that has examined substrate utilization during prolonged exercise in wheelchair athletes with spinal cord injury under simulated conditions in the laboratory. The evidence (Skrinar et al. 1982) indicates that during forty to sixty minutes of submaximal wheelchair exercise at approximately 60 to 70 percent of peak aerobic power, the primary substrates utilized are intramuscular glycogen (based on depletion levels in the deltoid), blood glucose, free fatty acids, and glycerol. The proportion of free fatty acids and glycerol utilized increases with the exercise duration and is accompanied by a moderate decrease in blood glucose metabolism (Gass and Camp 1987; Hooker and Wells 1990; Skrinar et al. 1982). However, some evidence suggests that blood glucose is not utilized during prolonged exercise at these intensities (Campbell, Williams, and Lakomy 1997). The increased contribution of fat relative to carbohydrate is indirectly evident as a decrease in the respiratory exchange ratio

(ratio between carbon dioxide production and oxygen consumption) which is monitored non-invasively during exercise. The concentration of blood lactate increases significantly during the early stages of exercise and tends to decline towards the latter stages of the exercise bout (Campbell et al. 1997; Gass and Camp 1987; Hooker and Wells 1990). This is most likely due to an increase in lactate utilization by other tissues such as the heart and liver during exercise. Individuals with paraplegia accumulate a significantly higher concentration of blood lactate than those with quadriplegia during a simulated wheelchair race, implying that that the degree of anaerobic metabolism is greater in the former group. This is despite the fact that individuals with paraplegia sustain a higher relative intensity (i.e., a higher percentage of the peak oxygen uptake) during the race than those with quadriplegia (Bhambhani et al. 1994). In general, these observations in individuals with spinal cord injury suggest that the overall pattern of substrate utilization during prolonged exercise is consistent with that observed in able-bodied subjects.

---

1 Will carbohydrate loading improve wheelchair distance racing performance in wheelchair athletes?

Muscle Fibre Types and Their Relationship to Sports Performance

In human skeletal muscle, the motor units (functional part of the skeletal muscle which results in movement) are classified into two broad categories according to their morphologic (physical), contractile, and metabolic characteristics (Komi 1986; McComas 1996). The slow twitch, or Type I, motor units have a smaller axon than the Type II, or fast twitch motor units. As a result, the slow twitch motor units have a slower contractile speed than the fast twitch motor units. Because of their smaller innervation ratio, (i.e., the number of muscle fibres that are innervated by the anterior motor neuron) the slow twitch motor units develop a lower muscular force than the fast

twitch units. Metabolically, the slow twitch motor units have a considerably higher aerobic capacity, compared to the fast twitch motor units, but a lower anaerobic potential. Their higher aerobic potential is due to several reasons including: greater mitochondrial densities within the muscle cell (i.e., greater size and number of mitochondria), enhanced activities of the enzymes involved in aerobic metabolism, and larger capillary density ratios. Because of these differences in the metabolic and contractile characteristics, the slow twitch motor units have a greater endurance capacity (fatigue resistant) while the fast twitch motor units have a limited capacity for prolonged work (fast fatiguing).

The Type II motor units can be subdivided into two subgroups, namely, Type IIa and Type IIb. Based on their contractile and metabolic characteristics, the Type IIa motor units have properties that are between those of the Type I and Type IIb units; i.e., they are considered to be the intermediate fibres with a moderate contractile speed and moderate aerobic and anaerobic capacities. In general, the Type I motor units are described as slow oxidative, while the Type IIa and IIb are referred to as the fast oxidative glycolytic and fast glycolytic units, respectively.

It is well documented that able-bodied subjects who succeed in endurance (aerobic) events have a large proportion of Type I motor units in the exercising muscle, whereas those who excel in sprint or power events (anaerobic) have a high percentage of Type II motor units. While this characteristic can be attributed to the type of training that these subjects undertake, it is likely that their genetic predisposition is also more suited to these sporting events (Komi 1986). In humans, the upper extremity muscles have a greater proportion of fast twitch motor units than the lower extremity muscles (Johnson et al. 1973). According to published reports, the quadriceps muscle group has an equal distribution of the Type I and Type II motor units, whereas the biceps brachii and triceps brachii have approximately 40 percent slow twitch and 60 percent fast twitch motor units (McComas

1996). From a functional standpoint, this implies that the upper extremities that are involved in wheelchair propulsion may be more suited for anaerobic rather than aerobic events. Despite this, the world record time for completing a wheelchair marathon race is comparable to that of an able-bodied athlete running a marathon.

Individuals with spinal cord injury have a preponderance of Type IIb motor units in the paralyzed limbs with a concomitant reduction in the Type I motor units (Grimby et al. 1976; Martin et al. 1992; Mohr et al. 1997). In sedentary individuals with quadriplegia, this alteration is evident in the muscles of the lower extremities (vastus lateralis) and the upper extremities (deltoid) (Grimby et al. 1976). This shift in the motor unit characteristics is due to the lack or reduction of neurological stimuli to the paralyzed muscle as well as the sedentary lifestyle as a result of the injury. The overall effect is that the aerobic capacity of such individuals is compromised and they have a limited ability to participate in distance events that are dependent upon long-term sources of energy. Evidence from wheelchair athletes with paraplegia (Taylor et al. 1979) indicates a fairly large variation in the motor unit characteristics in the triceps muscle. The fibre areas of the slow and fast twitch motor units ranged from large to very large and, in some cases, exceeded those observed in able-bodied Olympic athletes. However, the metabolic characteristics of these motor units demonstrated average or below average activities of selected anaerobic and aerobic enzymes. The researchers suggested that, although wheelchair exercise was sufficient to induce hypertrophy of the triceps muscle, the intensity of training was not sufficient to alter their metabolic characteristics and influence energy utilization from the short-term and long-term energy sources. The relationship between motor unit characteristics and wheelchair racing performance was not evaluated in any of these studies.

Muscle glycogen depletion studies in able-bodied subjects have demonstrated that motor unit recruitment during exercise is based on the size principle. The Type I motor units have smaller axons and are recruited primarily during low intensity, long duration efforts, whereas the Type II units that have larger axons are activated during high-intensity, short duration efforts (Komi 1986; McComas 1996). These differences in recruitment patterns seem to be due to differences in the activation threshold between the two types of motor units. Based on these observations, it is likely that during short wheelchair races, such as the 100- and 200-metre sprints, the Type IIb motor units will be primarily recruited because they have a fast contractile speed and high glycolytic capacity. A limited number of Type I and Type IIa motor units may also be recruited, depending upon the demands of the exercise bout. The energy for these events will be derived mainly from the immediate and short-term sources, which have a limited capacity, and therefore the intensity of performance will be reduced as the race duration increases. In contrast, during long-distance events, such as the wheelchair marathon, the slow twitch motor units (Type I) will be initially recruited because of the lower intensity at which the race is performed. Since these motor units have a high aerobic potential, energy will be metabolized primarily from the aerobic pathways. However, as the race progresses, these motor units will become fatigued and a greater proportion of the fast twitch units (Type IIa followed by Type IIb) will be recruited. If the athlete increases the velocity towards the end of the race, it is likely that a greater number of Type IIb units will be recruited during this period. Research on wheelchair athletes with spinal cord injury (Skrinar et al. 1982) suggests that during 30 minutes of submaximal wheelchair exercise at 40 to 60 percent of peak aerobic power, the slow oxidative motor units in the deltoid muscle are selectively recruited. This observation is consistent with the trend described in able-bodied subjects. However, more research on motor unit recruitment patterns during different intensities and durations of wheelchair races is required to increase our understanding of this area.

Figure 28.2 Profile of the Wingate Anaerobic Test in an Athlete with Spinal Cord Injury

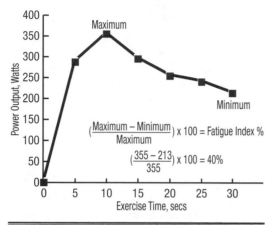

$$\left(\frac{Maximum - Minimum}{Maximum}\right) \times 100 = \text{Fatigue Index \%}$$

$$\left(\frac{355 - 213}{355}\right) \times 100 = 40\%$$

Figure 28.3 Influence of Lesion Level on Wingate Anaerobic Test Performance

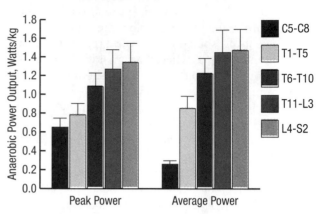

2 Identify the energy sources and motor unit recruitment patterns during a wheelchair race lasting two minutes.

Anaerobic and Aerobic Fitness in Wheelchair Athletes

ANAEROBIC POWER AND CAPACITY

Anaerobic *power* is defined as the maximum amount of power that can be generated using anaerobic (immediate and short-term) sources of energy production. Anaerobic *capacity* is defined as the average power that can be developed over a given period of time using the anaerobic energy sources (Bar-Or 1987; Maud and Foster 1995). While there are several tests that can measure these parameters in able-bodied individuals, the one most commonly used is the Wingate Anaerobic Test that was developed in Israel in the mid-1970s (Bar-Or 1987). This thirty-second test is performed on either a leg cycle or an arm-crank ergometer using a resistance that is proportional to the individual's body weight (usually 75 gm/kg body mass for men, 65 g/kg body mass for women during cycle exercise; 50 gm/kg body mass for men, 45 g/kg body mass for women during arm cranking). The objective is to complete as many revolutions as possible during the thirty-second interval. The maximum power developed over a five-second interval (usually the first five seconds)

is a measure of the anaerobic power, while the average power generated over the entire thirty seconds is considered to be an index of anaerobic capacity. The fatigue index is calculated in the following manner: (maximum power – minimum power)/maximum power. During the first few seconds of the Wingate test, energy is derived primarily from the immediate (alactacid) energy source. However, the energy for the latter portion is derived from the short-term source via anaerobic glycolysis, which results in a considerable degree of lactate production. The concentration of lactate can be measured in the blood using a finger prick, or venous sample, obtained within one to two minutes after the test. Studies on able-bodied athletes have demonstrated a strong relationship between Wingate test results and performance in sprint and power events that are dependent primarily upon anaerobic metabolism.

The Wingate test has been used to assess anaerobic power and capacity of individuals with a variety of disabilities. For nonambulatory individuals, such as those with spinal cord injury, the arm-cranking test is used for this measurement (Hutzler 1993). Researchers have also developed wheelchair ergometers that can quantify the power output using the Wingate protocol (Coutts and Stogryn 1987; Janssen et al. 1993; van der Woude et al. 1998; Veeger et al. 1991b). Currently there is no

Figure 28.4 Peak Anaerobic Power (Panel A) and Fatigue Index (Panel B) in Leisure and Competitive Athletes with Spinal Cord Injury

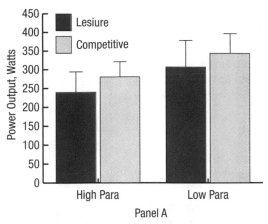

Panel A

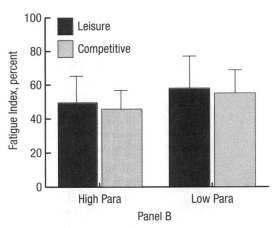

Panel B

standardized method for determining the resistance for the Wingate test protocol in individuals with spinal cord injury. The resistance applied is considerably lower than that used for able-bodied individuals because of the reduced muscle mass resulting from paralysis. The load setting for wheelchair users performing the Wingate test should be based upon the functionality, training status, and gender of the subjects (van der Woude et al 1998). A typical profile of the Wingate test in an athlete with spinal cord injury is provided in figure 28.2.

The test-retest reliability of the thirty-second Wingate wheelchair test in wheelchair athletes has been well established. In competitive wheelchair racers with paraplegia, the peak power, mean power, and maximum velocity demonstrated a high degree of stability over a five-week interval (Lees and Arthur 1988). Significant reliability coefficients have been reported for the peak power, mean power, peak velocity, mean velocity, and peak velocity fatigue index in older competitive male and female wheelchair basketball players (Hutzler, Vanlandewijck, and Vlieberghe 2000). Nonsignificant correlation coefficients were observed for the mean power and fatigue index of the peak power in these athletes. No significant differences were observed between the means of the two trials for each of these variables, except the mean velocity which was significantly higher in trial two and the

peak velocity fatigue index which was significantly lower in trial two. In general, the athletes performed better on the second test, which was most likely due to a learning effect from the first test. The researchers recommended that future Wingate anaerobic power studies include a complete habituation session prior to administration of the actual test.

In individuals with spinal cord injury, the peak anaerobic power and anaerobic capacity is inversely related to the level of lesion (Janssen et al. 1993; Veeger et al. 1991c). This implies that the lower the injury level the greater the anaerobic fitness, as indicated in figure 28.3. An athlete with low-level paraplegia (lesion levels between L4 and S3) can generate peak anaerobic power that is three to four times that of an athlete with quadriplegia (lesion level above C6) (Hutzler 1998; Hutzler et al. 1998; van der Woude et al. 1997; van der Woude et al. 1998). Significant differences between leisure and competitive athletes with high- and low-level paraplegia have been reported for the peak power and fatigue index during the Wingate test, as illustrated in figures 28.4A and 28.4B, respectively (Hutzler et al. 1998). Some evidence suggests that there is no significant difference between able-bodied subjects and those with low-level paraplegia (lesion at T8 or lower) for the absolute or relative values of anaerobic power during the Wingate test. However, the application of torque during wheelchair

Figure 28.5 Central and Peripheral Factors Influencing the Peak Aerobic Power in Subjects with Spinal Cord Injury

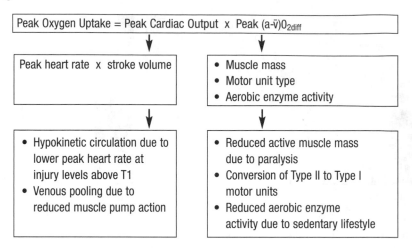

Peak Oxygen Uptake = Peak Cardiac Output x Peak $(a-\bar{v})O_{2diff}$

Peak heart rate x stroke volume

- Muscle mass
- Motor unit type
- Aerobic enzyme activity

- Hypokinetic circulation due to lower peak heart rate at injury levels above T1
- Venous pooling due to reduced muscle pump action

- Reduced active muscle mass due to paralysis
- Conversion of Type II to Type I motor units
- Reduced aerobic enzyme activity due to sedentary lifestyle

propulsion seems to be more effective in wheelchair dependent subjects than could be attributed to their specific training (Veeger et al. 1991c). Gender comparisons (Hutzler et al. 2000; Veeger et al. 1991c) indicate that (i) the absolute and relative values of the peak power, mean power, and mean velocity are significantly higher in male compared to female wheelchair athletes; (ii) the velocity fatigue index is significantly higher in females compared to males, suggesting a greater decline in force output during the test in females; and (iii) there is no significant correlation between peak power and body mass in either gender, suggesting that functional muscle mass plays a more important role in this assessment.

MAXIMAL AEROBIC POWER

The maximal aerobic power ($\dot{V}O_{2max}$) is defined as the maximum amount of oxygen that can be utilized per unit time. It is usually expressed as an absolute value in L/min or relative to body weight as ml/kg/min (Astrand and Rodahl 1986; McArdle, Katch, and Katch 1996). The $\dot{V}O_{2max}$ is dependent upon the overall ability to transport, deliver, and utilize oxygen and, therefore, is considered to be the best measure of maximal cardiorespiratory fitness. The $\dot{V}O_{2max}$ is calculated by the product of the maximal values of the cardiac output (central factor) and the mixed arterio-venous oxygen difference (peripheral factor), as depicted in figure 28.5. The maximal cardiac output is determined by the product of the maximal values of heart rate and stroke volume during exercise.

In able-bodied subjects, the $\dot{V}O_{2max}$ is normally assessed using a continuous incremental test protocol to voluntary fatigue on a cycle ergometer or treadmill. These exercise modes are selected because they utilize a large muscle mass and, therefore, it is possible to tax the cardiovascular system fully and attain true maximal values. During the test, the subject is connected to a computerized metabolic measurement cart which records the following key variables: oxygen uptake, carbon dioxide production, respiratory exchange ratio (ratio between carbon dioxide production and oxygen consumption), and ventilation rate. Heart rate is continuously monitored using an electrocardiogram, or wireless monitor, strapped to the chest. If the age-predicted maximum heart rate (220 – age in years) is attained towards the end of the test, it implies that the cardiovascular system has been fully stressed. Because the muscle mass utilized during upper body exercise is considerably smaller than that recruited during lower body exercise, it is difficult to tax the cardiovascular system fully and attain true $\dot{V}O_{2max}$ values.

Figure 28.6 Oxygen Uptake (Panel A) and Heart Rate (Panel B) Responses During Incremental Arm-cranking Exercise in Individuals with Quadriplegia, Paraplegia, and Cerebral Palsy

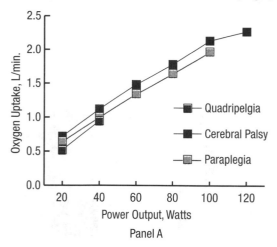

Panel A

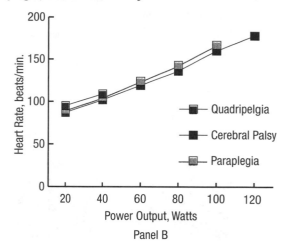

Panel B

Hence the term *peak oxygen uptake* (peak$\dot{V}O_2$) is commonly used instead of $\dot{V}O_{2max}$ when referring to these data. A review of numerous studies on able-bodied subjects has indicated that the peak $\dot{V}O_2$ and peak heart rate attained during upper body exercise are approximately 70 percent and 93 percent of the respective peak values attained during lower body exercise (Sawka 1986).

In individuals with spinal cord injury who are nonambulatory, the peak $\dot{V}O_2$ is assessed using an arm-crank or wheelchair ergometer. During arm-cranking, the subject performs synchronous or asynchronous incremental cycling exercise with the upper extremities. Although the synchronous method is perceived as being less stressful, research has indicated no significant differences in the peak physiological responses between these two methods of evaluation (Mossberg et al. 1999). In the case of wheelchair ergometry, the subjects perform synchronous upper body exercise that is specific to their normal mode of ambulation. Several methods have been used for evaluating the peak $\dot{V}O_2$ of subjects with spinal cord injury during wheelchair ergometry. The wheelchair can be mounted on a motor-driven treadmill (Coutts and Stogryn 1987; Gayle, Pohlman, and Glaser 1990; Lakomy 1987) or roller system

(Bhambhani, Eriksson, and Steadward 1991; Eriksson, Lofstrom, and Ekblom 1988) so that the velocity and/or slope of wheelchair propulsion can be controlled as desired. Other researchers have designed more sophisticated computer controlled ergometers that can quantify power output during exercise (van der Woude et al. 1990; Veeger et al. 1991). When testing untrained individuals with quadriplegia during arm-cranking or wheelchair ergometry, the optimal protocol is a work rate increment between two to six watts/minute. Work rate increments of eight watts/minute or higher will underestimate the peak $\dot{V}O_2$ in this population (Lasko-McCarthey and Davis 1991a, b). The test-retest reliability of the peak physiological responses (oxygen uptake, heart rate, oxygen pulse, and ventilation rate) during wheelchair roller exercise has been established (Bhambhani et al. 1991). As well, the validity of the peak physiological responses during different wheelchair-treadmill protocols has been demonstrated (Hartung, Lally, and Blancq 1993). The mechanical efficiency of wheelchair ergometry (7 to 8 percent) is considerably less than that of arm-cranking (17 to 18 percent), which in turn, is lower than that of cycle ergometry (23 percent) (Corcoran et al. 1980; Glaser 1985). The stress of wheelchair

Figure 28.7 Expected Peak Values of the Oxygen Uptake (Panel A), Cardiac Output (Panel B), Heart Rate (Panel C) and (a − v̄)O$_{2\text{diff}}$ (Panel D) in Able-bodied Subjects and Individuals with Quadriplegia and Paraplegia

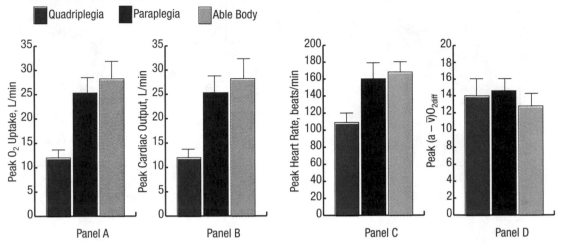

exercise is extremely high when the physiological responses are expressed as a percentage of the peak physiological capacity.

During incremental arm-cranking or wheelchair ergometry to volitional fatigue, the oxygen uptake and heart rate increase linearly with increasing power output until the peak values are attained at volitional fatigue. It has been reported (McLean, Jones, and Skinner 1995) that in some individuals with quadriplegia these physiological responses may not demonstrate a linear increase during incremental arm-cranking exercise. The physiological reasons for this are unclear. It is recommended that exercise testing in such individuals should be conducted with caution. Comparative responses for the oxygen uptake and heart rate during incremental exercise in individuals with quadriplegia, paraplegia, cerebral palsy, and able-bodied subjects are illustrated in figure 28.6. Expected values for the peak values of the oxygen uptake, cardiac output, heart rate, and (a − v̄)O$_{2\text{diff}}$ are depicted in Figure 28.7 Panels A to D, respectively. In untrained persons with spinal cord injury, the peak V̇O$_2$ is inversely related to the level of lesion (Eriksson et al. 1988; Van Loan et al. 1987). This means that the higher the level of injury, the lower the peak V̇O$_2$ and vice versa. This is due to alterations in the central and peripheral factors that determine the peak V̇O$_2$ during exercise (Hopman et al. 1993; Jehl et al. 1991).

At lesion levels above T1, the sympathetic stimulation to the myocardium is disrupted and the individual is physiologically unable to attain the age-predicted maximal heart rate. This reduces the cardiac output, thereby diminishing the overall capacity to transport oxygen to the tissues. At lesion levels below T1, the myocardium is fully innervated and the individual should theoretically be able to attain the age-predicted maximal heart rate (Figoni 1993; Glaser 1985). However, the degree of muscle mass that can be recruited for exercise is a major determinant of the amount of oxygen that can be extracted from the perfusing blood. Since this is also inversely related to the level of lesion, individuals with low-levels of paraplegia generally have higher peak V̇O$_2$ values that those with high-levels of paraplegia or quadriplegia (Van Loan et al. 1987; Wicks et al. 1983). At a given lesion level, the completeness of the injury also plays an important role in the ability to recruit muscle during exercise; more complete lesions will result in a smaller muscle mass available for exercise and vice versa (Eriksson et al. 1988). Recent cross-sectional evidence (Bernard et al. 2000) has indicated

Figure 28.8 Influence of Lesion Level (Panel A), Completeness of Lesion (Panel B), and Training Status (Panel C) on the Peak Oxygen Uptake in Individuals with Spinal Cord Injury

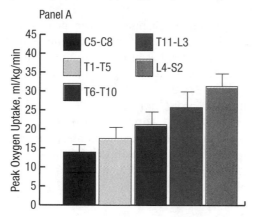

Panel A

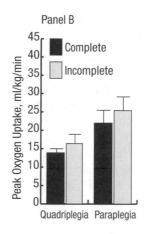

Panel B

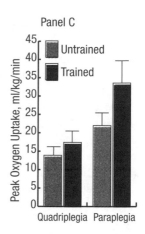

Panel C

that in well-trained wheelchair athletes with paraplegia the peak cardiorespiratory responses during incremental wheelchair ergometry may not be related to the lesion level. It is possible that training reduces the disparity among lesion levels that is normally seen in untrained individuals with spinal cord injury. The influence of lesion level, completeness of the lesion, and training status on the peak oxygen uptake in individuals with spinal cord injury is illustrated in figures 28.8a to 28.8c, respectively.

Cross-sectional studies have demonstrated that the peak $\dot{V}O_2$ of endurance-trained subjects with spinal cord injury is significantly greater than their untrained counterparts (Coutts and Stogryn 1987; Eriksson et al. 1988; Gass and Camp 1988; Huonker et al. 1998). While much of this increase can be attributed to the endurance training responses of these subjects, two other important factors must be considered (Shephard 1988): (a) the genetic predisposition of the subjects for aerobic metabolism (e.g., having a preponderance of Type I motor units) and (b) the fitness level of the subjects prior to the injury. It is likely that individuals who had high aerobic capacities prior to the injury would also adapt more readily to endurance training postinjury, which could result in their higher peak $\dot{V}O_2$ values.

Middle- and long-distance wheelchair races are usually performed at submaximal efforts. Research indicates that at the same absolute oxygen uptake during arm-cranking exercise, the cardiac output is significantly lower, while $(a - \bar{v})O_{2diff}$ is significantly higher in untrained individuals with quadriplegia compared to able-bodied subjects (Figoni et al. 1988). However, comparisons between individuals with paraplegia and able-bodied subjects indicate no significant differences in the cardiac output and $(a - \bar{v})O_{2diff}$ at the same absolute oxygen uptake (Hopman, Oeseburg, and Binkhorst 1992). Collectively, these observations suggest that the exercising muscles in individuals with quadriplegia have the capacity to increase oxygen extraction when blood perfusion is reduced. This is an interesting phenomenon in light of the fact that the aerobic capacity of the skeletal muscle is compromised in individuals with spinal cord injury (Grimby et al. 1976; Taylor et al. 1979). During submaximal exercise at the same relative intensity (i.e., percent of peak $\dot{V}O_2$), no significant differences have been reported between able-bodied subjects and individuals with paraplegia for the cardiac output and $(a - \bar{v})O_{2diff}$. With respect to the cardiac output, research has consistently demonstrated that this is attained by a lower stroke volume and proportionate increase in the heart rate in the subjects with spinal cord injury (Hopman et al. 1993; Hopman et al. 1992).

Unlike individuals with spinal cord injury, the sympathetic innervation to the myocardium in individuals with cerebral palsy is intact and, therefore, cardiac function is not directly compromised by the condition (Steadward 1998). Studies that have assessed the cardiorespiratory fitness of individuals with cerebral palsy during leg cycling (Bhambhani, Holland, and Steadward 1992; Lundberg 1976; Lundberg 1978), wheelchair egrometry (Bhambhani et al. 1992), and combination of arm and leg ergometry (Schwinn air dyne ergometer) (Fernandez and Pitetti 1993) have indicated that they can attain their age-predicted maximal heart rate (figure 28.6). In order to obtain valid measures of peak $\dot{V}O_2$, it is recommended that the testing mode utilized be specific to the mode of ambulation (Bhambhani et al. 1992). In other words, if the subject is able to walk independently without much difficulty, then a lower body exercise mode such as cycle ergometry should be used for assessment. However, if the person is nonambulatory, then an upper body exercise mode such as arm-cranking or wheelchair exercise is the preferred mode of assessment. Data pertaining to the stroke volume and cardiac output during exercise in individuals with cerebral palsy are not currently available. Both acute and chronic exercise studies need to be undertaken to understand fully their cardiovascular responses to exercise.

Direct measurement of the peak $\dot{V}O_2$ requires expensive laboratory equipment and technical expertise. However, coaches may not have access to such testing facilities for monitoring their athletes on a regular basis. In order to overcome this limitation, researchers have adapted valid field tests developed for able-bodied subjects to estimate the peak $\dot{V}O_2$ in subjects with spinal cord injury. Similar research on individuals with cerebral palsy has not been reported. The Leger and Boucher multistage incremental running test for able-bodied subjects has been validated for measuring the peak $\dot{V}O_2$ during wheelchair propulsion in male athletes with Class II to V paraplegia (Vinet et al. 1996). The short-term (three to ten days) and long-term (eight days to one month) reliability of the peak heart rate and maximal speed measurements of this adapted field test has also been demonstrated in male athletes with paraplegia (Poulain et al. 1999). The validity of the twelve-minute wheelchair propulsion distance (designed on the basis of the Cooper twelve-minute run-walk) against direct measurement of the peak $\dot{V}O_2$ has been demonstrated in individuals with paraplegia (Franklin et al. 1990; Rhodes et al. 1981) but not with quadriplegia. The correlation coefficient is stronger when the peak $\dot{V}O_2$ is expressed relative to body weight, suggesting that body mass plays an important role in determining wheelchair propulsion distance. The strength of the relationship is improved by including other variables such as blood pressure, age, and height of the subjects.

---

3 How will an increase in the amount of muscle mass available for exercise influence the peak values of the anaerobic and aerobic power in wheelchair athletes?

LACTATE OR VENTILATORY THRESHOLD

The *lactate threshold* is the lowest oxygen uptake at which a significant amount of lactate accumulates in the blood during a continuous incremental test to voluntary exhaustion (Wasserman 1986). Besides the normal units (L/min and ml/kg/min), the oxygen uptake at this threshold is also expressed as a percentage of the $\dot{V}O_{2max}$ (percent $\dot{V}O_{2max}$). The lactate threshold indicates the maximum amount of energy that can be derived from aerobic sources without the accumulation of lactic acid. This threshold is determined during the incremental $\dot{V}O_{2max}$ test using invasive and/or noninvasive methods. The invasive method involves the measurement of the lactate concentration from a blood sample that is withdrawn from a forearm vein or fingertip at each work rate during the incremental test. The exercise intensity (oxygen uptake) at which the lactate concentration increases exponentially is referred to as the lactate (anaerobic) threshold.

The lactate threshold can also be determined noninvasively from the respiratory gas exchange responses measured by the metabolic cart during the incremental exercise test (Wasserman 1986). It is generally accepted that when a significant amount of lactate accumulates in the blood an additional amount of carbon dioxide, above that formed as a result of aerobic metabolism, is released due to the buffering of lactate by bicarbonate in the blood. The increased carbon dioxide production elevates the arterial carbon dioxide tension which stimulates the peripheral chemoreceptors, thereby increasing the ventilatory drive. The net result is that the ventilation rate, carbon dioxide production, and respiratory exchange ratio all increase nonlinearly at the lactate threshold. Improved criteria for detecting this threshold from the respiratory gas exchange measurements are a systematic increase in the ventilatory equivalent for oxygen (ratio between ventilation rate and oxygen consumption), without a concomitant increase in the ventilatory equivalent for carbon dioxide (ratio between ventilation rate and carbon dioxide production). A typical trend of these variables during incremental exercise arm-cranking to volitional exhaustion is illustrated in figure 28.9. In the scientific literature, this exercise intensity is usually referred to as the *ventilatory threshold* because the exact physiological mechanism of the relationship between lactate accumulation and the respiratory gas exchange measurements is not completely understood.

The lactate (ventilatory) threshold is considered to be the best indicator of submaximal aerobic fitness because it represents the exercise intensity at which energy for muscular work can be produced aerobically with minimal utilization of anaerobic sources (McArdle, Katch, and Katch 1996). At this threshold, oxygen supplied by the central circulation is sufficient to meet the requirements of the muscle, resulting in the majority of energy being produced under aerobic

Figure 28.9 Detection of the Ventilatory Threshold During Incremental Arm-cranking Exercise Using Respiratory Gas Exchange Measurements

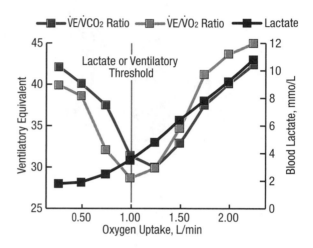

conditions. At exercise intensities below this threshold, the individual can continue exercising for prolonged periods because there is minimal accumulation of lactate, a metabolite that is implicated with muscular fatigue (Wenger and Reed 1973). At intensities above the threshold, blood lactate increases in an exponential manner with respect to exercise intensity, and performance is severely curtailed. Laboratory research on able-bodied subjects has indicated that the lactate threshold may be a better predictor of endurance performance than the $\dot{V}O_{2max}$. During prolonged treadmill running, individuals select a running velocity at which the oxygen uptake is closely related to that observed at the lactate (ventilatory) threshold (Coyle et al. 1988; Farrell et al. 1979). Hence, it is important that athletes competing in endurance events have a high lactate (ventilatory) threshold when the values are expressed relative to the $\dot{V}O_{2max}$.

A limited number of studies have evaluated the ventilatory threshold in individuals with spinal cord injury and cerebral palsy. One investigation (Flandrois et al. 1986) reported no significant differences in the absolute oxygen uptake at the ventilatory threshold between able-bodied subjects and those with paraplegia performing arm-crank exercise,

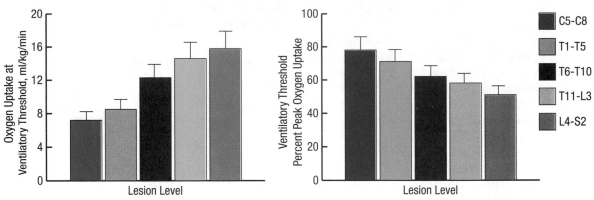

Figure 28.10 Influence of Lesion Level on the Ventilatory Threshold in Individuals with Spinal Cord Injury

whereas another (Lin et al. 1993) reported a significantly lower value in subjects with high-level paraplegia (lesion levels between T1 to T5). However, both these studies indicated that (a) the ventilatory threshold occurred at a significantly higher percentage of the peak $\dot{V}O_2$ in the subjects with paraplegia when compared to the able-bodied subjects, and (b) the values for the subjects with paraplegia were not related to the lesion level. Comparisons of the absolute oxygen uptake at the ventilatory threshold in subjects with quadriplegia (lesion levels C5 to C7) demonstrated significantly lower values than those with paraplegia (lesion levels T1 to S3) (Coutts and McKenzie 1995). However, when the values were expressed relative to peak $\dot{V}O_2$ the trend was reversed, as illustrated in figure 28.10. This could be due to loss of sympathetic control to the heart and/or loss of central innervation to the intercostal muscles in the subjects with quadriplegia, which could influence their respiratory response to incremental exercise.

The absolute oxygen uptake at the ventilatory threshold during simulated wheelchair exercise is significantly higher in competitive wheelchair marathon racers with quadriplegia compared to their untrained counterparts (Bhambhani et al. 1995a). As well, there is a strong correlation between the absolute oxygen uptake at the ventilatory threshold and the peak $\dot{V}O_2$ in both these groups of subjects, implying that subjects with a higher level of aerobic fitness are able to attain a higher oxygen uptake before the accumulation of significant amount of lactate during incremental exercise. When comparing the results by sport participation, track athletes demonstrate significantly higher values for the absolute oxygen uptake at the ventilatory threshold and peak exercise when compared to basketball players and other athletes (swimming, table tennis, and target shooting). No significant differences are observed among the athletes when the values at the ventilatory threshold are expressed as a percentage of peak $\dot{V}O_2$ (Vinet et al. 1997). Similar results are obtained when comparisons are made between track athletes and tennis players.

In athletes with cerebral palsy, the nonlinear increase in blood lactate during stepwise incremental cycle or wheelchair exercise does not coincide with the ventilatory threshold criteria outlined earlier (Bhambhani, Holland, and Steadward 1993), questioning the validity of this parameter in this population. The test-retest reliability of their gas exchange responses at the ventilatory threshold is also questionable, although the peak $\dot{V}O_2$ values can be determined with consistency. Therefore, when evaluating the cardiorespiratory fitness of athletes with cerebral palsy, it is recommended that the peak $\dot{V}O_2$ is used for analysis. Other observations (Dwyer and McMahon 1994) indicate that the absolute oxygen uptake at the ventilatory threshold in adults with cerebral palsy is similar during cycle ergometry and treadmill running. However, since the peak $\dot{V}O_2$ during treadmill exercise is significantly higher than that observed during cycle ergometry, the results suggest that the ventilatory threshold occurs at a higher percentage of peak $\dot{V}O_2$ during cycle ergometry compared to treadmill running. To date, the relationship between the lactate or ventilatory thresholds and wheelchair racing performance in athletes with spinal cord injury and cerebral palsy has not been examined. Given the importance of this parameter in endurance performance, it is important that such studies be undertaken in the future.

---

4 How does an increase in spasticity observed during exercise influence the lactate threshold in athletes with cerebral palsy?

Physiological Correlates of Wheelchair Racing Performance

There is limited research that has examined the physiological responses during wheelchair racing events and identified factors that are associated with performance in athletes with disabilities. The available evidence is controversial and questions the validity of using these physiological parameters to predict success in sprint- and distance-racing performance.

PREDICTION OF SPRINT-RACING PERFORMANCE

Research has demonstrated that the average power output during the Wingate test in elite athletes with a variety of disabilities is inversely related to performance time taken of a 200-metre race but not the marathon (van der Woude et al. 1997). In general, the Wingate test results varied considerably among the different disabilities and sports disciplines and was strongly influenced by the functionality, number of hours of training, and gender of the athletes. Other researchers (Lees and Arthur 1988) have also reported a strong correlation between wheelchair Wingate test results and performance during

a 400-metre race in wheelchair athletes. In contrast, one study (Hutzler 1993) indicated that measurements of anaerobic and aerobic power on an arm-crank ergometer in competitive wheelchair basketball players were not good predictors of success in three selected wheeling tasks: 400-metre race, slalom, and six-minute wheelchair endurance race. Interestingly, the maximum heart rate attained during the arm-cranking test correlated significantly with each of the wheeling tasks. The lack of association between the physiological parameters and performance in this study could be due to the difference in the testing modes: arm-cranking versus wheeling.

PREDICTION OF DISTANCE-RACING PERFORMANCE

A limited number of field studies have evaluated the physiological responses of wheelchair marathon racers during competitive events. In elite wheelchair racers with quadriplegia and paraplegia, the oxygen uptake and heart rate measured during distance-racing performance were approximately 90 to 95 percent of the respective peak values observed during incremental, exhaustive wheelchair exercise on a treadmill (Asayama et al. 1985; Crews 1982). The latter study reported that the relative intensity at marathon race pace was considerably higher in wheelchair marathoners with paraplegia compared to elite marathon runners. The wheelchair racers sustained an oxygen uptake and heart rate that corresponded to 94 percent and 96 percent of their respective peak values during incremental exercise, while the marathon runners sustained values of 78 percent and 85 percent, respectively.

The validity of simulated wheelchair racing performed on frictionless rollers in the laboratory has been demonstrated in athletes with quadriplegia and paraplegia (Bhambhani et al. 1994). These researchers reported significant correlations between an actual 3.2-kilometre race performed on a racing track and simulated race performed on the roller system for the following variables: racing time, velocity, heart rate, and blood lactate. They also documented that the athletes with paraplegia

Figure 28.11 Oxygen Uptake and Heart Rate during Simulated Wheelchair Racing in Individuals with Quadriplegia and Paraplegia

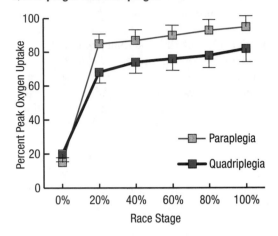

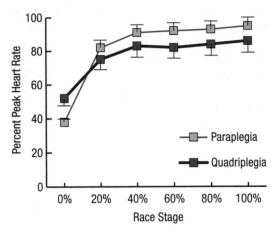

attained higher values of oxygen uptake and heart rate during the simulated race than those with quadriplegia. This difference in racing intensity was maintained when the values were expressed relative to the peak values that the athletes attained during the incremental wheelchair test to exhaustion, as illustrated in figure 28.11. The athletes with quadriplegia raced at 76 percent and 86 percent of their peak $\dot{V}O_2$ and peak heart rate, respectively, while those with paraplegia exercised at 95 percent of their peak values for both these variables. Another investigation (Lakomy 1987) documented that the average oxygen uptake during a simulated race in a group of mixed wheelchair athletes with paraplegia was approximately 76 percent of the peak $\dot{V}O_2$, while that attained by individuals with quadriplegia was approximately 90 percent. The findings of these studies, although descriptive in nature, are important from a training perspective as they indicate the extremely high intensity of wheelchair racing performance in well-trained athletes with disabilities.

Several studies have examined the relationship between measures of aerobic fitness and wheelchair distance-racing performance. Some evidence (Cooper 1992; Hooker and Wells 1992) indicates no significant relationship

between the peak $\dot{V}O_2$ and actual wheelchair racing velocity during a 10-kilometre road race in well-trained athletes with paraplegia. In contrast, other observations (Lakomy 1987) indicate a significant relationship between these two variables during a simulated 5-kilometre race in a similar group of athletes. In elite wheelchair athletes with quadriplegia, a significant correlation between the peak $\dot{V}O_2$ and time taken to complete a simulated 7.5-kilometre race has been reported (Bhambhani et al. 1994). These investigators also documented that racing performance was significantly related to the oxygen uptake, cardiac output, and stroke volume during the race, but not the $(a - \bar{v})O_{2diff}$, age, and lesion level of the athletes. These observations suggest that in athletes with quadriplegia (i) aerobic power is important for successful wheelchair distance-racing performance, and (ii) central factors related to oxygen transport play a more important role than peripheral factors in enhancing performance. Besides these metabolic and cardiorespiratory variables, other evidence indicates that, in elite wheelchair racers, arm power measured on a steel spring apparatus and total lung capacity play an important role in successful wheelchair marathon racing performance (Ide et al.

1994) In general, the differences in wheel-chair racing velocity of world-class athletes are dependent upon the race distances, as well as the gender and classes of the athletes (Coutts and Shultz 1988).

In summary, the research evidence pertaining to wheelchair racing performance in athletes with spinal cord injury does not support the generally accepted concept that high values of anaerobic and aerobic power are strongly associated with sprint and endurance racing performance, respectively, in this population. Besides these physiological factors, previous experience, motivation, tactics, and other variables can influence overall performance in wheelchair sport (Vanlandewijck, Spaepen, and Lysens 1995). Further research is needed to elucidate the factors that best predict performance in these events.

5 What is the physiological relationship between the lactate (ventilatory) threshold and distance-racing performance in wheelchair athletes?

6 How will an increase in cardiac output induced by lower body positive pressure affect wheelchair racing performance in wheelchair athletes with spinal cord injury?

Principles of Physical Training for Persons With Disabilities

Regular physical training enhances anaerobic and aerobic fitness in able-bodied subjects. However, in order to achieve these gains, the training programmes must be designed on the basis of valid scientific physiological principles. The following three training principles are generally recommended for developing training programmes for athletes: *progressive overload, specificity,* and *reversibility.* Although these principles have been utilized by rehabilitation professionals and exercise physiologists to enhance the physiological capacity of individuals with disabilities, it should be pointed out that well-controlled scientific information in many of these areas is lacking.

PRINCIPLE OF PROGRESSIVE OVERLOAD

According to this principle, a physiological system will improve its capacity if the exercise stimulus is higher than that to which the system is normally accustomed, provided it meets a minimum threshold intensity (Astrand and Rodahl 1986; McArdle, Katch, and Katch 1996). The exercise intensity is usually expressed relative to the physical fitness parameter that the exercise programme is designed to enhance. For example, if the objective is to increase the peak $\dot{V}O_2$, then the intensity of the training session is expressed as a percentage of the peak $\dot{V}O_2$ or another variable that is closely related to it such as the peak heart rate. Similarly, if the goal is to enhance muscular strength or endurance, then the intensity is expressed as a percentage of the maximum resistance that the individual can overcome a given number of times (i.e., repetitions maximum) for a specific movement of that muscle group. It is emphasized that in order to obtain continued gains in the fitness parameter it is imperative that the absolute exercise intensity be progressively increased in order to overload the system continually as it adapts to the training programme. If this practice is not followed, the initial gains in fitness will reach a plateau and performance may not improve. It is important, therefore, that athletes be tested on a regular basis so that adjustments can be made to their training programmes (Canadian Society for Exercise Physiology 1998; MacDougall, Wenger, and Green 1991; Maud and Foster 1995; Muller et al. 2000).

PRINCIPLE OF SPECIFICITY

The specificity of training refers to the adaptations in the physiological and energy systems that are specific to the type of overload imposed (Astrand and Rodahl 1986; McArdle, Katch, and Katch 1996). For example, if the cardiovascular system is stressed above the minimal intensity, then the aerobic power (e.g., peak $\dot{V}O_2$ during wheelchair exercise) is significantly increased as a result of improvements in both central circulation and/or peripheral oxygen extraction by the exercising muscle. The enhanced central circulation is due to an improvement in the peak values of cardiac output and stroke volume during exercise. Improved oxygen extraction capacity is due to significant increases in capillary density, mitochondrial volume (size and number), and activity of aerobic enzymes. This is evident as a widening of the $(a - \bar{v})O_{2diff}$. This type of training usually does not induce significant improvements in the muscular strength and endurance component of physical fitness. Similarly, if the musculoskeletal system is overloaded using resistance exercise, then significant gains in muscular strength and endurance will be attained with minimal changes in aerobic power. Reasons for the improvements in muscular strength and endurance include an increase in the number of motor units recruited, greater synchrony of motor units activated, and an increase in the size and number of myofibrils in the trained muscle. It should be pointed out that both these types of training when continued for prolonged periods usually result in significant changes in body composition: cardiovascular training will reduce percentage body fat primarily because fats are metabolized to produce energy during this type of exercise, whereas resistance training will increase lean body mass due to the synthesis of muscular proteins specific to this type of training.

The principle of specificity can also be extended to the energy systems that are overloaded during training. For example, high-intensity sprint training with short work-to-rest intervals (e.g., ten to thirty seconds) will enhance the capacity of the short-term source of energy with minimal effect on the intermediate and long-term energy sources (Gollnick and Hermansen 1973; Jacobs 1987). Similarly, long duration, low- to moderate-intensity endurance training will augment the capacity of the long-term energy sources of energy production but will not enhance the capacity of the immediate and short-term sources of energy production. This aspect of training is well illustrated in a research study that measured the metabolic responses of

Olympic athletes with disabilities (Veeger et al. 1991c). The track and field athletes who were more dependent upon aerobic metabolism had the highest values of peak $\dot{V}O_2$, while the target shooters whose sport did not stress the aerobic system had the lowest values.

Two other factors pertaining to the principle of specificity of training have been demonstrated: (a) the peripheral adaptations occur only in the muscle group(s) that are overloaded, and (b) the improvements in aerobic fitness (peak $\dot{V}O_2$) induced by training are usually evident during that particular exercise mode only with minimal transfer to other modes of exercise. These two findings have important implications for designing training programmes for wheelchair athletes. For example, a wheelchair marathon racer with quadriplegia or cerebral palsy would attain the maximum benefit by training on a wheelchair rather than an arm-crank ergometer, because the localized changes in aerobic capacity occur in the same muscle groups that are used by the athlete in the competitive event. As well, since the improvement in aerobic fitness is usually evident only during that particular mode of exercise, training on an arm-crank ergometer will most likely not have a significant impact on wheelchair racing performance.

PRINCIPLE OF REVERSIBILITY

Physiological improvements induced by training are reduced when there is a decrease in the intensity and volume of training over a period of time, or when training is temporarily stopped due to injury. While there is minimal research evidence to demonstrate this in athletes with disabilities, considerable research is available on able-bodied athletes, which suggests that improvements in the physical fitness parameters that occur with training decline quite rapidly upon the cessation of training. With respect to aerobic training, it is generally accepted that both the central and peripheral adaptations begin to decline within two to three weeks following bedrest in healthy subjects (Saltin et al. 1968). Because of the reversible nature of these physiological changes, it is important that wheelchair athletes continue to do some moderate intensity, sport-specific training during the off-season. This will minimize losses in physical fitness that could affect their ability to train during the in-season.

Designing Physical Training Programmes for Improving Wheelchair-racing Performance

COMPONENTS OF THE TRAINING PROGRAMME

When designing physical training programmes for enhancing sport performance, the following parameters must be considered: *frequency* of training, defined as the number of training sessions per week; *intensity* of the training session, commonly expressed as a percentage of the peak $\dot{V}O_2$ or peak heart rate for aerobic training programmes; *duration* of the training session, quantified as the number of minutes per training session; and *length* of the training programme, expressed in weeks or months of training. The total *volume* of training over a period of time is directly related to the above parameters. It is recommended that competitive athletes maintain a log that documents each parameter of their training regimen. It is also the responsibility of the coach to monitor closely these aspects of the training programme in elite athletes in order to optimize their performance.

THE MINIMUM TRAINING REQUIREMENTS

In the able-bodied population, the minimum training requirements for enhancing cardiorespiratory and musculoskeletal fitness have been well established (American College of Sports Medicine 1990). It is generally agreed that a training frequency of three times a week at a minimum intensity equivalent to 50 percent of $\dot{V}O_{2max}$, or 60 percent of the heart rate reserve, is necessary to induce significant improvements in cardiorespiratory fitness. The heart rate reserve is calculated as: (peak heart rate – resting heart rate). The training target heart rate is then determined as the specific percentage of the heart rate reserve

plus the resting heart rate. In order to obtain these benefits, the training should be performed continuously for at least twenty minutes so as to burn a minimum of 200 Kcals per training session. In competitive athletes training for sport performance, the training intensity is usually increased and can be as high as 85 percent of $\dot{V}O_{2max}$, or 90 percent of the heart rate reserve. In order to improve the lactate (ventilatory) threshold, it is suggested that the training intensity be above this threshold so that localized changes in aerobic capacity and tolerance to lactate during exercise can be enhanced. High-intensity interval training with long work-to-rest intervals (e.g., one minute work to one minute rest), performed at 100 percent of $\dot{V}O_{2max}$, can also induce significant improvements in aerobic fitness. With respect to the maintenance of aerobic fitness, it is generally accepted that one training session per week is sufficient, as long as the training intensity and duration are equivalent to that achieved during the regular training sessions.

Besides these objective physiological variables that necessitate direct measurement of the cardiorespiratory responses, the subjective degree of stress during exercise can also be used to prescribe aerobic training programmes. The Borg Scale for the Rating of Perceived Exertion (RPE) (Borg 1982) is a numerical scale that ranges from 6 to 20. The odd numbers on this scale have the following descriptors: 7 = very, very light; 9 = very light; 11 = fairly light; 13 = somewhat hard; 15 = hard; 17 = very hard; 19 = very, very hard. This scale has been validated against the cardiorespiratory responses during incremental exercise in a variety of healthy and clinical populations. When using this scale for exercise prescription, the individual is required to exercise at a specific RPE. In able-bodied individuals, an RPE of 13 or 14 usually corresponds to 70 percent of the maximum heart rate (Borg 1982), while a value of 11 corresponds to the lactate threshold in both untrained and trained subjects (Seip et al. 1991). This method of exercise prescription is found to correspond closely with objective measures such as the heart rate during exercise (Dishman et al. 1987). Alterations to the training programme are based on changes in the subjective feeling observed during the course of the training programme.

Limited research has been conducted to examine the minimum training requirements necessary to improve aerobic fitness in individuals with disabilities. It has been reported (Hooker et al. 1993) that the relationship between heart rate and oxygen uptake during incremental arm-cranking exercise in untrained subjects with quadriplegia and paraplegia was similar to that observed in able-bodied subjects. The researchers suggested that there was no need to modify the method of prescribing the intensity of training in individuals with spinal cord injury. However, another investigation (McLean, Jones, and Skinner 1995) questioned the validity of the relationship between the heart rate and oxygen uptake during incremental arm-cranking exercise in individuals with quadriplegia. The results indicated considerable variability in the relationship between these two variables to accurately prescribe a training intensity of 70 percent of peak heart rate in either the sitting or supine position. Within the limitations of their findings, the authors recommended that exercise training intensity for individuals with quadriplegia be based on 50 percent to 60 percent of the peak power output and/or an RPE of 10 to 12. Other research (Hooker and Wells 1989) that examined the effects of low- and moderate-intensity arm-crank training on the peak $\dot{V}O_2$ in subjects with quadriplegia demonstrated that moderate-intensity training at 60 to 75 percent of peak $\dot{V}O_2$ was necessary to improve the peak $\dot{V}O_2$, whereas low-intensity training at 40 to 50 percent of peak $\dot{V}O_2$ was ineffective. Many wheelchair athletes commonly train at specific percentages of their maximum speed attained during testing (Campbell, Williams, and Lakomy 1997). Research that has examined this method of exercise prescription has indicated that the physiological responses during sixteen minutes of wheelchair racing at 60 percent, 70 percent, 80 percent, and 90 percent of the

top speed did not match the corresponding values of the peak $\dot{V}O_2$ in well-trained male wheelchair athletes The practical implication of this observation is that wheelchair athletes should avoid using this training method if the assumption is that it corresponds to the same percentage of peak $\dot{V}O_2$.

---

7 How would you incorporate the principle of progressive overload in training programmes designed to improve anaerobic and aerobic fitness? Which physiological variables would you monitor to evaluate the success of these training programmes?

TRAINING ADAPTATIONS IN INDIVIDUALS WITH SPINAL CORD INJURY AND CEREBRAL PALSY

Longitudinal training studies designed to improve the anaerobic fitness in individuals with spinal cord injury and cerebral palsy have not been conducted. Although numerous studies have evaluated the anaerobic fitness in nonathletes and athletes with spinal cord injury, comparisons among studies are difficult because of the differences in testing modes (arm-cranking, wheelchair ergometry) and load factors used in these studies (Dallmeijer et al. 1994; Hutzler et al. 1998; van der Woude et al. 1998; Veeger et al. 1992). Moreover, the conclusions derived from cross-sectional evidence should be interpreted with caution because the differences in performance could be due to genetic factors and the pre-injury training level of the athletes (Shephard 1988).

Several studies that have examined the effects of *voluntary aerobic training* on the peak cardiorespiratory responses in individuals with spinal cord injury and cerebral palsy are summarized in Table 28.1. It is evident that significant increases in peak $\dot{V}O_2$ ranging from 7 percent to 30 percent are observed within eight to twenty-four weeks of arm-cranking or wheelchair exercise in untrained individuals with quadriplegia and paraplegia. An increase of 24 percent has been reported in well-trained wheelchair basketball players subsequent to eight weeks of wheelchair ergometry

Table 28.1 Effects of Training on Peak Cardiorespiratory Responses in Individuals with Spinal Cord Injury and Cerebral Palsy

Authors	Subjects/Lesion Level/Test Mode	Training Mode	Training Details		Percent Change/Statistical Significance			Other Findings/Comments
			Intensity/Duration	Frequency Length	Peak Power (Watts)	Peak Oxygen Uptake (ml/kg/min)	Peak Heart Rate (beats/min)	
Spinal Cord Injury								
Cooney and Walker, 1986	6M, 4F C5 to L1 ACE	HRE	60% to 90% of peak HR 30 to 40 mins	3x/week 9 weeks	36.7% $p<.01$	28.1% $p<.01$		
Davis, Plyley, and Shephard, 1991	24M T6 to L5 ACE	ACE	HL: 70% peak $\dot{V}O_2$ HS: 70% peak $\dot{V}O_2$ LL: 50% peak $\dot{V}O_2$ LS: 50% peak $\dot{V}O_2$	3x/week 24 weeks		16.1% 16.3% 20.5% Incomplete		Significant increases in submaximal stroke volume
DiCarlo, Supp, and Taylor, 1983	4M C5 to T8 ACE	ACE	60% to 80 % peak HR 30 mins	5 weeks	NS: 64.3%	NS: 60.3%		Non-significant findings due to small sample
Hooker and Wells, 1989	4M,4F WERG	ACE	L: 50 to 60% HRR M: 70 to 80% HRR 20 mins	3x/week 8 weeks	L: NS; 10% M: NS; 24%	L: NS; 12% M: NS; 13%		Submaximal heart rate reduced in M group
Jacobs, Nash, and Rusinowski, 2001	10M T5 to L1 ACE	CRT	40 to 45 mins	3x/week 12 weeks	16.1% $p<.01$	29.7% $p<.01$		
McLean and Skinner, 1995	7 Sitting 7 Supine ACE	ACE	60% of peak power 25 to 35 mins	3x/week 10 weeks	10.1% 16% $p<.001$	7.5% 9.8% $p<.01$	6.2% 1% NS	No significant change in stroke volume
Miles, Sawka, Wilde, Durbin, Gotshall and Glaser, 1982	8M WA WERG	WERG	80% of maximum HRR 30 mins	3x/week 8 weeks	30.7% $p<.05$	26% $p<.05$		
Taylor, McDonell, and Brassard, 1986	10M T6 to L4 ACE	ACE	80% of peak HR 30 mins	5x/week 8 weeks		15.5% $p<.05$	3% NS	Significant increase in slow twitch fibre area
Cerebral Palsy								
Fernandez and Pitetti, 1993	5M, 2F ambulatory SAE, ACE	SAE	40 to 70% of peak $\dot{V}O_2$ 30 mins	2x/week 8 weeks		SAE: 15% $p<.05$ ACE: NS	SAE: NS ACE: NS	No transfer effect between exercise modes

M = male; F = Female; ACE = arm-cranking exercise; HRE = hydraulic resistance exercise; HR = heart rate; HL = high-intensity, long duration, HS = high-intensity, short duration; LL = Low intensity, long duration, LS = low intensity, short duration; L = low intensity, M = moderate intensity; HRR = heart rate reserve, WERG = wheelchair ergometry, CRT = circuit resistance training; WA = wheelchair athletes, SAE = Schwinn air-dyne ergometry, NS = statistically non-significant.

at 60 percent of the maximum heart reserve (Miles et al. 1982). The increased peak $\dot{V}O_2$ is attained at a significantly higher power output post-training. Training does not seem to increase the peak heart rate during maximal exercise in individuals with spinal cord injury, implying that the ability to tax a greater proportion of the heart rate reserve does not occur. In individuals with quadriplegia, no significant increases in stroke volume have been reported following eight weeks of training in the sitting or supine position (McLean and Skinner 1995). However, in individuals with paraplegia, the stroke volume is significantly elevated following twenty-four weeks of arm-cranking exercise (Davis, Plyley, and Shephard 1991). These investigators suggested that the primary reason for the improvement in cardiorespiratory fitness in individuals with paraplegia was a significant increase in the oxygen transport capacity. This was most likely due to: (a) an enhanced cardiac preload resulting from improved muscle pump action and increased venous tone, (b) reduced afterload resulting from a decreased vascular impedance, and (c) increased myocardial contractility or structural hypertrophy of the left ventricle. Although cross-sectional evidence (Huonker et al. 1998) suggests that the cardiac dimensions are significantly larger in wheelchair athletes with paraplegia compared to their sedentary counterparts, these changes are not evident as a result of short-term aerobic training (Davis, Shephard, and Leenen 1987). Some evidence (Cooney and Walker 1986) suggests that hydraulic resistance training, which increases the strength and endurance of the upper body, is effective in enhancing the peak $\dot{V}O_2$ during arm-cranking exercise, provided that the intensity is within 60 percent to 90 percent of the peak heart rate. In general, the training responses observed in individuals with paraplegia are consistent with those observed in able-bodied subjects. However, the capacity to improve central circulation may be limited in individuals with quadriplegia due to their inability to tax a higher proportion of the peak heart rate.

In untrained individuals with cerebral palsy, eight weeks of aerobic training at an intensity of 40 percent to 70 percent of peak $\dot{V}O_2$ increases the peak oxygen uptake during combined arm and leg exercise (Schwinn airdyne ergometry) by 15 percent. This improvement, however, is not observed when the peak $\dot{V}O_2$ is assessed during arm-cranking exercise (Fernandez and Pitetti 1993). A six-year longitudinal study (Lundberg 1984) of children aged twelve to eighteen years with spastic diplegia and dyskinesia who were enrolled in physical activity (gymnastics) classes indicated that their aerobic power and physical work capacity increased at a slower rate than that of healthy age-matched children. However, no significant differences were observed between the groups for the change in the maximal values of the heart rate, ventilation rate, and blood lactate concentration during peak exercise over the six-year period. The net mechanical efficiency of submaximal work performed on a cycle ergometer declined in the children with diplegia but was unchanged in the healthy controls. Currently, it is not known whether regular aerobic training that increases the peak physiological responses also improves the lactate (ventilatory) threshold in individuals with spinal cord injury and cerebral palsy. Further research is necessary to examine the effects of regular aerobic training on concomitant changes in the physiological responses at both these exercise intensities in individuals with these disabilities.

8 How does regular aerobic training affect the lactate (ventilatory) threshold in individuals with spinal cord injury and cerebral palsy? How would you evaluate the relationship of these two variables with wheelchair racing performance?

9 What role does upper body muscular strength and endurance play in enhancing wheelchair racing performance?

THE TRAINING SEASON

From a planning perspective, the athlete's training year is usually organized into three main seasons: pre-season, in-season and off-season. The length of these seasons varies considerably. Usually, the in-season is the longest because elite athletes participate at international sporting events all year round. The primary objective in the pre-season is to enhance the overall fitness of the athlete with a specific focus on the component(s) that are most closely associated with improved performance. For example, if the person competes in middle- or long-distance wheelchair racing events, the goal would be to increase the aerobic capacity (peak $\dot{V}O_2$) because it is inversely related to racing time (Bhambhani et al. 1995b). The development of the optimal biomechanical techniques (van der Woude et al. 1990; van der Woude et al. 1998; Veeger, van der Woude, and Rozendal 1991a) for wheelchair propulsion during anaerobic and aerobic events is also a priority during the pre-season. During the in-season, the training should be designed to further increase the peak $\dot{V}O_2$ and refine the biomechanical skills so as to attain continued improvements in performance, with the athlete peaking at competitions that are considered to be most important. It is recognized that in order to attain peak performance the athlete's training must be closely monitored (Maud and Foster 1995; Muller et al. 2000). Usually, a tapering programme that involves a 50 to 70 percent reduction in the training volume for one or two weeks preceding the competition is implemented to attain this goal (Banister, Carter, and Zarkadus 1999; Neary et al. 1992). During the off-season, the athlete should take time off from the competitive sport. However, it is recommended that the athlete participate in other recreational activities so as to minimize the loss of fitness and possible increase in fat mass due to a reduction in physical activity. As observed in the able-bodied population, improvements in the various fitness parameters in individuals with disabilities are inversely related to the initial fitness level; i.e., those with lower fitness levels at the onset of training will most likely show the most improvement and vice versa. It is likely, therefore, that the magnitude of the improvement in fitness in competitive athletes will be quite low because of their high initial fitness levels.

Training programmes for competitive athletes should be designed by professionals who have expertise in the physiological, bio-mechanical, and psychological aspects of the specific sport. Recently, several studies that have combined the disciplines of physiology and biomechanics have been published (Boninger et al. 1997; O'Connor, Robertson, and Cooper 1998; van der Woude et al. 1990, 1998; Veeger et al. 1991a, b). The findings of these interdisciplinary studies have important implications for: (a) optimizing wheelchair propulsion techniques that minimize energy expenditure thereby improving performance, (b) designing physical training programmes specific for wheelchair racing, and (c) reducing the incidence of injuries to the upper extremities. A review of wheelchair racing performance times over the last several years has indicated considerable improvement in a large number of events (Tiessen 1997). It is likely that further improvements in performance of elite wheelchair racers will result from refinements in training techniques rather than increases in physical fitness because of the genetic limits resulting from training.

CONSEQUENCES OF OVERTRAINING

Currently, there is minimal research that indicates the optimum amount of training for peak performance. Some studies suggest that there appears to be an inverted U-shaped relationship between training volume and improvement in performance, implying that once training exceeds a certain volume, performance deteriorates quite rapidly. This phenomenon, commonly referred to as *overtraining*, arises when insufficient recovery is provided between regular bouts of exercise. Since the actual training adaptations occur during the recovery phase, this component of the training programme should be carefully monitored in elite athletes (Hartmann and Mester 2000; Kuipers 2000). Overtraining can be characterized in three ways, based on the pathogenesis and organ systems affected. *Mechanical* overtraining refers to the constant wear and tear on the locomotor system that can result from excessive training and/or rapid increases in training volume. Since the connective tissue and bone have relatively poor vascularization, recovery is usually delayed. This could lead to chronic sports injuries in the athlete (Kibbler, Chandler, and Straceber 1992). *Metabolic* overtraining usually occurs when athletes incorporate high volumes of intensive exercise into their training programme. This type of training rapidly depletes intramuscular glycogen stores that must be replenished during recovery. Insufficient rest between successive training sessions and inadequate amount of carbohydrate in the diet will result in premature fatigue and deterioration in performance (Lehmann, Foster, and Keul 1993). The third facet of overtraining, referred to as staleness, occurs as a result of dysfunction to the *neuro-endocrine* system and may be associated with changes in autoimmune function (Barron et al. 1985). Symptoms associated with this type of overtraining syndrome are classified as those affecting the sympathetic or parasympathetic systems. The sympathetic type of overtraining can result in an elevated heart rate at rest or during exercise, increased resting and systolic and diastolic blood pressure, delayed recovery from exercise, poor appetite resulting in weight loss, disturbed sleep, mental instability and irritability, and menstrual abnormalities in female athletes. Symptoms of the parasympathetic type of overtraining may be confused with those associated with good health: low or normal resting heart rate and blood pressure, reduced exercise heart rate, rapid recovery of heart rate from exercise, good appetite, normal sleep, and lack of lethargy and depression.

During the last decade, considerable research has been conducted on the overtraining phenomenon in able-bodied subjects. However, the exact mechanism for this phenomenon has not been elucidated and precise biological markers have yet to be identified. Many competitive wheelchair road racers accumulate a lot of mileage during the course of their year-round training programmes and could be susceptible to any of the three types of overtraining described above. Although research pertaining to overtraining in wheelchair athletes is not available, it is important that the athletes and their coaches recognize this possibility and prevent it from occurring by closely regulating all aspects of the physical training programme and dietary regimen during the season. Research on wheelchair athletes has documented their susceptibility to musculoskeletal and neurologic injuries due to overuse of the upper extremities (Curtis and Dillon 1985; Ferrara et al. 1992). Identifying the optimum design of a training programme to avoid the overtraining phenomenon is indeed a challenge for the sports medicine professional and should be the focus of research in athletes with disabilities.

Summary

Wheelchair racing is the most popular competitive sporting activity for athletes with a disability. In international competitions, athletes compete in wheelchair races based on their functional capacity and not on the basis of their medical disability. The anaerobic power and capacity, aerobic power, and the lactate/ventilatory threshold in wheelchair athletes with spinal cord injury have been well documented in the scientific literature. A limited number of studies have reported on these fitness parameters in athletes with cerebral palsy. However, research that has examined the relationship between these fitness parameters and racing performance in wheelchair athletes is limited. Current evidence suggests that the generally accepted concept that high values of anaerobic and aerobic power are strongly associated with sprint and endurance racing performance, respectively, are not necessarily true in wheelchair athletes. Physical training programmes for athletes with disabilities should incorporate the same basic principles used for able-bodied subjects: progressive overload, specificity of training, and reversibility of training. The minimum training intensity for improving cardiorespiratory fitness in individuals with spinal cord injury is approximately 60 to 75 percent of the peak $\dot{V}O_2$ or 50 to 60 percent of the peak power output. Aerobic training performed three times a week for five to twelve weeks can increase the peak $\dot{V}O_2$ by 10 to 15 percent in individuals with spinal cord injury and cerebral palsy. Training programmes of elite wheelchair athletes who do large volumes of training should be constantly monitored so as to avoid the phenomenon of overtraining, which could be detrimental to performance.

Study Questions

1. Briefly discuss the different energy systems during wheelchair exercise and how they apply to short and long duration wheelchair races.

2. Describe the metabolic characteristics of the different types of motor units. How are these motor units recruited during wheelchair sprint and endurance races?

3. Define anaerobic power and capacity. How are these fitness parameters measured in athletes with spinal cord injury?

4. Define maximal aerobic power and identify the methods that can be used to measure this parameter in athletes with spinal cord injury and cerebral palsy.

5. Discuss the central and peripheral factors that determine the maximal aerobic power. How do these factors affect the peak oxygen uptake in individuals with quadriplegia and paraplegia?

6. How accurate are standardized laboratory fitness tests in predicting wheelchair racing performance in athletes with spinal cord injury and cerebral palsy?

7. Use the principles and components of physical training identified in this chapter to develop a year-round fitness training programme to enhance the aerobic and anaerobic fitness in wheelchair athletes with spinal cord injury and cerebral palsy.

References

American College of Sports Medicine. (1990). Position stand on the recommended quantity and quality of exercise for developing and maintaining cardiorespiratory and muscular fitness in healthy adults. *Medicine and Science in Sports and Exercise, 22*, 265–74.

Asayama, K., Nakamura, Y., Ogata, H., Hatada, K., Okuma, H., and Deguchi, Y. (1985). Physical fitness of paraplegics in full wheelchair marathon racing. *Paraplegia, 23*, 277–87.

Astrand, P.O., and Rodahl, K. (1986). *Textbook of work physiology: Physiological bases of exercise* (3rd ed.). New York: McGraw-Hill.

Banister, E.W., Carter, J.B., and Zarkadus, P.C. (1999). Training theory and taper: Validation in triathlon athletes. *European Journal of Applied Physiology, 79*, 182–92.

Bar-Or, O. (1987) The Wingate anaerobic test: An update on methodology, reliability and validity. *Sports Medicine, 4*, 381–97.

Barron, G.L., Noakes, T.D., Levy, W., Smith, C., and Millar, R.P. (1985). Hypothalmic dysfunction in overtrained athletes. *Journal of Clinical Endocrinology and Metabolism, 60*, 803–6.

Bernard, P.L., Mercier, J., Varray, A., and Prefaut, C. (2000). Influence of lesion level on the cardioventilatory adaptations in paraplegic wheelchair athletes during muscular exercise. *Spinal Cord, 38*, 16–25.

Bhambhani, Y., Burnham, R., Wheeler, G., Eriksson, P., Holland, L.J., and Steadward, R. (1995a) Ventilatory threshold in untrained and endurance trained quadriplegics during wheelchair exercise. *Adapted Physical Activity Quarterly, 12*, 333–43.

Bhambhani, Y., Burnham, R.S., Wheeler, G.D., Eriksson, P., Holland, L.J., and Steadward, R.D. (1995b). Physiological correlates of wheelchair racing performance in trained quadriplegics. *Canadian Journal of Applied Physiology, 20*, 65–77.

Bhambhani, Y., Eriksson, P., and Steadward, R. (1991). Reliability of peak physiological responses during wheelchair ergometry in persons with spinal cord injury. *Archives of Physical Medicine and Rehabilitation, 71*, 559–62.

Bhambhani, Y., Holland, L., Eriksson, P., and Steadward, R. (1994). Physiological responses during wheelchair racing in quadriplegics and paraplegics. *Paraplegia, 32*, 253–60.

Bhambhani, Y., Holland, L., and Steadward, R. (1993). Anaerobic threshold in wheelchair athletes with cerebral palsy: Validity and reliability. *Archives of Physical Medicine and Rehabilitation, 74*, 305–11.

Bhambhani, Y., Holland, L., and Steadward, R. (1992). Validity and reliability of the maximal aerobic power in cerebral palsied wheelchair athletes. *Archives of Physical Medicine and Rehabilitation, 73*, 246–52.

Boninger, M.L., Cooper, R.A., Robertson, R.N., and Shimada, S.D. (1997). Three-dimensional pushrim forces during two speeds of wheelchair propulsion. *American Journal of Physical Medicine and Rehabilitation, 76,* 420–26.

Borg, G.A. (1982). Psychophysical bases of perceived exertion. *Medicine and Science in Sports and Exercise, 14,* 377–81.

Campbell, A.G., Williams, C., and Lakomy, H.K.A. (1997). Physiological responses of wheelchair athletes at percentages of top speed. *British Journal of Sports Medicine, 31,* 36–40.

Canadian Society for Exercise Physiology. (1998). Recommendations for the fitness assessment, programming and counselling for persons with a disability. *Canadian Journal of Applied Physiology, 23,* 119–30.

Chow, J.W., and Mindock, L.A. (1999). Discus throwing performances and medical classification of wheelchair athletes. *Medicine and Science in Sports and Exercise, 31,* 1272–79.

Cooney, M., and Walker, J.B. (1986). Hydraulic resistance exercise benefits cardiovascular fitness of spinal cord injured. *Medicine and Science in Sports and Exercise, 18,* 522–25.

Cooper, R.A. (1992). The contribution of selected anthropometric and physiological variables to 10K performance of wheelchair users: A preliminary study. *Journal of Rehabilitation Research and Development, 29,* 29–24.

Corcoran, P.J., Goldman, R.F., Hoerner, E.F., Kling, C., Knuttgen, H.G., Marquis, B., McCann, B.C., and Rossier, A.B. (1980). Sports medicine and the physiology of wheelchair marathon racing. *Orthopedic Clinics of North America, 11,* 697–716.

Coutts, K.D., and McKenzie, D.C. (1995). Ventilatory threshold during wheelchair exercise in individuals with spinal cord injuries. *Paraplegia, 33,* 419–22.

Coutts, K.D., and Shultz, R.W. (1988). Analysis of wheelchair track performances. *Medicine and Science in Sports and Exercise, 20,* 188–94.

Coutts, K.D., and Stogryn, J.L. (1987). Aerobic and anaerobic power of Canadian wheelchair track athletes. *Medicine and Science in Sports and Exercise, 19,* 62–65.

Coyle, E.F., Coggan, A.R., Hopper, M.H., and Walters, T.J. (1988). Determinants of endurance in well-trained cyclists. *Journal of Applied Physiology, 64,* 2622–30.

Crews, D.L. (1982). Physiological profile of wheelchair marathon racers. *Physician and Sports Medicine, 10,* 243–49.

Curtis, K.A., and Dillon, D.A. (1985). Survey of wheelchair athletic injuries: Common patterns and prevention. *Paraplegia, 23,* 170–85.

Dallmeijer, A.J., Kappe, Y.J., Veeger, H.E.J., Janssen, T.W.J., and van der Woude, L.H.V. (1994). Anaerobic power output and propulsion technique in spinal cord injured subjects during wheelchair ergometry. *Journal of Rehabilitation Research and Development, 31,* 120–28.

Davis, G., Plyley, M.J., and Shephard, R.J. (1991). Gains of cardiorespiratory fitness with arm-crank training in spinally disabled men. *Canadian Journal of Sport Sciences, 16,* 64–72.

Davis, G., Shephard, R.J., and Leenen, F. (1987). Cardiac effects of short-term arm-crank training in paraplegics: Echocardiographic evidence. *European Journal of Applied Physiology, 56,* 90–96.

Davis, G.M., and Shephard, R.J. (1988). Cardiorespiratory fitness in highly active versus inactive paraplegics. *Medicine and Science in Sports and Exercise, 20,* 463–68.

DiCarlo, S.E., Supp, M.D., Taylor, H.C. (1983). Effect of arm ergometry training on physical work capacity of individuals with spinal cord injuries. *Physical Therapy, 63,* 1104–07.

Dishman, R.K., Patton, R.W., Smith, J., Weinberg, R., and Jackson, A. (1987). Using perceived exertion to monitor and prescribe exercise training heart rate. *International Journal of Sports Medicine, 8,* 208–13.

Dwyer, G.B., and McMahon, A.D. (1994). Ventilatory threshold and peak exercise responses in athletes with CP during treadmill and cycle ergometry. *Adapted Physical Activity Quarterly, 11,* 329–34.

Eriksson, P., Lofstrom, L., and Ekblom, B. (1988). Aerobic power during maximal exercise in untrained and well-trained persons with quadriplegia and paraplegia. *Scandinavian Journal of Rehabilitation Medicine, 20,* 141–47.

Farrell, P.A., Wilmore, J.H., Coyle, E.F., Billing, E.F. and Cosill, D.L. (1979). Plasma lactate accumulation and distance running performance. *Medicine and Science in Sports and Exercise, 11,* 338–44.

Fernandez, J.E., and Pitetti, K.H. (1993). Training of ambulatory individuals with cerebral palsy. *Archives of Physical Medicine and Rehabilitation, 74,* 468–72.

Ferrara, M., Buckley, W.E., McCann, B.C., Limbird, T.J., Powell, J.W., and Robl, R. (1992). The injury experience of the competitive athlete with a disability: Prevention implications. *Medicine and Science in Sports and Exercise, 24,* 184–88.

Figoni, S.F. (1993). Exercise responses and quadriplegia. *Medicine and Science in Sports and Exercise, 25,* 433–41.

Figoni, S.F., Boileau, R.A., Massey, B.H., and Larsen, J.R. (1988). Physiological responses of quadriplegic and able-bodied men during exercise at the same VO_2. *Adapted Physical Activity Quarterly, 5,* 130–39.

Flandrois, R., Grandmontagne, M., Gerin, H., Mayet, M.H., Jehl, J.L., and Eyssette, M. (1986). Aerobic performance capacity in paraplegic subjects. *European Journal of Applied Physiology, 55,* 604–9.

Franklin, B.A., Swantek, K.I., Grais, S.L., and Johnstone, K.S. (1990). Field test estimation of maximal oxygen consumption in wheelchair users. *Archives of Physical Medicine and Rehabilitation, 71,* 574–78.

Gass, G.C., and Camp, E.M. (1988). Physiological characteristics of trained Australian paraplegic and tetraplegic subjects. *Medicine and Science in Sports and Exercise, 11,* 256–59.

Gass, G.C., and Camp, E.M. (1987). Effects of prolonged exercise in highly trained traumatic paraplegic men. *Journal of Applied Physiology, 63,* 1846–52.

Gayle, G.W., Pohlman, R.L., and Glaser, R.M. (1990). Cardiorespiratory and perceptual responses to arm-crank and wheelchair exercise using various handrims in male paraplegics. *Research Quarterly for Sports and Exercise, 61,* 224–32.

Glaser, R.M. (1985). Exercise and locomotion for the spinal cord injured. In R.L. Terjung (Ed.), *Exercise and Sports Sciences Reviews, Vol. 13,* pp. 263–303. New York: Macmillan.

Gollnick, P., and Hermansen, L. (1973). Biochemical adaptation to exercise: Anaerobic metabolism. In J. Wilmore (Ed.), *Exercise and Sport Sciences Reviews, Vol. 1,* pp. 1–39. New York: Academic Press.

Grimby, G., Broberg, C., Krotkiewska, I., and Krotiewska, M. (1976). Muscle fibre composition in patients with traumatic cord lesion. *Scandinavian Journal of Rehabilitation Medicine, 8,* 37–42.

Hartmann, U., and Mester, J. (2000). Training and over-training markers in selected sport events. *Medicine and Science in Sports and Exercise, 32,* 209–15.

Hartung, G., Lally, D., and Blancq, R. (1993). Comparison of treadmill exercise testing protocols for wheelchair users. *European Journal of Applied, 66,* 362–65.

Hooker, S.P., Greenwood, J.D., Hatae, D.T., Husson, R.P., Matthiesen, T.L., and Waters, A.R. (1993). Oxygen uptake and heart rate relationship in persons with spinal cord injury. *Medicine and Science in Sports and Exercise, 25,* 1115–19.

Hooker, S.P., and Wells, C.L. (1989). Effects of low- and moderate-intensity training in spinal cord injured persons. *Medicine and Science in Sports and Exercise, 21,* 18–22.

Hooker, S.P., and Wells, C.L. (1990). Physiologic response of elite paraplegic road racers to prolonged exercise. *Journal of the American Paraplegia Society, 13,* 72–77.

Hooker, S.P., and Wells, C.L. (1992). Aerobic power of competitive paraplegic road racers. *Paraplegia, 30,* 428–36.

Hopman, M.T.E. (1994). Circulatory responses during arm exercise in individuals with paraplegia. *International Journal of Sports Medicine, 15,* 126–31.

Hopman, M.T.E., Oeseburg, B., and Binkhorst, R. (1992). Cardiovascular responses in paraplegic subjects during arm exercise. *European Journal of Applied, 65,* 73–78.

Hopman, M.T.E., Pistorius, M., Kamerbeck, I.C.E., and Binkhorst, R. (1993). Cardiac output in paraplegic subjects at high exercise intensities. *European Journal of Applied Physiology, 66,* 531–35.

Huonker, M., Schmid, A., Sorichter, S., Schmidt-Trucksab, A., Mirosek, P., and Keul, J. (1998). Cardiovascular differences between sedentary and wheelchair-trained subjects with paraplegia. *Medicine and Science in Sports and Exercise, 30,* 609–13.

Hutzler, Y. (1993). Physical performance of elite wheelchair basketball players in arm-cranking and in selected wheeling tasks. *Paraplegia, 31,* 255–61.

Hutzler, Y. (1998). Anaerobic fitness testing of wheelchair users. *Sports Medicine, 25,* 101–13.

Hutzler, Y., Grunze, M., and Kaiser, R. (1995). Physiological and dynamic responses to maximal velocity wheelchair ergometry. *Adapted Physical Activity Quarterly, 12,* 344–61.

Hutzler, Y., Ochana, S., Bolotin, R., and Kalina, E. (1998). Aerobic and anaerobic arm-cranking power outputs of males with lower limb impairments: Relationship with sport participation intensity, age, impairment and functional classification. *Spinal Cord, 36,* 205–12.

Hutzler, Y., Vanlandewijck, Y., and Van Vlierberghe, M. (2000). Anaerobic performance of older female and male wheelchair basketball players on a mobile wheelchair ergometer. *Adapted Physical Activity Quarterly, 17,* 450–65.

Ide, M., Ogata, H., Kobayashi, M., Tajima, F., and Hatada, K. (1994). Anthropometric features of wheelchair marathon race competitors with spinal cord injuries. *Paraplegia, 32,* 174–79.

International Paralympic Committee. (2000a). *The Paralympian: Newsletter of the International Paralympic Committee, No. 4.*

International Paralympic Committee. (2000b). *International Paralympic Committee Handbook* (2nd ed.), Part I, Section II. Bonn: Author.

Jacobs, I. (1987). Sprint training effects on muscle myoglobin, enzymes, fibre types, and blood lactate. *Medicine and Science in Sports and Exercise, 19,* 368–74.

Jacobs, P.L., Nash, M.S., and Rusinowski, J.W. (2001). Circuit training provides cardiorespiratory and strength benefits in persons with paraplegia. *Medicine and Science in Sports and Exercise, 33,* 711–17.

Janssen, T.W., Van-Oers, C., Hollander, A., Veeger, H., and van der Woude, L. (1993). Isometric strength, sprint power, and aerobic power in individuals with spinal cord injury. *Medicine and Science in Sports and Exercise, 25,* 863–70.

Jehl, J., Gandmontagne, M., Pastene, G., Eysette, M., Flandrois, R., and Coudert, J. (1991). Cardiac output during exercise in paraplegic subjects. *European Journal of Applied Physiology, 62,* 356–60.

Johnson, M.A., Polgar, J., Weightman, D., and Appleton, D. (1973). Data on the distribution of fibres in thirty-six human muscles: An autopsy study. *Journal of Neurological Science, 18,* 111–29.

Jones, J.A. (Ed.). (1988). *Training guide to cerebral palsy sports: The recognized guide of the United States Cerebral Palsy Athletic Association* (3rd ed.). Champaign, IL: Human Kinetics.

Kibbler, W.B., Chandler, E.S., and Straceber, E.S. (1992). Musculoskeletal adaptations and injuries to overtaining. In J. Holloszy (Ed.), *Exercise and Sport Sciences Reviews, Vol. 20*, 99–126. Baltimore: Williams and Wilkins.

Komi, P.A.V. (1986). Muscle fibre types in humans. *Acta Physiologica Scandinavica, 23*, 1–45.

Kuipers, H. (2000). Overtraining: A nightmare for sport practice and a challenge for sport science. In *Pushing the Limits: Proceedings of the Fifth Scientific Congress Sydney 2000 Paralympic Games* (pp. 1–16).

Lakomy, H.K.A. (1987). Treadmill performance and selected physiological characteristics of wheelchair athletes. *British Journal of Sports Medicine, 21*, 130–33.

Lasko-McCarthey, P., and Davis, J.A. (1991a) Protocol dependency of VO_{2max} during arm cycle ergometry in males with quadriplegia. *Medicine and Science in Sports and Exercise, 23*, 1097–101.

Lasko-McCarthey, P., and Davis, J.A. (1991b) Effect of work rate increment on peak oxygen uptake during wheelchair ergometry in men with quadriplegia. *European Journal of Applied Physiology, 63*, 349–53.

Lees, A., and Arthur, S. (1988). An investigation into anaerobic performance of wheelchair athletes. *Ergonomics, 31*, 1529–527.

Lehmann, M., Foster, C., and Keul, J. (1993). Overtraining in endurance athletes: A brief review. *Medicine and Science in Sports and Exercise, 25*, 854–62.

Lin, K., Lai, J., Kao, M., and Lien, I. (1993). Anaerobic threshold and maximal oxygen consumption during arm-cranking exercise in paraplegia. *Archives of Physical Medicine and Rehabilitation, 74*, 515–20.

Liow, D.K., and Hopkins, W.G. (1996). Training practices of athletes with disabilities. *Adapted Physical Activity Quarterly, 13*, 372–81.

Lundberg, A. (1976). Oxygen consumption in relation to workload in students with cerebral palsy. *Journal of Applied Physiology, 40*, 873–75.

Lundberg, A. (1978). Maximal aerobic capacity of young people with spastic cerebral palsy. *Developmental Medicine and Child Neurology, 20*, 205–10.

Lundberg, A. (1984). Longitudinal study of physical work capacity of young people with cerebral palsy. *Developmental Medicine and Child Neurology, 26*, 328–34.

MacDougall, J.D., Wenger, H.J., Green, H.J. (Eds). (1991). *Physiological testing of the high-performance athlete* (2nd ed.). Champaign, IL: Human Kinetics.

Martin, T.P., Stein, R.B., Hoeppner, P.H., and Reid, D.C. (1992). Influence of electrical stimulation on the morphological and metabolic properties of paralysed muscle. *Journal of Applied Physiology, 72*, 1393–400.

Maud, P.J., and Foster, C. (Eds). (1995). *Physiological assessment of human fitness.* Champaign, IL: Human Kinetics.

McArdle, W.D., Katch, F.I., and Katch, V.L. (1996). *Exercise physiology: Energy, nutrition and human performance* (4th ed.). Baltimore: Williams and Wilkins.

McComas, A.J. (1996). *Skeletal muscle form and function.* Champaign. IL: Human Kinetics.

McLean, K.P., Jones, P.P., and Skinner, J.S. (1995). Exercise prescription for sitting and supine exercise in subjects with quadriplegia. *Medicine and Science in Sports and Exercise, 27*, 15–21.

McLean, K.P., and Skinner, J.S. (1995). Effect of body training position on outcomes of an aerobic training study on individuals with quadriplegia. *Archives of Physical Medicine and Rehabilitation, 76*, 139–50.

Miles, D.S., Sawka, M.N., Wilde, W., Durbin, R.J., Gotshall, R.W., and Glaser, R.M. (1982). Pulmonary function changes in wheelchair athletes subsequent to exercise training. *Ergonomics, 25*, 239–46.

Mohr, T., Andersen, J.L., Biering-Sorensen, F., Galbo, H., Bangsbo, J. Wagner, A., and Kjaer, M. (1997). Long-term adaptation to electrically induced cycle training in severe spinal cord injured individuals. *Spinal Cord, 35*, 1–16.

Mossberg, K., Willman, C., Topor, M.A., Crook, H., and Patak, S. (1999). Comparison of asynchronous versus synchronous arm-crank ergometry. *Spinal Cord, 37*, 569–74.

Muller, E., Benko, U., Raschner, C., and Schwameider, H. (2000). Specific fitness training and testing in competitive sports. *Medicine and Science in Sports and Exercise, 32*, 216–20.

Neary, J.P., Martin, T.P., Reid, D.C., Burnham, R., and Quinney, H.A. (1992). The effects of a reduced exercise duration taper programme on performance and muscle enzymes of endurance cyclists. *European Journal of Applied Physiology, 65*, 30–36.

O'Connor, T.J., Robertson, R.N., and Cooper, R.A. (1998). Three-dimensional kinematic analysis and physiologic assessment of racing wheelchair propulsion. *Adapted Physical Activity Quarterly, 15*, 1–14.

Poulain, M., Vinet, A., Bernard, P.L., Varray, A. (1999). Reproducibility of the Adapted Leger and Boucher Test for wheelchair-dependent athletes. *Spinal Cord, 37*, 129–35.

Rhodes, E.C., Mckenzie, D.C., Coutts, K.D., and Rogers, A.R. (1981) A field test for the prediction of aerobic capacity in male paraplegics and quadriplegics. *Canadian Journal of Applied Sport Sciences, 6*, 182–86.

Saltin, B., Blomqvist, B., Mitchell, J.H., Johnson, R.L., Wildenthal, K., and Chapman, C.B. (1968). Response to submaximal and maximal exercise after bed-rest and training. *Circulation 38*(Suppl. 7).

Sawka, M.N. (1986). Physiology of upper body exercise. In K. Pandolf (Ed.), *Exercise and Sport Science Reviews, Vol. 14*, 175–211, Baltimore: Williams and Wilkins.

Seip, R.L., Snead, D., Pierce, E.F., Stein, P., and Weltman, A. (1991). Perceptual responses and blood lactate concentration: Effect of training state. *Medicine and Science in Sports and Exercise, 23*, 80–87.

Shephard, R.J. (1990). *Fitness in special populations.* Champaign, IL: Human Kinetics.

Shephard, R.J. (1988). Sports medicine and the wheelchair athlete. *Sports Medicine, 4,* 226–47.

Skrinar, G.S., Evans, W.J., Ornstein, L.J., and Brown, D.A. (1982). Glycogen utilization in wheelchair-dependent athletes. *International Journal of Sports Medicine, 3,* 215–19.

Steadward, R. (1998). Musculoskeletal and neurological disabilities: Implications for fitness appraisal, programming and counselling. *Canadian Journal of Applied Physiology, 23,* 31–165.

Taylor, A.W., McDonnell, E., Royer, D., Loiselle, R., Lush, N., Steadward, R. (1979). Skeletal muscle analysis of wheelchair athletes. *Paraplegia, 17,* 456–60.

Taylor, A.W., McDonnell, E., and Brassard, L. (1986). The effects of an arm ergometer training programme on wheelchair subjects. *Paraplegia, 24,* 105–14.

Tiessen, J.A. (Ed.). (1997). *The triumph of the human spirit: the Atlanta paralympic experience.* Disability Today.

van der Woude, L.H.V., Bakker, W.H., Elkhuizen, J.W., Veeger, H.E.J., and Gwinn, T. (1997). Anaerobic work capacity in elite wheelchair athletes. *American Journal of Physical Medicine and Rehabilitation, 76,* 355–65.

van der Woude, L.H.V., Bakker, W.H., Elkhuizen, J.W., Veeger, H.E.J., and Gwinn, T. (1998). Propulsion technique and anaerobic work capacity in elite wheelchair athletes. *American Journal of Physical Medicine and Rehabilitation, 77,* 222–34.

van der Woude, L.H.V., Veeger, H.E.J., Rozendal, R.H., Van Ingen Schenau, G.J., and Rooth, R. (1990). Wheelchair racing: Effects of rim diametre on physiology and technique. *Medicine and Science in Sports and Exercise, 20,* 492–500.

Van Loan, M.D., McCluer, S., Loftin, J.M., and Boileau, R.A. (1987). Comparison of physiological responses to maximal arm-cranking exercise among able-bodied, paraplegics, and quadriplegics. *Paraplegia, 25,* 397–405.

Vanlandewijck, Y.C., Spaepen, A.J., Lysens, R.J. (1995). Relationship between the level of physical impairment and sports performance in elite wheelchair basketball athletes. *Adapted Physical Activity Quarterly, 12,* 139–50.

Veeger, H.E.J., Hadj Yahmed, M., van der Woude, L., and Charpentier, P. (1991c). Peak oxygen uptake and maximal power output of Olympic wheelchair dependent athletes. *Medicine and Science in Sports and Exercise, 23,* 1201–9.

Veeger, H.E.J., Lute, E.M., Roelveldt, K., van der Woude, L.H.V. (1992). Differences in performance between untrained and trained subjects during a 30-s sprint test in a wheelchair ergometer. *European Journal of Applied Physiology, 64,* 158–64.

Veeger, H.E.J., van der Woude, L.H.V., and Rozendal, R.H. (1991a). Wheelchair propulsion technique at different speeds. *Scandinavian Journal of Rehabilitation Medicine, 21,* 197–203.

Veeger, H.E.J., van der Woude, L.H.V., and Rozendal, R.H. (1991b). Within-cycle characteristics of the wheelchair push in sprinting on a wheelchair ergometer. *Medicine and Science in Sports and Exercise, 23,* 264–72.

Vinet, A., Bernard, P.L., Poulain, M., Varray, A., Le Gallais, D., Micallef, J.P. (1996). Validation of an incremental field test for the direct assessment of peak oxygen uptake in wheelchair-dependent athletes. *Spinal Cord, 34,* 288–91.

Vinet, A., Le Gallais, D., Bernard, P.L., Poulain, M., Varray, A., Mercier, J., Micallef, J.P. (1997). Aerobic metabolism and cardioventilatory responses in paraplegic athletes during incremental wheelchair exercise. *European Journal of Applied Physiology, 76,* 455–61.

Wasserman K. (1986). The anaerobic threshold: Definition, physiological significance, and identification. *Advances in Cardiology, 35,* 1–23.

Wenger, H.A., and Reed, D.C. (1973). Metabolic factors associated with muscular fatigue in anaerobic and aerobic work. *Canadian Journal of Applied Sports Sciences, 1,* 25–31.

Wicks, J.R., Oldridge, N.B., Cameron, B.J., and Jones, N.L. (1983). Arm-cranking and wheelchair ergometry in elite spinal cord injured athletes. *Medicine and Science in Sports and Exercise, 15,* 224–31.

CHAPTER 29

Technological Developments in Disability Sport

Stéphane Perreault

Learning Objectives

- To understand the place of technology in disability sport.
- To define and differentiate between an orthosis, a prosthesis, and a wheelchair.
- To describe the social factors that have influenced technological changes in disability sport.
- To describe the consequences of technological changes with respect to prostheses and wheelchairs.
- To cite the evidence relating the role of technology on performance in disability sport.
- To be knowledgeable of the ethical concerns related to technology and performance in disability sport.

Introduction

More and more athletes are turning to technology to find that elusive fraction of a second that can make the difference between a gold or a silver medal. As athletes strive towards fulfilling the *Citius, Altius, Fortius* (Swifter, Higher, Stronger) ideal, ethical questions are now being raised with respect to the application of technology in sport (Freeman 1991; Froes 1997). The purpose of this chapter is to show how this issue applies to disability sport. More precisely, we will try to show how technology has evolved in the field of prosthetics and wheelchair design. Furthermore, we will attempt to show how technological improvements have influenced disability sport performance. Finally, we will attempt to show how continued technological improvements in sport might ultimately influence disability sport.

Technology and Disability Sport

"It looks good at NASA One." *Flight Com*

"Roger." *B-52 Pilot*

"BCS Arm switch is on." *B-52 Pilot*

"Okay, Victor." *Flight Com*

"Lining Rocket Arm switch is on." *B-52 Pilot*

"Here comes the throttle." *B-52 Pilot*

"Circuit breakers in." *B-52 Pilot*

"We have separation." *Steve Austin*

"Roger." *SR-71 Chase Plane Pilot*

"Inboard and outboards are on." *B-52 Pilot*

"I'm comin' forward with the side stick." *B-52 Pilot*

"Looks good." *Flight Com*

"Ah, Roger." *B-52 Pilot*

"I've got a blow-out in damper three!" *Steve Austin*

"Get your pitch to zero." *SR-71 Chase Plane Pilot*

"Pitch is out! I can't hold altitude!" *Steve Austin*

"Correction, Alpha Hold is off. . . Turn selectors… Emergency!" *B-52 Pilot*

"Flight Com! I can't hold it! She's breaking up, she's break—" *Steve Austin*

"Steve Austin. Astronaut. A man barely alive." *Narrator (Harve Bennett)*

"Gentlemen, we can rebuild him. We have the technology. We have the capability to make the world's first bionic man. Steve Austin will be that man. Better than he was before. Better… stronger… faster." *Oscar Goldman*

Every Sunday in the early 1970s, these words served as the introduction to a television series entitled *The Six Million Dollar Man* (Bennett 1973). Steve Austin, a man barely alive as a result of the crash described above, was fitted with two bionic legs, a bionic arm, and a bionic eye, in order to replace the loss of his legs, right arm, and left eye. These cybernetic implants enabled Steve Austin to run faster and jump higher than any human. With the help of his right arm, he also could lift an incredible amount of weight and bend steel with the greatest of ease. His bionic eye gave him the opportunity to see further and with more precision than the normal human eye, and it was so technologically advanced that he could even see at night.

Let us now move forward in time. In *Star Wars: The Empire Strikes Back* (Kershner, 1980), Luke Skywalker must battle the dark forces of the Empire. Towards the end of the movie, he fights his evil father Darth Vader. During this duel, Luke Skywalker's hand is severed by Darth Vader's lightsabre. Luke Skywalker narrowly escapes, is rescued by the crew of the *Millennium Falcon*, and is immediately taken to a medical facility to mend his injuries. The movie ends with a robot testing the sensitivity of Luke's new cybernetic hand.

> **1** What do *The Six Million Dollar Man* and *Star Wars* have to do with technological developments in disability sport?

These two examples underscore three important points with respect to the relationship between technology and disability. The first is that, in both examples, advanced technology is used to replace various body parts. Technology in these examples is portrayed as a tool that can help people regain the functional use of an arm, a leg, or even an eye. Thus, the use of technology is intimately associated with the idea of functionality. Although important technological changes have occurred in disability sport, they are slowly approaching those portrayed in our two examples. Still, technological improvements in the area of disability sport are now

Figure 29.1 The Functionality Continuum

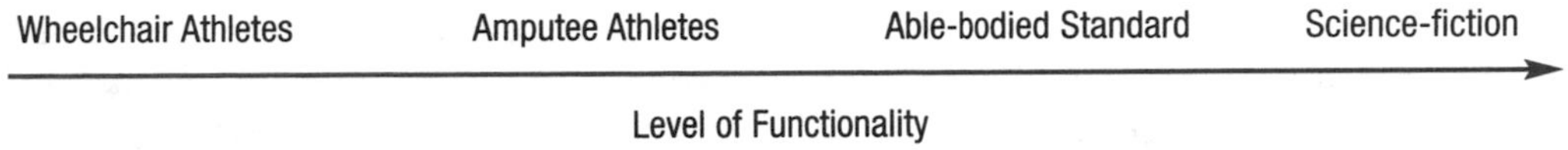

Wheelchair Athletes   Amputee Athletes   Able-bodied Standard   Science-fiction

→

Level of Functionality

permitting more and more people to take part in physical activity. With recent technological advances, one can even wonder if, someday, technology will be sufficiently advanced to perform the feats shown on certain TV shows (e.g., *Dark Angel* [Cameron 2000] and *Star Trek: The Next Generation* [Roddenberry 1987] and in certain science-fiction movies (e.g., *Terminator 2: Judgment Day* [Cameron 1991]).

A second point of interest which is related to the first is that, in both examples, prosthetic devices are fitted to mimic or even surpass human biomechanical standards. Both examples hint at the idea that technology can reproduce or even extend human capabilities. Put another way, these examples suggest that technology could even make a person more functional than an individual without a disability. Thus, these examples suggest that technology has an effect on adapted sport performance. Although the technological changes highlighted in these examples are ahead of their time, they point to an important question. With respect to modern day technology, how has technology influenced adapted sport performance? For example, are track and field athletes who have an amputation as functional as track and field athletes who are able-bodied? Do today's athletes who use a wheelchair push their wheelchairs faster than athletes did twenty years ago? Based on the preceding questions, it thus seems important to ascertain the impact of technology on adapted sports participants.

Finally, in our two introductory examples (and in most science-fiction novels, TV series, or movies) an 'able-bodied standard' is used to evaluate what is functional. By able-bodied standard we mean that the so-called "able-bodied individual" (i.e., person with two legs,

two arms, two ears, etc.) is used to define what is functional (see figure 29.1).

Notice that the creators of *The Six Million Dollar Man* did not choose to portray Steve Austin as an individual who is in a wheelchair. Implicitly, these science-fiction series are informing people that future technology will help individuals attain (or even surpass) the able-bodied standard and possibly create a new category of individuals. See Chapter 5 (Shogan). A closer inspection of figure 29.1 suggests that athletes who use a wheelchair are at the lower end of the continuum. Although talk of neural regeneration has surfaced in medicine (Nichols 2000) and popular television series such as *Star Trek: The Next Generation*, medicine cannot make individuals who have experienced a spinal cord lesion as functional as individuals who have experienced an amputation. No prosthesis has been developed to counter this type of injury. However, individuals who have experienced a spinal cord injury can still take part in physical activity by using various apparatuses such as wheelchairs, sleds, and adapted bicycles. Technological improvements (especially in the area of materials used to design these devices) have occurred in the area of wheelchair and prosthetic design. Individuals who have a disability can run and play baseball with specially designed prostheses. Also, wheelchair users can also play a variety of sports such as basketball, rugby, and tennis. These changes are now making individuals more and more functional in their respective sports.

In summary, the two examples presented in our introduction suggest that technology is associated with the idea of functionality. More precisely, a positive linear relationship between technology and functionality seems to be postulated in these examples. As can be

Figure 29.2 Linear Relationship between Technology and Functionality

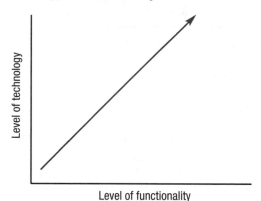

seen in figure 29.2, the more technology a society has, the more functional it can make individuals who have various medical conditions or who have experienced certain types of injuries.

To show how technology has influenced disability sports across time, this chapter will be divided into four sections. In the first section, various terms will be defined in order to provide the reader with a clear conceptual foundation. In the second section, historical changes will be used to generate a model that explains four technological changes which have arisen in the field of prosthetics and wheelchair design. In the third section, track and field results (i.e., double amputee 100-metre race and wheelchair marathon results) from the past twenty years will be presented to demonstrate how technology has influenced the athletic performance of individuals who have a disability. In the final section of this chapter, we will attempt to show how continued technological improvements in disability sport raise some important ethical questions (Freeman 1991; Froes 1997). For example, if technology could adequately mimic human biomechanical standards, should technologically equipped athletes perform side-by-side against athletes who are able-bodied? The purpose of this section will not be to try to answer such questions but rather to try to present some of the potential repercussions of technological advances in disability sport, in order to foster classroom discussion.

Definitions of Key Concepts

Before we proceed to explain how prosthetics, wheelchairs, and technology are linked, we would like to define the terms *orthosis*, *prosthesis*, *wheelchair*, and *technology*.

Some of you may have worn an orthosis. For example, if you have sprained your ankle often enough while practicing a particular sport and are still competing in that sport, you may be playing with a specially designed ankle brace. Thus, an orthosis refers to a brace. A brace serves to assist a particular body part in alleviating a motor deficiency. A prosthesis does not serve this function. Rather, a prosthesis serves as a replacement for a particular body part. A prosthesis can thus be defined as an external artificial body part. In short, an orthosis supplements while a prosthesis replaces.

Another concept that needs to be defined is the term *wheelchair*. It is probably safe to say that everyone knows what a wheelchair is. A wheelchair is a chair mounted on two large bicycle-like wheels. Two smaller wheels are usually placed in front of the chair in order to assure stability. What might not be as clear is who uses a wheelchair. Most of you would probably agree that wheelchairs are used by individuals who have a disability. Thus, a variety of groups such as rugby players, track and field athletes, individuals who have cerebral palsy, and basketball players all take part in disability sport with this particular apparatus. However, you might be surprised to find that, in Canada, wheelchairs are not strictly reserved for individuals with disability. Wheelchairs are also being used by able-bodied individuals who play wheelchair basketball. Wheelchairs, at least in wheelchair basketball, are no longer only associated with individuals who have a disability. In the sport of wheelchair basketball, the wheelchair has become a tool which can be used by all to compete in this sport.

The final concept that needs to be defined is *technology*. According to the *American Heritage Dictionary* (1985), technology can be defined as "the application of science, especially to industrial or commercial objectives."

Figure 29.3 A Model of Technological Changes Associated with Prostheses and Wheelchairs

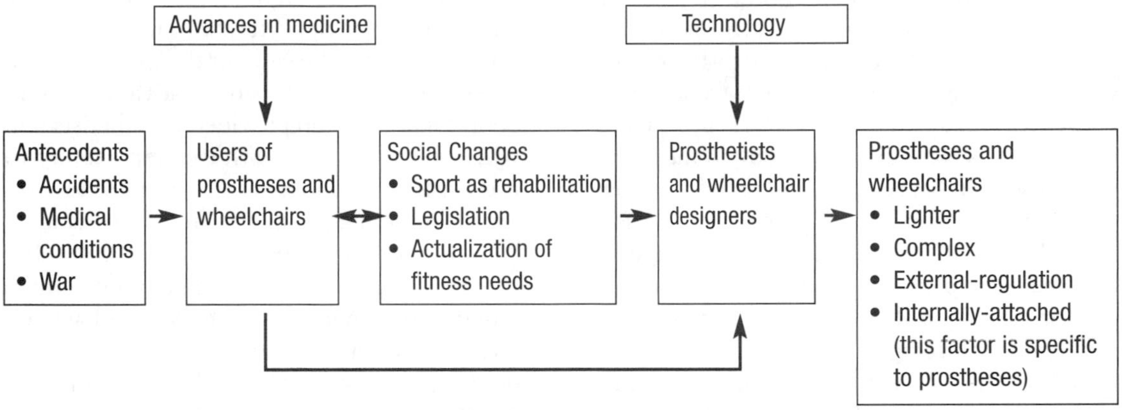

This definition is broad but it will help us to better understand the link between technology and functionality. Recall our two examples in the introduction. We hinted at the idea that technology and functionality are strongly associated. Although there is no denying that technological changes in the field of adapted physical activity have a commercial aim, the main objective of technology in adapted physical activity is to make individuals more functional (i.e., increase participation and performance to similar levels as athletes who are able-bodied). It is therefore not surprising to find that these two concepts are so intertwined. Thus, when we use the term *technology* in this chapter, we are referring to the application of science (i.e., various scientific methods and knowledge about materials) to orthoses, prostheses, and wheelchairs with the objective of making the users of these devices more functional.

Having defined our concepts, we will now concentrate our attention in the upcoming section on the relationship between prosthetics, wheelchairs, and technology. Undoubtedly, technological changes have also occurred in the area of orthotics, but due to space limitations we have chosen to direct our attention to the relationship between prosthetics, wheelchairs, and technology.

A Model of Technological Changes Associated With Prostheses and Wheelchairs

In this section, specific historical events will be presented to highlight how technology has influenced prostheses and wheelchairs. By using key historical events, we will try to demonstrate the impact of various events on prosthetists and wheelchair designers. In order to achieve this objective, a model of technological change associated with prostheses and wheelchairs will be presented (see figure 29.3). According to this model, specific antecedents events (i.e., accidents, certain medical conditions, and war) have caused individuals to become users of prostheses and wheelchairs. It should also be noted that advances in medicine have increased the survival rate of the users of these devices. In turn, this increase in the survival rate of individuals using these devices has sparked the development of new attitudes (i.e., sport as a rehabilitation tool, new laws, and the actualization of fitness needs of adapted sport participants). Finally, these social changes have influenced designers of prostheses and wheelchairs.

Based on figure 29.3, three important changes have occurred to prostheses and wheelchairs across time as a result of prosthetists and wheelchair designers using various technological advances. Prostheses and wheelchairs have become lighter, more complex, and externally-regulated. By externally-regulated, we mean that some prostheses and wheelchairs are now being controlled with computer chips and motors. The onus of using these devices is no longer directly in the hands of the users. In some instances, technology has taken over the burden of propelling the user (i.e., electric wheelchair for individuals who have cerebral palsy) or modifying the response of a prosthetic foot as it lands on the ground. A fourth technological change, which seems to only apply to the area of prosthetics, is that more and more prosthetists are now considering attaching prostheses internally. We will expand on this notion later in the chapter.

ANTECEDENTS TO DISABILITY

There are three causes of diability and of the resulting need for people to use prostheses or wheelchairs: accidents, medical conditions, and war injuries. Farm accidents claim many limbs, and car accidents are often responsible for spinal cord injuries. Children who play in train yards sometimes get their limbs severed when a train departs unexpectedly. Various medical conditions (see Chapter 4 (Squair and Groeneveld)) can force individuals to rely on prostheses or wheelchairs. War exposes people to gun fire, bomb shells, and land mines which can result in the loss of limbs or spinal cord injuries.

While these antecedents to disability directly influence the use of prostheses and wheelchairs, it is important to consider how medical advances enter the equation. Two hundred years ago, individuals who underwent an amputation usually died as a result of the infection generated by the surgery. Since very few people survived this ordeal, there was no real need for prostheses. For those who survived, simple prostheses were created to meet their needs. A similar story can be told about wheelchair design. Prior to the end of World War II, the life expectancy for a spinal cord injury victim was approximately two to three years (Higgs 2000a). Generally, patients were expected to die from an infection of the paralyzed bladder or kidney failure.

Individuals with spinal cord injuries were not surviving long enough to give designers of wheelchairs the opportunity to use new technologies, as was the case for designers of prostheses. As a result of medical advances, more people survived and provided prosthetists and wheelchair designers with the opportunity to use existing technologies in order to develop more functional prostheses and wheelchairs.

Although the sheer increase in the number of users of prostheses and wheelchairs induced designers of prostheses and wheelchairs to work on their respective endeavours, we believe that the designers of such adapted sport equipment were motivated to perfect prostheses and wheelchairs as a result of important social changes. The promotion by Sir Guttmann of the idea that sport could be used as a rehabilitation tool greatly influenced the world of adapted sport (see Chapter 26 (Steadward and Foster)) and led to the creation of the Stoke Mandeville Games in 1948. More importantly, the Stoke Mandeville Games became an international event in 1952, resulting in more and more participants taking part in adapted sport, which, in turn, once again influenced designers of prostheses and wheelchairs.

Legislation (see Chapter 6 (McPherson, Wheeler, and Foster)) and the need to be physically fit (see Chapter 22 (Seidl)) also affected designers of prostheses and wheelchairs. Legislation helped individuals with a disability get access to more sporting facilities (see Chapter 6 (McPherson, Wheeler and Foster)). Furthermore, as users of prostheses and wheelchairs grew in number, these two groups developed the need to compete and to partake in daily leisure activities. Both of these factors promoted modifications in the sport environment (i.e., make existing physical education facilities more accessible) in order to welcome individuals with a disability. For example, at the Université de Sherbrooke the weight room is completely accessible and adapted to the needs of wheelchair track and field athletes. In turn, changes in the sporting environment and attitudes impacted on prosthetists and wheelchair designers.

DESIGNING PROSTHESES AND WHEELCHAIRS

In this section, we will highlight specific technological changes that have occurred in disability sport and the consequences of those changes. According to Froes (1997), one of the most important technological changes in disability sport is the use of advanced materials such as polymers, ceramics, carbon fibres, and so on, which have mechanical and physical characteristics well in excess of conventional materials such as steel or aluminium. These materials are stronger, last longer, and withstand more punishment than steel or aluminium. For example, many Paralympic athletes run with high-tech prostheses made of these materials. Froes (1997) states that Paralympic athlete "Volpentest runs on carbon-graphite feet bolted to carbon-composite sockets (built by Flex-Foot) that encase his legs." The material in Volpentest's prostheses propels him forward as he punches the track with the specially designed prostheses. Froes (1997) claims that this technology catapults users more efficiently than if they were running on two human feet. Finally, another advantage of using such materials is that prostheses can be made to be springy for sprinters or shock-absorbing for long-distance runners.

A second important technological change in disability sport is the use of computers to help design prostheses and wheelchairs. Once again, this is quite apparent in the field of prosthetics where computers are now being used to help carve sockets. Computer chips are also being integrated into the prosthesis itself to help regulate walking. Another important technological change which seems to be specific to prosthetics is osseointegration, where titanium-based prostheses are attached directly to residual limbs. More information with respect to these changes will be presented later on in this section.

Before we proceed to explain the consequences of technological changes in disability sport, it is important to note that prosthesis and wheelchair designers are constructing these devices with technology that has been around for thirty to forty years. For example, the endolite adaptive prosthesis has successfully integrated hydraulics, pneumatics, and computer technology. According to Pike (2000a),

> In the Adaptive Prosthesis from Blatchford, a hydraulic and pneumatic system is controlled by two stepper motor valves operated by the microprocessor. The hydraulic part of the system controls stance, flexion, and terminal impact. The pneumatic part of the system controls swing phase and extension assistance.

Technological changes are occurring in the field of prosthetics and wheelchair design but they are not as rapid as many believe (*American Online Amputee Journal* 2000). Thus, what seems new can be old at times. For the purpose of this chapter, we will try to point out how existing or new technology is helping individuals who have a disability to take part in disability sport.

CONSEQUENCES OF TECHNOLOGICAL CHANGES

Four changes have occurred to prostheses and wheelchairs as a result of designers using technology. Prostheses and wheelchairs have become lighter, more complex, and externally-regulated. The fourth technological change which seems to only apply to the area of prosthetics is that more and more prosthetists are now attaching prostheses internally (i.e., osseointegrated prostheses).

When Lighter Is Better

The materials used to design prostheses and wheelchairs have changed tremendously. According to the historical sketch provided by Pike (2000b), the first record of an iron prosthesis was written between 3500 and 1800 BC. During the Dark Ages, knights were fitted with prostheses made by their armorers. From the 1600s to the early 1800s, prostheses remained heavy and bulky, but new and lighter materials progressively appeared as prostheses evolved. For example, in 1696 a wooden foot was attached to non-locking below-knee prosthesis. In 1863, the rubber foot was patented. In 1912, Charles and Marcel Desoutter constructed the first aluminium prosthesis.

Wheelchairs have also undergone similar changes. The first wheelchairs were made of wood, but today wheelchairs are being made of different metals such as chrome moly, T6 aircraft aluminium, and titanium. By changing the materials used to construct prostheses and wheelchairs, they have become lighter. How much lighter? If we use wheelchairs as an example, the athletes who competed in the first wheelchair games at Stoke Mandeville in 1948 did so in all-purpose wheelchairs that weighed approximately fifty pounds (22.5 kg). Modern track chairs now weigh between ten to twelve pounds (5.5 kg) and are often equipped with carbon fibre spoked wheels (Paciorek 1993).

The changes in the materials used to make prostheses and wheelchairs has had a considerable impact on the users of these devices. For example, early prostheses were made of iron and were quite heavy. Knights fitted with this type of prosthesis could fight but could not perform every-day activities such as walking. The prosthesis was cosmetic rather than functional. As materials became lighter, functionality was greatly improved. It is much easier to walk with a prosthesis weighing four pounds than with one that weighs twenty pounds. Still, lighter materials are only one technological factor which has contributed to greater functionality on the part of individuals using prostheses and wheelchairs.

When Complexity Becomes Synonymous with Functionality

A second important change in prostheses and wheelchairs as a result of technology is that these devices have become more complex. The first prostheses were relatively simple and consisted of wooden legs and hand hooks. Modern prostheses are articulated and responsive (Michael 1989) as a result of advances in biomechanics (i.e., the application of physical laws of motion to the study of biological systems) and kinematics (i.e., the branch of dynamics that deals with acceleration,

displacement, velocity without reference to the forces responsible for motion). For example, in 1956 the SACH (solid ankle cushion heel) foot was developed. The rigid toe lever in the SACH foot permitted rapid acceleration which was very useful for sprinting at that time (Michael 1986). Still, the SACH foot did not respond well to inclines or uneven surfaces. This situation led to the development of the SAFE in 1980 (solid ankle flexible endo-skeleton) foot. The SAFE foot was one of the first energy-storing feet. According to Michael (1986), the flexible plastic spring built into the SAFE foot helps store and use energy when walking or running. More precisely, Michael (1986) states that: "At flat foot, it compresses and stores energy generated as the amputee's body moves forward. At toe off, the energy is released, providing a gentle push similar to that of a normal foot." Today, modern prosthetic feet such as the Flex-Foot utilize graphite composite fibre technology to store energy. They have very large energy potential because they use the entire distance from the tip of the toes to the end of the residual limb for function (Michael 1986).

Prosthetists have adapted existing prostheses to respond to the increased participation in sport of individuals who have an amputation (Michael, Gailey, and Bowker 1990; Radocy 1988). For example, according to Saadah (1992), most individuals who have a below-knee amputation can swim without a prosthesis. However, some of the individuals who have a below-knee amputation find swimming with one leg displeasing because of the imbalance they feel in the water. In response to this situation, prostheses can be adapted by attaching a flipper to the socket of the prosthesis. Prostheses have also been modified for baseball (Truong, Erickson, and Galbreath 1986), rock climbing (Lévesque and Gauthier-Gagnon 1987), and a variety of other sports (Engstrom and Van de Ven 1999; Michael et al. 1990).

Wheelchair designers have made wheelchairs more complex in response to increased demands by wheelchair users. Although the Stoke Mandeville Games became an international event in 1952, wheelchair athletes continued to use an all-purpose wheelchair for the next twenty-eight years. However, in 1980, the first sport wheelchair appeared. Furthermore, with increasing specialization in wheelchair sports, athletes needed wheelchairs that could meet the demands of their sport. The 'simple', all-purpose wheelchair gave way to more complex wheelchairs such as the throwing chair, the racing chair, and the ball game chair (Higgs 1995). In essence, the configuration of the all-purpose chair was altered to meet the demands of particular sports. For example, the throwing chair has no wheels and is fixed to the ground. This modification enables the athlete who uses this piece of equipment to throw further. The racing chair is composed of three wheels and looks like an elongated tricycle. The sleek design permits the athlete to generate more speed. Brakes and a steering mechanism can also be found on this particular sport chair. The ball game chair is the closest relative to the old all-purpose chair. However, some ball game chairs now have five wheels (for basketball) in order to avoid tipping over. This modification also permits greater range of motion for pass reception. This type of chair is also constructed with materials that will be able to sustain a great deal of pounding. For example, wheelchair rugby players are constantly colliding with each other, and wheelchairs have to be constructed to withstand this particular aspect of the game. Finally, athletes who use wheelchairs can also ski and play hockey using specially designed sleds (Porreta 1995). They can also partake in a variety of sports such as mountaineering, cycling by way of arm-cranking, and even racquetball (Sherill 1998).

In summary, wheelchairs and prostheses have evolved to meet the requirements of various sports. Furthermore, prostheses and wheelchairs have evolved even further in that these devices are now being fitted to meet the particular requirements of specific individuals. For example, wheelchair basketball players who have a low classification (i.e., 1 or 2) will have wheelchairs that have an elevated back to enhance stability; this may not be necessary for a player with a high classification (i.e., 4 or 4.5). In short, present-day wheelchairs are very different in comparison to the old standard wheelchair. Still, it is important to note that prostheses and wheelchairs have changed because advanced materials are permitting designers to apply technologies that have been around for quite some time. Once again, what looks new is, in fact, inspired by the past.

When Computers Start Doing the Work

A third technological factor, which we have termed *type of regulation*, is related to the idea that prostheses and wheelchairs have become more complex. As we discussed earlier, the first prostheses and wheelchairs were quite simple, heavy, and required a great deal of work from their users. Specifically, the first prostheses were relatively straight and required the user to adjust his or her walking (or running) pattern accordingly. As prostheses became more articulated in that they better mimicked walking and running patterns, users of these devices gave less thought to these activities. When you walk or run, you don't really pay attention to these activities because they have become automatic. Early prostheses forced users to be active cognitively when they used these devices. In short, early prostheses required internal-regulation (or self-regulation) on the part of their users.

Modern prostheses still require some internal-regulation on the part of their users but not to the same extent as early prostheses. So-called new 'intelligent' prostheses have been created. Individuals who have an amputation can now walk more efficiently with the help of a computer chip. This type of technological change also applies to some extent to wheelchair design. Although most wheelchair athletes who take part in disability sport still regulate the use of their wheelchairs themselves (i.e., individuals still push and control how their wheelchair turns), some adapted physical education participants, such as children with cerebral palsy, may use an electric wheelchair (i.e., external regulation) to move about when they play soccer.

Becoming Attached for Life

Technology has also changed how prostheses are measured and attached to remaining limbs. Prostheses used to be attached to their users with various types of straps. These days, advances in medicine have caused dramatic changes in this area. Computers design and carve models for prosthetic sockets. In order to produce a socket with computer technology, a prosthetist will pass a specially designed pen over the residual limb of an individual who has an amputation. This pen will relay information to a computer that, in turn, will help generate a template of the socket. After the template is generated, the socket can be produced very quickly. According to Ian Jones (personal communication, October 3, 2001), creating a transtibial socket can take less than hour.

Doctors can attach prosthetic devices to residual limbs (i.e., osseointegrated prostheses). This technological change resulted from work done in the field of dentistry. Researchers in this field discovered that it was possible to place titanium cylinders into the jawbone in order to support replacement teeth. This discovery led researchers to attempt to apply this method to other types of prostheses. Although this technique is not for all individuals who have an amputated limb, it has been successfully used in Sweden. Unlike prostheses that rely on a socket for attachment, bone-anchored prostheses are attached directly to the recipient's bone. Thus, this type of prosthesis is not in direct contact with the recipient's skin, which makes it more comfortable to wear (i.e., less pressure, sores, and pain). Research by Brånemark, Bergh, Gunterberg, Rydevik, and Brånemark (2000) indicates that users of such devices state that they walk better, feel more comfortable when sitting, and find it easier to attach and detach their prostheses.

In summary, advances in computer science and medicine are improving the way by which prostheses are attached to individuals who have an amputation. By applying these new technologies, prosthetists have, once again, made the users of such devices more functional.

SUMMARY

The model presented in this section shows how different factors have played a role in the production of technologically advanced prostheses and wheelchairs. The model postulates that medicine and various social attitudes have impacted on prosthetists and wheelchair designers. In turn, designers of these devices have responded by using technology to make prostheses and wheelchairs lighter, more complex, externally-regulated, and prostheses internally-attached.

Technology is continually evolving; no limit appears in sight. Computer and medical sciences are progressing at a rapid pace and their effect on the field of prosthetics and wheelchair design remains to be seen. Regardless of how these sciences evolve, one can clearly see with this brief historical sketch that, by making prostheses and wheelchairs lighter, more complex, externally-regulated, and internally attached (in the case of prostheses), prosthetists and wheelchair designers have improved the functionality of individuals using these devices.

2 To what extent has technology made athletes functional?

3 Where will it all end?

We will address this question in the last section by raising ethical concerns related with the use of technology in sport.

Technology and Performance

In the previous section, we tried to show how various technological trends helped users of prostheses and wheelchairs become more functional. The question that now needs to be asked is to what extent has technology made *individuals* more functional? More precisely, how has technology influenced adapted physical performance?

4 If you were in our position, how would you try to demonstrate this point?

In order to show how technology has influenced performance in disability sport, it might be useful to use time as a comparison factor.

5 Are athletes who have a disability performing better today than twenty years ago?

Another way that might help us to understand how technology has influenced performance in disability sport is by comparing athletes who take part in disability sport with athletes who are able-bodied.

Let us now take a look at various track and field results. In order to ascertain the impact of prosthetic technology in sport, results were taken from the 1980 and 2000 Paralympic and Olympic games for the men's 100-metre dash. The results are plotted in figure 29.4 where Paralympics winning times are plotted against Olympic winning times.[1]

Figure 29.4 reveals that winning times for the 100-metre dash have changed greatly for T44 Paralympic athletes competing in the 100-metre race. In 1980, Denis Lapalme, a Canadian Paralympic athlete, won the event in a time of 16.96 seconds. In 2000, Marlon Ray Shirley, an American Paralympic athlete, won this race in a world record time of 11.09 seconds. If we subtract Shirley's time from Lapalme's time, we see that the time for this particular event has improved by 5.87 seconds (i.e., a 35 percent improvement) in the past twenty years. If we perform the same mathematical operation with the winning times from the Olympic games, times in this event have improved by 0.38 seconds (i.e., a 4 percent improvement).

Another way to look at this graphic is by a making a direct comparison between the two groups (athletes who have an amputation

Figure 29.4 Winning 100-metre Dash Paralympic and Olympic Times

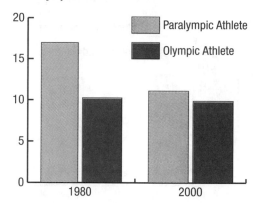

vs. athletes who are able-bodied). How fast do you run the 100-metre dash? Remember that Marlon Ray Shirley is running with a specially designed prosthesis. Could you beat him in the 100-metre dash? It is also possible to compare these times by dividing the Paralympic times by the Olympic times. If we divide British sprinter Allan Wells' winning time in the 1980 Olympic games by Denis Lapalme's 1980 Paralympic time, we end up with a ratio of 0.60. If we apply this rationale once again to the 1996 results (i.e., divide Maurice Green's winning time by Marlon Ray Shirley's time), we end up with a ratio of .89. Notice how this ratio has increased in the last twenty years. Based on these results, one could argue that performances by Paralympic athletes are nearing those of Olympic athletes.

6 Have similar changes occurred in wheelchair sports?

The answer seems to be "yes." Higgs (1995) reports that in 1975 Bob Hall completed the Boston Marathon in a wheelchair in unofficial time[2] of time of 2:40:46 while his winning able-bodied counterpart finished in a time of 2:20:46. He further reports that by

---

1 For the purpose of this section, Paralympic athletes classified as T44 were used (i.e., single below-knee amputation or athletes who can walk with moderately reduced function in one or both legs). It is important to know that this particular system did not exist in 1980 (see Chapter 26 (Steadward and Foster)). After consultation (A. Dean, personal communication, October 3, 2001) we chose to use the winner of the C1 100-metre race.

2 No official time was kept at this race because wheelchair athletes were not allowed to take part in it.

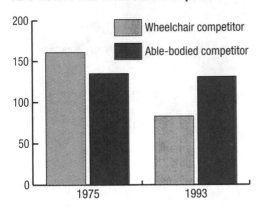

Figure 29.5 Winning Boston Marathon Times for Able-bodied and Wheelchair Competitors

1993 runners who were able-bodied had improved their time by four minutes and thirteen seconds (i.e., 2:16:33); athletes who use a wheelchair in this event improved their time by more than seventy-eight minutes. Based on these results, one can see that athletes who use a wheelchair have exceeded the performance of athletes who are able-bodied in the Boston Marathon.

All of the results shown above suggest that technology has increased adapted physical performance to a great extent. By having lighter, more complex prostheses and tailor-made sport-specific chairs, individuals who use this type of equipment are performing much better today than twenty years ago. In some events, such as the Boston Marathon race, athletes who use wheelchairs have even surpassed runners who are able-bodied.

7 But are we correct in our interpretation? What seems to be missing in our analysis?

Rather than taking a twenty-year span to answer the question of how technology is influencing performance, let us take a shorter time period. More precisely, let us compare the 1996 Paralympic (11.36 seconds) and Olympic (9.84) 100-metre winning times with the 2000 (11.09 seconds) and Olympic (9.87) 100-metre winning times. In 1996, Anthony Volpentest won the event in 11.36 seconds. In

2000, Marlon Ray Shirley won his race in a world record time of 11.09 seconds. If we subtract Shirley's time from Volpentest's, we see that the time for this particular event has improved (i.e., a 2.5 percent improvement) by .27 seconds in a four-year span. The same mathematical calculations with the winning times from the Olympic games show that times in this event have not improved. There has been a negligible drop of 0.03 seconds. Furthermore, if we divide Donovan Bailey's winning time in the 1996 Olympic games by Anthony Volpentest's Paralympic time, we end up with a ratio of 0.87. If we apply this rationale once again to the 2000 results (i.e. divide Maurice Green's winning time by Marlon Ray Shirley's time), we end up with a ratio of .89. Although the results still show some (minimal) improvements for this particular group of Paralympic athletes, caution seems to be warranted in our interpretations.

Undoubtedly, technology has played a role in helping athletes who have a disability perform to new heights. However, it is difficult to ascertain exactly what impact technology has had on performance. Take the average Paralympic track and field athlete. This athlete competes with very sophisticated and expensive prostheses. However, this individual trains, competes regularly, and is probably sponsored. He also weight trains and is likely supported by family and coaches. Now the question is, "Which of these factors can account for the fact that a Paralympic athlete such as Marlon Ray Shirley holds the world record for the 100-metre dash?" Most likely all of them. Still, this statement forces us to ponder the real impact of technology in sport.

A similar claim can also be made for wheelchair sports. Paciorek (1993) has argued convincingly that technology played a smaller part than could be expected in the setting of many Paralympic and world records in the 1992 Paralympic Games held in Barcelona. According to this author, technology was only part of the story, as world records fell in the 1992 Paralympic Games. Greater crowd support, better coaching, and increased opportunities for competition for athletes were some of the main reasons which athletes and coaches gave to explain such a great number of records falling.

Arguments proposed by Higgs (2000b) also support the idea that technology is only part of the story. In two chapters written on his web site, Higgs (2000b, 2000c) summarizes research with respect to wheelchair fundamentals and wheelchair design. These two chapters provide fascinating nuances with respect to how wheelchair parametres can influence performance. For example, Higgs (2000b) notes that wheelchairs are becoming lighter as result of technological advances in materials, a point we made earlier. However, he goes on to state that if we apply one of Newton's famous laws, we can arrive at the following conclusion: "If the same force is applied to different weights, the lightest will accelerate most rapidly." Thus, it seems that having a lighter wheelchair might be beneficial for an athlete. However, it is also important to consider who is exerting the force. For example, you can have the best wheelchair in the world from a technological point of view, but if you are incapable of generating any force owning such a chair will prove pointless.

Research by de Groot et al. (1999) suggests that it also seems warranted to qualify the effect of technology on performance in wheelchair basketball. Earlier in the chapter, we mentioned that costly, customized wheelchairs are now being constructed to meet the specific needs of wheelchair athletes. In the de Groot et al. (1999) study, seventeen wheelchair basketball players participated in a battery of physiological (e.g., maximum aerobic power), biomechanical (e.g., chair stability), and field (e.g., shooting performance) tests, once using their personal wheelchair and once using a prototype wheelchair; all tests were completed twice. The wheelchair basketball players also completed a questionnaire that measured their perceptions of the performance and characteristics of the type of wheelchair used. Results indicated that no significant differences were found between the personal and prototype wheelchair on any of the tests. However, the prototype chair was rated significantly superior concerning weight, maneuverability, rolling resistance, and footrest stability but rated significantly inferior concerning height of the chair and backrest. These results cast doubts with respect to the perceived need for special fitting. By making a few simple adjustments, a prototype chair can be made to fit a variety of users. Furthermore, the questionnaire results are fascinating because they point to an interesting hypothesis. Notice that the new wheelchair is perceived as better than one's personal wheelchair on a number of performance-related indicators. Is it possible that when athletes use a new piece of technologically-advanced equipment they feel they are performing or going to perform better? What we are saying is that what might be affecting performance is the belief in the idea that technology influences performance and not the actual technology itself. By using a new chair, wheelchair basketball players might perceive the new chair to be more technologically advanced. This perception may, in turn, lead to the belief that athletes are performing at a higher level. Sometimes giving a sugar pill to alleviate a particular malady is just as effective as a real pill. Consider this little anecdote. When you buy a new pair of shoes, do you feel as if you could jump higher? Nike has made millions by making people believe they can be like Mike!

In conclusion, one needs to be aware that we have chosen track and field events, which rely on technology, to demonstrate the influence of technology on performance. Although these results seem to suggest that technology is beneficial, it remains unclear to what extent. Technology has changed over time but so have coaching and training methods (see Chapter 28 (Bhambhani)), the number of competitions, crowd support, sponsorship, and the external environment in which events take place. Thus, with so many factors involved, it is difficult to clearly identify the contribution of technology in the enhancement of adapted physical performance.

ETHICS AND TECHNOLOGY

Technology is progressing at an incredible rate. More and more scientific breakthroughs are being applied to prostheses and wheelchairs everyday in an attempt to make individuals more functional. In this part of the chapter, we feel it is important to tackle ethical issues concerning the relationship between technology and disability sport by asking ourselves: where will it all end?

Before we proceed to look to the future, let us take time to reflect on present-day ethical questions surrounding technology and disability sport. According to York Chow, International Paralympic Committee vice-president, the technological explosion related to disability sport raises the issue of "technological boosting." In essence, the questions behind technological boosting are:

8 Should athletes from all countries use the same technology? If not, are athletes from wealthy countries unfairly advantaged? Or, is this no different than able-bodied sport and therefore not an issue?

These are interesting questions because they seem to suggest that technology influences disability sport performance. However, the underlying factor which is now being used as a comparison point is nationality and not a particular time or a certain type of athlete. It is important to note that the 100-metre Paralympic winners we used as examples in the previous section all came from Canada or the United States. By using a third comparison point, we come up with a completely new interpretation of the data we presented in the previous section. The technological improvements we highlighted seem to be specific to wealthy countries. Finally, the questions raised by the issue of technological boosting seem to be based on the assumption that technology does influence performance. We are not here to dispute this assumption. Still, we are left to wonder, as we have already stated in the chapter, to what extent this is a true statement. Debates often occur because problems are ill-defined. As

Froes (1997) states, "Lots of questions, few answers. What do you think?"

Let us now jump ahead in time and try to tackle this delicate issue with the help of another science-fiction example. In our introduction, we suggested that technology is often pictured in the science-fiction media as being able to reproduce or even extend human capabilities. Imagine for a moment that some company was able to construct a leg prosthesis that could reproduce able-bodied walking and running patterns to perfection (i.e., meet the normative standard).

9 What would be the social consequences of such an invention?

This question is somewhat addressed in the film *Bicentennial Man* (Columbus 1999). In this movie, Robin Williams plays a robot whose programming is altered by a twist of fate (i.e., it falls out of a window). As a result of this accident, the robot becomes an inventor and creates a series of prostheses in order to become human. After much research, the robot modifies itself to such an extent that it asks to be considered human. *Bicentennial Man* is an intriguing movie because it asks the question "Can I be human?" from the perspective of a machine.

Let us now reverse the equation, as the Robin Williams character does at one point in the movie. If someone used such a highly evolved prosthesis, should we still consider that person to be human? We presume so, but where do we draw the line? Imagine for one second that you are a world class athlete running the 100-metre dash. You have trained all your life and the Olympic Committee has just agreed to let athletes who have prostheses compete against athletes who are able-bodied. How would you feel? Imagine yourself warming up the day before your event. You are enjoying yourself as you test the new track. Unfortunately for you, you fail to notice a wet spot on the track and fall to the ground breaking your leg. You are rushed to the hospital only to be told that your leg will take two weeks to heal. Your dreams are shattered.

What if we replaced you with an individual wearing a Bicentennial Man-type prosthesis similar to the previous scenario? Would that individual have encountered such a problem? Maybe, but it would probably take less time to fix a broken prosthesis than to wait for a broken limb to heal. Who knows? This unlikely scenario raises a strange question:

10 What if many individuals were equipped with prostheses designed to correspond to the able-bodied standard? Would they be allowed to compete against individuals who are able-bodied? Should separate games be held for individuals who use prostheses and individuals who are able-bodied?

In essence, these questions all deal with the idea that rules might be needed with respect to the application of technology in sport (Freeman 1991). We have rules for performance enhancement drugs. Why not have rules about the application of technology in sport?

Another important potential consequence of technology is the disappearance of wheelchair culture as we know it. Imagine if a company could design prostheses which could alleviate spinal cord injuries. Once again, this reality is clearly portrayed in *Bicentennial Man*. The able-bodied standard is fully met in the movie. It is not for us to judge whether striving for this standard is appropriate or not. However, attaining such a standard will mean the disappearance of wheelchairs, wheelchair designers, and of a variety of services (e.g., adapted physical education teachers) associated with the users of these devices. Surely, records will be kept. Still, wheelchair sports would become a thing of the past.

One might think that losing wheelchair culture is a small price to pay if prostheses could be made to counter spinal cord injuries. However, please consider the following story before arriving at such a conclusion. If you were deaf and could be fitted with a prosthesis that could help you hear better, would you have surgery to implant a specially designed prosthesis in your ear? Such a device now exists. A cochlear implant is a device which is positioned in the inner ear and helps

amplify sounds. It is still somewhat experimental but it has been shown to help individuals who have never heard before. Great news, is it not? It depends on where you stand with respect to the debate on cochlear implants. At the time this type of prosthesis was first used, designers of this device believed it could improve the quality of life of people with a hearing disability. This expectation revealed itself to be partially true in that only some individuals who have a hearing disability praised the value of the implant. Contrary to what had been expected by the designers, some individuals who have a hearing disability felt threatened by the implant in that they believed that the widespread use of such a device would certainly lead to the disappearance of sign language and, possibly, of deaf culture (see Chapter 26 (Steadward and Foster)). No one is at fault here. The designers of such a device had noble intentions, but little did they expect that individuals who have a hearing disability who identify to their group would respond so strongly to this new technological advance. It just goes to show that, at times, culture (or traditions) and technology may not mix very well.

A FINAL THOUGHT

In conclusion, there is no doubt that science will continue to progress and, as a result, so will technology. There is also no doubt that technology will keep influencing disability sport. To what extent remains to be seen. This point brings us to the question "When will this progression stop?" There is no simple answer to this question. Still, this question opens the door to another question. In this last section, we did not chose to deal with the idea that technology could in fact extend human capabilities such as in *The Six Million Dollar Man*. If technology were to reach such a pinnacle, it may significantly alter our definition of what being human is like. A new category of individuals may likely be created as a resulted of such technological advances. Although these are speculative statements, these are issues that adapted physical students, teachers, and coaches may need to tackle some day.

Study Questions

1. Define and differentiate between an orthosis, a prosthesis, and a wheelchair.
2. Define each of these terms: *orthosis*, *prosthesis*, and *wheelchair*.
3. What is the key difference between an orthosis and a prosthesis?
4. Describe the social factors that have influenced technological changes in disability sport.
5. Explain the difference between an *antecedent* and a *consequence* of technological change.
6. Explain how social factors influenced the design of wheelchairs and prostheses.
7. Describe the consequences of technological changes with respect to prostheses and wheelchairs.
8. Name the consequences of technological changes associated with respect to prostheses and wheelchairs.
9. Do these changes apply equally to wheelchairs and prostheses?
10. Cite the evidence relating the role of technology on performance in disability sport.
11. What is the evidence with respect to the effect of technology on sport?
12. What conclusions can you reach based on this evidence?
13. Pick various Paralympic sports and find out if the trends expressed in this chapter are similar in other sports. Check if the trends presented herein are also true for women.
14. Discuss the ethical concerns related to technology and performance in disability sport.
15. What is technological boosting?
16. Should we have rules against technological boosting?

Acknowledgements

The author would like to thank Sheri Foster, Robert Steadward, Jane Watkinson, and Garry Wheeler for their helpful comments on a previous version of this chapter. We also would like to thank Alan Dean, Donald Royer, Mike Frogley, Ian Gregson, and Ian Jones for providing us with information concerning the relationship between technology and disability performance.

References

American Heritage Dictionary (2nd ed.). (1985). Boston: Houghton Mifflin.

American Online Amputee Journal. (January, 2000). *The future of amputation and limb loss: The science.* [On-line]. Available: http://amputee-online.com/amputation/jan00/Jan00.html (URL on December 17, 2002).

Bennett, H. (Executive Producer). (1973). *The six million dollar man.* United States: MCA/Universal studios. [Television series].

Brånemark, R., Bergh, P., Gunterberg, B., Rydevik, B., and Brånemark, P.I. (2000). *Bone anchored amputation prostheses.* Paper presented at the 5th Scientific Congress, Sydney 2000 Paralympic Games, Sydney, Australia.

Cameron, J. (Director). (1991). *Terminator 2: Judgment day.* United States: TriStar Pictures. [Motion picture].

Cameron, J. (Executive Producer). (2000). *Dark angel.* United States: 20th Century Fox Television. [Television series].

Columbus, C. (Director). (1999). *Bicentennial man.* United States: Touchstone Pictures. [Motion picture].

de Groot, S., Coppoolse, J.M., Wheeler, G.D., Bhambhani, Y., Gervais, P., Malone, L., Nelson E., and Steadward, R.D. (1999). Evaluation of a new sports wheelchair design. In L.H.V. van der Woude, M.T.E. Hopman, and C.H. van Kemenade (Eds.), *Biomedical aspects of manual wheelchair propulsion: The state of the art: II* (pp. 183–86). Amsterdam: IOS Press.

Dean, A. (October 3, 2001). Personal communication.

Engstrom, B., and Van de Ven, C. (1999). *Therapy for amputees.* Edinburgh: Churchill Livingstone.

Freeman, W.H. (1991). *Sport and technology: Ethics on the cutting edge.* Paper presented at the Sport Philosophy Academy Session American Alliance for Health, Physical Education, Recreation and Dance, San Francisco.

Froes, F.H. (1997). Is the use of advanced materials in sports equipment unethical? *JOM, 49,* 15–19.

Higgs, C. (1995). Enhancing wheelchair sport performance. In Joseph P. Winnick (Ed.), *Adapted Physical Education and Sport* (pp. 421–33). Champaign, IL: Human Kinetics.

Higgs, C. (2000a). *Chapter 1: History, classification, and performance.* [On-line]. Available: http/www.ucs.mun.ca/~chiggs/NewFiles/Chapter1.pdf (URL on December 17, 2002). St. John's: Memorial University, School of Human Kinetics and Recreation.

Higgs, C. (2000b). *Chapter 2: Wheelchair fundamentals.* [On-line]. Available: www.ucs.mun.ca/~chiggs/NewFiles/Chap2a.pdf (URL on December 17, 2002). St. John's: Memorial University, School of Human Kinetics and Recreation.

Higgs, C. (2000c). *Chapter 3: Wheelchair design.* [On-line]. Available: http/www.ucs.mun.ca/~chiggs/NewFiles/Chapter3.pdf (URL on December 17, 2002). St. John's:

Memorial University, School of Human Kinetics and Recreation.

Jones, I. (October 3, 2001). Personal communication.

(Kershner, I. (Director). (1980). *Star wars: The empire strikes back*. United States: Lucasfilms. [Motion picture].

Lévesque, C., and Gauthier-Gagnon, C. (1987). An above-knee prosthesis for rock climbing. *Orthotics and Prosthetics, 40*, 41–45.

Michael, J.W. (1986). Prosthetic feet for the amputee athlete. *Palaestra, 5*, 21–22; 32; 34–35.

Michael, J. W. (1989). New developments in prosthetic feet and sports for recreation. *Palaestra, 5*, 21–22; 32; 34–35.

Michael, J.W., Gailey, R.S., and Bowker, J.H. (1990). New developments in recreational and adaptive devices for the amputee. *Clinical Orthopaedics and Related Research, 256*, 64–75.

Nichols. J. (2000). *Why does the central nervous system not regenerate after injury?* Paper presented at the 5th Scientific Congress, Sydney 2000 Paralympic Games, Sydney, Australia.

Paciorek, M.J. (1993). Technology only part of the story as world records fall. *Palaestra, 9*, 14–17.

Pike, A.C. (2000a). *New high tech prostheses.* [On-line]. Available: http/www.amputeeresource.org/ High%20tech%20prostheses.htm (URL on December 17, 2002). Amputee Resource Foundation of America.

Pike, A.C. (2000b). *History and Prosthetics.* [On-line]. Available: http/www.amputeeresource.org/ History%20and%20prosthetics.htm (URL on December 17, 2002). Amputee Resource Foundation of America.

Porreta, D.L. (1995). Team sports. In Joseph P. Winnick (Ed.), *Adapted Physical Education and Sport* (pp. 421–33). Champaign, IL: Human Kinetics.

Radocy, B. (1988). Hands for all seasons: Upper-extremity sports prosthetics. *Palaestra, 4*, 24–29, 46.

Roddenberry, G. (Executive Producer). (1987) *Star trek: The next generation.* United States: Paramount Pictures. [Television series].

Saadah, E.S.M. (1992). Swimming devices for below-knee amputees. *Prosthetics and Orthotics International, 16*, 140–41.

Sherill, C. (1998). *Adapted physical activity, recreation and sport.* Boston: WCB McGraw-Hill.

Truong, X.T., Erickson, R., Galbreath, R. (1986). Baseball adaptation for below-elbow prosthesis. *Archives of Physical Medicine and Rehabilitation, 67*, 418.

CHAPTER 30

Physical Activity and Sport for Individuals With Intellectual Disability

Jennifer B. Mactavish
Maureen J. Dowds

Learning Objectives

- To enhance your knowledge and/or understanding of concepts and issues in defining intellectual disability and its effects on physical activity and sport.
- To enhance your knowledge and/or understanding of your role as physical activity professionals in working with individuals with intellectual disability (i.e., the importance of your attitudes).
- To learn about instructional strategies for supporting and promoting participation in physical activity and sport.
- To understand the conceptual foundation of sport for persons with intellectual disability.
- To become aware of sport organizations that serve athletes with intellectual disability (Special Olympics International and the International Sports Federation for Persons with Intellectual Disability).
- To understand the key issues affecting the delivery of sport for these individuals.

Introduction

Sport is meaningful and important in the lives of many people, including those with intellectual disability. Like other members of society, some individuals with intellectual disability participate in sport for purely recreational reasons–to develop skills and fitness and to have fun socializing with other people. For others, the transition from recreational sport to intensive training and competition is a natural progression for testing personal limits and pursuing athletic dreams and goals. Whatever the individual's ultimate aim–be it recreation or competition–you, as a physical activity professional, play a key role in promoting and supporting the inclusion of individuals with intellectual disability in sport. Furthermore, the importance of your role remains consistent, independent of where you might work in the field (e.g., school, community recreation, or sport).

This chapter is an introduction to essential information for service providers who, directly (e.g., coaches) or indirectly (e.g., physical education teachers), contribute to people's involvement in sport.

Intellectual Disability

The term *intellectual disability* refers to the condition formerly known as *mental retardation* (Chapter 4 (Squair and Groeneveld)). Before refreshing your memory about this state of functioning, we first need to consider two questions: (a) why the change in terminology from mental retardation to intellectual disability, and (b) what is meant by the term *people first language*?

TERMINOLOGY

For individuals familiar with the history of disability, *mental retardation* is a controversial label that is inextricably linked with outdated and negative stereotypes (Hastings 1994). Consequently, this term is used infrequently outside the medical profession and legal statutes in the United States. In its place, different countries popularized alternative terms—*mental disability, mental handicap, learning disability,* and *developmental disability*. Over time, it became apparent that these alternatives were understood to have different meanings in different parts of the world, which proved more confusing than helpful (Hastings 1994). Recognizing this concern, the merits of various options have been debated in an effort to identify a single, internationally recognized term (Baroff 1991; Goldfarb 1990; Sandieson 1998). This debate has not been resolved. In Canada, Australia, and many Western European countries, however, *intellectual disability* has emerged as the most consistently used alternative to the term *mental retardation*—hence its use in this chapter (Gething 1997; Seidl 1998).

Another important issue related to terminology is the use of what is known as *people first language*. People first language is based on the recognition that the words we choose and how we use them communicate powerful messages about underlying attitudes towards people with disabilities and their value as human beings. As such, when terms such as the *intellectually disabled* or simply *the disabled* are used, we create and inappropriately reinforce the idea that all individuals who carry this label are exactly the same. This leads to stereotyping, which fails to acknowledge the diversity of personalities, strengths, and capabilities that are unique to each individual with intellectual disability. People first language, therefore, emphasizes the person first, followed by the description of his or her disability (e.g., we first say "people," "individual," or "person," followed by "who are…" or "who have…" or "with…."). By using this type of phrasing we are communicating and acknowledging, respectfully and with dignity, that individuals with a disability are, first and foremost, people. The person's disability, if it is relevant to mention at all, is of secondary importance.

DEFINITION OF INTELLECTUAL DISABILITY

What is the basis for determining that a person has intellectual disability? Parallel to the controversy that led to the emergence of the term *intellectual disability*, the definition of what it means to have this condition has engendered considerable debate (Reiss 1994). Much of this stems from differences in opinion about the value and usefulness of IQ scores, the extent to which IQ scores provide accurate measures of cognitive functioning, and the relationship between adaptive behaviours and cognitive skills (Batshaw 1997; Gould 1981; Parmenter 2001).

Looking beyond these differences, there is general agreement that three elements are essential to the definition of intellectual disability: (1) significantly subaverage intellectual functioning, (2) impairment in the performance of adaptive skills, and (3) evident before age eighteen. The American Association on Mental Retardation (AAMR), the oldest and one of the most respected authorities in this area of disability, formally linked these elements in their most recent definition:

Mental retardation[1] is a disability characterized by significant limitations in both intellectual functioning and adaptive behavior as expressed in conceptual, social, and practical adaptive skills. This disability originates before age 18 (American Association on Mental Retardation 2002, p. 1).

CHARACTERISTICS

What is the effect of intellectual disability and what is the role of sport? Intellectual disability affects different individuals in different ways. Many individuals experience learning difficulties, which are particularly evident in learning abstract concepts, complex rules, and transferring learning from one setting to another (Eichstaedt and Lavay 1992). Social skill development is another area that is sometimes affected by a person's intellectual disability. Some individuals have well-developed social skills, while others, because of limited opportunities for learning and use, may exhibit inappropriate or immature social interaction skills (Abery and Fahnestock 1994; Schleien, Ray, and Green 1997). Related to social skill development, some people with intellectual disability rely on nonverbal forms of communication (e.g., sign language, symbols) to express themselves; however, most are able to communicate verbally (Jones 1994).

While these challenges may affect participation in sport, two additional factors are of particular importance in this context. Specifically, slower rates of motor skill acquisition and lower levels of physical fitness have been identified when individuals with intellectual disability are compared to those who do not have a disability (Fernhall, Tymeson, and Webster 1988; Pitetti, Rimmer, and Fernhall 1993; Seidl 1998). Research, however, demonstrates that these outcomes are not inherent aspects of a person's intellectual disability but, generally, are associated with inadequate instruction and limited opportunities in the physical domain (Seidl 1998).

Susan's story, told in the following vignette, helps to illustrate this point. Additionally, for some individuals low levels of fitness and delays in motor development (not to mention other facets of learning) are further complicated by low motivation. This comes about when repeated efforts to perform a skill or task are unsuccessful, which reduces subsequent interest and willingness to persist until a skill or task has been mastered (Switzky 1997).

Susan's Story

When Susan was a baby, over twenty-five years ago, she was involved in an accident that resulted, ultimately, in a diagnosis of intellectual disability. Since that time, her family has worked tirelessly, spending hours and hours on learning and practicing life-long physical activity skills. Although having difficulty differentiating between hot and cold, selecting clothing appropriate for the weather, learning new ideas, and sometimes having outbursts that might be considered socially inappropriate, Susan is one of the premier Nordic skiers in Canada. She has competed in two Paralympic Games and numerous World Special Olympic Games in both skiing and athletics. Strong family support, lots of training, and competitive experiences have contributed greatly to Susan's development as a fiercely competitive and highly trained athlete. These skills also help Susan hold down a full-time job, which includes all the benefits enjoyed by her co-workers who do not have a disability. Susan is a respected member of her community—a community that follows her many accomplishments with great interest.

In sum then, the extent to which people may be affected by their disability varies widely and is largely dependent on the origin of disability, level of impairment, life experiences, and opportunities for developing skills and competencies. Furthermore, the preceding

---

1 *Mental retardation* is the term used in the official AAMR definition and, as such, it is used in this context. It should be noted, however, that AAMR has acknowledged concerns about usage of this term and appears supportive of efforts to identify an accurate and agreeable alternative (American Association on Mental Retardation, 1992, p. xi).

discussion illustrates that physical activity and sport can and do play instrumental roles in enabling individuals with intellectual disability to maximize their potential.

IMPLICATIONS FOR PHYSICAL ACTIVITY PROFESSIONALS

How does the information presented so far relate to your role? AAMR's new definition of intellectual disability, while criticized by some for continuing to use the term *mental retardation* (Gething 1997), is accepted widely—largely because it reflects a shift away from a deficit-based model of disability to one that places greater emphasis on people's abilities and their support needs across different settings (Batshaw 1997; Hastings 1994; Reiss 1994). This shift in perspective represents a radical change in the way we typically have thought about intellectual disability. Under the old deficit-based model, the learning difficulties of a person with intellectual disability often were attributed to the disability and, as such, provided a built-in excuse for failing to achieve instructional aims and a rationale for excluding these individuals from interactions with their peers without disabilities. The new support-model view recognizes that the consequences of a person's disability come about because of complex interactions between the individual and his or her environment (American Association on Mental Retardation 2002). It is implicit in this perspective that people with intellectual disability have the potential to learn and the ability to perform socially appropriate adaptive skills when supported in ways that are consistent with their needs.

Applying these notions to sport, we know that the interests and skills required for participation in sport are shaped by experiences in physical activity. These experiences may take place within the context of family activities, but more often than not are the result of participation in school-based physical education and/or community recreation programmes. As a professional likely to work in these areas, your ability to provide effective instruction will have a tremendous influence on a person's future interest and participation in sport. Your influence is likely to assume even greater importance for people with intellectual disability because these individuals typically have fewer options for experiencing and learning about sport outside of school settings. Furthermore, opportunities to enact this influence are no longer exclusive to special educators or other professionals specifically interested in working with individuals with a disability (Snell 1988). Instead, passage of the Canadian Charter of Rights and Freedoms in 1982 and ongoing movements towards inclusion mean that all physical activity professionals will have roles to play (Magsino 1993).

So, with this knowledge in mind, what can you do to fulfill your responsibility for promoting positive physical activity experiences that may lead to on-going involvement in sport? Although it may sound clichéd, the first step really comes down to attitude—what are your values and beliefs about the aims of physical activity and who should and/or can benefit from instruction in this area (Rizzo and Kirkendall 1995)?

While there are many possible responses to this question, contemporary education and recreation programming tend to be dominated by an inclusive, or zero-exclusion, perspective (Block 2000; Krebs and Block 1992; Schleien, Green, and Heyne 1993). From this perspective, physical activity is viewed as essential and beneficial for all individuals, independent of whether or not they have a disability. This does not mean that everyone will participate in exactly the same way, or that targeted goals will be consistent for all participants and/or readily achieved at all times. Instead, a zero-exclusion approach focusses on challenging all people to perform to their fullest potential and on ensuring that instruction supports progress towards individual, age-appropriate, and functional (i.e., relevant and important in real-life) goals.

Typically, an inclusive approach occurs within the context of programmes that welcome and encourage participation by individuals with and without a disability (i.e., integrated programmes). Other programme formats also may be appropriate, depending on the needs of the participants with a disability and the goals they are working towards. For example, an eighteen-year-old high school student with intellectual disability, along with her classmates without a disability, have just completed an introduction to golf during physical education class. Enjoying the activity immensely and in keeping with her goal of developing life-long pastimes, the young woman continues to practice her golf at the local driving range, while the rest of the class moves onto another unit. She may do this with an aide, a small group of classmates without a disability, or in the company of other students who also have intellectual disability (e.g., segregated).

In enacting the zero-exclusion approach to programming, physical activity professionals must be patient and willing to experiment with a number of different strategies and instructional techniques. A full accounting of all the approaches worth trying is beyond the scope of this chapter; however, most of the strategies required for effective instruction in general are applicable, as are many of the ideas presented elsewhere in this text (e.g., ecological task analysis, leisure education, abilities-based instruction, holistic learning). The following suggestions are offered as examples that will get you started in developing a 'bag of effective strategies' for assisting individuals with intellectual disability to acquire physical activity and sport skills.

PLANNING THE PROGRAMME, SETTING EXPECTATIONS, AND PROMOTING DECISION MAKING

Effectively including all participants in high quality programmes does not just happen; it is the product of careful planning. The key considerations in planning—goal setting, activity selection, lesson or activity plan preparation, instructional methods and strategies, and evaluation—are consistent with the requirements of any programme, independent of the participants' abilities or the setting (e.g., school or community).

How the programme plan is documented or recorded, however, may vary according to the setting. For example, in community sport or recreation, programme plans typically are written down but are less formal than those found in schools. In schools, an individual education plan (IEP) is used formally to document each student's unique learning needs, the supports and services required to address these needs, and goals for each area of instruction—including physical education. The plans are usually developed via a process that includes parents, school personnel (e.g., teachers, administrators), related service professionals (e.g., speech and physical therapists), and, sometimes, the student. Physical education teachers are not always included in this process, which often leads to inappropriate goals in this area or lack of awareness about what is contained in the IEP. Consequently, as a physical educator you should ask to be involved in this process, specifically in goal-setting for physical education. Additionally, you should have access to, and an understanding of, the contents of a student's IEP to facilitate your planning and to ensure that this supports progress towards the stated goals.

Goal-setting, for an IEP or any other type of programme plan, often proves more challenging than any other aspect of planning because of uncertainty about what can reasonably be expected of individuals with intellectual disability. All too often this uncertainty leads to limited expectations, which do not encourage people to achieve their maximum potential. To avoid this pitfall, it is essential that you learn as much as possible about the needs and abilities of the individuals in your programme. Conducting skill and fitness assessments, being knowledgeable about chronologically age-appropriate skills, knowing about any medical issues or concerns, talking with others (e.g., teachers, professionals, parents) who know your participants, and reviewing the IEP (if you are working in a school setting) are all steps that may prove useful in developing reasonable expectations. In turn, this information can be used for setting goals that stimulate development by building on an individual's current needs and abilities.

Programme goals will vary, obviously, depending on the focus of the unit or the programme and the strengths and needs of the individual student. As a general rule, however, goals should focus on one or more of the following:

- physical skill acquisition
- physical fitness
- social skill development
- decision making
- knowledge, understanding, and appreciation of physical activity

In designing programmes to address one or more of these goal areas, it is important to select activities that are consistent with the participants' interests and preferences (Davis 1989). To do this, a range of activity choices should be presented and participants should be taught and encouraged to consider the merits of each alternative, weigh the consequences of each, and choose one that meets their interests and needs. More than simply making choices then, decision making is about facilitating the individual's ability to evaluate alternatives in order to select the activity or activities consistent with their preferences and needs (Mahon 1994). By enhancing your participants' skills in this area, you will be fostering their ability to make decisions about different physical activity options that they may, in turn, be able to apply in different contexts and settings.

STRUCTURING THE ENVIRONMENT AND ESTABLISHING ROUTINES

A large open space, bright lights, colourful posters, interesting equipment, noise, other people–all of these factors present distractions that make it difficult for some students, particularly those with intellectual disability, to attend to learning tasks in a gymnasium (Block 2000). Being aware of this possibility and making efforts, where possible, to reduce these distractions may enhance learning.

Additionally, establishing a routine may prove helpful, as many individuals with intellectual disability learn most effectively when

instruction is presented in a consistent manner. Disruptions in routine may cause an individual to act out or tune out to instruction. To avoid this possibility, you might establish a 'contract' (see table 30.1) with an individual participant and/or develop a routine for your programme that includes:

- selecting an activity that signals the beginning of each class or session
- establishing standardized cues for starting and stopping activities
- developing and clearly communicating behavioural expectations and the consequences of not meeting those expectations
- using landmarks in the gym for structuring activities (e.g., using court markings to denote playing boundaries)
- assigning students to groupings/teams based on visual cues (e.g., coloured shirts)

Among these considerations, setting and clearly communicating expectations about behaviour and the consequences of not meeting these expectations is perhaps the most important (Amado 1988). Involving the programme participants in this process is often helpful in ensuring that they understand what is expected and what will happen if they do not fulfill these expectations.

FACILITATING UNDERSTANDING, LEARNING, AND PARTICIPATION

Following directions, learning abstract concepts, and performing complex skills are examples of some areas in which students with intellectual disability may experience difficulties. Sometimes these difficulties can be resolved by adjusting the way that information is presented. For example, when providing verbal instructions or directions:

- Be specific.
- Use brief and precise language.
- Use words that are in keeping with the student's level of understanding.
- Check to ensure understanding by asking the student to repeat the instructions or directions.

Table 30.1 What Is a Contract?

A contract is a useful strategy for helping an individual monitor his/her behaviour, make decisions, and identify consequences. An instructor usually helps an individual write simple statements that describe what the person, to fulfil his/her commitment, will do. The individual, teacher/coach/instructor, and, if appropriate, the parent/caregiver then signs the document to signal that everyone is aware of and agrees with the contents of the contract.

The following example is for a school-based physical education class, but it can easily be modified for use in a community recreation and/or sport context.

This is an agreement between me, (student's name), and my teacher that:

> I will be on time for my physical education class.
> I will change into the proper clothing for physical education.
> I will try my best every time I am in the gymnasium.
> I will assist my fellow students when I can.
> I will listen and pay attention to my teacher.
> I will work hard on improving my physical fitness.

If I follow through on all of my promises, I will get five minutes of free time at the end of class to shoot baskets (student's favourite physical activity).

If I do not follow through on my promises, I will not get free time to shoot baskets at the end of class (student's preferred activity).

_____   _____   _____
(student's signature)   (teacher's signature)   (parent/caregiver's signature)

Date _____

When teaching abstract concepts and complex skills, a number of strategies in tandem or alone may be effective. For example, using instructional prompts to tell, show, or physically assist a student in performing a task can be useful (Haney and Falvey 1989). Reinforcing efforts to engage in learning and rewarding the outcomes, no matter how small or large, also may be effective approaches for motivating learners with intellectual disability (French and Lavay 1990). Verbal praise, a physical gesture (e.g., a 'high five'), and/or the opportunity to engage in a preferred activity are commonly used reinforcements and rewards.

For other individuals, prompts and rewards coupled with breaking a complex skill into smaller parts may be required to stimulate learning and/or participation (Davis and Burton 1991). Breaking a complex skill into its component parts and developing a sequence for teaching these components is a strategy known as *task analysis*. In using this strategy, it is important to start by demonstrating or assisting the student to do the entire skill before teaching the component parts so that they have some understanding of the ultimate skill they are working towards. Ongoing practice and repetition of the component parts and the overall skill also are essential for supporting and facilitating learning in this way.

Another important consideration in promoting learning of abstract concepts and complex skills is the idea of teaching for *generalization* or *transferability* (Bishop and Falvey 1989; Edelstein 1989). This means that skills and activities must be introduced and practiced in the different settings that a participant would be expected to perform them. For example, if you initially introduce the game of soccer indoors in the gymnasium, you will need to provide a re-introduction to the game and provide opportunities for practicing once you move outdoors. Otherwise, the participants may experience difficulties in transferring the skills and concepts they learned in the gymnasium to the outdoor setting.

Modifying the equipment or the activity also may be useful approaches for promoting learning (Liberty 1985; Wehman and Schleien 1981). Examples of modifications to equipment include using a larger ball for learning catching skills, lowering the height of nets (e.g., volleyball or badminton) or basketball backboards, and using shorter racquets or bats, or ones with smaller grips. Activity modifications might involve altering the rules to eliminate complex concepts (e.g., the off-side rule in soccer), decreasing the size of the playing area, and changing the number of players on each team (e.g., five-a-side soccer versus eleven-a-side). Modifications of either variety are intended to encourage successful participation and, as such, should only be used when absolutely necessary and to the extent needed. Ideally, modifications should be eliminated, if possible, as the participants' skills improve.

A final consideration in facilitating learning and participation involves avoiding the use of instructional approaches that result in elimination of participants (Block 2000). For example, having participants select their own teammates or assigning team captains to pick teams often leads to the exclusion of less skilled participants. To counter this possibility, you, as the instructor, could assign teams based on any number of factors (e.g., eye colour, colour of the participants' t-shirts, month of birth).

In general, regardless of the specific strategy used, students should be encouraged to learn with the minimal amount of assistance needed to foster successful learning and participation. In this way, the individual's independence and self-confidence also will be promoted.

SENSITIZING OTHER PARTICIPANTS

While applicable to quality programming in general, the concepts and strategies discussed to this point focus on promoting learning and participation by individuals with intellectual disability. The inclusive or zero-exclusion approach to school and community programming means that individuals with and without disabilities will participate, more often than not, in programmes together. As such, it is also important to consider how these two participant groups can be included, successfully, within the same programme.

One premise for supporting the zero-exclusion approach to programming is that social interactions shared by individuals with intellectual disability and their peers without a disability will produce mutually beneficial outcomes (Stainback and Stainback 1992). Social interactions, positive or otherwise, are unlikely to occur, however, if the participants without a disability are not prepared. Consequently, as much as your awareness of the needs and abilities of individuals with intellectual disability will influence the success of their inclusion, so too will the awareness of other participants in the programme.

In preparing other participants, an awareness session is often very useful (Stone and Campbell 1991). When planning this session, you might want to enlist the support and assistance of parents, knowledgeable colleagues, and representatives from community organizations (e.g., a Special Olympics coach). Also, you must secure parents' approval before discussing anything about their children or their disability within your session.

The specific topics of discussion in the awareness session will vary depending on the age of the participants and the setting. The following are among the range of topics often covered in these sessions and are presented as ideas you might consider including:

- general information about individuals with intellectual disability
- tips on how to interact with individuals with this type of disability

- introduction of participants with intellectual disability (if appropriate–do not embarrass the participant)
- introduction of assistants or paraprofessionals (if there are any) and an explanation of their role in the programme
- explanation of any programme strategies that might be included to promote interactions among the participants (e.g., the buddy system)
- question and answer sessions in which participants are encouraged to ask questions or express any concerns they have about interacting with their peers with intellectual disability

Building on the enhanced awareness that a session such as this is intended to produce, programme strategies for promoting peer interactions are often instituted. Among the most common of these strategies is what is known as *peer tutoring*. In this approach, a participant without disability is paired with a peer who has intellectual disability (Houston-Wilson et al. 1997). Acting as a friend and helper, the participant without disability provides peer support, which, in the process, is intended to heighten awareness and appreciation of individual differences, perceptions of competence, and sense of responsibility. Participants with intellectual disability also benefit as these interactions increase interdependence, decrease reliance on adults, and provide critical opportunities for socializing with peers of the same age.

Participants without disability are sometimes reluctant to become peer tutors, especially by the time they reach adolescence. In these instances, making a peer tutoring system part of the programme structure and routine may require:

- talking privately with the 'reluctant' participant and communicating your confidence in his/her ability to be an effective buddy
- establishing a rotating schedule for buddies

- enabling participants to join an existing buddy pair until they feel more comfortable

If, after trying these approaches, an individual does not want to take part in peer tutoring, this decision must be respected. Peer tutoring works best when participants are willing participants.

SUMMARY OF IMPLICATIONS FOR PHYSICAL ACTIVITY PROFESSIONALS

Physical activity professionals who work in school and community settings provide the experiences and instruction that are essential for developing the interests and skills that promote participation in sport by individuals with intellectual disability. This starts with adopting an attitude that recognizes the value of physical activity and sport for all individuals. Translating this attitude into action requires effective programme planning, which includes setting reasonable yet challenging goals, using instructional strategies (e.g., prompting, reinforcement and rewards, task analysis, modifications) to facilitate achieving these goals, fostering positive interactions, and encouraging the participants' decision-making skills and independence.

The concepts and strategies discussed in this section of the chapter do not reflect everything you need to know about quality programming, but provide the basics that will get you started. It is also important to recognize that every strategy presented will not be effective in all situations and settings. Your commitment to trying these approaches, your willingness to experiment with others, your receptiveness to learning from your experiences, and your openness to the suggestions of other professionals ultimately will dictate your success in including participants with intellectual disability in physical activity and sport.

Sport for Persons With Intellectual Disability

Complementing and extending opportunities in school and community programmes, two international organizations–Special Olympics (SOI) and the International Sports Federation for Persons with Intellectual Disability (INAS-FID)–provide sport training and competitive outlets for individuals with intellectual disability. Before discussing these organizations, it is necessary to understand the conceptual foundation upon which both are based. This understanding is imperative as it provides the rationale that drives the delivery of sport for individuals with intellectual disability.

THE CONCEPTUAL FOUNDATION FOR THE DEVELOPMENT AND DELIVERY OF SPORT

Historically, full participation in mainstream society–never mind sport training and competition–was not an option for individuals with intellectual disability. This began to change over thirty years ago with the emergence of the *principle of normalization* (Nirje 1992). Grounded in the human rights movement of the 1960s and concepts central to quality of life and equality, the principle of normalization was originally introduced by Nirje (1969) as a means of advancing the rights of individuals with intellectual disability to experience, to the fullest degree possible, culturally normative patterns of life and conditions of everyday living.[2]

Culturally normative patterns of life and conditions of everyday living refer to the customs and routines that form the essence of people's lives. Apply this idea to your own life–think about the activities you do on a regular or daily basis. You probably start most days by getting out of bed, deciding what you are going to eat for breakfast, and going to school or work. Later, you might work out or visit with family and friends. All of these are examples of possible activities and interactions that, when repeated day after day, help create your life pattern. This pattern, while uniquely your own, is likely to include engagements that are similar, if not the same, as other members of your community. This is not surprising, as the people around us and the values and traditions in our culture influence much of what we do in life. Simply put then, the principle of normalization is about ensuring that individuals with intellectual disability have opportunities in life–to make decisions, attend school, have a job, participate in sport, be a member of a family–that mirror, whenever possible, those enjoyed by other members of society.

While this view reflects the original intention of the principle of normalization, Wolfensberger (1972) offered an alternative perspective in defining normalization as the "utilization of means which are as culturally normative as possible, in order to establish and/or maintain personal behaviours and characteristics which are as culturally normative as possible" (p. 28). In further explaining this position, Wolfensberger openly discussed 'normalizing' people with a disability through "eliciting, shaping, and maintaining normative skills and habits" (1972, p. 32) and that measures to support these aims "can be *offered* in some circumstances and *imposed* in others" (1972, p. 28).

Clearly, this conceptualization is less concerned with individual rights than with providing services and interventions that promote normative behaviours and skills. By focussing on these outcomes, critics contend that Wolfensberger is falsely perpetuating the notion that normalization is about transforming individuals with a disability into 'normal' people. In supporting this criticism, it also has been argued that 'normal' and, by extension, normative behaviours and skills are impossible standards to define given the diversity of human expression, even within a single community or culture (Dybwad 1982; Parmenter 2001).

Without distinguishing between Nirje and Wolfensberger's definitions, others have charged that the principle of normalization is inappropriate and impractical because it does not support the provision of special services. Countering this misconception, Perrin and Nirje (1985, p. 90) noted "the normalization principle, on the contrary, supports, indeed insists upon the provision of whatever services,

---

2   The principle of normalization originally focussed on individuals with intellectual disability, but since its inception has been expanded to include all individuals with a disability.

training, and support are required" for including individuals with intellectual disability in community life.

Debates such as these have raged for years about the relative merits of Nirje and Wolfensberger's definitions of normalization. Philosophically, there appears to be little chance of reconciliation and, as such, it is important to understand the differences between these two schools of thought. On a practical level, however, both definitions have played pivotal roles in the development and delivery of services for individuals with intellectual disability.

Applied to the context of sport for persons with intellectual disability, Nirje's view, with its emphasis on human rights and freedoms, has elevated awareness of the value of sport for these individuals and has stimulated greater access and opportunities in this area. Supporting these advances, Wolfensberger's position has been instrumental in increasing the availability of programmes and services that enable people's efforts to participate and compete in sport.

The Special Olympics (SO) Movement

Driven by the principle of normalization, Special Olympics began in the 1960s when opportunities for individuals with intellectual disability to pursue sport, whether it be for recreational or competitive purposes, seldom existed. Since that time, Special Olympics has become the single largest worldwide movement of sport for these individuals.

Usually, discussions about Special Olympics concentrate on the origins of this movement in the United States and its current applications in that country. The contributions of other countries to the evolution of Special Olympics and the different forms it assumes in various parts of the world, therefore, is not widely understood. In particular, the significant contributions of Canadians to the emergence of Special Olympics has gone largely unacknowledged as has Canada's distinctly unique version of this movement. As such, the present discussion includes information specific to Special Olympics International,

but concentrates on Special Olympics as it evolved and is implemented in Canada.

HISTORY OF SPECIAL OLYMPICS

The concept of Special Olympics originated in the early 1960s from the work of Dr. Frank Hayden, a Canadian researcher. This work revealed that children with intellectual disability were substantially less physically skilled and fit than their peers without a disability. Instead of assuming, as many did at the time, that low fitness and poor skill development were direct consequences of intellectual disability, Hayden argued that they were by-products of insufficient physical activity and the absence of opportunity. Instituting an intense fitness and skill-building programme with a group of children, he demonstrated that, with opportunity and appropriate instruction, individuals with intellectual disability could develop the physical skills that would enable them to participate in sport.

Inspired by his discoveries, Hayden searched for ways to develop a national sports programme for Canadians with intellectual disability. It was a goal he eventually achieved, albeit in the United States initially. His work came to the attention of the Kennedy Foundation in Washington, DC, and led to the creation of Special Olympics International (SOI). The first sport competition under SOI's banner occurred in 1968 at Soldier's Field in Chicago. Over one thousand athletes from the United States and a floor hockey team from Canada participated in these games.

Canada, led by the late Harry "Red" Foster, held its first Special Olympics event in Toronto in 1969. In doing so, Canada became the first country outside of the United States to host an event and to create a Special Olympics organization, Canadian Special Olympics (CSO). (In the fall of 2002, CSO changed its name to Special Olympics Canada (SOC).) From this modest beginning, Special Olympics has grown into a worldwide movement that provides sport training and competitive opportunities for people with intellectual disability in over one hundred and fifty countries (Special Olympics International 1999).

ORGANIZATIONAL STRUCTURE

Special Olympics International, located in Washington, DC, is the international coordinating body of Special Olympics. SOI's primary role lies in accrediting Special Olympic organizations around the world and in coordinating international winter and summer, multisport competitions. Within the United States, SOI also serves as the national body that supports state efforts to provide programmes and competitions at the local, district, and state levels.[3]

In Canada, Special Olympics includes four organizational levels: national, provincial/territorial, regional, and local. Special Olympics Canada, out of its office in Toronto, represents the national level of the organization. The national office accredits the provincial and territorial bodies, known as chapters, and supports their efforts to provide year-round Special Olympic programmes and competitions. In supporting programming, one of SOC's primary contributions has been the development of a national coaching education programme. This initiative is composed of two technical courses that address the competencies that coaches require to provide quality training for athletes with intellectual disability. These courses were developed in conjunction with Canada's National Coaching Certification Programme (NCCP) and are delivered regularly by certified course conductors across the country. SOC's other major responsibilities include coordinating national games in summer and winter sport, which take place on an alternating two-year schedule, and national teams (training and travel) that compete at international Special Olympic events.

All ten provinces and the Yukon have Special Olympic chapters. These chapters employ staff to coordinate and support sport training and competitive opportunities, which are delivered almost exclusively by volunteers and unpaid coaches at local, regional, and provincial levels. Over twenty thousand Canadians with intellectual disability participate in these grass roots initiatives on a regular basis (Special Olympics Canada, November 2001).

SOI MISSION

The mission of SOI is

> to provide year-round sports training and athletic competition in a variety of Olympic-type sports for individuals with mental retardation, giving them continuing opportunities to develop physical fitness, demonstrate courage, experience joy, and participate in a sharing of their gifts, skills, and friendship with their families, other Special Olympic athletes, and the community. (Special Olympics International, November 2001)

In Canada, the various organizational levels within SOC work together to fulfil a common goal or mission, which is consistent with SOI's but stated in different terms: "Enriching the lives of Canadians with a mental disability through sport" (J. Jordan, personal communication, October 25, 2001; approved by CSO Board of Directors, September 2, 2001). This mission is supported by nine guiding principles (see table 30.2) that reflect an athlete-centred approach to programme development and delivery, coaches' responsibilities in this process, and SOC's commitment to supporting involvement in other community-based sport training and competitive opportunities.

The second to last guiding principle, the practice of competition divisioning, is not specific to Special Olympics in Canada. Dividing athletes into categories based on age, sex, and ability is one of the defining elements of Special Olympic competitions around the world. In Canada, however, this principle has been extended whereby the performance of athletes in their respective divisions is part of a standardized process for selecting athletes for various levels of competition (for further details on divisioning and its use in selection, see section on Eligibility and Competition Classifications).

---

3 To date, the United States does not offer national level competitions. Instead, these usually occur within the context of International Winter and Summer Games.

Table 30.2 Guiding Principles to Support SOC's Mission Statement

- Special Olympics provides sport opportunities directly for athletes with intellectual disability.

- The athlete is all-important in Special Olympics. It is critical that coaches, parents, and caregivers encourage and provide athletes with intellectual disability with every opportunity to reach their highest level of athletic achievement.

- Special Olympics is a sport programme. Sport involves the matching of strength, endurance, and physical skills in formalized settings with structured rules and determined outcomes.

- Training and preparation are essential to meaningful participation in sport and are an indispensable element of any Special Olympics programme.

- Every Special Olympic athlete deserves the right to a certified coach.

- Special Olympics supports and promotes a fair and safe environment for both athletes and coaches.

- Special Olympics also links these athletes with other sport organizations that provide additional sport training and competitive opportunities.

- The practice of divisioning athletes for competition based on their abilities is fundamental to the Special Olympics programme. This practice ensures that all athletes experience equitable competition.

- Special Olympics uses the medium of sport to assist persons with intellectual disability to become all that they can be–physically, mentally, socially, emotionally–and to become accepted, respected, and productive members of society.

SOURCE: From the *Canadian Special Olympics Policy Manual*, by Special Olympics Canada, n.d., Toronto: Canadian Special Olympics. Reprinted with permission.

OFFICIAL SPORTS AND THE SPORT DELIVERY MODEL

SOI officially sanctions fourteen individual and five team sports (see table 30.3) (Special Olympics International 1996-1999; Special Olympics International 1999-2001). The popularity of these sports vary in different regions of the world, so programming and competitive events are not always offered in every country; however, all official sports are included in international competitions. In addition, SOI recognizes seven national sports, which are sports that enjoy high rates of participation in some, but not all, parts of the world (e.g., team handball) (see table 30.3). As a result, while training and competition is available in some of these sports in some countries, competition at the international level may or may not be provided.

In Canada, training and competitive opportunities are officially recognized in eleven individual and three team sports (table 30.3) *(Special Olympics Canada Policy Manual)*.

Curling also is recognized as a demonstration sport. This designation is used to denote a sport that is not available in all SOC chapters and competitions–usually, because of regional variations in popularity and participation *(Special Olympics Canada Policy Manual)*. In other words, a demonstration sport is SOC's equivalent of what SOI calls a national sport.

SOI does not have an official framework for delivering their programmes and competitions. In Canada, the delivery of these services is guided by SOC's sport model, which is illustrated in diagram 30.1 on p. 573. The outer circle of the model depicts the Canadian amateur sport system, of which Special Olympics is a part. Sport Canada, the federal government department that funds amateur sport in Canada, recognizes SOC as a national sport governing body.

The inner circle of the model reflects the athlete-centred nature of programmes and competitions (i.e., programmes are designed to meet athletes' needs and to offer training

Table 30.3 SOI and SOC

	Official Individual and Team Sports, and National/Demonstration Sports		
	Individual	Team	National/Demonstration
Special Olympics International			
Summer	Athletics	Basketball	Badminton
	Cycling	Softball	Bocce
	Diving	Soccer	Golf
	Equestrian	Volleyball	Powerlifting
	Gymnastics (rhythmic and artistic)	Sailing	
	10-pin Bowling	Table Tennis	
	Roller Skating	Team Handball	
	Swimming		
	Tennis		
Winter	Alpine Skiing	Floor Hockey	
	Nordic Skiing		
	Figure Skating		
	Speed Skating		
Special Olympics Canada			
Summer	Athletics	Soccer	
	Aquatics	Softball	
	5-pin Bowling		
	10-pin Bowling		
	Powerlifting		
	Rhythmic Gymnastics		
Winter	Alpine Skiing	Floor Hockey	Curling
	Nordic Skiing		
	Figure Skating		
	Speed Skating		
	Snowshoeing		

Figure 30.1 Canadian Amateur Sport System

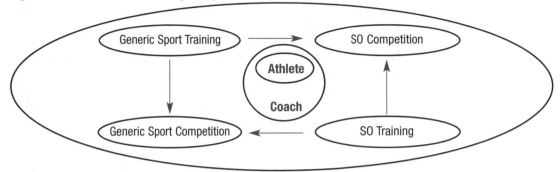

Note: Adaptation of the sport model based on the *Special Olympics Canada Policy Manual.*

and competitive options that enable them to achieve their maximum level of athletic performance). The coach circle indicates the central importance of coaching in promoting athlete development through training and competition.

The four interconnected ovals (e.g., SO Training, SO Competition), nested within the Canadian amateur sport context and encasing the athlete and coach, show the various training and competitive options that an athlete might access within Special Olympics or the broader community. The sport training circles suggest that athletes may choose to participate in generic and/or Special Olympic programmes. soc training options include athletic clubs, sport clubs, provincial, and/or national team training programmes. An athletic club, similar to a physical education class, provides exposure to and instruction in a number of different sport activities, which may or may not lead to competition. Sport clubs focus on training in a particular sport (e.g., athletics, swimming, floor hockey)–usually in preparation for local, regional, and/or provincial competitions. Extending the sport club concept, provincial and national team training programmes that provide high-intensity, sport-specific training have become the norm for athletes who aspire to or have been selected for higher levels of competition (i.e., provincial and national team members).

Paralleling the range of available training options, athletes may participate in generic and/or Special Olympic competitions. Participation in generic events might occur in the form of inclusive-open or parallel competitions. In inclusive-open competition, athletes with and without disabilities directly compete with one another. Although there are individual examples of athletes with intellectual disability who compete in these types of events (especially at high school or local levels), opportunities of this nature continue to be rare. Parallel competition, in which athletes with intellectual disability compete within a separate division in an event that includes athletes without disability, is the most common mode of generic competition. Recent examples of events of this type include Western Canada Games and Canada Games. soc-sponsored events encompass local, regional, provincial, national, and international competitions.

The soc sport model, in sum, is grounded in several fundamental concepts. Primary among these is the principle of normalization. Namely, the model supports the rights of individuals with intellectual disability to engage in sport training and competition, whether it is in Special Olympic or generic options. These rights are exercised by the decisions of individuals with intellectual disability. In turn, quality coaching that maximizes athletes' efforts to achieve personal excellence in training and competition supports these decisions.

ELIGIBILITY AND CLASSIFICATIONS FOR COMPETITION

Eligibility for participation in all levels of SOI is contingent on a person having intellectual disability. Sometimes participants have other, associated, disabilities (e.g., physical and/or sensory) as well, but the person's primary condition must be diagnosed as intellectual disability. Laws of confidentiality make it extremely difficult, if not impossible, for sport organizations (e.g., SOC) to access diagnostic information. Often, therefore, eligibility is determined according to whether a person receives services from other agencies (e.g., school, supported employment) that require a formal diagnosis of intellectual disability. Alternatively, identification by parents and/or caregivers that their child has intellectual disability also is accepted as a basis for eligibility.

Among the many conditions that may result in a person having intellectual disability, Down's syndrome is one of the most common. Approximately 17 percent of these individuals have a related condition that may affect eligibility–atlanto-axial instability. This is an orthopaedic problem that involves laxity in the ligaments supporting the first and second cervical vertebra, which, if present, may preclude a person with Down's syndrome from activities that involve excessive extension and/or flexion of the head and neck (e.g., butterfly stroke in swimming, diving, high jump, squat lifts, soccer, alpine skiing, tumbling activities). Within Canada, permission to participate in these types of activities can be secured by having: (a) a physician determine that an individual does not have atlanto-axial instability (determined by x-ray views of the neck in full flexion and extension),[4] or (b) parents and/or caregivers grant permission, after being made fully aware of this condition and its potential risks (Special Olympics Canada Policy Manual).

Within Canada, athletes are required to meet three additional standards (i.e., age, training, and qualification) in order to qualify for *competition*. Each of these standards serves a distinct purpose. The first standard, minimum age requirements, varies depending on whether the event occurs at the regional (age eight), provincial (age ten), national (age thirteen), or international (age fourteen) level. Minimum training standards are intended to ensure that athletes are adequately prepared for competitions. For example, athletes at the national level must engage in a minimum of two seasons of training, while those competing in international games must have trained for a minimum of three seasons. Performance in qualification events, the third and final standard, means that athletes' achievements at local, regional, provincial, and national competitions determine eligibility for successively higher levels of competition (i.e., local events are qualifiers for regional, regional for provincial, provincial for national, and national for international). A standardized system is used for awarding points for performance in each event and/or discipline that an athlete enters (e.g., within athletics ten points are awarded for each first place finish, eight for second, six for third, etc). A pool of eligible participants is identified through this process. Selection for a particular level of competition (e.g., provincial or national games) is based, in turn, on those who have earned the highest points in their respective events.[5]

To ensure equitable opportunities for earning points towards selection (and equitable competition in general), a classification system based on sex, age, and ability divisions is used. In individual sports this is done by separating male and female athletes and then further sub-dividing them, whenever possible, according to the following age groupings: eight to eleven, twelve to fifteen, sixteen to twenty-one, twenty-two to twenty-nine, and

---

4   Emerging evidence suggests that atlanto-axial may manifest itself at any point in a person's life and, as such, periodic retesting may be required to determine whether or not this condition is a factor (Batshaw 1997).

5   Selection of coaches also is governed by nationally standardized criteria (e.g., minimum requirements of national level coaches in most sports include: NCCP theory level 1, SOC/NCCP level 1, and a SO-based practical).

thirty plus. Ability is based on actual scores, times, or distances recorded in qualifying events and/or practice (seeding) rounds that take place immediately before the official competition. To verify the accuracy of the ability groupings, the 10 percent rule is used as a guideline. This means that the performances of athletes within a single division should be within 10 percent of one another. For example, if the average qualifying time in a 100-metre race division is 17 seconds, individual competitor's times should fall between 15.3 and 18.7 seconds (i.e., 10 percent plus and minus the average qualifying time). Divisioning for team sport follows the same general principles.

SUMMARY OF THE SPECIAL OLYMPICS MOVEMENT

Special Olympics is an international sport movement dedicated to promoting and providing training and competitive opportunities for individuals with intellectual disability. SOI is the international body that accredits national Special Olympic organizations in different countries of the world (e.g., SOC), coordinates international winter and summer games, and serves as the national body that oversees programme development and delivery in the United States. A classification system based on sex, age, and ability divisions (i.e., divisioning) is used to ensure equitable competition.

Canadians contributed significantly to the evolution of the Special Olympics movement and continue to do so today in a manner unique to Canada. Specifically, the principles that guide the mission, the sport delivery model, the philosophies it embodies (i.e., normalization and individual choice), and the use of standardized selection criteria for competition distinguishes Canada's version of Special Olympics.

The International Sports Federation for Persons With Intellectual Disability

Beginning in Europe in 1986, a second sport movement, separate and distinct from Special Olympics, emerged for persons with intellectual disability. This organization, which is now worldwide, is known as the International Sports Federation for Persons with Intellectual Disability (INAS-FID).[6] Founded on the principle of normalization, this movement evolved out of the belief that athletes dedicated to intense training and elite performance goals were not adequately served within SOI (B. Nirje, personal communication, November 20, 1999). Consequently, while supporting sport that includes participants at all levels of ability, INAS-FID is committed primarily to serving the competitive needs and aspirations of high-performance or elite athletes.

At its inception, INAS-FID became the organization representing athletes with intellectual disability on the International Coordinating Committee (ICC), the precursor to the International Paralympic Committee (IPC). The IPC, a body composed of national Paralympic committees (NPCs) and international sport organizations representing athletes with a disability (e.g., International Wheelchair Basketball Federation), is responsible for coordinating the involvement of these groups and the athletes they represent at the highest levels of international competition. These competitions include athletes with a wide range of disabilities (e.g., physical, sensory, neurological) in multisport Paralympic summer and winter games and sport-specific World Championships. The scheduling and location of these events parallels the cycle for the Olympic Games (summer and winter) and generic World Championship events.

As can been seen in the historical overview presented in table 30.4, athletes affiliated with INAS-FID have not always been part of IPC-sponsored events. Initially, athletes with

---

6 In 1986 INAS-FID was known as the International Sports Federation for Persons with Mental Handicaps (INAS-FMH); however, the name was officially changed in 1999 to reflect current terminology.

Table 30.4 A Brief History of INAS-FID

1989	INAS-FID World Championships in Athletics and Swimming, Harnosand, Sweden. This event only included athletes with intellectual disability (from here on described as an "INAS-FID-only event").
1999	INAS-FID Paralympic Games (summer), Madrid, Spain. INAS-FID-only event, competitions in athletics, swimming, five-a-side indoor soccer, table tennis, and basketball. This event occurred shortly after the IPC Paralympic Games in Barcelona, which did not include athletes with intellectual disability.
1994	IPC Paralympic Games (winter), Lillehammer, Norway. Competing in Nordic skiing demonstration events, this is the first time athletes with intellectual disability were included in an IPC event.
1994	IPC World Championships in athletics, Berlin, Germany, and IPC World Championships in swimming, Malta. First IPC World Championships to include athletes with intellectual disability.
1996	IPC Paralympic Games (summer), Atlanta, US. First Paralympic Games in which athletes with intellectual disability competed with full medal status.
1996	IPC World Championships in cross-country, Lisbon, Portugal. First event in which athletes with intellectual disability were fully included.
1998	IPC Paralympic Games (winter), Nagano, Japan. Athletes with intellectual disability competed with full medal status in Nordic skiing (five- through twenty-kilometre events).
1998	INAS-FID World Championships in basketball, (Brazil), and soccer (United Kingdom). These two events were INAS-FID only.
1999	INAS-FID World Championships in athletics (Spain), swimming (Czech Republic), and table tennis (Portugal). These events were INAS-FID-only.
1999	ParaPanamerican Games, Mexico City, Mexico. First IPC-sponsored event in the Americas region that included competition in athletics and swimming for athletes with intellectual disability.
2000	IPC Paralympic Games (summer), Sydney, Australia. Athletes with intellectual disability competed in an expanded range of events, i.e., in addition to athletics and swimming, men's basketball, and men's and women's table tennis were included.
2001	IPC suspended membership of INAS-FID (international body) and banned all athletes with intellectual disability from all IPC activities.
2001	INAS-FID World Championships in cross-country (Portugal), athletics (Tunisia)
2002	INAS-FID World Championships slated in rhythmic gymnastics (Belgium), cross-country (Poland), tennis (Czech Republic), basketball (Portugal), football (eleven-a-side, Japan)

intellectual disability only competed in separate INAS-FID World Championships and Paralympic Games. The Lillehammer Paralympic Games and the Berlin World Championships in athletics, both held in 1994, were the first IPC events that involved athletes with intellectual disability—albeit in limited numbers and in demonstration events (i.e., not included in medal standings). In 1996, the athletics and swimming competitions at the Paralympic Games in Atlanta signaled the first games in which INAS-FID athletes were officially included and afforded full medal status. Between 1996 and 2000, these athletes gradually gained access to an expanded array of IPC competitions (i.e., Paralympic Games and IPC World Championships). This progress was reversed in 2001 when the IPC suspended INAS-FID's membership and banned all athletes with intellectual disability from IPC activities (see "The Sydney Affair: Is Eligibility or Cheating the Issue?" on p. 582). Consequently, while consultations are presently underway, uncertainty surrounds the future of this organization and the athletes it represents within the IPC. INAS-FID, however, continues to host World Championship events in a variety of sports.

Also evident in table 30.4 is that athletes with intellectual disability, whether in INAS-FID- or IPC-affiliated events, compete in a limited range of individual and team sports. Individual sport options include athletics, swimming, Nordic skiing, and table tennis. Basketball, indoor five-a-side soccer, and outdoor eleven-a-side soccer are the current team sport offerings.

ORGANIZATIONAL STRUCTURE OF INAS-FID

INAS-FID includes organizational structures at three levels: international, regional, and national. The international body is the overall coordinator of regional and national INAS-FID activities and hosts sport-specific world championships. Prior to its suspension, the international body also represented INAS-FID on the IPC and worked collaboratively with this organization to access competitive options for athletes with intellectual disability at Paralympic Games. At the regional level,

INAS-FID includes organizations representing five areas of the world: Europe, Middle East, Africa, Asia/South Pacific, and the Americas (including South, Central, and North America). These organizations liaise with the international body, coordinate the activities of member nations within the region, and provide regional competitions.

Currently, eighty-six countries have national associations that are affiliated with INAS-FID (i.e., twenty-eight nations in Europe, ten from the Middle-East/North Africa, nineteen from Africa, thirteen in Asia/South Pacific, and sixteen from the Americas) (International Sports Federation for Persons with Intellectual Disability, November 2001). Within North America, Canada, the United States, and Mexico are members of INAS-FID. The Canadian body [i.e., Canadian Association of Sport for Athletes with Intellectual Disability, (CAAID)] is a member of the Canadian Paralympic Committee (CPC), which is the umbrella organization that represents sport organizations for athletes with disabilities in that country. CPC also is a member of the IPC. A similar organizational structure is in place in Mexico.

In the United States, the national Olympic Committee is responsible for all Olympic and amateur sport that includes athletes with and without disabilities (as per the Amateur Athletic Act 1998). Within this structure, the US Paralympic Committee represents all organizations that serve athletes with disabilities. This body also holds membership in INAS-FID, and as such, is responsible for US athletes with intellectual disability who qualify for, and access IPC and INAS-FID sanctioned events (J. Mulder, personal communication, November 7, 2001).

The national organizations of INAS-FID, including Canada's, typically do not provide grass roots training. Instead, national affiliates participate in identifying athletes who meet INAS-FID's eligibility standards and coordinating the inclusion of these athletes on national teams that represent their respective countries at Paralympic Games and World Championships. As such, athletes who compete in INAS-FID-affiliated events usually are products of intensive training programmes offered by other sport governing bodies in their home countries and communities. In Canada, most athletes are trained in generic sport programmes and, in some cases, are former members of provincial or national team training programmes sponsored by Special Olympics. To date, only athletes in swimming, athletics, and Nordic skiing have represented Canada internationally.

ELIGIBILITY AND COMPETITION CLASSIFICATIONS

Eligibility for inclusion in INAS-FID competitions requires that all athletes be certified as having intellectual disability (i.e., IQ in the 70–75 range, limitations in adaptive behaviour, manifested by age eighteen; *Bollnas Declaration* 1998). The word *certified* is imperative, because it means that athletes must go through a process of demonstrating their eligibility before being granted a license for competition. This process is largely the responsibility of national member organizations and involves securing official documentation that substantiates the diagnosis of intellectual disability by a qualified professional (e.g., certified psychologist) and/or eligibility for support services (e.g., educational, vocational) that require such a diagnosis. Once reviewed by the national body, this material is forwarded to INAS-FID at the international level, where it is evaluated and, if appropriate, a license is issued.

Beyond needing a license to compete, athletes must meet the minimum age requirement set by the appropriate international sport federation (e.g., IAAF, FINA, FIBA) and the qualification standards (i.e., performance standards) for their sport. The technical committee of INAS-FID sets the performance standards that athletes must achieve to qualify for INAS-FID-sponsored World Championships in athletics and swimming. This committee, in tandem with the IPC technical committee, establishes the competition standards that govern eligibility for the IPC-sponsored Paralympic Games and World Championships. Performance standards are published two years before the targeted event. Athletes then have this period of time in which to reach the standards for their event in a competition sanctioned by the national or international body of INAS-FID.

Athletes in team sports also are required to meet licensing and age requirements. For teams competing in Paralympic Games, regional competitions serve as qualifying events. For example, the Americas would host a tournament including national teams from countries within the region, and the winning team from this tournament would move on as the regional representative to the Paralympic Games. World Championships in a team sport involve a different qualifying process because these are strictly INAS-FID-governed events at this point (i.e., IPC does not offer World Championships in team sport). Teams that compete in these events qualify by winning national championships hosted by the INAS-FID body in their home countries (e.g., the Brazilian national champions in basketball would represent that country at the INAS-FID World Basketball Championships).

INAS-FID uses an open, performance-based system of classification at competitions. This means that, other than separating athletes by sex, competitions include a single category for each event and/or discipline. For example, in the 100-metres a single male and female winner would be awarded. Similarly, in team sports, gold, silver, and bronze medallists ultimately are determined through competition within one division. In individual sports, INAS-FID also maintains world rankings of the top performances in a given year, and records of best-ever performances (i.e., world records in athletics and swimming). At IPC World Championships and Paralympic Games, athletes with intellectual disability compete with one another in their own section. Once again, open competition within separate male and female categories produce a single winner in each event and/or discipline.

SUMMARY OF THE INAS-FID MOVEMENT

INAS-FID is an organization dedicated to furthering competitive opportunities for high-performance athletes with intellectual disability.

To access these opportunities, athletes must satisfy the minimum age requirement for international competition in their sport (as mandated by the appropriate international sport federation), have a license certifying that they have intellectual disability, and meet established qualification or performance standards. Male and female athletes and teams compete separately under an open system of classification. Ultimately, this leads to the awarding of medals (gold, silver, bronze) to the top male and female athletes and teams in each competition.

INAS-FID-sponsored events only include athletes with intellectual disability. Generally, these events involve individual (e.g., athletics, swimming) and/or team (basketball, soccer) competitions at the World Championship level. IPC events include athletes with a range of different disabilities (e.g., physical disabilities, sensory impairments)—each competing with athletes who have similar abilities. The IPC hosts sport-specific World Championships and multisport Paralympic Games that include athletes with a variety of disabilities.

Up to and including the Sydney 2000 Games, progress had been made in involving athletes with intellectual disability in IPC activities. This progress ceased with the IPC-imposed ban in 2001. While some may take issue with the rate of inclusion and concerns surrounding the ban, most agree that INAS-FID has come a long way in its short history and that cooperation and collaboration with member nations and the IPC may revive future progress.

Issues in Sport for Individuals with Intellectual Disability

So far, the discussion has concentrated on describing the two main international sport organizations (SOI and INAS-FID) that serve individuals with intellectual disability. Shifting focus, the following section addresses some of the key issues surrounding the organization and delivery of sport in this area. Specific issues to be examined include the relationship between SOI, INAS-FID, and the IPC; eligibility;

perspectives of other sport organizations for athletes with disability; and the segregated nature of sport for athletes with intellectual disability.

SOI, INAS-FID, AND THE IPC

> **1** Thinking back to the discussion of SOI and INAS-FID, do you have questions about how these organizations relate to one another and the IPC? If so, you are not alone, as questions of this nature are sources of considerable confusion. To clarify confusion, it is useful to consider the main characteristics of SOI and INAS-FID (see table 30.5).

While SOI and INAS-FID are driven by beliefs grounded in the principle of normalization and a shared commitment to sport for individuals with intellectual disability, table 30.5 shows that the two organizations are separate and distinct. SOI is the international body of the Special Olympics movement, which hosts its own competitive events in the form of World Winter and Summer Special Olympic Games. The Paralympic movement, governed by the IPC, provides multisport Paralympic Games and sport-specific World Championships for athletes from various disability groups. INAS-FID, as a member of the IPC, accesses these events. In addition, INAS-FID exclusively hosts World Championships for athletes with intellectual disability.[7]

Table 30.5 also illustrates the different aims of SOI and INAS-FID. SOI's goal is to provide sport *training and competition* for individuals with intellectual disability at *all ability levels*. INAS-FID, while philosophically in support of sport for individuals of all abilities, is primarily concerned with promoting and accessing *competitive opportunities* for athletes who have achieved *high performance standards*. The distinction between these aims is apparent in the way competitions are structured in the two organizations. Special Olympics uses a *divisioning system*, whereby participants are grouped according to age, sex, and ability.

---

7   In 1992 an INAS-FID Paralympic Games was hosted, however, it is unlikely that future INAS-FID exclusive games of this type will be hosted as the IPC moves towards full inclusion of athletes with intellectual disability.

Table 30.5 SOI and INAS-FID

	Comparative Summary of Main Characteristics	
	SOI	INAS-FID
History	• 1968, North America	• 1986, Europe
Conceptual/ philosophical foundation	• Principle of normalization	• Principle of normalization
Main goal	• Training and competition for athletes of all abilities	• Promoting competitive opportunities, primarily at the international level, for high performance athletes
Eligibility	• Intellectual disability • Age (minimum eight)	• Intellectual disability • Age (minimum as per appropriate international sport federation) • INAS-FID competition license
Competition classification	• Divisioning system	• Open system
Competitive events	SOI World Winter and Summer Games (multisport)	• INAS-FID World Championships • IPC Paralympic Games (multisport) • IPC World Championships (sport-specific)
Sponsors	• SOI	• IPC and/or INAS-FID
Levels	• Local to international	• World regions and international

This leads to awards for athletes in multiple ability groups in the same event and/or discipline. In INAS-FID-affiliated events, athletes are separated by sex, but otherwise an *open competition* approach is employed. Open competition means that men compete with men, and women compete with women to determine their respective standings within a single classification for each event and/or discipline.

In summary, to fully understand the sport delivery system for athletes with intellectual disability, it is important that you are knowledgeable about the similarities and differences between SOI and INAS-FID. Both organizations serve athletes with intellectual disability, but fundamentally differ in their purpose (i.e., sport for athletes of all abilities versus sport for elite level athletes) and system for competitive classification (i.e., divisioning versus open-competition).

ELIGIBILITY

What is the concern about eligibility and why is it an issue in sport for individuals with intellectual disability? The first step toward answering this question lies in understanding that equitable competition is a central premise of sport, whether it is in SOI, INAS-FID, or any other organization. To achieve equity in sport for persons with intellectual disability, a valid assessment and diagnosis of this state of functioning is essential. Internationally, this has been a challenging standard to satisfy because of the following:

- Not all countries in the world use exactly the same diagnostic procedures or have well-developed systems of assessment.
- Even when standard procedures and appropriate assessment systems are in place, sport organizations' access to this information often is severely limited, particularly in nations with stringent privacy laws (e.g., Sweden).

These challenges have led to charges that, in some instances, competitions include athletes who do not have intellectual disability. This criticism is less frequently applied to Special Olympics, largely because it uses a divisioning system (i.e., categorizing athletes according to age, sex, and ability) as a means of providing equitable competition for athletes of all ability levels. Within INAS-FID, the licensure requirement reflects the importance of a valid diagnosis as a foundation for equitable competition. This requirement, however, has not eliminated concerns about the eligibility of athletes who compete in INAS-FID and IPC events. In some cases, this concern seems to stem from stereotypic assumptions about the ability (e.g., individuals with intellectual disability are incapable of high levels of athletic achievement) and/or appearance of people with intellectual disability (e.g., individuals who manifest no visible signs of disability cannot be disabled). In other cases, eligibility has become a euphemism for other issues (see "The Sydney Affair: Is Eligibility or Cheating the Issue?" on p. 582).

Divisioning (SOI) and licensing (INAS-FID), although imperfect, are two strategies that have been used in an effort to resolve concerns about eligibility. The effectiveness of either approach requires that appropriate national and international organizations are committed to ensuring, and able to substantiate, that only athletes with intellectual disability are granted membership. Additionally, there is a great need for systematic education—at all levels of sport and within the general community—to dispel the myths and stereotypes that are often applied to individuals with intellectual disability.

PERSPECTIVES OF OTHER SPORT ORGANIZATIONS FOR ATHLETES WITH A DISABILITY

With the focus of this chapter on individuals with intellectual disability, there has been limited mention of sport organizations that serve athletes with other types of disabilities. As a result, you may be wondering about the relationship between these organizations and those geared towards athletes with intellectual disability. The simplest and most honest response is that sport organizations that serve different constituency groups have not always enjoyed harmonious relationships.

The Sydney Affair: Is Eligibility or Cheating the Issue?

In an exposé first published in *Capital* magazine (December 2000), Mr. Carlos Ribagorda reported that some events for athletes with intellectual disability at the 2000 Games included competitors without intellectual disability or, for that matter, any disability at all. These allegations were based on his first-hand experience as a member of the Spanish basketball team.

An investigation by the Spanish Paralympic Committee, the body responsible for Spain's delegation to the Games, confirmed that their basketball team for athletes with intellectual disability included members without disability (i.e., ten of the twelve members of the team did not have intellectual disability). Furthermore, it was revealed that no effort was made to comply with INAS-FID eligibility and licensing standards and procedures—they were simply ignored by the Spanish Paralympic Committee and the national body of INAS-FID. In an apparent endorsement of these findings, the president of the Spanish body of INAS-FID (who was also the president of the international body of INAS-FID at the time) charged that other contingents also included ineligible athletes.

The IPC responded by striking an investigation commission (in December 2000) to determine the extent of the problem. Before concluding this investigation, the IPC Management Committee suspended INAS-FID and banned all athletes with intellectual disability from future IPC events (IPC media release, January 27, 2001). The IPC and INAS-FID, at the international level, are presently continuing consultations to resolve this matter (IPC Newsflash, 5/2001). How and when a resolution may be reached, however, remains unclear.

One reason for this uncertainty is that the international leadership of the IPC and INAS-FID appear to have different interpretations about what transpired in Sydney. The IPC contends that eligibility is the central concern and that the events in Sydney are directly attributable to gross mismanagement of the "process of assessment and certification of intellectually disabled [sic] athletes" by all levels of INAS-FID (IPC, media release, March 9, 2001). From INAS-FID's perspective, unethical conduct in sport—cheating—is the primary issue at hand (J. Mulder, personal communication, February 2, 2001; and various INAS-FID member nation media releases). While acknowledging that the licensure process could be improved, advocates of this perspective point out that the Spanish delegation made no effort to comply with the standards and procedures required for proving eligibility.

What do you think about these competing points of view? What is the critical issue, eligibility or unethical conduct in sport? Who is responsible for what happened in Sydney? Who should be held accountable—athletes with intellectual disability, the ineligible athletes, and/or the national organizations that included these individuals in their delegation? Should all athletes with intellectual disability be banned based on the actions of a single team, from a single country? Are there other, more equitable, alternatives? What are they? Ultimately, the future of INAS-FID and the status of athletes with intellectual disability in ipc events will be contingent on answers and actions with respect to questions such as these.

One of the main reasons for this lack of harmony is directly related to the Special Olympic movement and the extent to which it has garnered media attention. Often times, so events are depicted as human interest stories that are described by adages such as "everyone's a winner." Little attention focusses on the unique nature of these participants' disability or the training that has preceded their involvement. It is not surprising, therefore, that other sport organizations for athletes with disabilities and their membership are left believing the following:

- Athletes with intellectual disability are 'Special Olympians' and not 'real' athletes committed to intensive training and high performance goals.
- The nature of intellectual disability renders it impossible for a person to engage in the level of training or mental preparation required for the highest and most intense levels of competition.
- If athletes are highly skilled, athletically, and their intellectual disability is not readily obvious (visible), sport opportunities outside of mainstream generic sport are unwarranted.

By now, your knowledge should help you to see that these beliefs are misguided; however, they have been the root of controversies and debates among proponents of sport for athletes with intellectual disability and sport organizations for athletes with other types of disabilities. In fact, each of the above-stated beliefs has been advanced, at one point or other, as arguments for excluding athletes with intellectual disability from IPC competitions. The recent movement towards full inclusion of these athletes in IPC events had put discussions of this nature to rest. Unfortunately, the scandal involving the Spanish basketball team at the 2000 Sydney Paralympic Summer Games and the subsequent banning of athletes with intellectual disability from IPC competitions seems to have reignited the debate (Naylor 2001). Now, perhaps more than ever, there is a need for collaborative efforts that will promote the mutual aims of all sport organizations for athletes with a disability—increased awareness, access, equity, and opportunity at all levels of sport for all athletes.

One priority area for collaboration needs to be public awareness about sport for athletes with a disability. The media coverage of Special Olympics also has had a tremendous influence on public perceptions, similar to its effect on sport organizations and athletes with *nonintellectual* disabilities. While these depictions have contributed positively to awareness, they also have left many members of the general public with several perceptions:

- They believe the incorrect assumption that Special Olympics is 'the' sport movement for athletes with all types of disabilities.
- They hold the idea that all people with a disability have intellectual disability (or, at least some degree thereof).
- They have a limited understanding of what it means to have intellectual disability and the challenges it presents.
- They have a lack of awareness of, or appreciation for, the intensity of training and competitiveness that underlies sport as it is pursued by high-calibre international athletes with all types of disability.

An entrenchment of these public perceptions is clearly problematic. Of particular concern, especially at the IPC level, is that these notions will infiltrate the corporate world (Cole 1999). If this occurs, if it has not already, corporations may assume that by sponsoring Special Olympics they are supporting sport for athletes with a disability in general. Obviously, this mistaken assumption may have serious ramifications for the funding of IPC Paralympic Games and World Championships, not to mention funding to support athletes training for these events. A systematic and broad-based approach to public education, which should involve all sport organizations that serve athletes with a disability, is needed to balance the media's over-emphasis on Special Olympics as the flagship of sport for athletes with disabilities.

SEGREGATED SPORT

Special Olympics, INAS-FID, and, indeed, most sport organizations for athletes with disability are segregated. This means that a person's disability is the primary basis for involvement and, typically, individuals without disability are not granted full membership in these organizations. Providing training and competition in this way has been the subject of considerable criticism over the years. Supporting this criticism, proponents of integration (i.e., programmes that include participants with and without disabilities) argue that segregated programmes are inconsistent with the principle of normalization and, as a result, should not be offered. Reflecting on the discussion of normalization, you should recall that specialized programmes—including sport—for individuals with a disability are not contrary to this principle and, in fact, may be used alone and/or in conjunction with other types of services (Perrin and Nirje 1985).

Despite this point, the criticism continues—particularly in application to SOI for providing segregated sport training and competition (Hourcade 1989; Wehman and Moon 1985). SOI, however, has acknowledged and attempted to address concerns about its segregated nature by introducing the concept of *unified team sports*. These programmes, offered primarily in the United States, bring participants with and without disabilities together in training and competition through Special Olympic sports (e.g., softball, soccer, sailing). These efforts, however, have not satisfied the critics who contend that these programmes are simply attempts to retain participants with intellectual disability who would be served, more appropriately, in integrated community programmes.

Extending these arguments, the success of Special Olympic programmes and their widespread growth has been charged with undermining the need for, and emergence of other, nonsegregated, options in the community. Special Olympics has been consistent in promoting itself as *one* option for individuals with intellectual disability and, in fact, advocating the need for opportunities beyond those available through their organization. As such, it is interesting that critics of Special Olympics have not devoted as much attention to generic providers of recreation and sport services who are mandated to, but do not always, offer options that are accessible to all members of their communities.

INAS-FID is also a segregated sport movement, but it has not been the target of the same degree of criticism as SOI. Why do you think this is the case? While there are many possible explanations (e.g., a newer organization, less well known), it seems likely that INAS-FID's emphasis on high-performance, international-level sport makes it less vulnerable to this type of criticism. Sport at the highest levels always has been exclusionary. Stop and think about this statement for a moment. No matter how much an athlete aspires to, dreams about, and trains in the hopes of reaching the Olympic Games—ability and performance ultimately play significant roles in determining whether an athlete makes it to this level. In other words, if INAS-FID is to be criticized for being segregated and exclusionary so, too, must sport in general. This is not a new idea, but it is probably the main reason that INAS-FID has not been judged as harshly on the segregation issue as SOI.

SUMMARY OF ISSUES IN SPORT

The preceding section presents four key issues that affect sport for athletes with intellectual disability: the relationship between SOI, INAS-FID, and the IPC; eligibility; perspectives of other sport organizations for athletes with a disability; and the segregated nature of sport for athletes with intellectual disability. These issues reflect what we believe to be the central concerns affecting the delivery of sport in this area. Your knowledge of these issues is an important part of the process that will lead to their resolution.

Summary and Conclusions

Sport is a valued tradition in most cultures of the world; however, as with many other facets of life, it was not widely accessible to individuals with intellectual disability until relatively recently. In the early 1960s this began to change as we came to appreciate that sport—recreational and competitive—is also a valued and important part of many of these individuals' lives. As a physical activity professional, you play a key role in promoting and supporting the inclusion of individuals with intellectual disability in sport and the activities that lead up to it (e.g., physical activity, physical education).

With these thoughts in mind, this chapter included a comprehensive introduction to a number of key concepts, strategies, and issues that are essential to the delivery of quality physical activity and sport opportunities for these individuals. The discussion started with an overview of appropriate terminology and the meaning of intellectual disability, an understanding of which is the first step towards effective programming. To assist in translating this understanding into action, the next section addressed your role as a physical activity professional in facilitating and supporting the participation of individuals with intellectual disability in school and community programmes—which are the precursors to involvement in sport. Also in this section, you were prompted to think about your attitude and how it might influence, positively and/or negatively, your practice as a professional and participation opportunities for these individuals. Suggestions that have been useful in facilitating learning and participation in physical activity and sport were presented as a start for developing your personal 'bag of effective instructional strategies'. As a transition to examining sport opportunities for individuals with intellectual disability, the principle of normalization was presented. This was followed by detailed descriptions of the two main sport movements that include athletes with intellectual disability, Special Olympics and INAS-FID (e.g., history, mission, organization, and competition structuring). In the final section, four key issues were presented that affect the delivery of sport.

Personal reflection and exposure to experiences that include individuals with intellectual disability are two approaches that you can use to further your understanding of the topics discussed in this chapter. To stimulate your efforts to learn more, we leave you with the following questions to think about and activities to try.

Activities to Try

- Make a personal commitment to provide programming that includes participants of all abilities and focusses on systematic instruction, positive reinforcement, opportunities for practice, play, competition, success, and enjoyment.
- Volunteer for a local recreation or sport programme that includes participants with an intellectual disability.
- Shadow a physical education teacher, instructor, and/or coach who is known for effectively including participants with intellectual disability or participants of all abilities in their programme, class, or club.
- Have interschool athletes serve as buddies or mentors for individuals with intellectual disability in school-based physical education. This could involve students from the same school or interschool athletes from secondary schools assisting middle or primary school students with a disability.
- Watch the next television programme or movie that focusses on sport or the lives of persons with a disability.
- Look for new and reliable information that will help you become as knowledgeable as possible about persons with intellectual disability (e.g., read books, journals, magazines, search the Internet, talk to other people).

Study Questions

- What does it mean to have intellectual disability?
- What does this mean for me as a physical activity professional?
- What are my attitudes towards and my assumptions about people with intellectual disability? Do these have a positive and/or negative affect on what I do as a professional?
- Do I use approaches to instruction and learning that help participants to be successful?
- Are there other strategies I could try?
- Am I knowledgeable about opportunities in sport training and competition that a student or participant with intellectual disability might be interested in accessing?

References

Abery, B., and Fahnestock, M. (1994). Enhancing the social inclusion of persons with developmental disabilities. In M.F. Hayden and B. Abery (Eds.), *Challenges for a service system in transition: Ensuring quality community experiences for persons with developmental disabilities* (pp. 83-119). Baltimore, MD: Paul H. Brookes.

Amado, R. (1988). Behavioral principles in community recreation. In S. Schleien and M.T. Ray (Eds.), *Community recreation and persons with disabilities: Strategies for integration* (pp. 79-90). Baltimore, MD: Paul H. Brookes.

American Association on Mental Retardation. (2002). *Mental retardation: Definition, classification, and systems of supports* (10th ed.). Washington, DC: Author.

Baroff, G.S. (1991). What's in a name? A comment on Goldfarb's guest editorial. *American Journal on Mental Retardation, 96*, 99-100.

Batshaw, M. (1997). *Children with disabilities* (4th ed.). Baltimore, MD: Paul H. Brookes.

Bishop, K.D., and Falvey, M. (1989). Transition issues and strategies. In M.A. Falvey (Ed.), *Community-based curriculum: Instructional strategies for students with severe handicaps* (2nd ed., pp. 189-228). Baltimore, MD: Paul H. Brookes.

Block, M. (2000). *A teacher's guide to including students with disabilities in general physical education* (2nd ed.). Baltimore, MD: Paul H. Brookes.

Bollnas Declaration. (1998). Unpublished proceeding from the Conference on Eligibility in the International Sports Federation for Persons with Intellectual Disability, Bollnas, Sweden, September 11-12, 1998.

Cole, C. (1999, August 28). Faster, higher, poorer. *The National Post*, pp. A15, A18.

Davis, W.E. (1989). Utilizing goals in adapted physical education. *Adapted Physical Activity Quarterly, 6*, 205-16.

Davis, W.E., and Burton, A.W. (1991). Ecological task analysis: Translating movement behaviour theory into practice. *Adapted Physical Activity Quarterly, 8*, 154-77.

Dybwad, G. (1982). Normalization and its impact on social and public policy. In *Advancing your citizenship: Normalization re-examined*. Eugene, OR: Rehabilitation Research Training Institute.

Edelstein, B.A. (1989). Introduction to mini-series: Generalization and maintenance of behavior change. *Behavior Therapy, 20*, 309-10.

Eichstaedt, C., and Lavay, B. (1992). *Physical activity for individuals with mental retardation: Infancy through adulthood.* Champaign, IL: Human Kinetics.

Fernhall, B., Tymeson, G., and Webster, G. (1988). Cardiovascular fitness of mentally retarded individuals. *Adapted Physical Activity Quarterly, 5*, 12-28.

French, R., and Lavay, B. (1990). *Behaviour management techniques for physical educators and recreators.* Kearney, NE: Educational Systems.

Gething, L. (1997). *Person to person: A guide for professionals working with people with disabilities.* Baltimore, MD: Paul H. Brookes.

Goldfarb, M. (1990). Guest editorial. *American Journal on Mental Retardation, 95*(3), v-vi.

Gould, S.J. (1981). *The mismeasure of man.* New York: Norton.

Haney, M., and Falvey, M. (1989). Instructional strategies. In M. Falvey (Ed.), *Community-based curriculum: Instructional strategies for students with severe disabilities* (2nd ed., pp. 63-90). Baltimore, MD: Paul H. Brookes.

Hastings, R. (1994). On "good" terms: Labeling people with mental retardation. *Mental Retardation, 32*, 363-65.

Hourcade, J. (1989). Special Olympics: A review and critical analysis. *Therapeutic Recreation Journal, 23*, 58-65.

Houston-Wilson, C., Lieberman, L., Horton, M., and Kasser, S. (1997). Peer tutoring: A plan for instructing students of all abilities. *Journal of Physical Education, Recreation, and Dance, 68*(6), 39-44.

International Sports Federation For Persons with Intellectual Disability. (November, 2001). [On-line]. Available: http://www.inas-fid.org/ (URL on December 4, 2002). [INAS-FID home page]. Amsterdam: Author.

Jordan, J. (October 25, 2001). Personal communication.

Krebs, P., and Block, M. (1992). Transition of students with disabilities into community recreation: The role of the adapted physical educator. *Adapted Physical Activity Quarterly, 9*, 305-15.

Jones, M. (1994). *Mental Retardation and Developmental Disabilities Prism Series: Vol. 1. Within our reach: Behavior prevention and intervention strategies for learners with mental retardation and autism.* Reston, VA: Division on Mental Retardation and Developmental Disabilities of the Council for Exceptional Children.

Liberty, K.A. (1985). Enhancing instruction for maintenance, generalization, and adaptation. In K.C. Lakin and R.H. Bruininks (Eds.), *Strategies for achieving community integration of developmentally disabled citizens* (pp. 29-71). Baltimore, MD: Paul H. Brookes.

Magsino, R. (1993). Teacher and pupil rights and the courts: An exploration of stability and change. In L. Stewin and S. McCann (Eds.), *Contemporary educational issues: The Canadian mosaic* (2nd ed., pp. 3-20). Toronto: Copp Clark.

Mahon, M. (1994). The use of self-control techniques to facilitate self determination skills during leisure in adolescents with mild and moderate mental retardation. *Therapeutic Recreation Journal, 28*, 58-72.

Mulder, J. (November 7, 2001). Personal communication.

Naylor, D. (2001, January 31). Officials suspend disabled athletes. *The Globe and Mail*, pp. S1, S2.

Nirje, B. (1969). The normalization principle and its human management implications. In R. Kugel and W. Wolfensberger (Eds.), *Changing patterns in residential services of the mentally retarded*. Washington, DC: President's Committee on Mental Retardation.

Nirje, B. (1992). *The normalization papers*. Uppsala, Sweden: Uppsala University Centre for Handicap Research.

Parmenter, T. (2001). Intellectual disabilities: Quo vadis? In G.L. Albrecht, K.D. Seelman, and M. Bury (Eds.), *Handbook of disability studies* (pp., 267-96). Thousand Oaks, CA: Sage.

Perrin, B., and Nirje, B. (1985). Setting the record straight: A critique of some frequent misconceptions of the normalization principle. *Australian and New Zealand Journal of Developmental Disabilities, 11,* 69-74.

Pitetti, K., Rimmer, H., and Fernhall, B. (1993). Physical fitness of adults with mental retardation: An overview of current research and future directions. *Sports Medicine, 16,* 174-77.

Reiss, S. (1994). Issues in defining mental retardation. *American Journal on Mental Retardation, 99,* 1-7.

Rizzo, T., and Kirkendall, D. (1995). Teaching students with mental disabilities: What affects attitudes of future physical educators? *Adapted Physical Activity Quarterly, 12,* 205-16.

Sandieson, R. (1998). A survey on terminology that refers to people with mental retardation/developmental disabilities. *Education and Training in Mental Retardation and Developmental Disabilities, 33,* 290-95.

Schleien, S., Green, F., and Heyne, L. (1993). Integrated community recreation. In M.E. Snell (Ed.), *Instruction of students with severe disabilities* (4th ed., pp. 526-55). New York: Macmillan.

Schleien, S., Ray, T., and Green, F. (1997). *Community recreation and people with disabilities: Strategies for inclusion* (2nd ed.). Baltimore, MD: Paul H. Brookes.

Seidl, C. (1998). Considerations for fitness appraisal, programming, and counseling of people with intellectual disabilities. *Canadian Journal of Applied Physiology, 23,* 185-222.

Snell, M.E. (1988). Gartner and Lipsky's beyond special education: Toward a quality system for all students: Messages for TASH. *Journal of the Association for Persons with Severe Handicaps, 13,* 137-40.

Special Olympics Canada Policy Manual. Toronto, ON: Special Olympics Canada.

Special Olympics Canada. (November, 2001). [On-line]. Available: http://www.soc.on.ca/CanadianSpecialOlympics (URL on December 4, 2002). [Special Olympics Canada home page].

Special Olympics International. (1996-1999). *The official Special Olympics summer sport rules* (rev. ed.). Washington, DC: Author.

Special Olympics International. (1999-2001). *The official Special Olympics winter sport rules* (rev. ed.). Washington, DC: Author.

Special Olympics International. (November, 2001). [On-line]. Available: olympics.org [Special Olympics International home page]. (URL December 4, 2002). Washington, DC: Author.

Stainback, S., and Stainback, W. (1992). *Curriculum considerations in inclusive classrooms: Facilitating learning for all students.* Baltimore, MD: Paul H. Brookes.

Stone, J., and Campbell, C. (1991). Student to student: Curriculum and the development of peer relationships. In G. Porter and D. Richler (Eds.), *Changing Canadian schools: Perspectives on inclusion disability.* Toronto: G. Allen Roeher Institute.

Switzky, H. (1997). Mental retardation and the neglected construct of motivation. *Education and Training in Mental Retardation and Developmental Disabilities, 32,* 194-200.

Wehman, P., and Moon, M.S. (1985). Designing and implementing leisure programmes for individuals with severe handicaps. In M.P. Brady and P.L. Gunter (Eds.), *Integrating moderately and severely handicapped learners.* Springfield, IL: Charles C. Thomas.

Wehman, P., and Schleien, S. (1981). *Leisure programs for handicapped persons: Adaptations, techniques, and curriculum.* Austin, TX: PRO-ED.

Wolfensberger, W. (1972). *The principle of normalization in human services.* Toronto: National Institute on Mental Retardation.

CHAPTER 31

The Female Athlete in Paralympic Sport

Lisa M. Olenik

Learning Objectives

- To discuss and consider ways in which the Paralympic movement compares to the Olympic movement in regard to gender.
- To think critically about and discuss the gendering of sport in general and the impact on the female Paralympic athlete.
- To discuss the under-representation of women in Paralympic sport and indicate the possible reasons for continued low participation rates.
- To appreciate the representative narratives of the elite female athlete and examine means by which the Paralympic movement can reproduce and sustain the successful experiences of women in disability sport.

Introduction

At the 2000 Paralympic Games in Sydney, Australia, the number of female athletes participating was expected to increase from previous events. The number of events for women was higher than ever before. For the first time, women competed in powerlifting. Of the 561 gold medal events scheduled on the Sydney 2000 programme, 321 were available for men, 197 for women, and 43 mixed (Reiff 2000). In the final tally, however, less than 25 percent of the athletes in Sydney were women.

Despite the efforts by sport governing bodies and academic groups to initiate research on the female athlete in elite disability sport, most research attempts still lack a female perspective, and they focus primarily on the physiological and psychological gains of male athletes who take part in competition (Cowell, Squires, and Raven 1986; Jackson and Davis 1983; Shepherd 1991; Valliant, Bezzubyk, Daley, and Asu 1985). Some studies relative to the sociological aspects of participation by the athlete with disability provide descriptive information about the athlete (Brandmeyer and McBee 1986; Cooper, Sherrill, and Marshall 1986; Hopper 1984; Sherrill, Rainbolt, Montelione, and Pope 1986). These initial studies acknowledge a relationship between the categories of *athlete* and *disability*, without considering the implications of gender, race, ethnicity, disability type, or socio-economic status. Of the studies that do include gender in their examination (Watkinson and Calzonetti 1989; Sherrill, Silliman, Gench, and Hinson 1990; Sherrill, et al. 1990) very few acknowledge the complex sociological context of sport or its relationship to physical activity (Kolkka and Williams 1997). Similar to inquiry in disability sport, there is very little research from the field of therapeutic recreation. Two recent studies, however, do explore some of the experiences of women with disability who are involved in physical activity and recreation (Blinde and McCallister 1999; Henderson and Bedin, 1995). In response to the shortage of gender-based sociological research, there has been a small but well-documented effort by adapted physical activity professionals to promote scholarship that acknowledges the multi-dimensionality of the athlete with a disability and thus expand the research agenda (Sherrill 1997a; Williams 1994a 1994b; Sherrill 1993; Olenik, 1998; DePauw 1994). According to Sherrill (1997a),

> Disability is a multidimensional identity that is specific to culture and history, is socially constructed, and is mediated by time of onset, nature of impairment, socio-economic status, gender, ethnicity, and the multitude of roles, expectancies, aspirations, and perceptions that each individual incorporates into the self. (p. 257)

In addition to low participation numbers and a limited amount of research on the female athlete, there is also a marked under-representation of women participating in the administrative levels of disability sport (DePauw and Gavron 1995; Olenik, Matthews, and Steadward 1995).

With regard to the low participation numbers, Sherrill (1993) states that the barriers that the female athlete faces in elite disability sport far exceed those described in sport for the nondisabled. The purpose of this chapter is to highlight the involvement of the female athlete in Paralympic sport and engage the reader in discussion regarding the lack of representation of women in the Paralympic Games.

Paralympic Context

Elite disability sport today is largely identified with the Paralympic movement, specifically the Paralympic Games. Although little documented evidence exists on organized disability sporting events before 1924, historical accounts confirm the participation of people with disabilities in physical activity and movement exercise in China dating back to 2700 BCE (DePauw and Gavron 1995). The Olympic model, which has to this point largely influenced the Paralympic model, has made only small gains in the area of women's sport development (Sherrill 1998). A study by Wilson (1996) on the status of women in the Olympic movement exposed the continued exclusion of women as first designed and supported by Pierre de Coubertin, founder of the modern Olympic games. The cultural meaning and issues surrounding the systematic exclusion of women in these games have only recently been questioned. It was not until 1973 that the first female International Olympic Committee (IOC) member was elected, and only since the election of President Juan Antonio Samaranch that the IOC formed a working group on women and sport. According to Wilson (1996), despite efforts over the past twenty years of the Samaranch presidency, women comprise just 7 percent of the IOC, hold 3 percent of the National Olympic Committee (NOC) presidencies, and, 6 percent of the Olympic International Federation presidencies. He also estimates that 36 percent of the athletes in the Atlanta Olympic Games were women and that women participated in 40 percent of the events (Wilson 1996).

The Paralympic effort to further gender equity has been similar to the Olympic efforts, yet while the Olympic movement has evolved over a hundred years, the Paralympic movement is much younger and it has made greater strides in promoting diversity on the sporting field than has the Olympic movement (Sherrill 1998).

Unfortunately, reliable statistical information on gender, disability type, age, and sport affiliation is unavailable for games prior to the 1994 Lillehammer Winter Paralympics. Paralympic Games organizers estimate that women now make up 25 to 30 percent of participants (International Paralympic Committee 1992, 1994; Sherrill 1993, 1997.) In Lillehammer, of 625 competitors from 31 countries, 481 were male and 144 female (International Paralympic Committee 1994). In the 1996 Atlanta Paralympics, the gender ratio was approximately 4 males to 1 female. Of the 104 participating countries, 49 had no female representation (Sherrill 1997b). According to International Paralympic Committee (IPC) Web site, it was estimated that there were 3,195 athletes competing in Atlanta, 2,415 male and 780 female.

Although the Paralympic Games continue to grow in size (122 countries participated at Sydney), of the total number of athletes who participated (4,032) only 1,109 were women. Similar to Atlanta, nearly three times as many men as women participated (Craft, 2001). This number may be due to the lack of representation of women from traditionally Muslim countries; however, the US team brought twice as many men (195) as women (93) to compete.

Sport for athletes with disability at the international level is the responsibility of, and is sanctioned, supervised, and coordinated by, the IPC. The IPC is the organizational equivalent of the IOC, and is a democratically-based organization with national representation, including more than 170 member nations, athlete representation, regional representation, twenty-three sport committee representatives, and representation from the five international sport organizations. Instead of being organized around specific sporting events, the international sport organizations (IOSDs) are established according to disability type and are gender-inclusive in their missions. These organizations include Cerebral Palsy-International Sport and Recreation Association (CP-ISRA), International Blind Sport Association (IBSA), International Sport Organization for the Disabled (ISOD), International Stoke Mandeville Wheelchair Sport Federation (ISMWSF), and the International Federation for Athletes with an Intellectual Disability (INAS-FID).

The Gendering of Paralympic Sport

According to the qualitative findings of a recent study, *Women, Disability, and Sport and Physical Fitness Activity: The Intersection of Gender and Disability Dynamics*, women with physical disabilities experience the intersection of two socially devalued roles (those of having a disability and being a woman) in a sport context which, by definition, is constructed to run counter to both of these roles (Blinde and McCallister 1999). In this study, several gender-related questions presented distinct differences between the way men and women perceived the role of physical activity in their lives. The study did not include the perception of men with physical disabilities in its analysis, but focussed instead on the perception of women regarding the male sport experience. Although the study included some mention of elite sport participation in the analysis, the focus was on the outcomes associated with regular sport-like physical activity by women. Those outcomes included the use of sport/physical activity to maintain functionality, to increase social relationships, to enhance the athlete's view of her capabilities, to use the body as a source of strength, and to increase control over one's life. These outcomes were very similar to those discussed in a qualitative study by Olenik et al. (1995) on elite female Paralympic athletes in the VI Winter Paralympic Games in Lillehammer in 1994. This study examined the participatory issues of the female athlete competing in elite winter Paralympic sport, with the intent of gaining insight into the barriers female athletes face relative to their participation. Although small in scope, this qualitative study highlighted some of the issues which should be analyzed in further detail. Important participatory issues expressed by these athletes included:

1. a perceived lack of competitive opportunities
2. a lack of acceptance by society of their sport
3. a lack of awareness of their needs on the part of the sport system
4. a need to validate their experiences with other female athletes

Also noteworthy in the development of elite disability sport for women are the choices researchers make as individuals who study the Paralympic movement, and their own relationship to the economic, social and political issues of those we study (Cole 1994). These choices include assumptions embedded in the theoretical framework, method, analysis, and reporting techniques used by researchers. In most sport sociological research using the feminist perspective, the dominant belief is that sport is socially constructed and gendered– as male or masculine. Often this construction has led to a perceived discrepancy between being both a female and an elite athlete. In other words, the elements associated with the dominant elite sporting experience have historically been used to reinforce social values, power relations, and conflicts between dominant groups and less powerful groups. It is this emphasis on social and cultural contexts that has placed feminist theory at the forefront of research on women in Paralympic sport and contemporary analysis of elite sport and culture.

Researchers using feminist theory argue that the experience of the female athlete in able-bodied sport differs from that of the male athlete because of the way in which society constructs gender and applies this construction to sporting contexts (Hall 1993). Historically, the dominant perspective in research related to the social construction of gender and sport has been based on a presumed "role conflict," or paradox, between female athleticism and femininity (Allison 1991). Assuming that the characteristics associated both with being a woman and an elite athlete were in conflict, many studies examine the ways in which female athletes could adapt or improve their sporting behaviour in order to "fit in" to sport in a male-dominated environment (Theberge 1985).

Messner's (1992) *Power at Play: Sports and the Problem of Masculinity* examines the masculine characteristics of sport using a feminist frame of analysis. He states that the historical influence of initial sporting events in the 1800s in both Europe and North America prepared the 'character' of young men to be better soldiers, leaders, citizens, and rulers. Rather than defining masculinity as some "buried biological essence of manhood," Messner maintains that this definition is socially constructed, and thus the concept of masculinity varies historically and cross-culturally. This social construction of sport that prepares individuals to be 'instrumental', 'aggressive', and 'dominating' has extended to the female's sporting arena. On most playing fields, the female athlete is considered a superior athlete if she can maintain a persona that reflects stereotypical masculine attributes. For many female athletes, the highest praise received on the playing field is that "she throws like a boy" or "she has a cool head." As sport sociologists began to notice this phenomenon in able-bodied sport, they developed a conceptual framework to examine the "role conflicts" that female athletes experience when they are expected to be both an athlete and a woman (Allison 1991). While researchers continue to evaluate women athletes based on this role conflict model, they have developed an image of the traditional female athlete: one who is struggling with her femininity and, equally, her athleticism (Hall 1988). Boutilier and San Giovanni (1983) describe the social construction of this theory:

> Underlying most analyses of role conflict is
> an uncritical acceptance of the traditional
> role of woman and the conventional

arrangement of sport. To ask if a woman can remain a woman and still play sports means that one has in mind a view of women and of sport that accepts the socially constructed definition of these two realities as contradictory and conflicting. (p. 117)

This view is especially relevant when exploring how the female elite Paralympic athlete's experience does or does not fit with the dominant sporting experience, that of the male athlete. The assumption that males, especially able-bodied males, are the standard for the entire population has been ingrained in most scientific disciplines and is a critical issue in current feminist and qualitative scholarship (Boutilier and San Giovanni 1983; DePauw 1994).

Elite sport itself is also socially constructed as able-bodied, so that being both a person with disability and an elite athlete places the female athlete with disability in her second perceived role conflict dilemma. The outcome is that these athletes are then challenged to treat physical difference such as gender and disability as obstacles to overcome. Reinforcing this assumption is research in disability sport that has been traditionally grounded in the rehabilitative and biomedical sciences in which sport or physical activity is used to overcome the limitations of disability (Williams 1994b). This biomedical orthodoxy in the literature is not surprising, since sport for people with a disability was first provided as an avenue for men to overcome the disabling conditions they sustained in World War II (DePauw and Gavron 1995; Jackson and Davis 1983; Steadward 1996).

---

1 Discuss methods the Paralympic movement could employ to achieve gender equity when planning for the Paralympic Games.

---

2 What is the evidence that Paralympic sport is socially constructed to be a traditionally male sporting domain?

---

3 What are alternatives to the perceived "role conflict" model when teaching physical activity and sport skills to the female athlete?

Identifying the Female Athlete Experience

In 1993, Hall examined the meaning, potential, and prospects of feminist cultural studies of sport. Specifically, she exposed many of the underlying assumptions driving the discourse surrounding gender and sport as "malestream" theories that do not take into account the production and reproduction of traditional gender roles. Assuming that sporting practices are historically produced, socially constructed, and culturally defined to serve the interests and needs of the dominant group, Hall proposes a "new set of scientific tools" necessary to understand the relationships between gender, class, race, and ethnicity in the construction of sport and sport practices. Moreover, the assumption that a homogeneity of experience exists among women involved in sport and physical activity, regardless of race, ethnicity or socioeconomic status, is called into question (Birrell 1990).

Interestingly, Birrell (1990) and Hall (1993) have not extended the discussion to include the social construction of disability and how it shapes, disguises, or impacts the lived experience of the female involved in sport and physical activity. Perhaps disability and the plethora of issues surrounding the lives of women with disability seem too vast, complex, or overwhelming to include in the discourse surrounding women and sport. Or perhaps the associated malestream theories that have driven the field of disability studies seem insurmountable to feminist researchers in able-bodied sport.

Because generalizing, from sport for athletes without disability to disability sport, ignores or erases the significance of the athlete's experience within disability sport, the participatory issues for both groups may be dissimilar. Simply accepting current theoretical models based upon the participatory issues of able-bodied female athletes and applying them to women with disability negates the experience of the female athletes with disability and overlooks the historical and political context of that experience. Furthermore, the trend to accept current models of male participation in disability sport and generalize them to the participatory experiences of the female denies her the right to name her own experience and also her own reality when it differs from the norm. In order to address the prevalence of role conflict and malestream research within sport sociology, feminist scholars and researchers have called for women-centred research that acknowledges the unique experiences of women within sport (Allison 1991; Cole 1994; Hall 1985, 1988; Theberge 1981). In other words, research that is informed by the unique perspective of the female participant and acknowledges the production of gender roles in sport. Bar On (1993) argues that feminist claims have emerged as counterpoints to the Enlightenment strategies for claiming authority. As such, feminist arguments have been framed within the Enlightenment's terms of discourse and replicate its repressive mechanisms for claiming the authority and privilege to silence others. For example, in the application of feminist theory, researchers have falsely universalized the experiences and concerns of white, middle-class, able-bodied, young, heterosexual women in sport to all other female populations (Dewar 1993). Likewise, Dewar (1993) argues that standpoint theory has been used in ways to suggest the existence of "generic women" with generic experiences of oppression in sport. Additionally, in order to provide a more inclusive feminist research agenda that contains both a critique of traditional scientific practices and recommendations for change, the relative privilege of the researcher must be recognized.

DePauw (1997) shows how the traditional scientific view of the body as dismembered is challenged via feminist critiques and is replaced by feminist understandings of the body as holistic and socially constructed.

> Although the body has been central to our field, we have studied it in parts and not necessarily as a whole or in relation to society. We have argued nature/nurture and relied mostly on biological essentialism. This reliance on biological essentialism has reinforced our traditional views of the body and the quest for the 'ideal' body. It is only recently that the body and bodies have become a focus of scholarly inquiry and has been aided by feminist theory. (p. 419)

While not all feminist research and advocacy efforts have been conscious of their own limitations and social context, recent work reveals that, with such self-consciousness, feminist theory can be used successfully with other perspectives without losing its critical essence. Also noteworthy is that, despite the complexity of the experience, sociological research addressing participation and disability sport is somewhat atheoretical, or if theoretical underpinnings are identifiable, the majority of research is grounded in positivism, and especially *structural functionalism* (Williams 1994a). Structural functionalism is often used in many organizational studies where the sociological perspective is based on an assumed a priori social structure, one that contains inherent meaning or function which is detached from the participants. When gender is included as a variable, it is in an attempt to show the difference in participation patterns and to identify socializing agents (e.g., parents, schools, peers) of sport and physical activity (Sherrill and Williams 1996; Williams 1994b). The need for feminist theory in the study of gender in disability sport has been discussed in several works (DePauw 1994; Kolkka and Williams 1997; Sherrill 1993). However, Begum (1992) and Wendell (1993) acknowledge that the feminist theory paradigm is often inadequate when examining disability. Wendell (1993) argues that, in order to build a feminist theory of disability that takes adequate account of experiential differences, we will need to know how experiences of disability and social oppression of people with disabilities interact with sexism, racism, and class oppression (p. 51). The tapestry of experience becomes more tightly woven with each variable considered and thus more difficult to discern.

The constitution of the IPC states that, as a governing body, it will promote sports for athletes with disability without discrimination for political, religious, economic, gender, or racial reasons, and, further, that it will seek expansion of the opportunities for persons with disabilities to participate in sports (International Paralympic Committee, 1994). In other words, the opportunity to participate at the elite sport level is an IPC constitutionally supported opportunity afforded to all elite level athletes with disability.

As we have seen, adapted physical activity scholars have speculated about the barriers that exist for women in disability sport. Some of the barriers reported in the literature include the classification systems that are not sensitive to women, that too few women are involved in the power structure of the disability sports movement, and that an under-representation of women athletes occurs in wheelchair sport (which often receives the most attention by the able-bodied media).

It is necessary to move beyond the speculation about barriers that limit women's participation and to focus on the experiences of women who are successful participants in elite sport in order to link theory to practice. According to Boutilier and San Giovanni (1983), a qualitative approach, rather than the traditional quantitative analysis, enables researchers together with informants to explore and describe "women's ways of knowing," ways of ascertaining and verifying truth in the domain of sport. As there exists little cumulative knowledge regarding the socializing agents that influence participation by women in elite disability sport, more first-hand knowledge is needed. Moreover, to understand women in disability sport adequately, the social context in which the activity occurs must be taken into consideration, specifically, the level of competition and sport discipline. Increasing the involvement of female athletes may depend on the sport system's ability to reproduce or increase the circumstances in which women choose to

participate. In response to this argument, IPC President Dr. Robert D. Steadward (1989–2001) and his executive council formed the first Commission on Women in Sport. This commission is an IPC unit, given the authority and mandate to develop for approval by the executive committee and the general assembly, the philosophy, policy, strategy, and action plans for specific IPC objectives related to the female athlete. It is important to note that membership on this committee includes women with disability, former Paralympic athletes, and IOC representation.

4 How are the outcomes in sociological research related to the choices made by researchers regarding whom to study and what to study?

5 What is the relationship between research results and real world applications when studying gender and disability?

6 What strategies could international sport governing bodies use to address the issue of under-representation of women in Paralympic Sport?

The Voice of the Female Athlete

The following statements of two former athletes and one up-and-coming female athlete are examples of the impact that the female athletic experience can have on women with disabilities, both personally and professionally. The first two athletes, Ann Cody and Ronda Jarvis-Ray, represent those women who, despite the perceived gender and disability barriers in Paralympic sport, have achieved great success both on and off the playing field. After discussing the present-day status of these athletes, they were asked to respond to a series of four questions related to their initial experience with sport: the sustainment of their athletic careers, the decisions made regarding their lifestyle and career choices, and the advice they would give to young female athletes. The third interview took place with a newly competitive athlete, Lauren Woolstencroft, who was just beginning to create her own narrative regarding her experiences with disability sport. Lauren responded to similar questions regarding her experience with competition; however, she primarily provided descriptive information relative to the evolutionary status of her involvement. Much of the discussion provided by these athletes lends support to some of the preliminary findings in research on women in disability sport. It is important to note that each athlete participated in a different sport (track and field, basketball, and downhill skiing).

ANN CODY—UNITED STATES

Ann Cody lives in Washington, DC, and works with Sagamore Associates, providing planning, advocacy, and governmental affairs services to organizations in the areas of amateur sports, health, and disability. She has competed in the Olympic and Paralympic games. In addition to her gold, silver, and bronze Paralympic medals in track and field, Ann is a clinically-trained therapeutic recreation specialist. With eleven years experience working with the nonprofit sector on disability issues, she is a key player on Sagamore Associates' health and disability practice teams. She earned her bachelor of fine arts and master of science degrees from the University of Illinois.

Ann is involved with amateur sports governance, programmes, and event management as an active volunteer. She has served on the United States Olympic Committee's subcommittee on Paralympic team selection criteria. She is a board member of the American Association of Adapted Sports Programs, which provides competitive sports leagues for youth with disabilities.

Ann Cody on the Athletic Experience

WHAT FACTORS INFLUENCED YOUR DECISION TO ENTER ELITE DISABILITY SPORT?

Attending the University of Illinois, where I received excellent coaching and training enabling me to make it to the elite level.

Also the idea of setting performance goals in sport and meeting those goals demonstrating that disability isn't necessarily a limiting factor in achieving goals.

WHAT SUSTAINED YOUR INVOLVEMENT?

The relationships I developed with my team-mates and my coaches sustained me as did the support of my family and friends. Additionally, the health benefits and high level of fitness, which gave me greater physical mobility, were incredible motivators.

HOW HAS YOUR ATHLETIC EXPERIENCE INFORMED YOUR LIFESTYLE AND CAREER CHOICES?

My athletic experience led me to seek a graduate degree which led me to a series of career-building jobs. The investment of time and resources [in elite sport] has paid off in ways I couldn't have imagined. I trusted that my demonstrated success in sport would pay off in my career, and it has!

WHAT ADVICE DO YOU HAVE FOR FEMALE ATHLETES REGARDING THEIR COMPETITIVE CAREERS?

Work toward a professional/academic degree. Build a network of people who can help support you in your training, travel, emotionally, and eventually as you transition from elite athlete to career person. The bonds you build in this competitive environment will be invaluable in your future, if you work with people who can support you beyond the athletic field.

RONDA JARVIS-RAY—UNITED STATES

Ronda Jarvis-Ray was a member of the 1996 Bronze Medal US Women's Paralympic Wheelchair Basketball team in Atlanta, Georgia, and the 1992 Silver Medal US Women's Paralympic Wheelchair Basketball team that competed in Barcelona, Spain. She has five consecutive National Championship titles as a member of the University of Illinois

Women's Wheelchair Basketball Team. Ronda also has a gold medal from the 1990 World Championship Games in France. She was two-time recipient of the George Huff Award for academic excellence while earning a varsity letter in athletics. Ronda received a bachelor of science degree in psychology and a master's degree in social work. After college Ronda pursued a career in the field of rehabilitation medicine as a case manager. She went on to find a unique balance for her career endeavors and athletic aspirations when she began directing outreach efforts at the Lakeshore Foundation in Birmingham, Alabama, one of the largest nonprofit organizations dedicated to improving the health and wellness of people in Alabama with physical disabilities.

Ronda Jarvis-Ray on the Female Athlete

WHAT FACTORS INFLUENCED YOUR DECISION TO ENTER ELITE DISABILITY SPORT?

The single most influential moment was watching the 800-metre women's track event at the 1984 Olympic Games in Los Angeles and seeing Sharon Hedrick win the gold medal. This was my first exposure to disabled sports and what a powerful one! I knew at that moment that I wanted to be an elite wheelchair sport athlete. Prior to that time, athletics were always a central part of my life as an able-bodied child. I was actively involved in several sports including basketball, swimming, volleyball, and track.

WHAT SUSTAINED YOUR INVOLVEMENT?

Primarily, I continued my involvement in athletics because of my competitive spirit and the enjoyment I derive from competition. Sports involvement has always been a tremendous source of focus, strength, and motivation for me in my life aspirations.

HOW HAS YOUR ATHLETIC EXPERIENCE INFORMED YOUR LIFESTYLE AND CAREER CHOICES?

Athletics have undoubtedly shaped several of my life choices. Through my involvement in a collegiate athletic programme [University of Illinois] and the importance placed on athletic achievement within the context of academic excellence, I gained tremendous discipline, focus, and clarity. In addition, my experiences preparing for the Paralympics and involvement in international competition provided me with a strong work ethic which has allowed me to excel in all aspects of life.

WHAT ADVICE DO YOU HAVE FOR FEMALE ATHLETES REGARDING THEIR COMPETITIVE CAREERS?

I would strongly encourage young women who are interested in pursuing competitive athletics to use sport as a vehicle to achieve greater success in one's life; however, I do not believe elite sport and all of the accolades that can accompany competition should be pursued as a means in and of themselves. Furthermore, while sports can provide a wonderful avenue to broaden and enrich one's life, I would advise that one should not so narrowly identify or define oneself as an athlete. I strongly believe in the importance of cultivating other aspects of self such as one's intellect, emotional, and spiritual well-being. Balance is often difficult to achieve, but is essential to strive for!

LAUREN WOOLSTENCROFT—CANADA

Lauren Woolstencroft participates in downhill skiing as an up-and-coming elite Paralympic athlete. For the first few years of her development, she was lucky enough to ski with an instructor who was familiar with teaching people with disability how to ski. At the age of six, her parents enrolled her in the learn-to-ski programme for the disabled at Canada Olympic Park in Calgary. This programme is within CADS (Canadian Association for Disabled Skiing). She skied recreationally through elementary and junior high. She went on to compete on an annual basis where she participated in ski school as a 'normal' kid.

Lauren Woolstencroft on the Female Athlete

I definitely enjoyed skiing; however, I bet I didn't ski more than ten to fifteen days in the year. I was lucky to be born with knees so I ski pretty normal. I use only one pole, but the rest of my equipment is the same. I have special ski legs that allow for specific angulation in the ankle, as well as stabilization for my knees. They are somewhat complex and it took until I was sixteen to find what works best for me. This, for me, is one of the hardest parts of disabled skiing. There was not a single person out there that I met that was a double below the knee amputee and skiing competitively, and it would have been helpful to know other skiers with similar issues to obtain possible solutions to my equipment problems. It has always been trial and error which is time-consuming. Not only do I have to worry about my boot buckles breaking on race day, but I have to worry about my artificial legs breaking too. Each year, however, we seem to get better at solving these problems and issues seem to become more infrequent.

In the beginning of grade ten (1996), a friend of Lauren's whom she had met through the CHAMP programme asked her to try out for the Alberta Disabled Team. The provincial team is a feeder team to the national team. She agreed but really didn't know what it meant.

I had never heard of the Alberta Disabled Team, but I knew I enjoyed skiing and figured it would just add some structure to that. The Alberta team was certainly a mixed bag when I joined. Not only was it a mixed bag of personalities, but there was a wide variety of abilities. My friend and I were the only female members, and while

it was a small team of only about six people, it was certainly male-dominated with skiers ranging from age eight to twenty-eight! Our programme consisted of Saturday and Sunday ski days, as well as a structured dryland programme. My skiing ability improved dramatically and I logged in about forty-five ski days over the first year.

She competed in a few able-bodied Alberta races that season where, much to her surprise, she achieved exceptional results. She competed in the Western Disabled Canadians in February 1997 and, at the end of that month, the team travelled to Winter Park, Colorado, for the Columbia Crest Cup.

This was definitely my first real introduction to the world of disabled skiing. There is a very large disabled skiing programme in Winter Park and I was amazed with the number of people involved. While I did win the giant slalom and slalom in the junior category, I wouldn't say it was due to any amazing talent on my part. The junior women's field was only four women at that event! It was clear that the real competition lay in the senior category and I still had a ways to go. The Canadian Nationals were at the end of March in Kimberley, BC. This, too, was a great experience as the entire Canadian team was there, as well as the US team and some other countries. It was a great feeling to go in entirely unknown and manage to do as well as I did. The one thing that I did notice at these nationals was the severe lack of women. There were definitely only a quarter as many women as men, which played a large factor in me breaking in so easily. As nationals marked the end of the racing season, I was more than pleased with my improvement as a skier, and with all of the results that I had achieved.

By year three of her ski racing career, grade twelve in 1998, she was placed on the national team. She trained with two other women members of the team who had similar disabilities. The higher level of competitive training certainly improved her skiing. It has thus become clear how necessary it is to train with a group of athletes with similar abilities, as everyone is constantly pushing each other to the next level.

> I was also the youngest and definitely least experienced member of the team and had so much to learn from everyone. That year there were nine men and four women on the team. Some teams, however, had no women members at all. But while the field was small (only fifteen to twenty girls), we were all very competitive. We travelled to Europe, Colorado, and within Canada, and I definitely saw my skiing improve dramatically throughout the year. I was so happy with all of my results that year and I was honoured to receive the Athlete of the Year award for our team.

Fall 1999 marked the beginning of her second year on the national team. While she planned to travel full-time with the team that year, her training was limited as she was attending her first year of university at the University of Victoria. Taking a full engineering course load did not promote great training for the fall or winter. She managed to train hard over the Christmas break and pull it all together for when it really mattered at the world championships in late January in Anzere, Switzerland. All of her results over the past two years are far more than she had ever expected. The field of women remained much the same that year as it was the year before with perhaps only one or two new faces.

> Even though I have only been involved in this sport on a very active basis for four years, I have definitely seen it become more competitive every year. At the beginning my wins sometimes felt more like default then true talent, whereas now they feel much more like an accomplishment. The women's field on the international scene is still small, but there is a very strong group of ten to twelve women where it could be anyone's game. As mentioned before, having the small field of women played a factor in me achieving great results so early. Competing in a larger field would be

better; however, I'm never out there feeling without a challenge. I am also encouraged to feel that the size of the field is increasing and thus becoming more competitive. I have hardly lived a long life on this circuit and I remain one of the youngest people on the circuit. I'm certainly not ready to quit yet and am now focussing on the 2002 Paralympics in Salt Lake City and the upcoming 2000/2001 season.

Discussion

In linking theoretical discussion to practice, it is necessary to examine the practical efforts made by sport governing bodies along with the response of the female athlete to those changes. The former president of the IPC, Dr. Robert D. Steadward, along with Carol Mushett, the technical officer of the IPC, indicated a strong commitment to developing opportunities for female athletes in Paralympic sport. In October 1999, some formally proposed sports technical development initiatives were reported, including:

1. Rule Change by the IPC Sports Council Executive Committee–The IPC Sports Council Management Committee (SCMC) has agreed to evaluate women's opportunities in the Paralympics by event criteria, rather than criteria for sport disciplines. The significance of this decision is that women's opportunities could be more effectively and systematically preserved on the Paralympic Programme.
2. Changes in the Budget Allocation Process for Sport–The new budget funding formula "rewards" sports which have active and measurable initiatives to promote opportunities for women.
3. Seed Money–Paralympic and IPC Championship Sports are eligible and are encouraged to apply for small seed grants which promote women's initiatives.
4. Powerlifting–Perhaps the most successful initiative in the development

of women's Paralympic Sport was organized by Pol Wautermartens, chairman of IPC Powerlifting. In less than two years, IPC powerlifting has gone from 0 to over 50 countries which widely practice women's powerlifting.
(Mushett, C., personal communication, October 4, 1999)

Despite these attempts, there continues to exist a lack of measurable outcomes or research-based explanations related to the female athlete's participation in elite disability sport. This lack may be because of the complexity of issues surrounding disability and gender. We know that representations of gender and the way that gender operates in the world of sport are not static. According to Adams (1993), gender is an ideological construct that is an integral part of all aspects of social, economic, and political life. The meanings of femininity and masculinity are constantly challenged and negotiated within a larger nexus of social relations (p. 164). Participation in the sporting world is often guided by socially reinforced gender roles, or culturally accepted gendered sports. Football, baseball, hockey, and rugby are the most apparent examples of male-gendered sports, while rhythmic gymnastics, figure skating, field hockey, and synchronized swimming are perceived as being more appropriate for women. Wheelchair basketball, or goalball, has not entered the gender specific discussion, and, instead, dialogue surrounding 'difference' within these Paralympic sports is related to levels of injury and extent of visual impairment.

When professionals and athletes in the disability sport field are asked to comment on the reasons that women are not participating in elite disability sport, they are often additionally questioned on whether the situation is related to the athlete being female or due to her disability. If practitioners could attribute the lack of participation to one variable such as gender or disability or even examine the variables in isolation, they would be fulfilling the desire of some researchers and sport administrators who believe that this is a discrete issue that may be person-centred or biologically-based. Many choose not to answer this question directly, but refocus the question to examine the context of elite disability sport and the ideological assumptions embedded in the disability sport movement. Can one empower the elite female athlete to participate? Do we know what she needs to sustain her involvement? This dialogue provides a basis for asking these questions; however, answers for these questions require further thought on the specific changes we need to make in elite disability sport to meet the needs of all of athletes.

Because the Paralympic movement is founded on the creed that all people have a right to participate in elite sport and because it is committed to the concept and celebration of diversity, to extend this consideration to the female athlete would be natural. Yet, to decentralize traditional gender-based notions in the sport forum is not without cost. Dewar (1993) examined the historical trend among feminist scholars to produce the "generic women," which resulted in the construction of generic experiences of oppression in sport. In a similar statement, Birrell (1990) also argued for better acknowledgment of parallel, but very different, experiences between and among women participating in sport, specifically women of colour.

> If we are to understand gender and racial relations in sport, particularly as they relate to women of color, we cannot remain in our old theoretical homes. Instead we need to increase our awareness of issues in the lives of women of color as they themselves articulate these issues. (p. 195)

Although these researchers have yet to apply their epistemological lenses to the female athlete with disability, as Dewar (1993) states, "We are showing signs that we are learning to find ways of moving away from the relative safety and comfort of our old theoretical homes."

In December 1995, a group of researchers and female athletes met in Berlin at the invitation of Professor Gudrun Doll-Tepper and Freie University of Berlin in order to discuss the merits of collaborative research and professional development in the area of women and disability sport. The group included women from a variety of academic and sporting backgrounds, but more apparent were the cultural and political differences among the participants. After three days of discussion, this group developed a goals and purpose statement and agreed to support and actively pursue them in their home countries. Entitled "Breaking the Barriers to Participation: Women with Disabilities in Sport–A Cross Cultural and Interdisciplinary Perspective," this document represented one of the first attempts at linking academia to change efforts regarding equity and the disability sport movement. The following statements were to assist in the development of dialogue between disability sport professionals and female athletes:

1. Develop a broader awareness and understanding of the social and cultural world of disability sport.
2. Develop a deeper awareness and understanding of gender and disability in the context of sport.
3. Identify resources and persons currently participating in the field of disability sport (participants, coaches, teachers, administrators, researchers, etc.).
4. Develop a network of persons and organizations involved in the field of women and disability sport.
5. Develop a network of individuals involved in the research of gender and disability sport.
6. Initiate strategies within relevant organizations to implement the guidelines set out within the Brighton Declaration on Women and Sport.
7. Facilitate the clarification and recognition of the identity of the disability sport movement.

In considering the future of the female athlete's progression in Paralympic sport, it is important to acknowledge the speed at which the Paralympic movement has addressed issues of diversity as compared to its Olympic counterpart. The female athlete has made great strides in performance and in obtaining inclusion within Paralympic events. The issues surrounding the female athlete with disability, however, are far from resolved. Given that nearly half of the countries participating in the Atlanta Paralympic games did not bring female athletes, it may be necessary to put direct pressure on the sport governing bodies within those countries to increase the female athletes' involvement. Hall (1994) provides very useful discussion regarding the feminist activism in sport and external relations by examining strategies from Canada, the United States, Australia, and the United Kingdom which may, if applied, prove useful to disability sport.

> External relations concern the nature, intensity, and content of an organizations's ties to its environment or to individuals, groups, and organizations (including the state) beyond its boundary. The relationship between an organization and its environment is one that centers power with the environment (e.g., controls an organization's resources), or locates power with members. (p. 57)

The organizational structure of the International Paralympic Committee locates power to create Paralympic sport with its members. Yet, often the female athlete's experience with the system actively deters her from participating by not allowing her the power to shape the forces that shape her. The Paralympic movement has made great strides in securing a more equitable playing field for athletes with disabilities. In order to be more effective when initiating, supporting, or facilitating the representation of the female athlete in elite disability sport, the athlete should play an active part in the creation of those systems that govern her participation.

Resources

Women's sport organizations in Canada and US
- CAWS—Canadian Association of Women and Sport
- NAGWS—National (US) Association of Girls and Women in Sport
- Australian Sports Commission—National Programmes Women
- Center for Research on Girls and Women in Sport—Minneapolis, Minnesota
- Women's Sports Foundation—New York

International sport organizations that focus on women
- International Working Group on Women and Sport—Department of Canadian Heritage

Study Questions

1. In light of the success of the women Paralympians at the 2000 games in Sydney, is it realistic to assume that each new Paralympics will see more female entrants or more events for women?
2. Discuss gender roles in the new millennium. Will there be more women administrators, coaches, and athletes, or will men continue to dominate the Paralympic arena?
3. Discuss the "generic woman" in sport and express how women's oppression in general has decentralized the experience of women with disabilities in sport.
4. Review the suggested steps suggested by the group of women practitioners, athletes and researchers who met in Berlin. Prioritize these steps and indicate what you feel would help accomplish these items in an efficient manner. Justify your priorities.
5. Describe the achievements of the three female athletes highlighted in this text. Describe those aspects of their involvement in Paralympic sport that could be used to direct future discussion by organizing members of the Paralympic games.

References

Adams, M.L. (1993). To be an ordinary hero: Male figure skaters and the ideology of gender. In T. Haddad (Ed.), *Men and masculinities: A critical anthology* (pp. 163–81). Toronto: Canadian Scholarly Press.

Allison, M.T. (1991). Role conflict and the female athlete: Preoccupations with little grounding. *Journal of Applied Sport Psychology, 3,* 49–60.

Bar On, B. (1993). Marginality and epistemic privilege. In L. Alcoff and E. Potter (Eds.), *Feminist epistemologies.* New York: Routledge.

Barcelona Paralympic Organizing Committee. (1992). *Barcelona Paralympic official report: Barcelona Paralympic Organizing Committee.* Barcelona: International Paralympic Committee.

Begum, N. (1992). Disabled women and the feminist agenda. *Feminist Review, 40,* 70–84.

Birrell, S.J. (1990). Women of color, critical autobiography, and sport. In M.A. Messner and D.F. Sabo (Eds.), *Sport, men, and the gender order: Critical feminist perspectives.* Champaign, IL: Human Kinetics.

Blinde, E.M., and McCallister, S.G. (1999). Women, disability, and sport and physical fitness activity: The intersection of gender and disability dynamics. *Research Quarterly for Exercise and Sport, 70*(3), 303–12.

Boutilier, M., and San Giovanni, L. (1983). *The Sporting Woman.* Champaign, IL: Human Kinetics.

Brandmeyer, G.A., and McBee, G.F. (1986). Social status and athletic competition for the disabled athlete: The case of wheelchair roadracing. In C. Sherrill (Ed.), *Sport and disabled athletes.* Champaign, IL: Human Kinetics.

Cole, C.L. (1994). Resisting the canon: Feminist cultural studies, sport, and technologies of the body. In S. Birrell and C.L. Cole (Eds.), *Women, sport, and culture.* Champaign, IL: Human Kinetics.

Cooper, M.A., Sherrill, C., and Marshall, D. (1986). Attitudes toward physical activity of elite cerebral palsied athletes. *Adapted Physical Activity Quarterly, 3,* 14–21.

Cowell, L.L., Squires, W.G., and Raven, P.B. (1986). Benefits of aerobic exercise for the paraplegic: A brief review. *Medicine and Science in Sports and Exercise, 18*(5), 501–8.

Craft, D.H. (2001). Impressions from Australia: The Sydney 2000 Paralympic games. *Palaestra, 17*(1), 20–35.

DePauw, K.P. and Gavron, S.J. (1995). *Disability and Sport.* Champaign, IL: Human Kinetics.

DePauw, K. (1994). A feminist perspective on sports and sports organizations for persons with disabilities. In R.D. Steadward, E.R. Nelson, and G.D. Wheeler (Eds.), *The outlook: Proceedings from Vista '93: An International Conference on High Performance Sport for Athletes with Disabilities.* Edmonton, AB: University of Alberta Rick Hansen Centre.

DePauw, K. (1997). The (in)visibility of disability: cultural contexts and "sporting bodies". *Quest, 49*(4), 416–30.

Dewar, A. (1993). Would all the generic women in sport please stand up? Challenges facing feminist sport sociology. *Quest, 45,* 211–29.

Hall, M.A. (1985). Knowledge and gender: Epistemological questions in the social analysis of sport. *Sociology of Sport Journal, 2,* 25–42.

Hall, M.A. (1988). The discourse of gender and sport: From femininity to feminism. *Sociology of Sport Journal, 5,* 330–40.

Hall, M.A. (1993). Gender and sport in the 1990s: Feminism, culture, and politics. *Sport Science Review, 2*(1), 48–68.

Hall, M.A. (1994). Women's sport advocacy organizations comparing feminist activism in sport. *Journal of Comparative Physical Education and Sport (JCPES), 16,* 50–59.

Henderson, K.A., and Bedini, L.A. (1995). "I have a soul that dances like Tina Turner, but my body can't": Physical activity and women with mobility impairments. *Research Quarterly for Exercise and Sport, 66*(2), 151–61.

Hopper, C.A. (1984). Socialization of wheelchair athletes. In C. Sherrill (Ed.), *Sport and disabled athletes: The 1984 Olympic Scientific Congress Proceedings* (pp. 197–202). Champaign, IL: Human Kinetics.

International Paralympic Committee. (1994). *Lillehammer Paralympic Official Report. Lillehammer Paralympic Organizing committee.* Lillehammer: Author.

International Paralympic Committee. (1992). *Barcelona Paralympic Official Report. Barcelona Paralympic Organizing Committee.* Barcelona: Author.

Jackson, R.W., and Davis, G.M. (1983). The value of sports and recreation for the physically disabled. *Orthopaedic Clinics of North America, 14*(2), 301–15.

Kolkka, T., and Williams, T. (1997). Gender and disability sport participation: Setting a sociological research agenda. *Adapted Physical Activity Quarterly, 14*(1), 8–23.

Messner, M. (1992). *Power at play: Sports and the problem of masculinity.* Boston: Beacon Press.

Mushett, C. (October 4, 1999). Personal communication.

Olenik, L.M. (1998). *Women in elite disability sport: Multidimensional perspectives.* Unpublished doctoral dissertation, University of Alberta, Edmonton.

Olenik, L.M., Matthews, J., and Steadward, R. (1995). Women, disability and sport: Unheard voices. *Canadian Woman's Studies Journal, 15*(4), 54–57.

Reiff, S. (2000). Sydney 2000: The pace heats up. *The Paralympian, 3.* [On-line]. Available: http://www.paralympic.org/default.asp (URL December 4, 2002).

Shepherd, R.J. (1991). Benefits of sport and physical activity for the disabled: Implications for the individual and for society. *Scandinavian Journal of Rehabilitative Medicine, 23*(2), 51–59.

Sherrill, C. (1993). Women with disability, Paralympics, and reasoned action contact theory. *Women in Sport and Physical Activity Journal, 2*(2), 51–60.

Sherrill, C. (1997a). Disability, identity, and involvement in sport and exercise. In K.R. Fox (Ed.), *The physical self: From motivation to well-being.* Champaign, IL: Human Kinetics.

Sherrill, C. (1997b). Paralympic Games 1996: Feminist and other concerns: What's your excuse? *Palaestra, 13*(1), 32–38.

Sherrill, C. (1998). Philosophical and ethical aspects of paralympic sports. In R. Naul, K. Hardman, M. Pieron, and B. Skirstad (Eds.), *Physical activity and active lifestyle of children and youth* (pp. 19–28). Schorndorf, Germany: Verlag Karl Hoffman.

Sherrill, C., Gench, B., Hinson, M., Gilstrap, T., Richir, K., and Mastro, J. (1990). Self-actualization of elite blind athletes. *Journal of Visual Impairment and Blindness, 84*(2), 55–60.

Sherrill, C., Rainbolt, W., Montelione, T., and Pope, C. (1986). Sport socialization of blind and of cerebral palsied elite athletes. In C. Sherrill (Ed.), *Sport and disabled athletes* (pp. 189–95). Champaign, IL: Human Kinetics.

Sherrill, C., Silliman, L., Gench, B., and Hinson, M. (1990). Self-actualization of elite wheelchair athletes. *Paraplegia, 28,* 252–60.

Sherrill, C., and Williams, T. (1996). Disability and sport: Psychosocial perspectives on inclusion, integration and participation. *Sport Science Review, 5*(1), 42–64.

Steadward, R.D. (1996). Integration and sport in the paralympic movement. *Sport Science Review, 5*(1), 26–41.

Theberge, N. (1981). A critique of critiques: Radical and feminist writing in sport. *Social Forces, 60,* 341–53.

Theberge, N. (1985). Toward a feminist alternative to sport as a male preserve. *Quest, 37*(2), 193–202.

Valliant, P.M., Bezzubyk, I., Daley, L., and Asu, M.E. (1985). Psychological impact of sport on disabled athletes. *Psychological Reports, 56*(3), 923–29.

Watkinson, E.J., and Calzonetti, K. (1989). Physical activity patterns of physically disabled women in Canada. *CAHPER Journal,* November-December, 21–26.

Wendell, S. (1993). Toward a feminist theory of disability. In A. Minas (Ed.), *Gender basics: Feminist perspectives on women and men.* Belmont, CA: Wadsworth.

Williams, T. (1994a). Disability sport socialization and identity construction. *Adapted Physical Activity Quarterly, 11,* 14–31.

Williams, T. (1994b). Sociological perspectives on sport and disability: Structural functionalism. *Physical Education Review, 17*(1), 14–24.

Wilson, W. (1996). The IOC and the status of women in the Olympic movement: 1972–1996. *Research Quarterly for Exercise and Sport, 67*(2), 183–92.

ADDITIONAL WEB SITES
(URLs JANUARY 13, 2003)

Women and Sport Sites

Active Australia
   http://www.activeaustralia.org/women/

Canadian Association for the Advancement of Women and Sport
   http://www.caaws.ca

National Association of Girls and Women in Sport
   http://www.aahperd.org/nagws/

Olympic Women in Sport
   http://www.olympicwomen.co.uk

Disability Sport Sites

American Association of Adapted Sport Programs
   http://www.aaasp.orgInternational Disabled Sport
   USA: http://www.dsusa.org

National Disabled Sport Alliance
   http://www.ndsaonline.org

National Sport Center for the Disabled
   http://www.nscd.org

Paralympic Committee:
   http://www.paralympic.org

Research and Education Sites

International Council of Sport Science and Physical Education
   http://www.icsspe.org

Northeastern Research Initiative on Sport and Society
   http://www.sportinsociety.org

Palaestra Magazine
   www.palaestra.com

Steadward Centre for Personal and Physical Achievement
   http://www.steadwardcentre.org

CHAPTER 32

Athletes in Transition

Garry D. Wheeler

Learning Objectives

- To recognize the difference between the terms *transition* and *retirement*.
- To define *transition* and describe essential elements of transition theory.
- To describe methodological problems associated with able-bodied research in athlete transition and retirement.
- To describe factors associated with satisfactory and unsatisfactory transition from sports.
- To describe aspects of the athlete career and transition experiences which may lead to difficulties.
- To discuss the duties and responsibilities of the institution of sport (able-bodied and disability sport) towards its athletes during and after their careers and during the transition phase.
- To list recommendations for coaches and young professionals working with athletes with a disability in relation to facilitating a smooth transition from disability sport to retirement.

It was the most emotionally draining, upsetting time I ever had in my life and I wouldn't wish it on anybody. It was awful, absolutely awful.... I was mad for a really long time and then it kind of alternated from being mad to crying and being upset.... It's like somebody in your family died.... It's like a death in your family and this thing that was this person or whatever was so important to you must disappeared.... I think you go through all the grieving things you do when somebody dies. [An athlete with a disability describing the retirement experience.] (Wheeler et al. 1999, p. 228)

Introduction

The impact of retirement or transition from able-bodied high school, college, amateur, and professional sports has been the subject of a great deal of research. While the majority of athletes do well in their lives, most experience varying degrees of emotional difficulty on leaving sports. A small but significant percentage experience significant psychological problems, including clinical depression or prolonged periods of grieving. The degree of difficulty in retiring from sport seems to be associated with a number of factors, including voluntary versus involuntary retirement, perceived level of success, commitment and ego identification with sport, sense of personal control during career, and availability of support networks. It is now recognized that retirement from sport is not simply an acute event but rather a complex process or *transition*. Adjustment or adaptation to retirement is also a highly individual process and represents a complex interaction of many factors. Until recently, retirement experiences have not been studied in the athlete with a disability.

---

1 What factors do you think have resulted in our ignoring the study of the retirement experiences of the athlete with a disability *and* what assumptions have been made with regard to the athlete experience which may have led to the neglect of this issue?

The vast majority of research in the area of disability sport is associated with physiological and psychological effects of exercise and salient issues such as classification, doping and performance enhancement, technology and equipment design, athletic injury, and sports medicine.

Think for a moment about the concept of an athletic career. Moreover, think of the athletic career as a three-phase process of initiation, competition, and retirement. Between each phase there is a period of transition as the athlete adapts to each new experience (Wheeler et al. 1995). It is clear that we have essentially ignored the last phase of the career—retirement. In our research we have given less attention to questions regarding the duties and responsibilities of the institution of disability sport to the athlete. One of these *possible* duties may be assisting the athlete in retirement. Perhaps we have proceeded in research on the assumption that disability sports are inherently good for those who are involved, that the outcomes of sport by

definition must be beneficial to the athlete with a disability. Therefore, studying the athlete in retirement might seem redundant.

But, there are a number of reasons for examining the retirement process in the athlete with a disability.

The nature of disability sport has changed significantly in the latter part of the twentieth century and continues to change. Increased sophistication of organizations and technology, and increased profile and levels of sponsorship are, in turn, associated with increased levels of economic and personal investment of organizations, coaches, and athletes in disability sport. We have very little idea of the impact of total personal investment in sport on the athlete with a disability, particularly in relation to quality of life after sport. Chronic injuries acquired in sports can significantly affect quality of life after the sports career is over. For example, many athletes with a spinal injury who use wheelchairs develop chronic overuse problems in the shoulder. While this has been well described in the sports medicine literature (e.g., Burnham et al. 1993), we do not know what impact the acquisition of a *"secondary disability"* (e.g., a chronic shoulder injury in a spinal cord injured athlete) can have on the retirement period and future quality of life in this population.

---

2 Based on the reasons given for conducting research in the area of athlete retirement, consider these questions: Does the institution of sport in general have a duty and obligation towards preparing for and assisting them during retirement? On what do you base your answer? Is the athlete with a disability a special case?

You have now had a chance to think about and discuss the concept of retirement from sports. You have had the opportunity to consider whether the athlete with a disability constitutes a special case.

Athletes With a Disability in Transition

The purpose of the chapter is to review the issue of athlete transition in general and specifically with reference to the athlete with a disability. First, we will examine the limited amount of existing research. Then we will address the question of duties and responsibilities of disability sport towards its athletes, suggest possible interventions, and provide some guidance for the young coach working in the area.

The terms *transition* and *retirement* will be used since both are used in the literature. The term *transition* is used primarily and can be thought of as including the term *retirement*. Consider for a moment what these terms mean. Think of retirement as an event: the decision to leave sports. Retirement also describes the period of life after sport. The term *transition* is a more inclusive term which reflects the *process* of coming to the decision to retire, coping with the initial exit, adjusting to life after sport, and, finally, adapting to life without (the previous level of) sport. Athletes therefore make the transition from the athletic career to the retirement period. A brief description of transition theory will help you to appreciate the complexity of making transition from the sport environment. According to Schlossberg (1981, 1984) adults continuously experience transitions during their lifetimes. A transition can be said to occur if an event or nonevent results in a change in assumptions about oneself and the world and thus requires a corresponding change in one's behaviour and relationships (Schlossberg 1981). These transitions occur naturally in life and include marriage, getting a first job, and so forth. *Adaptation* may be defined as a process during which an individual moves from being totally preoccupied with the transition, to integrating the transition into his or her life (Schlossberg 1981). Adaptation to transition may be thought of as the balance between personal assets and liabilities and a function of pre- and post-transitional environmental factors (e.g., interpersonal and institutional support) and characteristics of the transition (e.g., on- or off-time, role gain or loss, positive or negative emotional responses). Schlossberg (1984) suggests that view of self, personal situation, support structures, and

problem-solving strategies are important predictors of adaptation to transition. Transition theory is a framework for examining life transitions in general but has also been considered a flexible and multidimensional model for examining transition from sports (Crook and Robertson 1991).

Transition From Able-bodied Sports

Early studies focussed on the concept of retirement. Reports of the impact of athlete retirement were often sensationalized in newspaper articles of a dramatic nature and were lacking in objectivity (e.g., Kaplan 1977). Researchers often described retirement as a traumatic event (Blinde and Stratta 1992; Ogilvie and Howe 1982, 1986; McLaughlin 1981; Bradley 1976; Hill and Lowe 1974; Mihovilovic 1968), an identity crisis (Hill and Lowe 1974), a role loss (Gordon 1988), an inevitable metathesis (Hill and Lowe 1974), and social (Lerch 1982; Rosenberg 1982) or career death (Blinde and Stratta 1992). It has been suggested that athletes pass through similar emotional stages to those described by Kübler-Ross (1969) in her stage theory of death and dying: denial, anger, bargaining, depression, and final acceptance (Blinde and Stratta 1992). McGown and Rail (1996) concluded that the exit from sports was often a "lonesome experience," abrupt, unplanned, and that athletes are often left "up the creek without a paddle."

Difficult transitions have been associated with total commitment to sport, ego involvement in sport, and the development of an athletic identity (Ogilvie and Howe 1986; Thomas and Ermler 1988; Baillie 1993; Hill and Lowe 1974), and with loss of autonomy and control of personal development during the sport career (Thomas and Ermler 1988; McGown and Rail 1996; Parker 1994). According to many authors, intense commitment to sport leads to an identity and sense of self-worth based exclusively on self as an athlete and on athletic performance. Once sport is over, the athlete may face the question, Who am I, if I am not an athlete? Identity issues and lack of perceived control over personal development leaves the athlete ill-prepared for an autonomous existence outside of sports (Thomas and Ermler 1988).

However, others have suggested that there is little evidence of emotional or adjustment difficulties (Coakley 1983), and that athletes generally make the transition out of sport successfully (McPherson 1978; Sinclair and Orlick 1993). Athletic transition has been described as a time of opportunity to explore new areas in life, as a rebirth (Coakley 1983), or a period accompanied by a sense of intense relief at no longer having to face the drudgery of training and travel (Blinde and Greendorfer 1985; Greendorfer and Blinde 1985).

---

3 What features of research studies might account for these apparently opposite research findings? (Consider level of participation, for example.)

Five features of research studies have likely contributed to this confusion. These include, (a) the population studied and level of athletic participation studied, (b) timing of the research (time since retirement), (c) theories or models informing and guiding researchers and research methods, (d) methodological approaches used, and (e) a gender bias in research.

LEVEL OF PARTICIPATION

Some reports have suggested that, as professional elite athletes make the transition from sport, they face significant adjustment problems associated with lack of career options, alcohol and drug abuse, identity crises, intense feelings of loss, and a devaluation in social status (Mihovilovic 1968; Hill and Lowe 1974; Bradley 1976). Conversely, others have concluded that the majority of former professional athletes adjust successfully to transition (McPherson 1978; Baillie 1992) although the second career is not perceived as rewarding as the athletic career (McPherson 1980), with adjustment taking up to ten years (Baillie, 1992).

Anecdotal reports in the media have painted a picture of the retired amateur athlete as being alienated from the real world,

feeling lost, and suffering from low levels of self-esteem (e.g., Kaplan 1977). Up to 83 percent of athletes experienced varying degrees of negative emotions at retirement (Ogilvie and Howe 1982) and as many as 32 percent experienced a very difficult time on leaving sports (Werthner and Orlick 1986). McGown and Rail (1996) suggested that retirement was an abrupt and a lonesome experience for retired elite women canoeists, and that athletes were, indeed, left up the creek without a paddle. However, Sinclair and Orlick (1993) concluded *"that adjustment to retirement from high-performance sports may not be as distressing or as liberating as previously suggested."*

Athletes cut from school teams or whose programmes had been cut have experienced significant emotional trauma similar to stages of grieving (Blinde and Stratta 1992). Former collegiate football players reported a sense of loss of control of self and future, and a "Now what?" reaction to retirement (Parker 1994). However, Greendorfer and Blinde (1985) suggested that there was little evidence of adjustment difficulties in their sample of college athletes. Parker (1994) reported athletes feeling a sense of relief from the pressures of intercollegiate sports.

To summarize, it would appear that different responses to retirement and the transition process in general are a function of the different types of athletes studied and the different levels of sport in which athletes participate.

TIME SINCE RETIREMENT

Retrospective reporting of emotional reactions may be inaccurate, since studies of transition experiences of athletes may involve athletes who have been retired for a number of months (Blinde and Stratta 1992) or those who have retired for up to twenty-five years (McGown and Rail 1996). Blinde and Stratta (1992) reported emotional problems analogous to the grieving process in the majority of their sample of intercollegiate athletes who were from four to nine months into retirement. Sinclair and Orlick (1993) suggested that 23 percent of their sample of elite amateur athletes were still not adjusted after four years. Werthner and Orlick (1986) reported that 32 percent experienced a very difficult time on leaving sports, and that adjustment was highly individual, taking up to three years. Baillie (1992) suggested that the adjustment process takes between two to ten years, and McGown and Rail (1996) suggest that some athletes may not have completely adjusted to leaving sports as long as twenty-eight years after leaving competitve sports.

However, it does appear clear that adjustment (a) takes a considerable amount of time, and (b) some athletes continue to experience difficulties long after the initial exit from sports.

EXAMINING THE TRANSITION PROCESS
In studying athlete transition, there has been a lack of consistency in the application of theoretical models (i.e., frameworks arising from observation or research studies which act as a guide for asking research questions) (Crooke and Robertson 1991). Gerontological (study of aging) and thanatological (study of death and dying) theories/models have often been used to study transition. These models may lead to a narrow interpretation of data based on pre-existing constructs (concepts/ideas) and tend to begin with the assumption that athletes in general experience a serious adjustment dilemma on exiting sports. The ability of such models to capture adequately the process of leaving sport has been questioned (Greendorfer and Blinde 1985; Blinde and Greendorfer 1985).

It is now generally understood that *retirement is not a discrete event.* Rather it is a *complex transition process* and must be examined in context with many other factors or variables which occur for a given person at a given time and for certain reasons (Coakley 1983, Sinclair and Orlick 1993). Thus, it has been suggested that the transition model (Schlossberg 1981, 1984) may provide the flexible model required for interpretation of athletic experiences (Crooke and Robertson 1991). A number of recent studies have focussed on the concept of transition, rather than treating retirement as an acute event (e.g., McGown and Rail

1996; Sinclair and Orlick 1993; Parker 1994; Werthner and Orlick 1986).

METHODS CHOSEN TO STUDY THE RETIREMENT ISSUE
Structured and unstructured interviews and specifically designed questionnaires or instruments have all been used to study transition (Werthner and Orlick 1986; Greendorfer and Blinde 1985; Blinde and Stratta 1992; Parker 1994; McGown and Rail 1996; Sinclair and Orlick 1993). A variety of research approaches often provide a confusing and fragmented view of the transition process, showing that what you find out may well depend on how you study it.

GENDER BIAS
It has been suggested that transition research has focussed mainly on male athletes (Greendorfer and Blinde, 1985; McGown and Rail, 1996), and that research findings may not be generalizable or transferable to female athletes. However, an examination of the recent literature would tend to refute, (a) the claim that women have been underrepresented in studies, and (b) that differences in the transition experience exist between men and women. Greendorfer and Blinde (1985) included 427 males and 697 females in their study of 1,124 former intercollegiate athletes. The authors reported no differences between perceptions of adjustment to the transition period. They concluded that there was little in either gender to suggest that athletes experienced life disruption, trauma, or severe difficulties in retirement. Werthner and Orlick (1986) included 14 males and 14 females in their study of the transition experiences of Canadian elite amateur athletes. No apparent attempt was made to distinguish between men and women during data analysis in this questionnaire-based study and no comment was made on male/female differences in adjustment experiences or difficulties. Blinde and Stratta (1992) included 11 male and 2 female athletes in their study of college athletes who had experienced an unanticipated exit from sports, and Sinclair and Orlick (1993) included

100 women among their sample of 199 athletes from thirty-one different sports. Responses to an athlete retirement questionnaire were apparently not analysed for gender-specific responses. However, they did note that males as compared to females tended to report both finding a job and finances as reasons for leaving sports. No other differences were reported.

The assertion that there is a *"dearth of information regarding women athletes,"* (McGown and Rail 1996, p. 119) may not be an entirely accurate reflection of the recent research in the area of athlete transition. As well, research to date does not offer strong support for differences between the transition response of men and women. Gender differences may not be as great a threat to generalizability or transferability of data as previously thought.

---

4 How can researchers improve studies in relation to the retirement and transition experiences of athletes?

What can be said about athlete transitions?

Despite methodological discrepancies, there is at least some consistency in the research findings. A number of factors have been clearly identified as affecting the nature of the transition experience. These include: (a) anticipatory socialization (including maintaining relationships outside of sport and finding a new focus in life after sports), (b) identity and self-esteem issues, (c) personal management skills, (d) social support of family and friends, (e) voluntary or involuntary retirement (including health-related and athletic injury-related factors), (f) sense of accomplishment, (g) political and personal relationships (including relationships with organizations and coaches), (h) finances, and (i) maintaining involvement in sport, coaching and/or training (Ogilvie and Howe 1986; Werthner and Orlick 1986; Crook and Robertson 1991; Sinclair and Orlick 1993).

In summary, athletes without problems tend to remain involved in sports, have an immediate new focus, and a readiness to move on with their lives. Key factors impacting on adjustment to transition in those with difficulties after sports are: intense commitment and ego involvement in sports, lack of anticipatory socialization, abandonment of other life interests including personal relationships and friendships during the athletic career, neglect of career and education, and lack of support during transition (Botteril 1981; Baillie 1993; Werthner and Orlick 1986).

Transition from Disability Sports

To date, the author is only aware of four research investigations and one theoretical paper on the transition process in the athlete with a disability. Details are provided in table 32.1. Two qualitatively-based interview studies have been completed in Canada (Wheeler et al. 1996; 1999) and two quantitative questionnaire-type studies were done in Israel (Schaefer and Bergman 1994; Makoff 1999). Data are preliminary in nature and must be examined critically. The Wheeler et al. (1996; 1999) investigations examined the athletic careers of two multisport samples of athletes with a disability using an interview format to develop an initial understanding of athlete experience. Schaefer and Bergman (1994) used a structured questionnaire to examine the transition process including preparation for retirement, reasons for retirement, feelings shortly before and after retirement, and issues of social support. Makoff (1999) examined issues of social support before, during, and after transition from sport. This work was based on the Wheeler et al. (1996; 1999) investigations in which it was suggested that athletes had an unfavourable view of institutional support systems (i.e., follow-up and post-athletic career support from coaches and athletic organizations). Finally, a paper by Martin (1996) examined unique and common predictors of difficulties in transition for the athlete with a disability. However, this was based on speculation rather

Table 32.1 Characteristics of Research Investigations into Transition and Retirement in Athletes with a Disability

Authors	Research Method	Subjects Informants Participants and Impairments	Gender	Time Since Retirement (range)	Sports
Wheeler et al. (1999)	• Grounded Theory • In-depth interviews • Iterative analysis and constant comparison • Development of a basic social process	9 Canada 3 USA 11 United Kingdom 17 Israel Retired elite international level athletes *Impairment:* SCI, spina bifida, amputee, polio, cerebral palsy	27 male 13 female	1 – 18 years	Basketball Fencing Skiing Swimming Table tennis Track and field Water polo

Wheeler et al. (1996)	• Transition Theory
	• In-depth interviews
	• Iterative analysis and constant comparison
	• Development of a basic social process
		10 Canadian retired athletes
		also:
		  (4 semi-retired)
		  (4 competing)
		Impairment: SCI, amputee, polio, spina bifida, cerebral palsy
			5 male
			5 female
				2 – 19 years	Swimming
					Track and field
					Basketball
					Cycling

Schaefer and Bergman (1994)	• 260-item questionnaire • Likert Scale responses and quantitative analysis	15 retired, elite, international level Israeli athletes *Impairment:* amputee, polio, SCI	10 male 5 female	2 – 10 years	Basketball Track and field Swimming
Makoff et al. (1999)	• In-depth interviews • Hierarchical class analysis	5 retired, elite, international level Israeli athletes *Impairment:* SCI, polio, blind	5 male	2 – 7 years	Track and field Water skiing Power lifting
Martin (1996)	• Theoretical paper	Reference to athletes with a disability in general	n/a	n/a	All sports

than research findings. The level of athletic participation, multiple sports environments, and representation of both genders is consistent across the research. All the athletes involved in the research had participated at the national and international levels.

You will recall that level of commitment, ego identification (degree to which the individual identifies self as athlete), failure to maintain outside interests or relationships, and lack of support during and after transition are important predictors of difficulties in transition for able-bodied athletes. The first question we must address is whether these factors are generalizable to the athlete with a disability.

---

5 What issues do you think might arise during the transition from sport to retirement? What impact might disability type have on the transition experience?

Are athletes with a disability totally committed to sports?

Baillie (1993) stated that:

> It is the salience that sports involvement has across a significant proportion of the life span of the athlete that makes retirement so potentially difficult for many [athletes]. Years of external evaluation and internal reinforcers associated with sports, help to form an identity in which physical competition is central to the athlete's sense of self, but such an identity may also be harmful in its consequence after retirement from the sports environment. (p. 401)

This total commitment may lead to the exclusion of all else. Werthner and Orlick (1986) stated that:

> Now in order to be a world class athlete in most sports, it is often impossible to be much else—their identity is often totally tied up in sport. They define themselves as an athlete. They concentrate totally on training and competition, which has a positive effect on performance but often this occurs to the exclusion of everything else in their lives. (p. 337)

Athletes with disabilities *are* highly committed to sports. Wheeler et al. (1996) found that this commitment was associated with identification as athlete; training while injured; and exclusion of other important aspects in life such as family, relationships, social activities, job/career, education, and personal health. For example, one athlete noted that:

> Now sport is my life—everything revolves around sport. When I am not racing I think about it all the time. It takes up at least 90 percent of my time. I love it. I spend all my time living, thinking, breathing it. I define myself as being an athlete. (p. 389)

Such comments were duplicated in a second study (Wheeler et al. 1999). In this study a *personal investment* analogy was employed to examine returns and losses on personal investment in sport. Clearly, commitment to disability sport was associated with many returns on investment, including developing a sense of personal competency, increased self-esteem, a sense of normalcy, sport as a place to demonstrate personal competency. The concept of personal competency and a sense of self-efficacy was confirmed by Makoff et al. (1999) who reported that athletes believed that sport was a way to *"show the society"* that an athlete with a disability can succeed. One of the athletes in the Makoff et al. (1999) study stated that *"I found something I am good at it,"* and another stated that he was involved in sports *"in order to prove (myself) and the society that a disabled person can also do things the same as a valid person."*

Do athletes with a disability develop a sense of athletic identity?

One of the most significant returns experienced by the athletes in both of the Wheeler et al. (1996; 1999) studies was the development of a new sense of identity: the development of identity as athlete, being defined by sport, identifying the self as able-bodied and not disabled, identifying self as athlete not disabled, or identifying self as super-normal. The development of a sense of athletic identity is clearly illustrated in the comments of athletes from the Wheeler et al. (1996) study:

> It was wonderful. When I started swimming, it allowed me the opportunity to find an identity. It brought out a whole bunch of personal characteristics that I think might not have come out had I not been swimming…. (p. 388)

> Swimming was a sport in which my disability didn't hamper me, since there was no need for lower body strength. I was excited when I discovered swimming gave me a way to compete…. I was in the water and I was just about an able-bodied person other than the fact that I couldn't move my legs and no one could notice that…until I got back out of the water and into my chair and then I am handicapped again. (p. 386)

> When we're on the track, I think we don't look at ourselves as disabled. When we're in our racing chair it is like putting on a uniform; it's like you are out of it now, you are out of the disability. It gives you that. It's like putting a Superman vest on. (p. 388)

These findings are consistent with Martin (1996), who suggested that "elite athletes with disabilities may be particularly susceptible to developing exclusive athletic identities due to reduced social contact and opportunity for career mastery experiences." (p. 131)

There was a downside to this total commitment. Many athletes incurred chronic injuries as a function of this total commitment and identification with sport, although injuries were often ignored. One athlete in the Wheeler et al. (1996) investigation noted:

> I never listened or respected my body and what it was doing. I swam through them [the injuries]…. I just had incredible pain…. It was winning or nothing. I was going to die trying, that was what I was going to do. (p. 389)

Athletes with disabilities are highly committed to their sports, identify strongly with sport or as being not disabled, and may be willing to pay a heavy price for such commitment.

Do athletes with disabilities neglect the maintenance of their social circle and relationships?

Athletes in the Wheeler et al. (1996, 1999) investigations often described the impact of total commitment on their lives. Athletes often stated that they did not have time for friends or relationships outside of sports, that they ignored their education, and that sport cost them a great deal of money or their careers. Athletes said that life literally "passed them by."

> Nothing other than sport interested me. As I got older, I pushed myself in sport and forgot education. I threw myself into sport…looking back this was silly… education was never high profile…my career was as an athlete! (1999, p. 225)

Many athletes do commit to and identify with sport, to the exclusion of other interests including career, education, and personal relationships outside of sports.

Do athletes perceive adequate sources of support during their careers and during the transition phase of their careers?

According to transition theory (Schlossberg 1981, 1984), personal and institutional support (e.g., church, community groups) systems are important for adapting to transition. A number of previously-cited authors studying able-bodied athletes referred to a sense of either dissatisfaction with, or lack of support of, coaching staff and the athletic institution during their careers and upon retirement (Baillie 1992; Sinclair and Orlick 1993; Parker 1994; McGown and Rail 1996). This is particularly relevant if other sources of support have been neglected during the career. One athlete in the Werthner and Orlick (1986) study summed it up in saying, "They sort of dump you off, throw you away" (p. 355).

Athletes who experienced extreme isolation or who lacked a support group (for example, athletes cut from teams), often revealed the most severe forms of depression, which led to unusual personality and behaviour changes as well as problems related to alcohol use (Blinde and Stratta 1992). Sinclair and Orlick (1993) observed that the most supportive groups during transition were spouse/mate and other family members. They found that institutional groups–national sports organizations, and the Olympic athlete career centre–provided the least support of all for the athlete. Coaches were perceived as providing little or no support for the athlete in transition.

With regard to the athlete with a disability, Martin (1996) suggested that difficulties in maintaining social support systems associated with sport might make transition problematic for the athlete. It was suggested that social support may be an issue in two ways. First, that leaving sports may mean access to less social support provided by team-mates. Second, by obtaining support from other athletes, the athlete may neglect to develop a support system outside of sport. Research in the area of athlete with a disability transition supports this notion.

Athletes in the Wheeler et al. (1996, 1999) investigations often admitted to neglecting relationships outside of sports. This may increase the athlete's expectations for support from his or her institution. However, as with able-bodied athletes, this support was clearly not perceived to be there for the athletes. Athletes referred to the inadequacy of support they received from their sports associations. This could leave athletes feeling that there was no one available to help them and that they were isolated. For example, consider the comments of these two athletes.

> It was very tough. The knowledge of that chapter of my career, and it was a very lengthy chapter of twenty-one years, and it's just over. I didn't really have a replacement for it. There wasn't anything exactly waiting for me…. I came back from the Olympics [1988] and I sat at home and that was not a very good feeling. More

than that, it's when I actually felt that there was nobody there helping me. (1999, p. 228)

> I would make the comment, and it's still in effect today…you are cut off from everyone. Everyone meaning the disabled community [in sport], and you know, should you happen to run into someone or meet up with someone…, you are not given the time of day. (1996, p. 392)

Athletes with a disability often felt that disability sport organizations were dominated by able-bodied administrators and often failed to consider the welfare of the athletes (Wheeler et al. 1999). This sense of abandonment during transition is captured in the statement of an athlete in the Wheeler et al. (1999) study.

> They don't even know me…they had no idea…they have never written me and asked whether I was interested in any kind of coaching, they have never asked me; they have never asked me to do anything. It's like my usefulness is done. I'm toast. (p. 231)

However, Schaefer and Bergman's (1995) findings suggest that the relationship with the sports association was not "extremely important" (see table 32.2).

It is unclear whether this perceived lack of importance was based on perceived lack of support. However, the data do support the importance of relationships with family and friends for adapting to transition. Makoff et al. (1999) identified fifteen potential support structures for athletes ranging from family to the sport organizations. Makoff et al. (1999) reported that the coach was still viewed as an important source of support between two and seven years post-retirement (although not as important as family), which became important on leaving sport and a sense of focus into which new energy was channelled. On retirement, the spouse became more important but was not the primary support structure cited. In particular, athletes in the Makoff et al. (1999) study were upset at the inequities in treatment and recognition of athletes by organizations once they reached elite levels.

Table 32.2 Ratings of Importance of Sources of Support at Various Points of the Athletic Career

Source of support	Percentage of athletes perceiving relationships as "extremely important"			
	During career	Shortly before retirement	Just after retirement	Two years later
Family and friends	65	55	46	40
Coaches/athletes/ managers	35	22	15	11
Sports associations	22	14	21	7

SOURCE: From unpublished research observations by Y. Schaefer and Y. Bergman, 1994, presented by Y. Hutzler at The International Symposium of Adapted Physical Activity, Oslo, Norway, May 22–26, 1995.

Finally, one athlete in the Wheeler et al. (1999) investigation, was not at all surprised at the lack of support during transition: *"I didn't see the federation doing enough for athletes that compete, so I didn't expect them to do anything for those that retire"* (p. 231).

It would appear that athletes with a disability do exhibit characteristics and behaviours that authors in the able-bodied sport retirement literature have linked to future difficulties. What difficulties do athletes with a disability face in retirement?

Do some or all athletes experience emotional difficulties on leaving sports?

Some able-bodied athletes experience emotional and other difficulties in making the transition from sports to the *"non-sport world,"* (e.g., Blinde and Stratta 1992; Werthner and Orlick 1986) *although* future outcome is generally positive. Werthner and Orlick (1986) referred to athletes hitting "rock bottom," and experiencing the "blackest two weeks of my life," and "a huge emptiness, a huge void." Werthner and Orlick (1986) cite one athlete as stating that she felt she "died" when the 1980 Olympic boycott was announced, marking the end of her international career. An athlete in the McGown and Rail (1996) investigation suggested that emotions associated with transition to retirement were similar to those associated with the death of a family member. Often, researchers describe a plethora of negative emotions experienced by athletes exiting sport. Emotions included bitterness, disappointment, anger, depression, loss, confusion, failure, fear, frustration, conflict, lack of purpose, and other reactions. What do athletes with a disability experience?

A variety of emotional reactions including shock, grief, hollowness/emptiness, anger, sadness, and mourning have consistently been reported by researchers in the area of athlete with a disability retirement (Schaefer and Bergman 1994; Makoff 1999; Wheeler et al. 1996, 1999). Episodes of depression meeting the major diagnostic criteria for a depressive episode (*Diagnostic and Statistical Manual of Mental Disorders* 1994) have been reported (Wheeler et al. 1996, 1999). Athletes have referred to transition as falling into a "black hole" following the "golden years" of participation. (Wheeler et al. 1996; Makoff 1999). This is consistent with Baillie's (1993) comment that, *"It seems clear that although many athletes make satisfactory transitions from sports, there are at the high school, college, elite and professional levels, significant numbers of athletes for whom the adjustment is difficult, incomplete and traumatic"* (p. 403).

Two comments from athletes in the Wheeler et al. (1999) investigations clearly outline the emotional stress or trauma of making the transition out of sports.

> It was the most emotionally draining, upsetting time I ever had in my life and I wouldn't wish it on anybody. It was awful, absolutely awful.... How come this happened to me? I was mad for a really long time and then it kind of alternated from being mad to crying and being upset.... It's like somebody in your family died.... It's like a death in your family and this thing that was this person or whatever that was so important to you just disappeared.... I think you go through all the grieving things you do when somebody dies. (1999, p. 228)

Perhaps most poignant was this comment from a woman returning from her final competition.

> I talked to a lot of my girlfriends–there were a lot of miscarriages. I honestly believe it is very closely related to it–as if you were to lose a baby–just like a miscarriage. It is just the sorrow inside and it is something that you have looked forward to and planned for and boom, it is taken away...all of a sudden you get back [from the last competition] and that focus in gone and guess what–so are you basically. If you are not involved with sports anymore you are really nobody–that is exactly how you are treated when you get back. (1996, p. 389)

Some researchers in able-bodied sports have described a sense of relief experienced by athletes no longer having to put up with the rigours of training, travel, and stress and a high degree of life satisfaction after the sport career even though negative emotions were present (Sinclair and Orlick 1993; Greendorfer and Blinde 1985; Coakley 1983). This apparent ambivalence in potential feelings brings into "question the intuitively attractive linkage between feelings such as sadness or unhappiness and psychological adjustment" (Blinde and Greendorfer 1985, p. 108).

Consistent with the observations of Blinde and Greendorfer (1985), athletes in the Wheeler et al. (1996, 1999) and Makoff et al. (1999) studies often experienced ambivalent emotions on leaving sports. Often reporting a sense of "sadness," "anger," "frustration," "loss," and "grief," athletes would also refer to a paradoxical sense of relief from the rigours of travel, training, diet, and so on. The range of emotional impact and degree of relief from training also varied and appeared to be consistent with the degree of commitment/investment of the athlete in sports and the salience of sports in his or her life. The following comments from athletes in the Wheeler (1999) study refer to this sense of relief and to time for other aspects of life.

> It was a sense of relief that you've just in one fell swoop removed all the responsibility, all the commitment you've put into the sport for the previous twenty-five years–it's gone. It's like a weight lifted off your shoulders. There wasn't any reason to be sad. I think it is a natural transition, it is something that is inevitable. (1999, p. 228)

> [I had] more time for other things... more time for the business and family. I wasn't so tired...my social life was better and I enjoyed recreational pursuits more. It's fantastic I am not training anymore. I have more time for my work...more social life...it has helped to improve the relationship [with spouse]. (1999, p. 226)

Makoff et al. (1999) also reported mixed feelings–a sense of ambivalence–in the athletes in her study. Although most of the athletes reported a certain sense of loss upon leaving sports, they did not regret the decision to retire, and all seemed to be well-adjusted to the transition process.

The evidence available in relation to disability sport therefore suggests that athletes may experience a range of ambivalent emotions on leaving disability sports. These may include anger, sadness, and grief which may attain clinical significance but are often accompanied by paradoxical feelings of needing to move on and a sense of relief from the stresses of sports.

What factors assist the athlete with a disability in coping with and adjusting to the transition from sports?

Martin (1996) speculated that a number of factors might impact on transitional experiences of the athlete with a disability, including an interaction between identity, social support, goal accomplishment, and post-athletic preparation factors.

COMMITMENT LEVEL

Although commitment to sport is very high in the athlete with a disability, maintaining a balanced perspective on the position of sport among other life domains was important in dealing with life after sports.

IDENTITY

Loss of athletic identity was a problem for some athletes in making transitions from sports. The maintenance of a diverse identity based on sports and other life domains is likely an important factor in coping with and adjusting to transition.

COPING STYLE

Coping styles that may be adopted by athletes include emotional style (What does this all mean? Who am I now?) or a problem-solving style (What shall I do next?). Successful copers often adopted a problem-solving or action-oriented strategy. They channelled their energies into other areas as a means of coping with transition from sport (Wheeler et al. 1996, 1999; Makoff et al. 1999). This *reinvestment* (channelling) of time and energy into other aspects of the life portfolio includes *paying back debts* (time to family, friends, education, and the bank), and *moving on in life*. Athletes often felt that they *owed a debt to their families* for neglecting them during their careers. In some cases they had accrued a great deal of financial debt and were still paying it off years later.

Makoff et al. (1999) also reported that channelling energies into other areas of life, including occupation, helped the athletes in this study overcome the emotionality of leaving sports. An athlete in the Wheeler studies sums this up well while reflecting on what might have been.

> Since I have given up sports I have channelled my energies into my career and now I look back and wonder what might have been if I had invested the same amount of energy. It was a loss of years. I might have been in a better position than I am now. (Wheeler et al. 1999, p. 225)

SUPPORT STRUCTURES

Support of family and friends is often referred to in the able-bodied retirement literature as important in coping with exiting sports (Werthner and Orlick 1986; McGown and Rail 1996).

Interestingly, Makoff et al. (1999) noted that coping with transition was relatively independent of perceptions of support variation. However, in both the Wheeler et al. (1996, 1999) studies it was evident that the family and/or spouse are important adjuncts to coping with the transition from sports as well as being important support mechanisms throughout the career.

REMAINING INVOLVED IN SPORTS

Remaining in sports in some other capacity than athlete (e.g., coaching, administration), is often referred to as a means of coping with the exit from sports and adjustment issues. (Greendorfer and Blinde 1985; Werthner and Orlick 1986; Baillie 1992).

Athletes in the Wheeler et al. (1996, 1999) and Makoff et al. (1999) studies often reported the importance of remaining in sports at some level as a means of dealing with the transition from sports. However, this did not apply to all athletes, particularly those struggling with the loss of sport.

Blinde and Stratta (1992) noted that some able-bodied athletes avoided sports and isolated themselves during the "shock and denial" stage of adjustment to retirement from sports. In their study, athletes who were cut from the team tended to isolate themselves since they felt they had little support. Athletes whose programmes had been cut, however, did not associate with this isolation strategy for coping since they had support of others in a similar situation. Some athletes with a disability behave in a similar manner.

An athlete in the Wheeler et al. (1999) study lamented,

> For a long time I missed it. I couldn't go and watch competition. I felt left on the shelf, no longer invited out to dinners, news interviews. It all just stopped. I felt really miserable, as if I wasn't worth anything…it hurt more by coming out [retiring] early.

What are the moral and ethical obligations of the institution of disability sport to the athlete in transition?

6 Based on your having read the chapter, review your response to the earlier question with regard to duties and obligations of the institution of sport towards the athlete in transition. Is your opinion the same or has it changed. If you have changed your position. provide a rationale for that change.

What level of responsibility does the institution of disability sports have towards its athletes in transition? At the Vista '99 conference in Cologne, Germany, Dr. Robert Steadward, president of the International Paralympic Committee, made the following statement: *"It is significant to recognize that the athlete cannot exist without the organization, neither can the organization exist without the athlete."* Thomas and Ermler (1988) suggest that this is simply not happening in able-bodied sports.

> What we see happening with the gifted athlete is not caring for the whole person but all too often caring for the athletic person. We allow the individual to define

the self in terms of athletic talent and to lose touch with the truer self. We allow the athlete to narrow his or her personal development and self concept and become identified only in terms of athletic development. (p. 138)

Parker (1994) poignantly captures the importance of transitional support for athletes.

> If anything is to be learned [from research] it is that former athletes have a lot to say and perhaps no one to tell. These unresolved feelings and emotions coupled with the lack of a safe forum of expression are potentially harmful to the mental health of these individuals. Transitional athletes need to be afforded the opportunity to vent and clarify their feelings about their sport careers without fear of reprisals. (p. 301)

Given the data available, we might at least conclude that athletes with a disability need access to similar services as those provided to able-bodied athletes.

What do athletes say they need?

Athletes in a number of studies of able-bodied athlete retirement have articulated the support they feel they need in transition. These are summarized in the following table (see table 32.3).

Little information is available regarding athletes with a disability, although athletes in the studies discussed previously do make a number of recommendations. These are summarized below.

COUNSELLING SERVICES

Athletes suggested that counselling be provided during the athletic career, in transition and post-transition phases. Education on maintaining a balance in life, including social, educational, and vocational aspects, and helping athletes prepare and deal with the emotionality of retirement were important. An important aspect of counselling includes the issue of training with injuries that may become chronic and affect future quality of

Table 32.3 The Needs of Athletes During Transition

Support—"needs" Domain	Specific Support	Authors
General	"Treat the retiring athlete with respect rather than as a disposable commodity."	Sinclair and Orlick (1993)
Needs during the career		
Planning	• Begin planning during the career • Lay plans for gradual retirement	Sinclair and Orlick (1993) McGown and Rail (1996)
Education	• Education of coaches and athletes regarding the issues of transition	Werthner and Orlick (1986)
	• Experiential literature (former athletes)	Sinclair and Orlick (1993)
	• Seminars with retired athletes	Sinclair and Orlick (1993)
	• Use of mental skills outside of sports	Sinclair and Orlick (1993)
	• Continue with education or career while competing	McGown and Rail (1996)
Social	Maintain alternative activities and friendships outside of sports	McGown and Rail (1996)
Athlete development	Development of the whole self	McGown and Rail (1996)
Support structures	Seek support for retirement transition	McGown and Rail (1996)
Needs during transition		
Counselling support	• Exit interview provision	Werthner and Orlick (1986)
	• Self-esteem and personal competency counselling	McGown and Rail (1996)
	• Maintenance of a positive perspective	Sinclair and Orlick (1993)
	• Detraining and counselling programmes made available to athletes	McGown and Rail (1996)
	• Use of sport psychologists during transition	McGown and Rail (1996)
Educational	Physiological and dietary training programme	Sinclair and Orlick (1993)
Continued involvement in sports	• Representation of athletes on boards • Maintain contact with sports assocations	Werthner and Orlick (1986) McGown and Rail (1996)
Retirement/Transition Programmes	• Federal retirement programme including bridging financial support and career counselling and placement services	Werthner and Orlick (1986)
	• Ongoing financial assistance	Sinclair and Orlick (1993)
	• Job and educational opportunity information	Sinclair and Orlick (1993)
	• Career focus and location assistance	Sinclair and Orlick (1993)
	• Treat athletes equitably in terms of financial assistance	McGown and Rail (1996)
Recommendations to institutions	• Increase contact and communication with retirees	McGown and Rail (1996)
	• Incorporation of alumni into national sports associations	McGown and Rail (1996)
	• Maintain athlete/institutional relationships through national coaches	McGown and Rail (1996)

life. This is consistent with suggestions in the able-bodied literature (Baillie 1993; Lanning 1982; Chartrand and Lent 1987; Taylor and Ogilvie 1984).

COMMUNICATION

Athletes believed that the relationship and communication with the organizational levels of sport had to be improved significantly.

RECOGNITION

Increased recognition of the athlete during and after his or her career. Suggestions included alumni associations, annual events, an athlete's hall of fame, and athlete of the year awards.

Are there retirement or transition programmes for the athlete with a disability?

To the knowledge of the author, there is no programme specifically targeted for the athlete with a disability. However, as athletes with a disability are increasingly integrated into able-bodied sports organizations, presumably athletes will be able to avail themselves of the same opportunities such as those provided by the Canadian and US Olympic programmes.

Who should provide intervention services for athletes with a disability in transition?

Werthner and Orlick (1986) reported that 35 percent of their sample of 199 retired Canadian athletes would consult with a sport psychologist following retirement while only 8 percent would consult with any other type of 'psychologist.' They then go on to observe that this *"sends an important message to the profession of applied sport psychology with regard to the growing debate on certification procedures and who possesses the credibility and expertise to develop and refine mental training and transition skills with athletes."*

Without launching into a debate about the legalities of the term *psychologist* and certification issues, it is clear that the transition experience is complex and likely requires a *team*

approach involving a clinical or counselling psychologist (screening for emotional issues), the sport psychology consultant (basic career counselling, development of mental skills in pretransition period, and adaptation of mental skills during and after transition), peer counsellors (former high level athletes who have experienced and adapted to the transition), and the athletes themselves.

RECOMMENDATIONS

Recommendations for the young professional working with athletes with a disability include the following points:

During the athletic career

- Emphasize balance during the athletic career and encourage athletes to maintain social, academic and/or vocational interests outside of sports.
- Carefully monitor athletes and encourage athletes to self-monitor in relation to the development of overuse injuries which may seriously impact on post-athletic career quality of life.

During transition and in retirement

- Encourage the athlete to talk about his or her feelings in relation to leaving sports with an appropriate support person to whom you refer the athlete (e.g. sport psychology consultant, clinical or counselling psychologist).
- Encourage the athlete to monitor any chronic injuries carefully and to seek ongoing medical attention.
- Encourage the athlete to remain involved in sports in some capacity— as a mentor, coach, or administrator.
- Encourage the athlete to remain physically active for physical and emotional health.

Summary

The author recognizes that there is a paucity of research in the area of retirement and transition from disability sport. However, there appears to be adequate justification for the national and international sports organizations, including the International Paralympic Committee, to consider developing some form of support structures for athletes before, during, and after the onset of transition. This demonstrates a commitment to the athletes without whom disability sport organizations could not exist. In addition, this would encourage more athletes to remain involved in sports rather than becoming lost resources. The exact nature of such support is to be determined, but a good start is to conduct initial discussions with experts in the field, including members of the helping profession with experiences in this matter–administrators, coaches, and athletes–retired and currently participating. Beginning the dialogue is an important step to setting up caring and effective programmes to assist the athlete in making the transition out of sport and facilitating fond memories of the athletic experience. Finally to quote Sinclair and Orlick (1993): "In sport it appears that most organisations have not paid the same attention to helping athletes move out of the organisational structure as they have to helping them move in." (p. 148)

Study Questions

1. Define *transition* as used in this chapter and describe the key elements of transition theory as described by Schlossberg (1981; 1984).

2. What are the factors that may contribute to satisfactory or unsatisfactory transition experiences in able-bodied athletes?

3. What unique characteristics of the disabled athlete transition experience differentiate the athlete with a disability from the able-bodied athlete?

4. Does the institution of sport and disability sport have a duty and obligation towards providing transition support for athletes? Justify your response.

5. As an experienced athlete with a disability who had undergone the transition experience, what advice might you give a young coach or professional who plans to work with elite athletes with a disability?

References

Baillie, P. (1992, October/November). *Career transition in elite and professional athletes: A study of individuals in their preparation for and adjustment to retirement from competitive sport.* Colloquium presented at the 7th Annual Conference of the Association for the Advancement of Applied Sport Psychology, Colorado Springs, CO.

Baillie, P. (1993). Understanding retirement from sports: Therapeutic ideas for helping athletes in transition. *The Counseling Psychologist, 21*(3), 399–410.

Blinde, E.M., and Greendorfer, S.L. (1985). A reconceptualization of the process of leaving the role of competitive athlete. *International Review for the Sociology of Sport, 20,* 87–94.

Blinde, E.M., and Stratta, T.M. (1992). The sport career death of college athletes: Involuntary and unanticipated sports exits. *The Journal of Sport Behaviour, 15,* 3–20.

Botteril, C. (1981). What "endings tell us about beginnings." In T. Orlick, J. Partington, and J. Salmela (Eds.) *Mental training for coaches and athletes.* Ottawa: Fitness and Amateur Sport.

Bradley, B. (1976). *Life on the run.* New York: Quadrangle/ *The New York Times.*

Burnham, R., Wheeler, G.D., Bhambhani, Y., Belanger, M., Eriksson, P., and Steadward, R.D. (1994). Intentional induction of autonomic dysreflexia among quadriplegic athletes for performance enhancement: Efficacy, safety and mechanism of action. *Clinical Journal of Sport Medicine, 4,* 1–10.

Burnham, R.S., May, L., Nelson, E., Steadward, R.D., and Reid, D. (1993). Shoulder pain in wheelchair athletes: The role of muscle imbalance. *The American Journal of Sports Medicine, 21*(2), 238–42.

Chartrand, J.M., and Lent, R.W. (1987). Sports counseling: enhancing the development of the student athlete. *Journal of Counseling and Development, 66,* 164–67.

Coakley, J.J. (1983). Leaving competitive sport: Retirement or rebirth. *Quest, 35,* 1–11.

Constantine, M. (1995). Retired female athletes in transition: A group counseling intervention. *Journal of College Student Development, 36*(6), 604–5.

Crook, J.M., and Robertson, S.E. (1991). Transitions out of elite sport. *Journal of Sport Psychology, 22,* 115–27.

Diagnostic and statistical manual of mental disorders (4th ed.). (1994). Washington, DC: American Psychiatric Association.

Duda, J.L., and Tappe, M.K. (1988). Predictors of personal investment among middle aged and older adults. *Perceptual and Motor Skills, 66,* 543–49.

Duda, J.L., and Tappe, M.K. (1989a). Personal investment in exercise among middle aged and older adults. In A. Ostrow (Ed.), *Aging and motor behaviour* (pp. 219–38). Indianapolis: Benchmark.

Duda, J.L. and Tappe, M.K. (1989b). Personal investment in exercise among adults: The examination of age and gender-related differences in motivational orientation.

In A. Ostrow (Ed.), *Aging and motor behaviour* (pp. 239–56). Indianapolis: Benchmark.

Gordon, R.L. (1988). Athletic retirement as role loss: A construct validity study of self as process and role behaviour. [Order No. DA8820299]. *Dissertation Abstracts International, 49*(8–B), 3469.

Greendorfer, S.L., and Blinde, E.M. (1985). Retirement from intercollegiate sport: Theoretical and empirical considerations. *Sociology of Sport Journal, 2,* 101–10.

Hill, P., and Lowe, B. (1974). The inevitable metathesis of the retiring athlete. *The International Review of Sport Sociology, 9,* 5–29.

Kaplan, J. (1977). What you do when you grow up. *Sports Illustrated, 47*(1), 30–32, 37–38.

Kübler-Ross, E. (1969). *On death and dying.* New York: Macmillan.

Lanning, J. (1982). The privileged few: Special counseling needs of athletes. *Journal of Sport Psychology, 4,* 19–23.

Lerch, S.H. (1982). *Athlete retirement as social death: An overview.* Paper presented at the 3rd annual meeting of the North American Society for the Sociology of Sport, Toronto.

Maehr, M.L., and Brasskamp, L.A. (1986). *The motivation factor: A theory of personal investment.* Lexington, MA: Lexington Press.

Martin, J.J. (1996). Transitions out of competitive sport for athletes with disabilities. *Therapeutic Recreation Journal, 30*(2), 128–36.

Makoff, D., Van den Auweele, Y., Van Landewijck, Y. (1999, May). *Transition out from elite disability sports: The social support aspect.* Paper presented at the 10th International Symposium of Adapted Physical Activity, Barcelona/Lleida, Spain. (Abstract).

McLaughlin, P. (1981). Retirement: Athlete transition. *Champion, 5,* 15–16.

McGown, E., and Rail, G. (1996). Up the creek without a paddle: Canadian women sprint racing canoeists' retirement from international sport. *Avante, 2*(3), 118–36.

McPherson, B.D. (1980). Retirement from professional sport: The process and problems of occupational and psychological adjustment. *Sociological Symposium, (30)* 126–43.

McPherson, B.D. (1978). Former professional athletes' adjustment to retirement. *The Physician and Sports Medicine, 6*(8) 52–59.

Mihovilovic, M. (1968). The status of former sportsmen. *International Review of Sport Sociology, 3,* 73–93.

Ogilvie, B.C., and Howe, M.A. (1982). Career crisis in sport. In T. Orlick, J.T. Partington, and J.H. Salmela (Eds.), *Mental training for coaches and athletes* (pp. 176–83). Ottawa: Sport in Perspective and Coaching Association of Canada.

Ogilvie, B.C., and Howe, M.A. (1986). The trauma of termination from athletics. In J.M. Williams (Ed.). *Applied Sport Psychology* (pp. 365–82). Palo Alto, CA: Mayfield.

Parker, K.B. (1994). "Has beens" and "wanna bes": Transition experiences of former college football players. *The Sport Psychologist, 8,* 287–304.

Pearson, R.E., and Petitpas, A.J. (1990). Transitions in athletes: Developmental and preventive perspectives. *Journal of Counseling and Development, 69,* 7–10.

Pemberton, C.L. (1986). *Motivational aspects of exercise adherence.* Unpublished doctoral dissertation, University of Illinois.

Rosenberg, E. (1982). Athletic retirement as social death: Concepts and perspectives. In N. Theberge and P. Donnelly (Eds.), *Sport in the life cycle* (pp. 243–58). Fort Worth: Texas Christian University Press.

Scanlon, T.K., Ravizza, K., and Stein, G.L. (1988). An in-depth study of former elite figure skaters II: Sources of enjoyment. *Journal of Sport and Exercise Psychology, 1*(1), 65–83.

Schaefer, Y., and Bergman, Y. (1995). Unpublished research observations presented by Y. Hutzler at The International Symposium of Adapted Physical Activity, Oslo, Norway, May 22–26, 1995.

Schlossberg, N.K. (1984). *Counseling adults in transition.* New York, Springer.

Schlossberg, N.K. (1981). A model of analyzing human adaptation to transition. *The Counseling Psychologist, 9,* 2–18.

Sinclair, D., and Orlick, T. (1993). Positive transitions from high performance sport. *The Sport Psychologist, 7,* 138–50.

Taylor, J, and Ogilvie, B.V. (1994). A conceptual model of adaptation to retirement among athletes. *Journal of Applied Sport Psychology, 6,* 1–20.

Thomas, C.E., and Ermler, K.L. (1988). Institutional obligations in the athletic retirement process. *Quest, 40,* 137–50.

Werthner, P, and Orlick, T. (1986). Retirement experiences of successful Olympic athletes. *International Journal of Sport Psychology, 17,* 337–63.

Wheeler, G.D., Malone, L., Steadward, R.D. (1995) *Retirement from disability sport: A qualitative study.* Paper presented at the 10th International Symposium of Adapted Physical Activity, Oslo, Norway, May 22–26, 1995.

Wheeler, G.D., Malone, L.A., Van Vlack, S., Nelson, E.R., and Steadward, R.D. (1996). Retirement from disability sport: A pilot study. *Adapted Physical Activity Quarterly, 13,* 382–89.

Wheeler, G.D., Steadward, R.D., Legg, D., Hutzler, Y., Campbell, E., and Johnson, A. (1999). Personal investment in disability sport careers: An international study. *Adapted Physical Activity Quarterly, 16,* 219–37.

Wolff, R., and Lester, D. (1989). A theoretical basis for counseling the retired professional athlete. *Psychological Reports, 64,* 1043–46.

Wilson, P.E., and Washington, R.L. (1993). Pediatric wheelchair athletics: Sports injuries and prevention. *Paraplegia, 31,* 330–37.

Index

* Boldface page numbers refer to charts and figures.

predictive validity in assessment, 170

predisposing risk factors in aging-disablement process, 432

PREP preschool play programme, 262–64, **263**

presage variables, APE conceptual framework, 197–98

preschool programmes
 benefits, 180–82
 GRIT programme, 182
 PREP programme, 262–64, **263**
 USA legislation, 86, 88–89

Pressley, M., self-determination, 221

pressure sores in SCI, 506

Principles for the Protection of Persons with Mental Illness and the Improvement of Mental Health Care (1991) UN, 81

privacy in assessment, 171–72

problem-solving process
 case study, troubled youth, 292–93
 in professional practice, 8–9
 self-determination, 218, 220–22
 strategic approach to motor skills instruction, 276–78

procedural knowledge, definition, 193

Proceedings of the Jasper Talks (1988), 38

process-product teaching model, 197–99

Prochaska, J.O., change model, 392, 394, **403**

professional fitness and lifestyle consultants (PFLC), inclusive fitness appraisals, 386, 394, 398

Professional Golfers Association (PGA), disability rights, 86

professional preparation, 1–10, 149–62
 definition, critical thinking, 5
 definition, teacher practices, 292
 advocacy, 144–45, 152–53, 367–69
 assumptions, 2, 256, 366–67
 athletes in transition support, 618
 competencies, 3–4, 367–69
 critical thinking, 5–9, 161
 historical overview, 34–36, 38
 Jasper Talks issues, 37–38
 power relationships, awareness, 291–93
 practicum placements, 159–61
 reflective practice, 5–6, 159–61, 293–95
 teacher attitudes and values, 200–202
 See also ethical issues and practice

proficiency barrier in developmental instructional approach, 265

programme planning and development
 Blueprint for Action, ALA, 37–41, 116–20, 184
 critical thinking approach, 8–9
 evaluation of service delivery, 158–61
 generalist and specialist competencies, 22, **23**
 intellectual disabilities, 563–64
 Jasper Talks, 37–38
 service delivery components, 155–61
 See also service delivery

progressive overload, 527

Project: Alive and Well, older adults, 443, 449

prompts
 assessment, 249, **249**, 251
 intellectual disability programmes, 565
 muscular endurance assessment, 397–98

prostheses
 definitions, prosthesis and orthosis, 544
 about, 543–45
 model of technological changes, **545**, 545–50
 technological boosting, 554–55
 See also technology and disability sport

Provan, Robert J., technology and disability rights, 86–87

Provincial/Territorial Initiative (PTI) partnerships, 117–19

psychological benefits of physical activity, 180–82

psychological empowerment. *See* empowerment and self-determination

psychological needs in self-determination theory, 337–41, **338**

psychological response to change. *See* athletes in transition

psychologists. *See* sports psychologists

PTI (Provincial and Territorial Initiatives) partnerships, 117–19

public awareness and publicity
 ALA resource materials, 40–41
 historical overview, 36–37, 40–41
 intellectual disabilities, 566–67, 583
 perpetuation of difference, 77–79
 programme promotion, 414
 Special Olympics movement, 583
 Viabilité fitness and active living campaign, 117, 119–20

punishment in behavioural instructional approaches, **268,** 268–69

quadriplegia, definition, 57
 See also spinal cord injuries (SCI)

quality of life
 definition, 347–48
 Harris Survey (1998), 346
 leisure education, 346–49, **348**, 358–59
 older adults and physical activity, 387, 443, 468–69
 policy development issue, 105–6
 PTI partnerships, 117–19
 See also athletes in transition

Quebec, disability rights, 85

questionnaires in fitness screening. *See* fitness appraisals, inclusive

Quetelet, Adolphe, normalization, 68–69

Raab, W., hypokinetic disease, 430

Rabinow, P., on Foucault, 66

race relations
 research, 590, 594, 600
 South Africa in Torontolympiad, 123–24
 whitestream discourse, 288

racing wheelchair, 549

Rail, G., athletes in transition, 607, 609, 615, 619

Rancourt, A.M., social role valorization, 351

Ransom, J.S., normalization, 70

readiness models in LRE, 139

Recommendations for the Fitness Assessment, Programming, and Counselling of Persons with a Disability (1998), CSEP, 394–98

recreation. *See* leisure and recreation; leisure education and services

score-keeping in physical education, 204–5

screening and informed consent, 396–97, 415, **427–28**, 457–58

screening in school assessments, 165

SDT (self-determination theory of motivation), 337–41, **338**

secondary disability, 606, 613

segregation by choice
definition, segregate, 408
active living continuum (inclusive/exclusive; integrated/segregated), **365**, 365–66
active living specialized programming model, 408–10, **409**
Deaflympics (formerly CISS), 472–76, **473**, **475–76**, 481
disability sport organizations, 584
Special Olympics movement, 143, 584
See also active living community programming; International Sports Federation for Persons with an Intellectual Disability (INAS-FID)

Seidl, Christine M., 397–98

self-control. *See* self-regulation and self-modification

self-determination and self-empowerment. *See* empowerment and self-determination; quality of life

self-injury, Web site, 290

self-regulation and self-modification
definitions, self-regulated behaviour, learning, strategies, 215, 217
strategic approach to learning, 276–78

self-report forms in assessment, **240**, 241, 248–51, 444

senility, 60, 218

seniors. *See* older adults

sensory disabilities, about, 57–59
See also blindness; deafness; hearing disabilities; visual disabilities

service-based paradigm
about, 15–17, 22
comparison of paradigms, **14**
as dependency model, 19
terminology, **16**

service delivery
definition, 152
assessment component, 153–54
critical thinking approach, 8–9
Jasper Talks recommendations, 37–38
policy development, 105–6
programme planning and development, 155–59
PTI partnerships, 117–19
sample policy analysis, recreation services, 108–10
See also abilities-based service delivery; inclusion

shaping in behavioural instructional approaches, **268**, 268–69

Shapiro, P.O., historical overview, 12

shared responsibility in teaching model, 199, 202–3

Shea, C.H., cognitive approaches, 272

Shebilski, W.L., cognitive approaches, 272

Shephard, R.J., 384, 386, **387**, 434, **531**

Sherrill, C., 72, 78, 258
definitions, 19, 163, 590
structured contacts, 340–41

Shirley, Marlon Ray, performance comparison, 551–52

Shoemaker, F.F., adopter characteristics, 454

shooting as IPC sport, 485

Shooting Federation of Canada, address, 129

Shumway-Cook, A., mobility, 434

Silent Games, World, 472–73

Simard, Clermont, 34–35, 42

Simpson, Al, 121–22

Sinclair, D., athletes in transition, 608–9, 614, 619, 621

skiing
CADS (Canadian Association for Disabled Skiing), 116, 120, 124, 128
female participation, 597–99
as IPC sport, 485
Moving to Inclusion resources, 41, 92, 116–17
sport injuries, 502

Skinner, J.S., training wheelchair athletes, **531**

Skrinar, G., exercise and mental illness, 183

sledge hockey
as gendered sport, 600
as IPC sport, 485
sport injuries, 502

Sledge Hockey of Canada (SHOC), 120, 129

small community partnerships, 118–19

Smith, J.D., disability paradigms, 12, 219

Smith, Murray, delivery system, 38

Smith, T.E.C., disability paradigms, 12, 219

SOC. *See* Special Olympics Canada (SOC)

soccer
as IPC sport, 485, 490
sport injuries, 501–2

social construction of disability, 65–74
definition, social construction, 65, 288
about, 12–13, 65, 76
discipline as social control, 66–69, 71–73
gender assumptions, 592, 600
normalization forces, 68–71
paradigms for disabilities, 12–13
social milieu, 155
troubled youth, 285–89
UN definitions of handicap, impairment, and disability, 69–71, 80
use of statistics, 68–69
whitestream discourse, 288, 295
See also classification of disabilities; language and disability terminology; normalization

social milieu, definition, 155

social role valorization, 151, 348, 351

socio-economic status in disability research, 590, 594

SOI. *See* Special Olympics Incorporated (SOI)

solvent use in troubled youth, 291

South Africa, in Torontolympiad, 123–24

South America, disability legislation, 90

Sowers, J., self-determination, 218

spastic cerebral palsy
about, 52
case study, physical education, 314–17

speaker's bureau, Activating Opportunities, 119

Special Committee on the Disabled and the Handicapped (1981) Canada, 100

Special Education Act (1961), PL 87–276, 88